Handbook of
Aging and Mental Health

An Integrative Approach

The Plenum Series in Adult Development and Aging

SERIES EDITOR:
Jack Demick, *Suffolk University, Boston, Massachusetts*

ADULT DEVELOPMENT, THERAPY, AND CULTURE
A Postmodern Synthesis
Gerald D. Young

THE AMERICAN FATHER
Biocultural and Developmental Aspects
Wade C. Mackey

THE DEVELOPMENT OF LOGIC IN ADULTHOOD
Postformal Thought and Its Applications
Jan D. Sinnot

HANDBOOK OF AGING AND MENTAL HEALTH
An Integrative Approach
Edited by Jacob Lomranz

HANDBOOK OF CLINICAL GEROPSYCHOLOGY
Edited by Michel Hersen and Vincent B. Van Hasselt

HANDBOOK OF PAIN AND AGING
Edited by David I. Mostofsky and Jacob Lomranz

HUMAN DEVELOPMENT IN ADULTHOOD
Lewis R. Aiken

PSYCHOLOGICAL TREATMENT OF OLDER ADULTS
An Introductory Text
Edited by Michel Hersen and Vincent B. Van Hasselt

Handbook of
Aging and Mental Health

An Integrative Approach

Edited by
Jacob Lomranz

Tel Aviv University
Tel Aviv, Israel

Plenum Press • New York and London

Library of Congress Cataloging-in-Publication Data

Handbook of aging and mental health : an integrative approach / edited
by Jacob Lomranz.
        p.   cm. -- (The Plenum series in adult development and aging)
    Includes bibliographical references and index.
    ISBN 0-306-45750-4
    1. Aging--Psychological aspects. 2. Aged--Psychology.
I. Lomrants, Ya'akov. II. Series.
BF724.8.H35 1998
618.97'689--dc21
                                                                  98-29824
                                                                  CIP

ISBN 0-306-45750-4

© 1998 Plenum Press, New York
A Division of Plenum Publishing Corporation
233 Spring Street, New York, N.Y. 10013

http://www.plenum.com

10 9 8 7 6 5 4 3 2 1

Printed in the United States of America

To my parents, Abraham and Ester,
and to my children, Liad and Roie

Contributors

DAN G. BLAZER, School of Medicine and the Divinity School, Duke University, Durham, North Carolina 27708

VICTOR C. CICIRELLI, Department of Psychological Sciences, Purdue University, West Lafayette, Indiana 47907

BERTRAM J. COHLER, Center for Health, Aging, and Society, The University of Chicago, Chicago, Illinois 60637-1603

GAYLE DIENBERG LOVE, Institute on Aging, University of Wisconsin–Madison, Madison, Wisconsin 53706

ANGELA S. EADS, Department of Psychology, Finch University of Health Sciences/ The Chicago Medical School, North Chicago, Illinois 60064

MARILYN J. ESSEX, Institute on Aging, University of Wisconsin–Madison, Madison, Wisconsin 53706

ROBERT P. FRIEDLAND, Department of Neurology, Case Western Reserve University, Cleveland, Ohio 44106

MARGARET GATZ, Department of Psychology, University of Southern California, Los Angeles, California 90089-1061

KARNI GINZBURG, The Bob Shapell School of Social Work, Tel Aviv University, Tel Aviv 69978, Israel

DAVID GUTMANN, Department of Psychiatry and Behavioral Sciences, Northwestern University Medical School, Chicago, Illinois 60657

HAIM HAZAN, Department of Sociology and Anthropology and the Herczeg Institute on Aging, Tel Aviv University, Tel Aviv 69978, Israel

STEVAN E. HOBFOLL, Applied Psychology Center, Department of Psychology, Kent State University, Kent, Ohio 44242

BOAZ KAHANA, Department of Psychology, Cleveland State University, Cleveland, Ohio 44115

ESTHER KAHANA, Department of Neurology, Barzilai Hospital, Ashkelon, Israel

EVA KAHANA, Department of Sociology, Case Western Reserve University, Cleveland, Ohio 44106

IRA KATZ, Department of Psychiatry, University of Pennsylvania, Philadelphia, Pennsylvania 19104

ROBERT KEGAN, Graduate School of Education, Harvard University, Cambridge, Massachusetts 02138 and Massachusetts School of Professional Psychology, Boston, Massachusetts 02132

AMOS D. KORCZYN, Sieratzki Chair of Neurology, Sackler School of Medicine, Tel Aviv University, Tel Aviv 69978, Israel

MORTON A. LIEBERMAN, Aging and Mental Health Program, Center for Social and Behavioral Sciences, University of California at San Francisco, California 94143

JACOB LOMRANZ, Department of Psychology and the Herczeg Institute on Aging, Tel Aviv University, Tel Aviv 69978, Israel

KEITH MEADOR, School of Medicine and the Divinity School, Duke University, Durham, North Carolina 27708

DAVID I. MOSTOFSKY, Department of Psychology, Boston University, Boston, Massachusetts 02215

GEORGE NIEDEREHE, Adult and Geriatric Treatment and Preventive Intervention, Research Branch, National Institute of Mental Health, Rockville, Maryland 20857

LEONARD I. PEARLIN, Department of Sociology, University of Maryland, College Park, Maryland 20742-1315

LAWRENCE C. PERLMUTER, Department of Psychology, Finch University of Health Sciences/The Chicago Medical School, North Chicago, Illinois 60064

HARVEY PESKIN, Department of Psychology, San Francisco State University, San Francisco, California 94132

FRIEDEL M. REISCHIES, Psychiatric Clinic, Freie Universität, 14050, Berlin, Germany

CAROL D. RYFF, Institute on Aging, University of Wisconsin–Madison, Madison, Wisconsin 53706

DOV SHMOTKIN, Department of Psychology and the Herczeg Institute on Aging, Tel Aviv University, Tel Aviv 69978, Israel

CATHERINE B. SILVER, Brooklyn College and the Graduate Center of City University of New York, 33 West 42nd Street, New York, New York 10036-8099

BURTON SINGER, Office of Population Research, Princeton University, New Jersey, New Jersey 08544

MARILYN M. SKAFF, Department of Sociology, University of Maryland, Maryland 20742-1315

ZAHAVA SOLOMON, The Bob Shapell School of Social Work, Tel Aviv University, Tel Aviv 69978, Israel

JENNIFER D. WELLS, Applied Psychology Center, Department of Psychology, Kent State University, Kent, Ohio 44242

Foreword

De cibo quod superest nobis sufficit; oportet gratias agere.

Some elders have accepted this proposition, although seldom with enthusiasm. Gerontologists also have been burdened with the adage: "Leftovers are good enough for us, and we should be grateful for them." I remember how a clerk tried to palm off a stale and cheap cigar to her octogenarian customer. He knew better and came away with a far superior smoke. The clerk fumed, "What does *he* need a good cigar for? Who is *he* to be particular!" In this and in many other ways, elders often have labored under the sociocultural expectation that they should be well content with whatever scraps and *shmattes* happen to come their way.

Gerontologists can identify with this situation. The systematic study of aging and the aged was a new enterprise at the midpoint of this century, but the concepts and methods were pretty much limited to those already on hand. What biological and sociobehavioral scientists had been doing for years was simply extended to the newly annexed territory. This as not only a convenient but also a cost-effective strategy. Data accumulated more rapidly by remaining within familiar frames of reference and relying on familiar designs and measures. The new gerontologists soon harvested a promising crop of descriptive findings. Within a decade after the establishment of the Gerontological Society of America (1947), it was possible to discern the outlines of a valuable new field of knowledge.

Nevertheless, the borrowed methodologies also had a constricting effect. These methodologies often were not sensitive to issues, phenomena, characteristics, and contexts that come to the fore in the later adult years. To cite one obvious example, measures of intellectual functioning established with young adult samples were unlikely to reveal much about judgment, integrative powers, and creativity in elderly adults. Likewise, studies of interpersonal relationships based on existing models and measures fell far short of encompassing intimate experiences that span the total life course. The extension of developmental psychology beyond the early adult years seldom involved a reconceptualization, and the same must be said for the investigation of psychopathology. With a few robust exceptions, aging and the aged were treated as add-ons to existing agendas and techniques, rather than as an opportunity to develop a more encompassing approach to understanding the human condition.

The theoretical foundations of gerontology were in a more dismal condition.

Although the borrowed methodologies were seldom up to the challenges of their subject matter, they were often applied vigorously and resulted in useful normative and building-block data. What about theory? Most sociobehavioral studies were essentially atheoretical. The concepts that did make their appearance were usually borrowed from fields of study that had given very little attention to age-related issues. Furthermore, these borrowings were seldom the most advanced and challenging concepts in their fields. Instead, those who were exploring gerontology for the first time seemed to take comfort in bringing along conceptual security blankets from their home disciplines. These leftovers did not inspire much in the way of theory-driven research. Very seldom were studies devised to evaluate competing theories or with the purpose of generating new theory. Within this dullish theoretical context, the skirmish between disengagement and activity theories took on the dimensions of a combined World Series–Superbowl–nuclear crisis. For the most part, gerontology chugged along without much attention to fundamental theoretical issues, although methodology and research design had made advances.

Handbook of Aging and Mental Health: An Integrative Approach provides a rousing demonstration of emerging theoretical vigor and sophistication. This contribution does not take the form of "set pieces" on this or that theory. Rather, every chapter is illuminated by fresh-minded approaches to the particular subject matter. Those who enter gerontology today as practitioners, researchers, policymakers, or educators are fortunate to have a number of first-rate reference works to consult for basic information. These are the books whose titles usually begin with *Handbook of …* or *Encyclopedia of…*. The handbook/encyclopedia genre excels in providing clear and reliable summaries of knowledge. The present volume also is built upon a strong base of expert knowledge. It offers something distinctive, however, something that is difficult to accommodate within the format of an encyclopedia, handbook, or textbook. Here are searching and often creative contributions. The well-chosen authors have been encouraged to interpret as well as report. Consequently, as readers, we will find ourselves encouraged to participate in the process of integrative thinking.

One can know a great deal about mental health issues in the later adult years and still find much that informs and stimulates in this volume. Newcomers to gerontology will find themselves immediately engaged in the state-of-the-art quest for understanding. Whether gerontological rookie or veteran, all are likely to return again and again to the creative contributions that abound in this volume, not the least of which is the editor's own innovative chapter.

How exciting it is to hear the sizzle of fresh thinking about such challenging and vital issues! Perhaps the diet of leftovers for both gerontologists and their subject matter is finally giving way to a more nourishing and spicy cuisine.

ROBERT KASTENBAUM
Professor of Gerontology
Department of Communication
Arizona State University
Tempe, Arizona

Preface

This volume grew out of our interest in advancing mental health theory in gerontology, thus expanding the understanding of theoreticians, researchers, and clinicians in gerontology at large and in the field of mental health and aging in particular. We felt that systematic efforts of a theoretical nature are required to promote clinical gerontology. Under the auspices of the Herczeg Institute of Aging at Tel Aviv University, we formed an international, multidisciplinary working group consisting of the foremost experts in the field of mental health and aging. We also invited those researchers who had developed original systems in the areas of development and mental health and were willing to apply them to the aged population. We began by corresponding with one another from our various worksites around the world and disseminated our working papers as drafts that cover the main themes presented in this volume. Finally, in the framework of the First Herczeg International Forum on Aging, under the title "Towards Theories on Mental Health and Aging," we met in the Shfayim guest house in Israel for a week of intense and enriching discussions and reflections on these themes, based on our preconference drafts, after which the final chapters for this volume were composed; the core of this volume is the written product of this process.

To enrich a book that stresses integrative conceptualization, we also included other leading scientists, prominent contributors to the field of mental health in the aged. The core of researchers participating in the forum has been tremendously enriched by those contributors—many of them initially invited—who did not participate in the forum but read some of the other predraft manuscripts. As editor, I feel privileged to have worked with such a senior group. This volume presents the cogent issues and main areas in mental health and aging. The novelty of this volume lies in the original contribution of its authors, who have integrated the knowledge and findings in their respective fields and provided new theoretical perspectives, models, and their empirical and applied implications.

Overall, I hope that this volume becomes an important handbook, stimulating and inspiring, for those interested in comprehensive knowledge and conceptualization as well as in the quality of life and well-being of elderly people. It should be of interest to those who study gerontology, those who wish to advance theory and research, and those who are engaged in clinical work with the elderly. I hope that both scientists and practitioners are aided by the chapters and can use them as stepping-stones to advance the theoretical and applied fields of mental health and aging.

Acknowledgments

I have many people to thank for making the first Herczeg International Forum on Aging, "Towards Theories on Aging and Mental Health," and this volume based on it, possible. The Herczeg Institute on Aging at Tel Aviv University funded and supported both projects. The publication of any book is a collaborative effort, with contributions from many individuals. Those who helped to establish and support the institute and the international forum should all be acknowledged. These include the president of Tel Aviv University, Yoram Dienstein, and its rectors, Dan Amir and Itamar Rabinowitz. Continuous support and encouragement have been provided by many colleagues. Particularly important are Ilana Ben Ami, Shimon Bergman, Gabriel Cohen, Nili Cohen, Nitza Eyal, Ariella Friedman, Haim Hazan, Stevan Hobfoll, Beno Giter, Shimon Giter, Dan Jacobson, Joshep Katan, Bob Lubow, Arie Nadler, Rina Shapira, Yonathan Shapira, Dov Shmotkin, Efraim Yaar, and Alik Joffe. Much overseas encouragement and advice has come from Irving Alexander, Margaret Gatz, David Gutmann, Michael Kahn, Martin Lakin, Mort Lieberman, David Mostofsky, Larry Perlmuter, Harvey Peskin, and Irving Rosow. At the institute, the help of Meira Beger in organizing the forum and helping prepare this manuscript for publication was indispensable.

The helpful hand and constant presence of Ziona Goldman proved to be a significant contribution to the completion of this volume. Finally, I am fortunate to have gained from the patience and encouragement of sympathetic editors Elliot Werner and Herman Makler at Plenum Press, and series editor, Jack Demick.

Contents

Introduction

Toward Theories in Mental Health and Aging

JACOB LOMRANZ

This chapter offers a perspective on the state of and need for theory in adult development generally and in the domain of mental health and aging particularly. Although gerontology is continuously making progress (Streib & Binstock, 1990), in many ways, the field of aging is still in the formative stages of collecting and accumulating data that are the basis for theory construction. In other respects, however, owing to the accumulation and availability of valuable research findings, gerontology has reached a point in its development as a science at which such data should be generalized between and across related fields to make it possible to embark upon theory construction. Decades ago, Wittgenstein (1953) wrote, "In psychology there are experimental methods and conceptual confusion" (p. xiv). This also seems to be true today of gerontology. The chapters in this volume present the state of knowledge, research, and integrative attempts toward theory construction in cogent areas of mental health and aging. Most of the chapters are based on the first international forum of the Herczeg Institute on Aging, convened under the title "Toward Theories in Mental Health and Aging." Despite the gains made in the realm of theory construction (e.g., Achenbaum, 1995; Bengtson, Burgess, & Parrot, 1997; Birren & Bengtson, 1988), the background to the Herczeg forum was the fact that gerontological theory, empirical research, and processes of aging in reality have not always been complementary and congruent. There may be a gap in what we know and what we think we know that influences our choices in research (Habermas, 1971) and perhaps has led to the present situation in which "the study of aging has become a field of knowledge that is data rich and theory poor, a vast collection of unintegrated pieces of information" (Birren, 1995, p. 1). Thus,

JACOB LOMRANZ • Department of Psychology and the Herczeg Institute on Aging, Tel Aviv University, 69978, Tel Aviv, Israel.

Handbook of Aging and Mental Health: An Integrative Approach, edited by Jacob Lomranz. Plenum Press, New York, 1998.

there has been insufficient progress in theory building in gerontology in general and specifically in the area of mental health and aging, which is the concern of this volume. Because gerontology is inherently a multidisciplinary field, due to its goals and subject matter (human beings), we should certainly strive for multidisciplinary theories of aging in general, including in the field of mental health. However, the reader of this volume may well ask: How can biological, sociological, economical, psychological, and medical approaches be combined? How can this be accomplished when these disciplines are not unified within themselves?

THEORIES IN SCIENCE AND GERONTOLOGY

The challenges that confront gerontology, namely, to explain aging processes and contribute to the improvement of the human quality of life, are tremendous. How can these challenges and goals be met? Obviously, by following the canons of science: theory and research. Since we emphasize theory, let us recall its definition.

Scientific Theories

How clear and strict are we in our use of the term *theory*? Theories, their construction, meaning, role, and functions, have been variously defined and approached on various levels of abstraction and according to the nature of their propositions. In *Webster's Dictionary* (1985), we find the root in the Greek term *theoria*, which means the act of viewing, contemplation, or consideration. The range of definitions is then catalogued to give a broad signification of the term, such as belief, policy, a body of generalizations, a body of mathematical theorems, a hypothetical entity or working hypothesis. *Theory*, like *hypothesis*, is a term belonging to everyday language, its meaning ranging from description to explanation, from the abstract to concrete hypotheticals (Turner, 1965). Mainly with the work of N. R. Campbell (1920), the term "theory in the language of science has come to designate connected sets of propositions' and operational derivatives which serve as the formal basis for the prediction and explanation of phenomena by empirical means" (p. 7). Propositions may be related to as *laws*, defined as statements expressing an exact invariance between two or more readily observable experimental properties under relatively well-defined conditions. Laws are *confirmed* by data if the data are consistent with every appropriate logical consequence of the law (Ackermann, 1970). We should also be aware of whether we are striving to establish nomothetic or idiographic laws and whether such laws are deterministic or probabilistic. Data collection and experimentation should be theoretically based; otherwise, researchers may find they have fulfilled their scientific program but have achieved meaningless results and are reduced to methodological sterility (Louch, 1969). The comprehensiveness of theories may be related to the available data or the scope of the phenomena it attempts to explain; hence, what may be called a theory in one branch of science may be considered a hypothesis in another. Psychological theories on aging and development should be differentiated as to their construction and evaluation (Baltes & Willis, 1977). Schroots (1995a) distinguishes between the terms *theory*, *model*, and *metaphor*, but these distinctions are not clear enough, because each of them can be conceived on various levels and as various types (e.g., of models), and they are in fact, unfortunately, used interchangeably.

The social sciences, especially psychology, view theory "as a coherent set of hypothetical conceptual and pragmatic (predictive) principles forming the general frame of reference for a field of inquiry. From this coherent entity, the theoretician deduces principles, formulates hypotheses, and then undertakes the actions necessary to validate these hypotheses" (Rychlak, 1968, p. 11). In gerontology, theory has been emphasized as the integration and explanation of knowledge, enabling prediction, providing a basis for intervention and applications (Bengtson, Parrot, & Burgess, 1996). However, a strict definition of theory, as indicated earlier, would not allow any of the conceptual approaches in gerontology (without belittling their value) to be termed theory, although that label is attached to them (e.g., "Disengagement/Activity Theory," or "Branching Theory"). George (1995) distinguishes between "Theory (with a capital T) and theory (with a lower-case t). Virtually all published articles include theory—in the form of testable hypotheses ... very few, however, include Theory—i.e., broad views of fundamental processes" (p. 1). We should also recognize that while humanistic or philosophical scholarship is often dichotomized as being apart from science, when we examine theory construction, such a dichotomy becomes far less impressive, as "scientist" and "humanist" operate upon similar principles (Holton, 1967). With Kuhn (1967), we note that a theory "is seldom or never just an increment to what is already known. Its assimilation requires the reconstruction of prior theory and the re-evaluation of prior fact" (p. 7). Do gerontologists acknowledge the ground-rule definitions of theory construction? Scientists should clarify their position regarding the relationships among theoretical principles, conceptual levels, and logical presuppositions in their research. We have to ask ourselves: Despite the variance in definitions of theories and their functions, where is gerontology positioned in regard to theories, and what theoretical progress has it made?

Theories in Gerontology

The history of gerontology is short (Riegel, 1977); yet this field is constantly expanding and breaking valuable new ground. Schroots (1995a) reviews theoretical trends in the psychology of aging since World War II, dividing them into three periods: "Classical" (e.g., theories based on developmental tasks, cognitive theory, activity theory), "Modern" (e.g., lifespan development, behavioral genetics), and "New" (e.g. gerotranscendence, gerodynamics). Increased methodological rigor and statistical sophistication have perhaps been the hallmark of research on aging during the past quarter century. However, the equivalent scientific effort in the sphere of conceptualization and theory building is lagging behind (Achenbaum, 1995), and there is an obvious lack of cumulative progress associated with these theories (Kastenbaum, 1965). Stevens-Long (1990) notes that "if we adopt the standard definition of *theory* ... then the study of adulthood has not yet produced rigorous theory" (p. 125). A number of characteristics portray past and present theoretical developments and problems in gerontology: Attempts to formulate "grand" theories have been abandoned; the focus is changing from specific mechanisms of aging to general concepts (e.g., "well-being"); researchers are concerned with methodological rigor rather than with theoretical issues; testing "goodness of fit" with statistically based models has become a major thrust; the positivistic scientific approach, while still dominant, has also given some room to the historical method and to interpretive and phenomenological approaches; basic research seems to have given way to applied, program-related research; most of the published research is atheoretical, presenting empirical results without adequate attention to theory (Bengtson et al., 1996); significant multidisciplinary research is still rare (George, 1995).

In the past few years, there has been a growing interest in theoretical issues in gerontology, and a decade ago, optimism increased, raising expectations of theory building in gerontology (e.g., Achenbaum, 1995; Birren, 1995; Birren & Bengtson, 1988; Hendricks, 1996; Marshall, 1980). These, however, have not been fulfilled, particularly in relation to the field of mental health, and progress has been hindered by pitfalls (Bengtson et al., 1996). Gerontologists await a momentum to further the theoretical state of affairs while they continue to accumulate "a vast collection of unintegrated pieces of information" (Birren, 1995, p. 1). They still lack unifying frameworks, clearer guidelines for future research, and coordination between research products and researchers, all of which make it increasingly difficult to relate to gerontology as a unified science. While this state of affairs may reflect the course of scientific development in which observational research, which characterizes most gerontological studies, often precedes theory, such a course is not deterministic. The present state may also reflect a Zeitgeist (Boring, 1950), a cultural ethos, an epistemological stance, a distinct mentality, or a paradigmatic orientation that favors experimentalism and neglects theory construction.

The heuristic value of science, even in the absence of comprehensive theories, or perhaps all the more so, is indispensable. One of its contributions lies in the formulation of broader theoretical questions. George (1995) notes that "the absence of attention to Theory in aging research also has costs, however, including a sense that knowledge is fragmented and that too many studies focus on trivial issues" (p. 2). The lack of capital Theories may lead to a parallel constriction of required theoretical questions. Furthermore, "there seem to be some large questions that shift in focus but never seem to be answered as more data accumulates" (Birren & Lanum, 1991, p. 124). For instance, the scientific breakthroughs of the great personality theories such as those of Freud, Adler, and Jung, cannot be found in empirical evidence but lie in their attempts to answer questions about human nature. When such theories are abandoned, the questions they asked about human nature do not disappear. In fact, after decades of focusing on the "variables" of personality, I believe it is time to supplement the present research with more basic questions about human nature, in personality theory as well as in the field of gerontology. Such attempts may spur theory building. Theory construction may demand more work of scientists. Empirical research has its frameworks, requirements, rules, and guidelines: Students are taught methodology and statistics to prepare them to conduct research. The ability to theorize may require a different education, conditions, and different kinds of scientists.

Theoreticians in gerontology confront a dual-aspect problem. On the one hand, they may strive to formulate grand theories, but on the other, many may understand that the process leading to grand theories is contingent on the unification of an extensive basis of background data, as the history and development of science have shown. I believe that while the former endeavor should not be abandoned, especially as it relates to the formulation of theoretical questions and constructs, concentrated efforts should be invested in integrating the background data. Conceptualization and theorizing in gerontology, even *within* subdisciplines such as social gerontology or clinical geropsychology, are still segmentalized, not to mention bridges *between* disciplines. Presently, I concur with Schroots (1995a), who points to the inadequate level of theorizing and detects little progress in the ability of the various subdisciplines to bridge knowledge and be genuine partners in theory construction in gerontology, a field whose hallmark is its interdisciplinary nature. Furthermore, one should caution against premature efforts to achieve a comprehensive, unified theory of gerontology. It this respect, we should heed Sacher (1980), who, after classifying theories of aging, states, "This reasoning process, whereby a part becomes equated to the whole, so that each *aspect-theory* pretends to be a *comprehensive theory* competing with all others, is detrimental to the healthy growth of gerontology" (p. 17, emphasis added).

Although the Zeitgeist presently encourages empirical work and application, there is nothing more practical then a theory, as Kurt Lewin noted (Marrow, 1969). Hence, I wish to counterbalance that Zeitgeist with a focus of conceptualization. This book is designed to focus on research to the extent that it serves fundamental ideas, problems, and attempts at integrative efforts in order to promote conceptualizations and contribute to theory construction in the field of the mental health of the aged. The authors of the present volume are concerned with achievements and gains within subfields. The elaboration of our present body of knowledge, its utilization as a coherent body of knowledge, its integration, the identification of central tendencies and generalizations, and its links to other relevant subfields, are prerequisites for progress toward theory construction.

THEORIES IN MENTAL HEALTH AND AGING

The task of clinical gerontology is to explain how adult development is both organized and disorganized. It should be noted that progress in some subdisciplines of gerontology is slower than in others. While, for instance, the biology of aging and social gerontology have become recognized fields, generating and producing extensive research, both *clinical gerontology* and *clinical geropsychology* are recent terms. Historically, the field of mental health has been a stepchild in gerontology. This may reflect the dismissive attitude with which gerontology traditionally viewed nonorganic, mental health elements, the insufficient number of interested researchers and clinicians (Santos & VandenBos, 1982), and the absence or inadequacy of mental health facilities for the elderly. We need to reconsider the underlying principles of health, social, and medical policy, and introduce changes in education and training. The colossal needs for mental health treatment for the elderly have not been met. It is my contention, however, that the barriers to progress in the field reside not only in the policy, medical, social, and cultural domains, but they also stem from the lack of appropriate theories that would attract and guide geroclinicians.

A review of mental health and aging textbooks reveals that there is hardly any mention of the term *theory* in the indexes or the content. Generally, mental health conceptualizations as well as treatment approaches are based on or refer to biological theories of aging, organicity, psychoanalytic and psychodynamic theory, cognitive and behavioral approaches, general psychiatric and psycho-pharmacological approaches, and adult developmental life-course approaches (e.g., Bienenfeld, 1990; Butler, Lewis, & Sunderland, 1991; Pollock & Greenspan, 1993; Woods, 1996).

However, the foundations of theoretical contributions are impressive and continuously growing. They could serve as cornerstones for future, more comprehensive theories of gerontological mental health. Major developmental, mental health–related, theoretical contributions may be found on three levels: (1) the important, almost "classical," theoretical bases found in the various lifespan developmental theories and concepts, such as those, of Jung (1960), Erikson (1963), Gould (1978), Havinghurst (1972), and Levinson, Darrow, Klein, Levinson, & McKee (1978); (2) initial presentations and reviews of fields and concepts found, for instance, in textbooks and the relevant clinical-related chapters such as those in the important volumes of Birren and Schaie (1977, 1985, 1990, 1996), Birren, Sloane, and Cohen (1992), Butler et al. (1991), Carlsen (1991), Gatz (1995), Kermis (1986), Neugarten (1977), Sadavoy and Leszcz (1987), Storandt, Siegler, and Elias (1978), Woods (1996), Zarit (1980), and Zarit and Knight (1996); (3) contributions that fall directly in the domain of theory construction. These theoretical, clinical, or adult-developmental works and may include, among others, the works of Gutmann (1994), who, by integrating various dimensions in psychology, psychiatry, gerontology, and anthropology, provides us with a "normal" theory of human development, personality, and change, a well as major contributions to pathology and clinical gerontology; Peskin (Peskin & Livson, 1981; Lieberman & Peskin, 1992), who develops a model of the uses of the past in adult psychological health and elaborates the concept of relational autonomy; Vaillant (1977, 1993), who elaborates the dual theoretical basis of adult personality development and creativity; as well as ego defenses and the influential works and volumes of Colarusso and Nemiroff (1981), Nemiroff and Colarusso (1985, 1990), and their contributors.

Other works conceptually relevant to mental health, in addition to those in the present volume, include the remarkable work of Kastenbaum (Kastenbaum, 1966; Kastenbaum et al., 1972) on temporality, which explicates the temporal world of the aged, its relation to the existential quality of psychological being and signifies to us that an inability to comprehend that world impoverishes our comprehension of the elderly and the meaning of aging; Basseches (1984) and Riegel (1975), who have provided dialectical models incorporating more sophisticated forms of thinking in adults; Hazan (1994, 1996), who attempts to comprehend the existential enigmas of aging through the prism of construction theory and the specific cultural language pertaining to the aged. Kegan (1982, 1994), who brings the work of Jean Piaget into the field of adult development, has provided us with a unique perspective of personality development of the evolving self, based on meaning-making and social processes, as well as an elaboration of culture's "hidden curriculum," which pressures us with cognitive and emotional demands, all perspectives that richly inform the process of therapy. The work of Moody (1992) integrates social structure and aging process with the histories of ideas and philosophy. Oldham and Liebert (1989) attempt to integrate the psychoanalytic perspective and object relations theory with the middle years of the lifespan.

The aforementioned, when interrelated, could provide a theoretical basis and derived clinical methodology for mental health in the elderly. Elaborated conceptualizations in gerontology and mental health should be sought not only in the domain of psychopathology, but also in the sphere of health, normal development, adjustment, resilience, and growth. These should be integrated with developmental theories in general and adult developmental, lifespan theories in particular. This is in keeping with the World Health Organization's (1964) definition of health as "a state of complete physical, mental and social well-being and not merely the absence of disease or infirmity" (p. 1). Furthermore, as the goals of mental health care shift to include a focus on prevention, the need to address normative events and behavior becomes more relevant to both theory and applications. Hence, in the present volume, we approach the problems of mental health in the aged not only manifesting themselves in senility and organicity but also in coping processes, stress, personality disorders, interpersonal difficulties, neuroticism, and psychosis. In such an approach, we must relate to difficulties in daily living and adjustment as well as to psychopathology and clinical methodology.

The area of mental health in gerontology needs to be further "opened" to diverse perspectives in order to broaden its conceptual basis. Fields such as behavioral medicine, medical anthropology, developmental constructivism, existentialism, stress and coping, narrative theory, phenomenological conceptions of the life course, as well as the more recent perspectives such as gerotranscendence (Tornstam, 1992) and gerodynamics/branching theory (Schroots, 1995b), together with the recent biological, psychiatric, psychoanalytic, and gerontological contributions, could all work to further the field of clinical adult theory. Conceptual frameworks that are more differentiated and process revealing on the personal, interpersonal, and psychosociological levels (Rosow, 1994) should be constructed. But first and foremost, we should further develop and integrate adult developmental theory with mental health approaches, so that adult developmental lifespan theory can play a role similar to the one personality theory (e.g., Freud, Sulivan, Rogers, etc.) played in providing the basis for clinical methodology in dynamic psychotherapy. In fact, the theoretical body of psychodynamics and its derived psychotherapy could serve as the basis upon which to build an elaborated conceptualization through which psychotherapeutic treatment of the elderly could be made more effective.

First steps in this direction of integrating psychotherapy and gerontology have already been taken (Knight, 1996; Muslin, 1992). While it is true that Freud himself rejected the elderly as a class and was pessimistic about their ability to change, an approach that led to the unfortunate neglect of the psychodynamic processes of later life by practicing psychoanalysts and psychotherapists (Kastenbaum, 1978), recent decades have witnessed developments in social gerontology and clinical psychodynamic theories that could lead to a psychodynamic conceptualization of the second half of life (Knight, 1996). The basis for such a multidimensional integration lies, to my mind, in four areas: the classic psychoanalytic–psychodynamic approach; the object relations approach, including its British and American branches (e.g., the work of Bion or Hans Loewald); psychodynamic ego theory that embodies social gerontology (e.g., the work of Neugarten) in clinical conceptualizations (e.g., the work of Gutmann); lifespan developmental psychology that modifies the concept of "development," elaborates the notions of change and time, and affords a potential for multidimensional integration of bio–psycho–social–historical areas (e.g., the work of Paul Baltes and his group). Such integrations can greatly advance the theoretical basis of clinical geropsychology and psychiatry.

Thomas Kuhn (1967) has portrayed for us the scenario of scientific progression:

> "Normal science" means research firmly based upon one or more past scientific achievements, achievements that some particular scientific community acknowledges for a time as supplying the foundation for its future practice…. Achievements I shall refer to henceforth as "paradigms," a term that relates closely to "normal science"…. Men (scientists) whose research is based on shared paradigms are committed to the same rules and standards for scientific practice. (Kuhn, 1967, pp. 10–11)

Such work, in itself a necessary condition, has to be followed by "anomalies that subvert the existing tradition of scientific practice" (p. 6). These will raise new questions not in line with the present paradigm, thus providing turning points in scientific development that may lead to scientific revolutions. Kuhn's description of the historical development of science may serve us by indicating the kind of scientific path we have taken, as well that which we have to seek. The above noted (p. 6) somewhat arbitrary (certainly omitting many other contributors and works) theoretical categorizations (1–3) may reflect the "normal" paradigmatic position of most of the scientific work in gerontological mental health (categories 1 and 2 especially). Mental health theoreticians and practitioners function on the basis of accepted concepts and language of mental health. Such a "common denominator" does not guarantee progress in the field of gerontological mental health. Only, I assume, after we have condensed, interrelated, and organized most of our research in mental health and aging under an encompassing conceptualization, as we attempt to do in the present volume, will we come closer to paradigmatic shifts and "theories."

Toward Theories: Integration of Knowledge

This volume, like the first International Forum of the Herczeg Institute on Aging, upon which it is based, has two anchors: the first in the domain of "Theories," and the second in the area of "mental health." The former aspect has focused the present discussion on the "scientific" modality and its place in gerontology in general, and specifically, in the area of mental health. The mental health discussion noted the various existing conceptualizations that, when complemented with the chapters in this volume, may provide a basis for future mental health theories in clinical gerontology.

The present resurgence of theoretical interest evokes discussions and debates that assume that perhaps there are "new waves," "transformations," or "paradigmatic shifts" in theories of aging. At the same time, the appropriateness of different theories is compared, for example, in biological theories of aging, should the cellular approach be preferred on the organismic level (Cristofalo, 1988)? Is "critical theory" (Moody, 1988) preferable to the life-course or social stratification perspective? Should priority be given to theoretical models that inform public discourse and policymaking on aging issues? Should preference be given to theoretical assumptions focusing on diversity, dispersion from the means, nonlinear development or, in contrast, on typical patterns, central tendencies, and linear patterns of change (Uhlenberg, 1988)? Is the interpretive framework more desirable than one that focuses on intervention, prediction, and control? Are limited-range conceptualizations more efficient than "grand" theorizing? Should mental health conceptualizations be biologically based? Or should they be based on social gerontology and the psychology of aging?

Although such discussions and debates have a certain heuristic value, they are, to my mind, somewhat premature. Because we are as yet unsure about which paradigmatic state we do our research in, it becomes untimely to talk about "paradigmatic shifts." Before we attempt to contrast theories, we have to be clear about whether we are in fact dealing with theories, and if so, what kind. We ought to recall Kuhn's (1967) statement that the ongoing work of science in the paradigmatic framework is done by "practitioners," and "gray workers." Is gerontology, including the field of mental health, perhaps at this stage? Or perhaps not even there yet?

In order to advance, we should simultaneously embark on the "normal science" route and try to construct integrating conceptualizations on various levels, thus coming closer to "rules" on our way *toward* theories. It is my belief that this *is* the present stage in theory building in gerontology. Therefore, scientists, without minimizing empirical research, should also be encouraged to "sit back, take a break from empirical research and devote more effort to integrating and synthesizing the knowledge base" (George, 1995, p. 2). Systematic efforts of a theoretical character have to be steady and constant. We await binding-together endeavors that portray the linkages between empirical results of discrete research findings in each of the various fields and subfields of gerontology (e.g., clinical gerontology and its subareas of stress, depression, personality, family, etc.) and clarify how and why empirically observed phenomena are related; only subsequently may we be able to incorporate the various fields under a broader scientific conceptualization. A main goal of the present volume is to provide linkages in the various subareas, thus establishing an advanced basis for broader theorizing.

An understanding of the process of aging appears to be one of the most challenging goals of scientific study. It is unquestionably an immensely difficult task to comprehend normal and pathological aging. Improvements in our models and concepts depend upon the state of acquired research, the kind of questions we ask of our data, and the methods used to answer them. The following chapters attempt to provide research-based conceptual products. It is my hope that they will provoke more creative and integrative efforts to link various aspects of research on mental health and aging into larger theoretical perspectives. They may not be final, but they lay the ground for the needed integrative frameworks and point toward the frontiers that may lead to novel questions, new conceptions, multidimensional models, and a comprehensive theory.

REFERENCES

Achenbaum, W. (1995). *Crossing frontiers: Gerontology emerges as a science*. New York: Cambridge University Press.

Ackermann, R. (1970). *The philosophy of science*. New York: Pegasus.

Baltes, P., & Willis, S. (1977). Towards psychological theories of aging and development. In J. Birren & W. Schaie (Eds.), *Handbook of the psychology of aging* (pp. 128–154). New York: Van Nostrand.

Basseches, M. (1984). *Dialectical thinking and adult development*. Norwood, NJ: Ablex.

Bengtson, V., Burgess, E., & Parrott, T. (1977). Theory, explanation and a third generation of theoretical development of social gerontology. *Journal of Gerontology: Social Sciences, 52B,* 72–88.

Bengtson, V., Parrott, T., & Burgess, E. (1996). Progress and pitfalls in gerontological theorizing. *Gerontologist, 36*(6), 768–772.

Bienenfeld, D. (Ed.). (1990). *Verwoerdt's clinical geropsychiatry* (3rd ed.). Baltimore: Williams & Wilkins.

Birren, J. (1995). Editorial: New models of aging: Comments on need and creative efforts. *Canadian Journal on Aging, 14*(1), 1–7.

Birren, J., & Bengston, V. (Eds.). (1988). *Emergent theories of aging*. New York: Springer.

Birren, J., & Schaie, W. (Eds.). (1977, 1985, 1990, 1996). *Handbook of the psychology of aging*. New York: Van Nostrand.

Birren, J., Sloane, R., & Cohen, R. (Eds.). (1992). *Handbook of mental health and aging* (2nd ed.). San Diego: Academic Press.

Birren, J., & Lanum, J. (1991). Metaphors of psychology and aging. In G. Kenyon, J. Birren, & J. Schroots (Eds.). *Metaphors of aging in science and humanities* (pp. 115–126). New York: Springer.

Boring, E. G. (1950). *A history of experimental psychology*. New York: Appleton.

Bugental, J. (1978). *Psychotherapy and process: The fundamentals of an existential–humanistic approach*. Reading, MA: Addison-Wesley.

Butler, R., Lewis, M., & Sunderland, T. (1991). *Aging and mental health: Positive psychosocial and biomedical approaches* (4th ed.). New York: Merrill.

Campbell, N. R. (1920). *What is science?* New York: Dover.

Carlsen, M. (1991). *Creative aging: A meaning-making perspective.* New York: Norton.

Colarusso, C., & Nemiroff, R. (1981). *Adult development.* New York: Plenum Press.

Cristofalo, V. (1988). An overview of the theories of biological aging. In J. Birren & V. Bengtson (Eds.), *Emergent theories of aging* (pp. 118–127). New York: Springer.

Elder, G., George, L., & Shanahan, M. (1966). Psychological stress over the life course. In Kaplan, H. (Ed.). *Psychological stress* (pp. 247–292). New York: Academic Press.

Erikson, E. (1963). *Childhood and society* (2nd ed.). New York: Norton.

Gatz, M. (Ed.). (1995). *Emerging issues in mental health and aging.* Washington, DC: American Psychological Association.

George, L. (1995). The last half-century of aging research—and thoughts for the future. *Journal of Gerontology, 50B*(1), S1–S3.

Gould, R. (1978). *Transformations.* New York: Simon & Schuster.

Gutmann, D. (1994). *Reclaimed powers: Men and women in later life.* Evanston, IL: Northwestern University Press.

Habermas, J. (1971). *Knowledge and human interests.* Boston: Beacon Press.

Havinghurst, R. (1972). *Developmental tasks and education.* New York: David McKay.

Hazan, H. (1994). *Old age: Constructions and deconstructions.* New York: Cambridge University Press.

Hazan, H. (1996). *From first principles: An experiment in aging.* London: Bergin & Garvey.

Hendricks, J. (1996). Where are the new frontiers in aging theory? *Gerontologist, 36,* 141–144.

Holton, G. (1967). *Science and culture.* Boston: Beacon Press.

Jung, C. (1960). The stages of life. *The collected works of C. G. Jung* (Vol. 8). Princeton, NJ: Princeton University Press.

Kastenbaum, R. (Ed.). (1965). *Contributions to the psycho-biology of aging.* New York: Springer.

Kastenbaum, R. (1966). On the meaning of temporality in later life. *Journal of Genetic Psychology, 109,* 9–25.

Kastenbaum, R. (1978). Personality theory, therapeutic approaches and the elderly client. In M. Storandt, C. Siegler, & M. Elias (Eds.), *The clinical psychology of aging* (pp. 199–224). New York: Plenum Press.

Kastenbaum, R., Derbin, V., Sabatini, P., & Artt, S. (1972). The ages of me: Toward personal and interpersonal definitions of functional aging. *International Journal of Aging and Human Development, 3,* 197–211.

Kegan, R. (1982). *The evolving self.* Cambridge, MA: Harvard University Press.

Kegan, R. (1994). *In over our heads: The mental demands of modern life.* Cambridge, MA: Harvard University Press.

Kermis, M. (1986). *Mental health in late life: The adaptive process.* Boston: Jones & Bartlett.

Knight, B. (1996). Psychodynamic therapy with older adults: Lessons from scientific gerontology. In R. Woods (Ed.), *Handbook of the clinical psychology of ageing* (pp. 545–560). New York: Wiley.

Kuhn, T. (1967). *The structure of scientific revolutions.* Chicago: University of Chicago Press.

Levinson, D. J., Darrow, N., Klein, E. B., Levinson, M. H., & McKee, B. (1978). *The season of a man's life.* New York: Knopf.

Lieberman, M., & Peskin, H. (1992). Adult life crisis. In J. Birren, R. Sloane, & R. Cohen (Eds.). (1992). *Handbook of mental health and aging* (2nd ed.) (pp. 119–143). San Diego: Academic Press.

Louch, A. (1969). *Explanation and human behavior.* Berkeley: University of California Press.

Marrow, A. (1969). *The practical theorist: The life and work of Kurt Lewin.* New York: Basic Books.

Marshall, V. (1980). State of the art lecture: The sociology of aging. In J. Cradford (Ed.), *Canadian gerontological collection,* (Vol. 3) (pp. 76–144). Winnipeg: Canadian Association of Gerontology.

Moody, R. (1988). Towards a critical gerontology: The contribution of the humanities to theories of aging. In J. Birren & V. Bengtson (Eds.), *Emergent theories of aging* (pp. 19–40). New York: Springer.

Moody, R. (1992). The meaning of life in old age. In N. Jecker (Ed.), *Aging and ethics* (pp. 51–92). Totowa, NJ: Humana Press.

Muslin, H. (1992). *The psychotherapy of the elderly self.* New York: Brunner/Mazel.

Nemiroff, R., & Colarusso, C. (1985). *The race against time.* New York: Plenum Press.

Nemiroff, R., & Colarusso, C. (1990). *New dimensions in adult development*. New York: Basic Books.
Neugarten, B. (1977). Personality and aging. In J. Birren & W. Schaie (Eds.), *Handbook of the psychology of aging* (pp. 626–649). New York: Van Nostrand.
Oldham, J., & Liebert, R. (1989). *The middle years*. New Haven, CT: Yale University Press.
Peskin, H., & Livson, N. (1981). Uses of the past in adult psychological health. In D. Eichorn, J. Clausen, N. Haan, M. Honzik, & P. Mussen (Eds.), *Present and past in middle life* (pp. 153–181). New York: Academic Press.
Pollock, G., & Greenspan, S. (Eds.). (1993). *The course of life: Late adulthood*. Madison, CT: International Universities Press.
Riegel, K. (1975). Towards a dialectical theory of development. *Human Development, 18*, 50–64.
Riegel, K. (1977). History of psychological gerontology. In J. Birren & W. Schaie (Eds.), *Handbook of the psychology of aging* (pp. 70–102). New York: Van Nostrand.
Rosow, I. (1994). Lessons from the museum: Claude Monet and social roles. *Gerontologist, 43*, 292–298.
Rychlak, J. (1968). *A philosophy of science for personality theory*. Boston: Houghton Mifflin.
Sacher, G. (1980). Theory in gerontology. *Annual Review of Gerontology and Geriatrics, 1*, 3–25.
Sadavoy, J., & Leszcz, M. (Eds.). (1989). *Treating the elderly with psychotherapy*. Madison, CT: International Universities Press.
Santos, J., & VandenBos, G. (Eds.). (1982). *Psychology and the older adult: Challenges for training in the 1980s*. Washington, DC: American Psychological Association.
Schroots, J. (1995a). Psychological models of aging. *Canadian Journal on Aging, 14*, 44–66.
Schroots, J. (1995b). Gerodynamics: Towards a branching theory of aging. *Canadian Journal of Aging, 14*, 74–81.
Stevens-Long, J. (1990). Adult development: Theories past and present. In R. Nemiroff & C. Colarusso (Eds.), *New dimensions in adult development* (pp. 125–165). New York: Basic Books.
Storandt, M., Siegler, I., & Elias, M. (1978). *The clinical psychology of aging*. New York: Plenum Press.
Tornstam, L. (1992). The quo vadis of gerontology: On the scientific paradigm of gerontology. *Gerontologist, 32*, 318–326.
Turner, M. (1965). *Philosophy and the science of behavior*. New York: Appleton-Century-Crofts.
Uhlenberg, P. (1988). Aging and societal significance of cohorts. In J. Birren & V. Bengtson (Eds.), *Emergent theories of aging* (pp. 385–404). New York: Springer.
Vaillant, G. (1977). *Adaptation to life*. Boston: Little Brown.
Valliant, G. (1993). *The wisdom of the ego*. Cambridge, MA: Harvard University Press.
Webster's Dictionary. (1985). Springfield, MA: Merrian Webster.
Wittgenstein, L. (1953). *Philosophical investigations*. Oxford, UK: Blackwell.
Woods, R. (Ed.). (1996). *Handbook of the clinical psychology of aging*. New York: Wiley.
World Health Organization. (1964). *Basic documents* (15th ed.). Geneva, Switzerland: Author.
Zarit, S. (1980). *Aging and mental disorders*. New York: Free Press.
Zarit, S., & Knight, B. (Eds.). (1996). *A guide to psychotherapy and aging*. Washington, DC: American Psychological Association.

Well-Being, Adjustment, and Growth Behaviors in Later Life

The chapters in Part I address cogent issues of stress, adjustment resilience, and growth. Personal evaluations of our own state have a serious impact on our existential condition, but, unfortunately, their meaning is often unclear. Focusing on the way people subjectively evaluate the quality of their lives, Shmotkin (Chapter 1) differentiates between various facets of well-being (see also Gatz, Chapter 4). Portraying the relationships between those facets, he integrates them through a topological model in which congruous and incongruous types of subjective well-being reveal specific characteristics. He notes the implications for the processes of well-being, adjustment, and aging (see Ryff et al., Chapter 3). Shmotkin's original work paves the way to further integration of the diversely used concept of well-being.

Well-being without a sense of control may actually be unrealizable. The question for the aged becomes how to enhance their sense of control, especially when they are often dependent, their lives determined by outside forces and caregivers. Perceived control and choice are potentially powerful and can be deployed to increase the quality of life of the aged. Cognizant of the limitations of self-reports, Perlmuter and Eads (Chapter 2) deal with the areas of control and their cognitive and motivational implications. They utilize experimental paradigms to examine how choice and control affect motivation and performance in individuals, both young and old. The authors develop criteria for making choice effective and propose principles that may be useful in enhancing the perception of control in the elderly, thus strengthening the linkage between the self-initiated efforts of individuals and their behaviors. Not only should this work contribute to the quality of research on control and choice, but also its further implications on education, clinical settings, therapy, styles of living, and living in institutions are obvious.

Ryff et al. (Chapter 3) propose a conceptualization of resilience in later life on the basis of psychological well-being and multidisciplinary resources. Their theoretical and empirical investigations expose strength and protective factors as well as vulnerabilities in the elderly population (see Gatz, Chapter 4). Illustrating their formulation with findings from longitudinal studies, the authors distinguish between resilience as a set of outcome criteria and as a dynamic process, thus providing a framework that addresses capacities which, in many cases, enable the aged person to stay well, cope constructively, or even improve in the face of adversity (see Silver, Chapter 17). This conceptualization advances our understanding of late-life resilience, directs future research of this construct, and suggests intervention programs to promote resilience in the aged population.

CHAPTER 1

Declarative and Differential Aspects of Subjective Well-Being and Its Implications for Mental Health in Later Life

Dov Shmotkin

Subjective well-being (SWB) refers to the overall evaluation that people make about the quality of their life, generally by summing up their essential life experiences along a positive–negative continuum. Though SWB is widely considered indicative of mental health (Bryant & Veroff, 1984; Gurin, Veroff, & Feld, 1960), the exact relationship between the two constructs is not yet settled. The definition of the DSM-IV (American Psychiatric Association, 1994) for mental disorder does not allude to SWB, but rather to "present distress" (p. xxi). In its definition since the 1940s, the World Health Organization (1996) states that "health is a state of complete physical, mental, and social well-being, and not merely the absence of disease or infirmity" (p. 1). Notably, this definition does not separate physical from mental health, and regards "well-being" in its broadest sense as an essential constituent of health. Thus, mental health can be conceptualized as composed of two inclusive elements, psychological distress and psychological well-being (Veit & Ware, 1983), which are not mutually reducible, but rather complementarily indicate the variations in a person's mental status (Lewinsohn, Redner, & Seeley, 1991). Although most scholars are concerned with the psychopathological and distressful aspects of mental health, the "positive mental health" approach (Johoda, 1958) attempts to better understand

Dov Shmotkin • Department of Psychology and the Herczeg Institute on Aging, Tel Aviv University, Tel Aviv, 69978 Israel.

Handbook of Aging and Mental Health: An Integrative Approach, edited by Jacob Lomranz. Plenum Press, New York, 1998.

the role of adaptive processes. It can reasonably be assumed that SWB plays a role in at least some of these processes.

References of major reviews on SWB (Chamberlain, 1988; Diener, 1984, 1994; Larson, 1978; Veenhoven, 1984, 1991) show that a great deal of the studies on the subject have been published in gerontological outlets. This probably reflects the fact that researchers of aging tend to regard SWB as usefully sensitive in assessing normative adjustment and positive mental health in a population where greater vulnerability to physical and mental deterioration must be considered. In order to further elaborate on this potential contribution of the SWB concept, the present chapter suggests a distinction between the more explicitly communicated *declarative* meaning of SWB self-reports and the more subtle *differential* combinations that such reports may constitute. These aspects of SWB will be considered here after a brief review of the structural characteristics of the concept. The differential approach to SWB will then be presented through a typological model and the results of a preliminary study that has examined the suggested typologies empirically.

GLOBAL APPROACH
TO SUBJECTIVE WELL-BEING

The term *global approach* is used here to refer to the study of SWB as a generalized concept that sums up one's core evaluations regarding happiness and satisfaction with life. The global concept ("life as a whole") is often separated from more specific evaluations of distinct life domains or concerns, such as family life, work, social life, housing, leisure, and health. This approach dominated the classical works of Andrews and Withey (1976) and Campbell, Converse, and Rodgers (1976), and was implemented in their large-scale, national surveys. Global SWB has been usually assessed by single-item, easily administered measures (Andrews & Robinson, 1991).

This conception of SWB might appear to be too simplified and lacking in a theoretical foundation. However, the measures have proved to be psychometrically sound and efficient in detecting differences between social groups. Moreover, the global and domain-specific evaluations, which often yield moderate to high intercorrelations, maintain a consistent structure across age groups and countries (Andrews & Inglehart, 1979; Herzog & Rodgers, 1981). The interplay between global SWB and specific satisfactions has raised a theoretical question as to the causal direction: Does global SWB predispose people to evaluate their life domains in a certain way (top-down theory), or do the domain satisfactions have a cumulative effect on global SWB (bottom-up theory)? The studies investigating this question (Brief, Butcher, George, & Link, 1993; Headey, Veenhoven, & Wearing, 1991) are also highly relevant to another theoretical question: Is SWB a consistent personality trait (Costa, McCrae, & Zonderman, 1987a), or is it merely a relatively stable characteristic that *is* sensitive to environmental effects (Veenhoven, 1994)? The findings indicate that neither of these two theoretical questions has yet been resolved.

The research on global SWB has taught us an interesting lesson. Protracted philosophical debates on the concepts notwithstanding, most people acquiesce to the request to rate their happiness and life satisfaction with surprising willingness, usually voicing no special difficulties in performing the task. Perhaps the scholarly conceptualizations of SWB should also attend to its heuristic and intuitive meaning.

MULTIDIMENTIONAL APPROACHES TO SWB

Positive versus Negative Affect Dimensionality

Bradburn (1969) presented a coherent two-factor conceptualization of SWB, proposing that happiness results from the balance between two independent affects—positive and negative. Numerous studies have investigated the generalizability of this conceptualization, and particularly the extent to which the independence of positive and negative affect is a methodological artifact or a genuine phenomenon, producing support for both options. On the one hand, the correlation between positive and negative affect has been found to depend on a variety of factors, such as measurement procedures (Green, Goldman, & Salovey, 1993; Kammann, Farry & Herbison, 1984) and the time frame (Diener & Emmons, 1984). On the other hand, the two affects have been found to be differentially associated with personality correlates (Costa & McCrae, 1980), representing two distinct, larger configurations, such as those termed "exterior" and "interior" well-being (Lawton, 1983) or "well-being" and "ill-being" (Headey, Holmstrom, & Wearing, 1985). Reviews of this debated issue (Diener, 1984, 1994) conclude that although positive and negative affect my not be strictly independent, they are separate entities with different antecedents and consequences. It should be noted that this conclusion applied to the frequency, or the relative amount of time, with which each affect is experienced. Where the intensity of positive and negative affect is concerned, the two maintain a strong positive correlation and may not represent the common quality of SWB because of the undesirable complications accompanying intense affects of both kinds (Diener, Larsen, Levine, & Emmons, 1985; Diener, Sandvik, & Pavot, 1991).

Cognitive versus Affective Dimensionality

The distinction between cognitive and affective dimensions of SWB is readily apparent from the two major sourcebooks of Campbell et al. (1976) and Andrews and Withey (1976). Campbell et al. (1976) noticed that ratings of satisfaction and happiness presented different meanings and were differentially associated with various correlates. Satisfaction referred to a cognitive–judgmental, long-term assessment of one's life, mainly as a function of the gap between one's level of aspirations and the presently perceived situation, whereas happiness referred to a spontaneous reflection of pleasant and unpleasant affects in one's immediate experience (Campbell, 1981; George, 1981). Andrews and Withey (1976) made the distinction between the components of cognition, positive affect, and negative affect on the basis of a factorial classification of numerous SWB measurement techniques, with further confirmation lent by subsequent structural modeling analyses (Andrews & McKennell, 1980; Horley & Little, 1985; Stock, Okun, & Benin, 1986). One must, however, be aware of certain terminological confusion in the literature: Although "happiness" may denote the subordinate, affective dimension of SWB (George, 1981; Okun, 1987), for some researchers it may also denote the general concept of SWB (Veenhoven, 1984). In the latter case, the affective dimension may be called the "hedonic level" or "affective well-being" (Diener, 1994).

Temporal Dimensionality

The conceptualization of SWB within a temporal framework was introduced by Cantril (1965), whose Self-Anchoring Scale consisted of three separate ratings of satisfaction with past, present, and future. His cross-national results, as well as those of Andrews and Withey (1976), depicted a lifespan pattern in which future was usually rated highest and past lowest, while ratings of past increased and ratings of future decreased with advancing age (Shmotkin, 1991a). This pattern points to the importance of time frames in SWB (Bryant & Veroff, 1984; Stock et al., 1986) and may be related to more general implications of time perspective in lifespan development and mental health (Kastenbaum, 1982; Lomranz, Friedman, Gitter, Shmotkin, & Medini, 1985). Although several systematic attempts have been made to assess SWB within temporal dimensions (Ryff, 1991; Staats & Skowronski, 1992), there is usually a great variability, and sometimes even confusion, regarding the time frames associated with SWB measures (Chamberlain, 1988).

Gerontological Studies of SWB Dimensionality

The study of SWB dimensionality in old age has relied largely on two main instruments: the Life Satisfaction Index A (LSIA; Neugarten, Havighurst, & Tobin, 1961) and the Philadelphia Geriatric Center Morale Scale (PGCMS; Lawton, 1975). Although both instruments have specifically addressed SWB in the older population, their orientations are different: LSIA was originally designed for community-dwelling older adults and emphasized positive affect and self-judgments; PGCMS was meant to better fit the institutionalized elderly and refers mainly to negative affect and states.

Factorial studies of LSIA (Hoyt & Creech, 1983; Liang, 1984; Shmotkin, 1991b) have usually delineated three factors: Mood Tone, referring to happiness and positive affect; Zest-for-Life, referring to positive outlook and optimism; and Congruence, referring to the degree to which one's desired goals have been attained. The factorial studies of the PGCMS (Lawton, 1975; Liang & Bollen, 1983) have also resulted in three factors, not necessarily analogous to those of the LSIA: Agitation, referring to manifestations of worries and anxiety; Attitude toward Own Aging, referring to self-perceived changes as one ages; and Dissatis-faction, referring to feelings of discontentment about life, with the possible addition of the notion of loneliness.

An integrative study of the LSIA's and PGCMS's combined item pools (Shmotkin & Hadari, 1996) has yielded five factors, labeled Reconciled Aging, Unstrained Affect, General Contentment, Present Happiness, and Past Self-Fulfillment. This study has confirmed that the thematic compositions of LSIA and PGCMS complement, rather than substitute for, each other. Notably, in both formulations, as well as in the integrative one, the attitude to old age and the ability to reconcile oneself to the negative implications of aging seem vital concomitants of maintaining SWB, and probably mental health, in later life. This finding, however, suggests a difficulty in the comparability of SWB measures in younger and older adulthood: While the ordinary epidemiological instru-ments do not address the aging issue, the gerontological instruments are not applicable to younger adults.

A general conclusion drawn from gerontological studies is that SWB con-sists of a two-level structure. On the lower level, the first-order factors present the basic themes of SWB, in which one can trace the three dimensions of positive versus negative affect, cognition versus affectivity, and past–present–future perspectives (Stock et al., 1986). On the higher level, a second-order factor presents SWB as a superordinate construct that retains its overall coherence. This two-level conceptualization has consistently been proposed in Liang's series of structural studies (e.g., Liang, 1984; Liang & Bollen, 1983) and has been found to fit the data well in other investigations (McNeil, Stones, & Kozma, 1986; Shmotkin, 1991b; Shmotkin & Hadari, 1996; Stones & Kozma, 1985).

DECLARATIVE ASPECTS OF SWB

The act of self-rating, as required in ordinary measures of SWB and indeed in most other measures of attitudes and personality, contains a *declarative* com-ponent. The term *declarative* indicates that the respondent is asked, whether in questionnaires or in oral interviews, to endorse some kind of personal statement that is addressed to a certain audience. While the audience usually consists of the research or assessment team, respondents often believe, either rightly or wrongly, that their statements will also be accessible to a larger public. In cases where anonymity is not guaranteed, respondents are likely to feel a higher commitment to the declarative impacts of their statement.

As in the measurement of other psychological constructs, researchers of SWB have expressed concern about the bias that may be engendered by the de-clarative component. Social desirability, which may reflect self-presentational tendencies, has in particular been suspected of being a threat to the validity of SWB measures (Carstensen & Cone, 1983). The response bias of acquiescence has been considered as another cause of a systematic error in SWB measures (Moum, 1988). It may also be assumed that the implications of reported SWB are some-times touchy enough to heighten the respondents' defensiveness, as typically reflected in the mechanisms of repression and denial, which result in concealing from oneself and from others distressful feelings regarding well-being. It has been argued that defense-driven reports probably portray illusory mental health (Shedler, Mayman, & Manis, 1993).

In addition to the understandable concerns over distortion in SWB measurement, it is suggested to consider the declarative aspects of SWB from another angle. Rather than viewing them as causing bias or nuisance, we would preferably regard them as inherent in SWB itself. Reporting one's SWB is indeed a social act of communication and sharing. In line with speech act theory (Austin, 1962), we are dealing here with an utterance that constitutes an act by virtue of something being said. Self-report of SWB may serve several functions that can operate jointly and complementarily: It may convey one's basic approach to life (*expressive* function), relate to perceived expectations as to how one should react (*self-presentational* function), communicate a tentative state of mind so that further feedback from inside or outside the self is generated to work it out (*self-orienting* function), maintain an anxiety-free mode of functioning where either internal or external threats are imminent (*defensive* function), or stage a certain mood or condition in order to explore or manipulate the resultant "as if" situation (*simulative* function). While the conception of declarative functions is being developed elsewhere (Shmotkin, 1996), the present reference to them suggests that the declarative aspects of SWB enable this basically introspective sentiment to be marked and communicated, thus facilitating various kinds of interactive reactions.

In line with this reasoning, several studies have shown that controlling individual differences in social desirability may *not* enhance the validity of SWB measures, probably because social desirability reflects a pertinent content of SWB (Diener, Sandvik, Pavot, & Gallagher, 1991; Kozma & Stones, 1987; McCrae, 1986). Moreover, situations that sensitize impression management needs, such as face-to-face interviews, may indeed influence one's reported level of SWB, but without lowering the validity of SWB measures as compared to anonymous settings (Diener, 1994). In the same vein, when the avowed SWB is a result of defensiveness and self-deception, it still remains a genuine product of a coping process that does not necessarily compromise any adaptive action, and often relates to culturally shared illusions that foster mental health rather than undermine it (Lazarus, 1991; Taylor & Brown, 1988). While various research indices demonstrated that typically defensive repressors were more anxious and stressful than they admitted by self-report, it was also evident that this repressive style was by no means easily reversed (Weinberger, 1990). Thus, there is evidence showing that the effects of both self-presentation and self-deception pose no external threat to the coherence of SWB, but rather play a certain role in its conceptual meaning. Indeed, the assessment of defensive or deceptive reports of SWB is still a challenge (Diener, 1994; Shedler et al., 1993), but it may also be seen as a part in the evaluation of the different declarative functions underlying SWB reports.

The empirical validation of the declarative functions is a task for future research. It would possibly begin with probing respondents for any intentions, feelings, associations, and expectations while reporting their SWB. Other feasible strategies would be to use standard SWB questionnaires accompanied by structured queries about the potential consequences of completing these questionnaires, or to content-analyze detailed reports of SWB in open-ended formats. Once delineated, declarative functions can be used to examine more thoroughly the relationships between SWB and other constructs or behaviors, and to detect more clearly the often implicit dialogues between respondents and their audience, or between different voices within the individual respondents themselves.

DIFFERENTIAL ASPECTS OF SWB
AND THE SUGGESTED TYPOLOGICAL MODEL

The term *differential* refers here to the use of various dimensions or attributes of a construct in order to derive configurations representing distinct modes of adjustment and behavior. Such combinations of multifaceted data are nothing new in psychological assessment, as evident from the classical examples of the scatter in the Wechsler intelligence scales, the profiles in the Multiphasic Minnesota Personality Inventory, and the structural summary in the Rorschach test. However, while the differential approach is now almost a prerequisite of large-scale evaluations, it must be proved theoretically justified and pragmatically useful for evaluating relatively limited constructs such as SWB. We have seen that research has demonstrated the usefulness of a multidimensional conception of SWB. The time is now ripe, therefore, for systematic explorations of whether the emerging dimensionality can facilitate formulation of the *differential* aspects of SWB, that is, the combinatory and interactive effects of relevant dimensions.

Several differential approaches to SWB have already been suggested. Prominent is Bradburn's (1969) aforementioned affect balance, which extracts a continuum of happiness out of the discrepancy between positive and negative affect. More elaborate is Michalos's (1985) discrepancies theory, which postulates that reported satisfaction is a function of a series of perceived gaps, such as those between what one has and wants, expects to have in the future, or believes that relevant others have. Another pertinent example is McKennell's (1978) SWB typology based on dichotomizing and cross-tabulating the ratings of happiness and satisfaction. There have been a number of attempts to apply this typology (de Haes, Pennink, & Welvaart, 1987; Michalos, 1980) as well as to propose further cross-classifications of SWB dimensions (Chamberlain, 1988). In a way, the study presented below is an extension of McKennell's idea.

The differential aspects of SWB are represented here by a typological model (see Figure 1–1) that cross-tabulates three pairs of relevant SWB dimensions: positive affect and negative affect as the two major affective components; affect balance and life satisfaction as the two basic constituents of emotion and cognition; and the two evaluations of present and future, which provide the temporal perspective.

These cross-tabulations formulate three sets of 2×2 typologies where each dimension is split into high and low. Note that negative affect is the only

A. Positive Negative Types — **Positive Affect**

Negative Affect	*Low*	*High*
High	Unhappy (4)	Inflated (2)
Low	Deflated (3)	Happy (1)

B. Cognitive Affective Types — **Life Satisfaction**

Affect Balance	*Low*	*High*
Low	Essentially Ungratified (4)	Satisfied-but Unhappy (2)
High	Happy-but Unsatisfied (3)	Amply Gratified (1)

C. Present Future Types — **Present Evaluation**

Future Evaluation	*Low*	*High*
Low	Reasonably Pessimistic (4)	Unreasonably Pessimistic (2)
High	Unreasonably Optimistic (3)	Reasonably Optimistic (1)

Figure 1–1. SWB differential types.

dimension in which "high" signals a *low* level of SWB and vice versa. Due to the usual correlations between SWB dimensions (positive and negative affect are often, but not always an exception), a distinction is made between *congruous types*, in which one is either high or low on SWB level according to *both* cross-tabulated dimensions (designated as cells 1 and 4 in Figure 1–1), and *incongruous types*, in which one is high on SWB level according to one dimension but low according to the other (cells 2 and 3). While the congruous types appear to indicate a definite higher (Type 1) or lower (Type 4) level of SWB, the incongruous types apparently indicate intermediate levels of SWB, with no prior expectation as to whether Type 2 or Type 3 is more advantageous. The labels given to the different types should be regarded as rudimentary.

The Positive–Negative Types (Figure 1–1, Section A)

Following Bradburn (1969), the congruous types reflect either the predominance of positive over negative (Happy) or negative over positive (Unhappy) affect. The incongruous types apply to people whose affective reactivity cannot be characterized by a dominant valence, but rather by a general arousal level. When both positive and negative affect are easily triggered and elevated (Inflated), one reacts with dense occurrences of seemingly contradictory moods; when both affects are flattened (Deflated), one reacts with lower emotional involvement of any sort. Although these incongruous types reflect different mechanisms of emotional adaptation, Bradburn's affect balance score fails to discriminate between them, since in both cases the discrepancy between positive and negative affect approaches zero.

The Cognitive–Affective Types (Figure 1–1, Section B)

The joint effect of life satisfaction and affect balance (Happiness) is very likely a potent one because it involves the combination of cognition and affect, the two major dimensions of SWB. Declaring oneself to be both satisfied and happy reflects a highly favorable position in which one's needs are largely met (Amply Gratified), whereas the opposite, stating that one is both dissatisfied and unhappy, bears the clear implication of distress and deprivation (Essentially Ungratified). The incongruous types occupy intermediate positions where higher satisfaction contains lower happiness (Satisfied-but-Unhappy) or vice versa (Happy-but-Unsatisfied), apparently representing two reverse modes where cognition and affect regulate or compensate for each other.

The Present–Future Types (Figure 1–1, Section C)

While evaluation of the present relies on an existing situation and tangible experience, evaluation of the future is a matter of anticipation and expectation. Thus, this typology deals with the ways in which the perception of the present provides a basis for visualizing the future either optimistically or pessimistically. In the congruous types, a high evaluation of the present causes one to reasonably expect a positive future (Reasonably Optimistic), while a low evaluation may justify a gloomy outlook on the future (Reasonably Pessimistic). In the incongruous types, one may be reluctant to trust in the future despite an admittedly good present (Unreasonably Pessimistic) or alternatively, may foster high expectations of the future unsubstantiated by the low-evaluated present (Unreasonably Optimistic). It is noted that the terms *reasonably* and *unreasonably* merely refer to the apparent congruity or incongruity between the temporal evaluations and should not be understood to imply any critical stand with regard to the appropriateness of these evaluations.

Any typological model, including the one suggested here, is in risk of falling into the trap of crude classification and oversimplification. Nevertheless, the present typologies have been designed to exemplify a differential approach by which different indices of SWB are not regarded just as correlated or even redundant, but as potentially contributing unique meanings that may be integrated into more elaborate schemes. The proposed model is also based on the following assumptions:

1. While SWB has various dimensions, certain dimensions seem more relevant to one another because of potentially mutual effects such as complementariness (e.g., only the combination of high positive affect and low negative affect may yield happiness), amplification (e.g., the joint effect of cognition and affect on SWB may be more potent than any effect of either separately), and compensation (e.g., SWB may be largely nourished by present zest even in the absence of optimistic outlook). The present taxonomy deals with three pairs of relevant dimensions, although other possible pairs (e.g., present and past evaluations) deserve further study.

2. The SWB structure appears to consist of first-order factors, or dimensions, with intercorrelations that are best explained by a second-order, superordinate factor of general SWB. It is this that has led to the distinction between congruous and incongruous types. While the former appear more expected and represent higher consistency within the SWB construct, the latter represent distinct ways of maintaining SWB within the construct's associated variability.

3. The raw material for the differential approach is self-ratings, or rather declarations, of SWB. It is by the combination of different ratings into certain configurations that the differential approach may provide extended, and often subtle, information on individual SWB. Thus, the declarative and the differential aspects constitute two levels of information, with the former incorporated in the latter. This implies, for example, that the declarative functions related to the SWB ratings may modify the meanings of the resultant SWB types, though it must await future research to be substantiated.

4. The actual classification into types is based on each respondent's position relative to the variability of his or her group. Thus, being relatively "high" or "low" on the relevant SWB dimensions introduces into the derived typology a normative basis and therefore also a social context.

5. The term *types* is not meant to imply that we are dealing here with trait-like predispositions. In fact, these types are ways of organizing one's SWB

structure and may serve as frames of reference for relating SWB to certain modes of adjustment. In this regard, the types that do not fit a person are as important as the type that does fit, because the unfit types represent available, though unused, options.

DIFFERENTIAL ASPECTS OF SWB AND MENTAL HEALTH ALONG THE LIFESPAN

The precise role of SWB in mental health processes is still obscure in many respects. As elaborated by Ryff (1989; Ryff & Keyes, 1995), research of SWB has lacked a sound theory and neglected important aspects of positive functioning. Ryff's conceptualization of *psychological well-being* explicitly relates to well-ness in terms of theory-guided functional dimensions. This formulation as well as other studies (Compton, Smith, Cornish, & Qualls, 1996; Waterman, 1993) require that SWB should not be confused with other core elements of positive mental health, such as personal expressiveness and growth.

There is, however, evidence to show that SWB dimensions are involved in maintaining psychological adjustment across the lifespan. Thus, Campbell et al. (1976) observed that ratings of life satisfaction *increased* with advancing age, whereas ratings of happiness *decreased*. The literature published since that observation (Shmotkin, 1990) shows that, beyond the inconsistencies of various findings, the cognitive dimension of SWB, especially as manifested in general assessments of life satisfaction, seems to be positively correlated with age, or at least yields similar levels across age groups. On the other hand, the affective dimension of SWB, especially when expressed in terms of positive *and* negative affect, seems to be negatively correlated with age, the decline of positive affect being somewhat more pronounced.

The explanations offered for this pattern reflect various modes of coping with aging. A major explanation proposed by Campbell et al. (1976) with regard to satisfaction is the adjustment of aspirations to present achievements. Thus, the elderly narrow the gap between expectations and actual reality, and so avoid dissatisfaction when unpleasant conditions prevail. This notion of perceived gaps as explaining satisfaction was extended into a multiple discrepancies theory (Michalos, 1985) that has been empirically confirmed in different age groups, including seniors (Michalos, 1986). Herzog and Rodgers (1986) at-tempted to substantiate the explanation of aspiration adjustment along with other explanations for the maintenance of satisfaction in older age, such as the prolonged habituation that makes older people more satisfied with situations they have long been exposed to, and the stronger use of denial as a potentially adaptive mechanism in old age.

Regarding the affective expression of SWB in older, as compared to younger, adults, Schulz (1985) noted that one would tend to expect the elderly to have lower positive affect and higher negative affect, which may be associated with the various losses of old age. This intuitive expectation is apparently in line with those studies that reported a higher incidence of depression in later life (Stenback, 1980). However, both positive *and* negative affect tend to decline with age, as found in cross-sectional comparisons (Bradburn, 1969; Costa et al., 1987b; Gaitz & Scott, 1972) and in a longitudinal design (Stacey & Gatz, 1991). Diener, Sandvick, and Larsen (1985) have contended that emotional intensity in general becomes weaker in old age, whether because of a biological decrease in autonomic arousal, the greater habituation of aging people to emotional life events, or cultural expectations that the elderly should not be too emotional. This affective decline appears less moderated by sociodemographic conditions than satisfaction level (Shmotkin, 1990), and more in line with studies that have found no clearly delineated increase in depression in old age (Gatz & Hurwicz, 1990; Newmann, 1989). The parallel decrease in positive and negative affect in old age may be adaptive, as it actually causes little change in the resultant affect balance (Stacey & Gatz, 1991) but permits the elderly to gain higher emotional control and moderation in coping with dependency, a slowing pace of activities, and lower engagement (Lawton, Kleban, Rajagopal, & Dean, 1992). In order to avoid a detrimentally excessive decline of positive affect in old age, there seem to be adaptive processes that help to coordinate resources and vulnerabilities by conservation of emotions or shifting from assimilative to accommodative strategies (Filipp, 1996). Stressing positive emotional balance in old age, Carstensen's socioemotional selectivity theory (Carstensen, Gross, & Fung, 1997) is stronger than others to suggest that emotion regulation improves among older people, most notably by pruning the social network in a way that focuses on closer relationships and thus assures emotionally meaningful and supportive experience.

It would appear, then, that the cognitive and affective dimensions play certain adaptive roles in aging. In an attempt to examine their differential impacts, McKennell (1978) suggested four types: Achievers (equivalent to the Amply Gratified in Figure 1–1, section B), Resigned (equivalent to the Satisfied-but-Unhappy), Aspirers (equivalent to the Happy-but-Unsatisfied), and Frustrated (equivalent to the Essentially Ungratified). McKennell's data showed that Aspirers had a higher proportion of younger participants (ages 18–34), resigned had a higher proportion of older participants (age 65+), and the two other types showed no consistent trend with age. Thus, the age-related effects were associated with the incongruous types in the present terminology: The younger adults were still critical of their achievements in life but could afford to express emotional vitality, whereas the older adults had lost some of this vitality but could rely on lifelong achievements.

The temporal dimension of SWB has also been strongly linked to coping with aging processes (Ryff, 1991). Older people have been depicted as increasingly "past-oriented" and decreasingly "future-oriented." The foreshortened future and often diminishing options in the present lead the aged to rely more heavily on the past (Kastenbaum, 1982). This seems true as far as the relative *levels* of evaluations attributed to one's past, present, and future are concerned. However, structural modeling analysis of five national samples in Israel (Shmotkin, 1991a) has shown that the relative *salience* (i.e., loading on the overall construct of satisfaction) of the future evaluation clearly increased from midlife (ages 51–60) onwards, eventually reaching its peak in the oldest group (age 71+);

the present maintained the highest salience throughout the lifespan; the past never reached the salience of the present and equaled that of the future only in the oldest group. These results suggest that the role played by each time referent of SWB should not be confused with the level of satisfaction attached to it, and that the conception of the future in particular continues to have considerable influence on the outlook of aging people.

Future evaluation is closely related to optimism, which represents people's tendency to hold positive expectancies for their future (Scheier & Carver, 1992). While this means that the construct of optimism is actually introduced into the temporal coordinates of SWB, Lucas, Diener, and Suh (1996) have found that optimism and SWB are nevertheless discriminable. We probably deal here with two correlated constructs that have mutual effects on one another, especially in the context of coping and adaptation (Scheier & Carver, 1992; Schwarzer & Jerusalem, 1995). Reker and Wong (1985) review the role of optimism in maintaining physical and mental health with particular reference to age. In their theory of personal meaning in aging (Reker & Wong, 1988), past-related reminiscence, present-related commitment, and future-related optimism provide a constant flow of meaning and a sense of time continuity that are essential to successful aging.

Thus, all the SWB dimensions, which constitute the differential types in the present model, have proved relevant to lifespan adjustment. On this basis, the suggested typological model might be a further step to explore the contribution of differential variants of SWB to age-related processes of mental health.

THE SWB DIFFERENTIAL TYPES:
AN EMPIRICAL EXAMINATION

The objective of the current study was to provide preliminary validation for the differential approach that is the focus of this chapter and is implemented in the taxonomy of SWB differential types. Specifically, the study sought to examine whether the threefold typology depicted in Figure 1–1 would be confirmed by the data with significant discrimination between the individual types. The discriminators chosen for this study were sociodemographic and descriptive variables that had appeared in the literature as relevant to SWB, at least for certain SWB dimensions. These included age, gender, place of birth (inside or outside the country), education, marital status, economic status, health, and religiosity. While some of these variables are not necessarily consistent predictors of SWB (Myers & Diener, 1995), they are definitely a starting point to characterize different types of people in terms of their most essential roles and social positions. Of particular importance was the attempt to differentiate the incongruous types as distinct from the congruous ones, thus shedding more light on the meaning of the apparent inconsistency among the SWB dimensions.

The database used in this study consisted of 4,081 Israeli adults aged 20 to 95. The data were collected from 1986 to 1994 by several dozen psychology students as a part of an ongoing large-scale study of SWB across the lifespan.

While dealing basically with a convenience sampling, the aim was twofold: to approach highly heterogeneous respondents in general, and to overrepresent certain target populations, such as older adults, residents of homes for the aged, and members of *kibbutzim*. Reference to the Israel Statistical Abstract (Israel Central Bureau of Statistics, 1994) suggests that the community-dwelling respondents corresponded fairly well to the national figures regarding gender and marital status but underrepresented people born in Asia or Africa, and those having a lower education level.

Method

Participants. Participants were drawn from the aforementioned database. The reported analyses were conducted on 3,185 noninstitutionalized residents of urban communities who were divided into four age groups: young adulthood (ages 20–39, $M = 27.8$, $Med = 27.0$, $SD = 4.9$); middle adulthood (ages 40–59, $M = 49.5$, $Med = 49.5$, $SD = 5.5$); later adulthood (ages 60–74, $M = 66.9$, $Med = 67.0$, $SD = 4.2$); and old age (ages 75–90, $M = 79.0$, $Med = 78.0$, $SD = 3.3$). Table 1–1 shows the percentage distributions of descriptive variables in the sample. As specified in the subsequent tables, the numbers of participants in the various analyses differed, mainly because some SWB measures were introduced into the study at a later time and thus completed by fewer respondents. Table 1–2 shows the number of participants with available data for each variable.

Instruments. The *Affect Balance Scale* (ABS), designed by Bradburn (1969), measures positive and negative affect. Each affect was tapped by five items referring to recent occurrences of feelings such as "pleased" and "proud" (Positive Affect Scale, or PAS) or "depressed" and "bored" (Negative Affect Scale, or NAS). In response to criticism of the original format (Brenner, 1975; Carp, 1989), the current adaptation referred to feelings in the "past week," and used a four-step scale with scores of 1 (*Never*), 2 (*Once*), 3 (*Several times*), and 4 (*Often*). Scores were the respective mean ratings of PAS and NAS items, and following Bradburn, the respondent's affect balance (AB) score was obtained by subtracting the NAS score from the PAS score. The Hebrew translation of the ABS (as well as the two following instruments) was agreed upon by seven judges using independent reverse translations. Alpha coefficients in the present sample were 0.71 (PAS) and 0.68 (NAS). The ABS has been widely used for measuring the affective components of SWB (Andrews & Robinson, 1991; Sauer & Warland, 1982), including in Israel (Shmotkin, 1990).

The *Satisfaction with Life Scale* (SWLS), constructed by Diener, Emmons, Larsen, and Griffin (1985), measures global life satisfaction as the cognitive aspect of SWB. It contains five items referring to general judgments of one's life (such as life being "close to one's ideal" or allowing one to have gotten "the important things" one wanted), and rated by respondents on a seven-step scale ranging from *Strongly disagree* (1) to *Strongly agree* (7). The score was the items' mean rating. Alpha coefficient in the present sample was 0.82. The instrument

Table 1–1. Percentage Distributions of Descriptive Variables in Four Age Groups

Variable	Group 1 Ages 20–39 N = 813	Group 2 Ages 40–59 N = 916	Group 3 Ages 60–74 N = 1031	Group 4 Ages 75–90 N = 425
Gender				
1 Men	51.8	44.9	48.4	57.6
2 Women	48.2	55.1	51.6	42.4
Place of birth[a]				
1 Israel	85.7	45.7	14.9	5.2
2 Europe–America	11.2	34.6	68.7	86.3
3 Asia–Africa	3.1	19.7	16.4	8.5
Education				
1 Elementary school	0.1	7.5	19.4	24.1
2 Some high school	1.7	14.1	23.8	21.5
3 High school graduate	23.2	16.6	20.1	22.6
4 Post high school studies	8.0	14.6	14.0	10.6
5 Some college	31.9	14.1	9.0	9.7
6 First academic degree	28.6	20.0	8.7	5.2
7 Higher academic degree	6.5	13.0	5.2	6.4
Marital status[b]				
1 Never married	60.3	1.5	1.3	1.9
2 Married	38.0	91.9	77.2	51.3
3 Divorced	1.6	4.9	2.8	1.9
4 Widowed	0.1	1.6	18.8	44.9
Self-rated economic status				
1 Below average	15.5	4.9	6.3	9.0
2 Average	63.5	66.7	74.3	76.7
3 Above average	21.0	28.4	19.3	14.4
Self-rated health				
1 Bad	10.6	1.8	3.4	10.4
2 Not so good	4.7	15.6	40.0	47.6
3 Good	84.7	82.7	56.5	41.9
Self-rated religiosity				
1 Secular	81.1	68.0	54.5	53.8
2 Traditional	15.0	25.6	39.4	40.1
3 Observant	3.9	6.4	6.0	6.1

[a]In order to include this variable in the analyses, it was dichotomized into 1 = born in Israel, 2 = born outside Israel.
[b]In order to include this variable in the analyses, it was dichotomized into 1 = not presently married, 2 = married.

has proved to have highly favorable psychometric properties (Diener, et al., 1985; Pavot & Diener, 1993).

The *Self-Anchoring Scale* (SAS), designed by Cantril (1965), measures global life satisfaction by addressing the person's own "anchors" or frames of reference. It presents a vertical ladder of 11 rungs, where the top (10) and the bottom (0) represent the best and worst possible lives, respectively, for each respondent. Respondents were asked to indicate on which rung they believed

Table 1–2. Means, Standard Deviations, and Intercorrelations for the Study Variables

Variable	N	M	SD	1	2	3	4	5	6	7	8	9	10	11	12	13	14
Descriptive variables																	
1 Age	3185	53.53	18.50	—													
2 Gender	3185	0.51	0.50	-03	—												
3 Place of birth	3180	0.59	0.49	62**	-00	—											
4 Education	3177	3.88	1.84	-38**	-05**	-33**	—										
5 Marital status	3183	0.68	0.47	20**	-12**	15**	02	—									
6 Economic status	3178	2.13	0.54	02	-02	-07*	18**	15**	—								
7 Health	3170	2.64	0.59	-22**	-04*	-17**	26**	12**	10**	—							
8 Religiosity	3179	1.41	0.59	18**	02	17**	-23**	05**	-04*	-11**	—						
SWB measures																	
9 PAS	1779	2.33	0.63	-25**	-03	-15**	18**	07**	07**	20**	03	—					
10 NAS	1779	1.74	0.62	-11**	08**	-05*	-08**	-24**	-17**	-19**	-01	-11**	—				
11 AB	1777	0.58	0.93	-10**	-07**	-07**	17**	20**	16**	26**	03	75**	-74**	—			
12 SWLS	1192	4.57	1.22	13**	-05	08**	08**	22**	26**	14**	01	31**	-47**	53**	—		
13 SAS-present	3132	6.78	1.76	-08**	-05**	-09**	16**	20**	25**	27**	-03	37**	-41**	53**	61**	—	
14 SAS-future	2788	7.14	2.29	-44**	-01	-29**	23**	03	16**	27**	-06**	36**	-26**	41**	32**	64**	—
15 SAS-past	3112	6.81	1.90	13**	-06**	05**	01	17**	14**	06**	05*	13**	-22**	24**	34**	48**	23**

Note: See Table 1–1 for the categories of the descriptive variables, and the Instruments section for the scales of the SWB measures. Decimal points omitted in the correlation coefficients. SWB = Subjective Well-Being; PAS = Positive Affect Scale; NAS = Negative Affect Scale; AB = Affect Balance; SWLS = Satisfaction with Life Scale; SAS = Self-Anchoring Scale.
*$p < .05$.
**$p < .01$.

they stood at the present time (SAS-present), had stood 5 years before (SAS-past), and would stand 5 years hence (SAS-future), thus constituting three separate scores. The SAS has been used extensively in numerous studies, usually providing satisfactory psychometric properties (Andrews & Robinson, 1991; Sauer & Warland, 1982). It has been administered in several national samples in Israel (Cantril, 1965; Shmotkin, 1991a).

Procedure.   The participants were interviewed individually or in small groups. They were approached at different public sites or in private homes throughout the country, were asked to participate in a study on feelings and attitudes, and were guaranteed anonymity. They first completed a sociodemographic questionnaire, and then various SWB measures in random order. The set of measures included additional SWB and psychological measures not reported in the current analyses. Where participants expressed difficulty in reading or understanding, the interviewers read the questionnaires aloud or supplied clarifications. Efforts were made to ensure minimal external distractions while the questionnaires were completed.

Results

Distributions of SWB Types.   The participants in each of the four age groups were divided into three 2×2 typologies (see Figure 1–1), division being made according to the group median on the relevant measures (the median score was included in either the lower or higher section so as to maximally approximate an even division). As expected, correlations between the pairs of cross-tabulated variables resulted in higher proportions of participants in congruous types (Cells 1 and 4) than in incongruous types (Cells 2 and 3). As Table 1–2 shows, the highest correlation (Pearson's r between the continuous variables) was found between SAS-present and SAS-future (.64, ranging from .53 to .75 in the different age groups). This led to a highly skewed Present–Future cross-tabulation, with the two incongruous types jointly constituting 28.2%, 28.4%, 17.4%, and 15.8% of the respective N's of this typology in the four age groups (corrected χ^2 with 1 df significant at the .00001 level in each age group). SWLS and AB also yielded a substantial correlation (.53, ranging from .49 to .62 in the different age groups), which similarly led to a skewed Cognitive–Affective cross-tabulation, with the incongruous types jointly constituting 32.6%, 33.6%, 30.2%, and 20.0% of the respective N's of this typology in the four age groups (corrected χ^2 with 1 df significant at the .00001 level in each age group). A different picture emerged with regard to PAS and NAS, which correlated relatively low (−.11, and respectively in the four age groups: −.13, −.02, −.14, −.31). Thus, in the Positive–Negative cross-tabulation, the incongruous types jointly constituted 47.2% in age group 1 (corrected χ^2 with 1 df was 1.79, nonsignificant), 54.3% in age group 2 ($\chi^2 = 2.71$, nonsignificant), 45.1% in age group 3 ($\chi^2 = 4.05$, $p < .05$), and 36.5% in age group 4 ($\chi^2 = 12.67$, $p < .001$). Out of 1,125 participants with available data for classification in all three cross-tabulations, 38.8% were classified into either incongruous type only once, 24.9% twice, and 6.1% all three times.

Discriminant Analysis of Types. In order to examine whether the suggested types could be differentiated by sociodemographic characteristics, a discriminant analysis of the four types was separately conducted in each of the three typologies for each of the four age groups, with the descriptive variables in Table 1–1 serving as predictors. Stepwise analysis (with the Wilks's Lambda criterion) was chosen to obtain parsimonious sets of predictors. To facilitate comparison between the age groups, age *within* each group served as a covariate by introducing it first into each equation (see Tabachnick & Fidell, 1989). The results for the three typologies are presented respectively in Tables 1–3, 1–4, and 1–5.

From these tables, it is clear that all 12 discriminant analyses yielded at least one significant discriminant function that explained most of the between-type variance, while eights analyses yielded a second significant function explaining 15.4%–37.7% of the variance. In two-thirds of the cases, the first function maximally separated between the congruous Types 1 and 4, as can be seen in the centroids, which are the mean scores of types on the discriminant function. In

Table 1–3. Results of Stepwise Discriminant Analyses of Cross-tabulated Positive–Negative Types in Four Age Groups

	Group 1 Ages 20–39 N = 726		Group 2 Ages 40–59 N = 440		Group 3 Ages 60–74 N = 428		Group 4 Ages 75–90 N = 176	
	F1	F2	F1	F2	F1	F2	F1	F2
A. Correlations of predictors with the discriminant functions[a,b]								
Age[c]	.64	−.18	−.00		−.39		−.08	
Gender	—	—	−.58		—		—	
Place of birth	—	—	—		—		—	
Education	—	—	—		—		.54	
Marital status	.72	−.70	—		.59		.47	
Economic status	—	—	—		.37		—	
Health	—	—	.80		.77		.69	
Religiosity	.71	.54	—		—		—	
B. Discriminant function information								
Canonical *R*	.18	.14	.24		.40		.43	
Variance explained (%)	62.1	37.2	91.5		89.6		89.1	
Centroids for:								
Type 1	0.32	−0.00	0.09		0.39		0.66	
Type 2	0.03	0.19	−0.07		−0.08		−0.26	
Type 3	0.05	−0.23	0.28		0.34		−0.28	
Type 4	−0.18	0.02	−0.37		−0.67		−0.40	
Pairs of types differing in Mahalanobis' D^2 ($p < .01$)	1#2,1#3,1#4, 2#3		1#4,3#4		1#2,1#4,2#3, 2#4,3#4		1#2,1#3,1#4	

Note: See Figure 1–1 (part A) for the specification of Types 1 to 4. *N*'s indicate valid cases after deleting respondents with missing data. F1 and F2 indicate the first and the second discriminat functions, respectively (functions are reported if they are significant at the .05 level).
[a]See Table 1–1 for the categories of the predictor variables.
[b]Reported are pooled within-types correlations of preditors entering the equation at the .05 level.
[c]Age within each group served as covariate by being entered first into each equation (see text).

Table 1–4. Results of Stepwise Discriminant Analyses of Cross-tabulated Cognitive–Affective Types in Four Age Groups

	Group 1 Ages 20–39 N = 609		Group 2 Ages 40–59 N = 264		Group 3 Ages 60–74 N = 232		Group 4 Ages 75–90 N = 80	
	F1	F2	F1	F2	F1	F2	F1	F2
A. Correlations of predictors with the discriminant functions[a,b]								
Age[c]	.42	−.78	.28	.66	.24	−.63	−.01	
Gender	—	—	—	—	−.64	.44	—	
Place of birth	—	—	—	—	—	—	—	
Education	.36	−.47	—	—	—	—	.53	
Marital status	.68	.42	—	—	.42	.55	.57	
Economic status	.72	−.09	.71	.51	—	—	—	
Health	—	—	.74	−.65	.65	.39	.53	
Religiosity	—	—	—	—	—	—	—	
B. Discriminant function information								
Canonical R	.24	.16	.30	.20	.31	.26	.62	
Variance explained (%)	67.1	29.6	70.1	29.6	55.0	37.7	95.3	
Centroids for:								
Type 1	0.26	0.12	0.33	0.03	0.24	0.17	0.82	
Type 2	0.18	−0.29	0.15	0.26	0.45	−0.40	−0.69	
Type 3	−0.16	0.20	0.01	−0.41	−0.26	0.38	0.28	
Type 4	−0.29	−0.04	−0.41	0.06	−0.38	−0.22	−0.82	
Pairs of types differing in Mahalanobis' D^2 ($p < .01$)	1#2,1#4,2#3, 2#4		1#4,3#4		1#4,2#3,2#4,		1#2,1#4	

Note: See Figure 1–1 (part B) for the specification of Types 1 to 4. *N*'s indicate valid cases after deleting respondents with missing data. F1 and F2 indicate the first and the second discriminat functions, respectively (functions are reported if they are signifificant at the .05 level).
[a]See Table 1–1 for the categories of the predictor variables.
[b]Reported are pooled within-types correlations of prediters entering the equation at the .05 level.
[c]Age within each group served as covariate by being entered first into each equation (see text).

all cases but one, the second function maximally separated between the incongruous Types 2 and 3. Using all discriminant functions to assess the general distance between each pair of individual types, Mahalanobis's D^2 indicated a frequently significant separation between all pairs, with the significant separation between Type 1 and 4 appearing in all analyses, and between Type 2 and 3 in two-thirds of the analyses (due to the multiple comparisons of pairs, only distances significant at the .01 level were considered).

In the analyses of the *Positive–Negative* types (Table 1–3), the loading matrix of correlations between predictors and discriminant functions (Section A) showed that the best predictor for distinguishing between Happy and Unhappy at age 60 and over (first function in Groups 3 and 4) was health (the former type reporting better health), while in younger adulthood (Group 1), the best predictors were marital status and religiosity (the former type being more frequently married and more traditional in religious orientation). Inflated was significantly distinguished from Deflated only in young adulthood (second

Table 1–5. Results of Stepwise Discriminant Analyses of Cross-tabulated Present–Future Types in Four Age Groups

	Group 1 Ages 20–39 N = 799		Group 2 Ages 40–59 N = 853		Group 3 Ages 60–74 N = 819		Group 4 Ages 75–90 N = 285	
	F1	F2	F1	F2	F1	F2	F1	F2
A. Correlations of predictors with the discriminant functions[a,b]								
Age[c]	.46	−.37	.10	.94	−.40	.81	.11	.24
Gender	—	—	—	—	—	—	—	—
Place of birth	—	—	—	—	—	—	—	—
Education	—	—	—	—	.54	.52	.34	.82
Marital status	.79	−.32	—	—	.52	.05	.37	.28
Economic status	.46	.86	.91	−.15	.50	−.01	.53	−.22
Health	.49	−.32	.50	.20	.69	.02	.80	−.25
Religiosity	—	—	—	—	—	—	—	—
B. Discriminant function information								
Canonical R	.28	.16	.29	.13	.40	.20	.43	.26
Variance explained (%)	73.2	22.8	79.8	15.4	80.8	17.3	75.6	24.2
Centroids for:								
Type 1	0.37	0.04	0.31	−0.01	0.40	−0.07	0.58	0.09
Type 2	0.28	0.18	0.40	0.17	0.20	0.45	−0.18	0.43
Type 3	−0.40	0.23	−0.22	−0.21	−0.14	−0.50	0.22	−0.81
Type 4	−0.13	−0.17	−0.32	0.14	−0.55	0.01	−0.45	−0.01
Pairs of types differing in Mahalanobis' D^2 ($p < .01$)	1#3,1#4,2#3, 2#4,3#4		1#3,1#4,2#3, 2#4,3#4		1#2,1#3,1#4, 2#3,2#4,3#4		1#3,1#4,2#3, 3#4	

Note: See Figure 1–1 (part C) for the specification of Types 1 to 4. N's indicate valid cases after deleting respondents with missing data. F1 and F2 indicate the first and the second discriminat functions, respectively (functions are reported if they are signififcant at the .05 level).
[a]See Table 1–1 for the categories of the predictor variables.
[b]Reported are pooled within-types correlations of prediters entering the equation at the .05 level.
[c]Age within each group served as covariate by being entered first into each equation (see text).

function), with the former type being less frequently married. Deflated was significantly distinguished from Unhappy in middle adulthood (first function in Group 2), mainly by better health in the former type.

In the analyses of the *Cognitive–Affective* types (Table 1–4), the best predictors for distinguishing between Amply Gratified and Essentially Ungratified (first function in Groups 1, 2, and 4) were economic status (the former type reporting a higher status in young and middle adulthood), marital status (the former type being more frequently married in young adulthood as well as in old age), and health (the former type reporting better health in middle adulthood and old age). Satisfied-but-Unhappy was significantly distinguished from Happy-but-Unsatisfied in all groups except old age (second function); after adjusting for the substantial effect made here by the age variability *within* the groups, the former type was found to be *more* educated in young adulthood, *less* healthy in middle adulthood, and *less* frequently married in later adulthood. Also, Satisfied-but-Unhappy was significantly distinguished from Essentially

Ungratified in later adulthood (first function), with the former type reporting better health and having a higher frequency of women.

In the analyses of the *Present–Future* types (Table 1–5), the best predictor for distinguishing between Reasonably Optimistic and Reasonably Pessimistic (first function in Groups 3 and 4) was health (the former type reporting better health). The best predictor for distinguishing between Unreasonably Pessimistic and Unreasonably Optimistic (second function in Groups 2, 3, and 4) was education (the former type having a higher education in later adulthood and old age), or no more than the within-group age in middle adulthood (this analysis of Group 2 was the only one to also yield a third significant function, explaining only 4.8% of the variance). Congruous types were significantly distinguished from incongruous types in Group 1 (first and second functions) and Group 2 (first function). Thus, married participants in young adulthood tended to be more Reasonably Optimistic than Unreasonably Optimistic, participants of higher economic status in young adulthood tended to be more Unreasonably Optimistic than Reasonably Pessimistic, and participants of higher economic status in middle adulthood tended to be more Unreasonably Pessimistic than Reasonably Pessimistic.

Discussion

The differential approach to SWB was implemented here in the formulation of SWB types by cross-tabulating three pairs of relevant measures. As the correlation between the cross-tabulated measures increased, more participants were concentrated in the two congruous types, scoring either high or low on SWB level on both measures. However, a sizable proportion of participants were represented by the incongruous types, scoring high on SWB level on one measure and low on the other, a finding deserving closer scrutiny. It should be noted that across the three typologies, the two incongruous types constituted lower proportions in the older age groups (age 60 and older) than in the two younger age groups. This trend reflects higher correlations and apparently lower differentiation between SWB attributes in older participants, as also found by Andrews and Herzog (1986). This finding is particularly important for the Positive–Negative types, because it suggests that the alleged independence between positive and negative affect (Bradburn, 1969) may be less applicable among the elderly.

The discriminant analyses revealed a largely consistent pattern of results: The first function indicated that the predictors were highly efficient in differentiating between the two congruous types, while the second function indicated that they could orthogonally differentiate, though less vigorously, between the two incongruous types as well. These results suggest that a combination of two relevant attributes of SWB makes people who are either congruously high *or* congruously low on these attributes much more distinct in their characteristics. Another important indication is that people who are incongruously high *and* low on such combined attributes also present a fairly distinguishable set of characteristics, depending on the specific attributes on which they are either high or low. Thus, the results confirm the expectation that the differential types can be empirically detected and characterized.

The analyses of the Positive–Negative types suggest that in this affective typology, the incongruous types are more relevant to younger and middle-aged adults, while the congruous types are more relevant to older adults. This finding conforms with the Diener et al. (1985) thesis that emotional reactivity is higher in younger than in older age, and thus the inflation or deflation of both positive and negative affect might have a stronger impact on regulating vitality and emotionality in younger age. The predictors of the affective types are best associated with what is apparently the main concern at each age—establishing the marriage bond in young adulthood, and maintaining one's health from middle-age on.

The analyses of the Cognitive–Affective types show that Amply Gratified, in contrast to Essentially Ungratified, is associated with better life conditions, such as higher economic status, being married (rather than single or widowed), and better health. This is not surprising according to the known literature (Diener, 1984; McNeil et al., 1986). The findings also suggest that the distinction between Satisfied-but-Unhappy and Happy-but-Unsatisfied, which might express different modes of regulation over cognition and affect, bears changing implications with the progress of age. Thus, the dominance of cognitive over affective constituents of SWB might be facilitated by formal education in young adulthood, signify the need to properly face more health concerns in middle adulthood, and provide adaptive coping with widowhood in later adulthood. These mere suggestions must be substantiated by further research.

The analyses of the Present–Future types point again to the importance of health in making distinctions among older adults, especially between congruous types. When incongruous types in older adults are concerned, higher education seems to make people more cautious about their future, thus preferring the Unreasonably Pessimistic to the Unreasonably Optimistic. The role of the incongruous types in the two younger groups suggests certain nuances in the temporal perspective: In young adulthood, sound conditions such as married life and higher economic status might strengthen the inclinations for a more optimistic stand, whereas in middle adulthood, higher economic status might cause people to evaluate their present, but not necessarily their future, more positively.

In examining the Present–Future types one should be aware that the response rates for future evaluation (SAS-future) were, respectively, 1.1% and 1.7% lower than for present evaluation (SAS-present) in the two younger groups, but notably, 18.7% and 30.8%, respectively, lower in the two older groups. In comparison, the response rates for SAS-past were approximately 1% lower in all age groups as compared to SAS-present. Thus, the Present–Future types did not include self-selected older respondents who avoided future evaluation, perhaps as a way of coping with the uncertainty of the future. This tendency among aged respondents to refrain from rating their future was explored in an earlier study (Shmotkin, 1992). It was found there that failing to rate one's future life satisfaction was associated with higher age, deteriorating health, widowhood, and higher proportion of women than men. Such failure was not necessarily linked to overall SWB, but rather to specific factors relating to time and aging. This phenomenon was questioned by Staats, Partlo, and Stubbs, (1993) but was also found elsewhere (Lowry, 1984; Ortiz & Arce, 1986).

The four most potent predictors in the discriminant analyses were health, marital status, economic status, and education. Gender and religiosity played a minor role in discriminating between types, and place of birth made no contribution at all. The role of gender is of particular interest because it has often been found to have relatively little or only a subtle effect on SWB (Haring, Stock, & Okun, 1984; Shmotkin, 1990), but on the other hand might relate to significant differences between men and women in developmental and aging patterns (Gutmann, 1987; Huyck, 1990). In the present results, men were found more frequently than women to be associated with types involving lower negative affect (Deflated) in middle adulthood, and higher cognitively based life satisfaction (Satisfied-but-Unhappy) in later adulthood. This may be just a hint of the reported trend of women to express more intense emotions, a feature not often manifested in general indices of SWB (Fujita, Diener, & Sandvik, 1991). Future research is still needed to examine gender effects in SWB types as associated with aging and adjustment.

The current study has considerable methodological limitations. To mention just a few: (1) The sample is not representative of the Israeli population; (2) the administration of some SWB measures began at different stages of the study, so that the three typologies were examined in different groupings of participants; (3) the cutoff point in the cross-tabulations could not prevent the possibly meaningless classification of participants whose scores were very close to the median on either side; (4) two typologies, namely the Positive–Negative and the Present–Future, cross-tabulated measures of the same format, thus perhaps introducing correlated error variance of "common method"; (5) in another typology, namely, the Cognitive–Affective, the affective dimension was operationalized in terms of a difference score (AB), which is unwarranted in most cases (Johns, 1981); (6) the measures applied here, particularly ABS and SAS, are indeed classical in the field but are not necessarily the best (Larsen, Diener, & Emmons, 1985). These limitations, of course, should be addressed in future studies and for the time being pose questions as to the generalizability of the current results. It is beyond the scope of the present chapter to report additional analyses of special groups (residents of homes for the aged, members of *kibbutzim*) or other instruments (LSIA and PGCMS), which generally provided more evidence for the delineation of the proposed types. Obviously, the whole typological model and its underlying assumptions are in need of further empirical validation that should address various personality variables as predictors of SWB types, the implications of these types for stress-related behaviors and health in general, and the possible replications of the model in both similar and different cultural contexts.

CONCLUSION

The study of SWB seems to have entered its third phase. In the first phase, during the 1960s and 1970s, the basic foundations were laid: The concept was defined and operationalized, epidemiological surveys were conducted, the subject proved particularly relevant to gerontological research, and the basic SWB dimensions emerged. In the second phase, during the 1980s, research on SWB largely involved increasing sophistication regarding the internal and external validity: Psychometric and structural studies required advanced methodologies, correlates of personality and adjustment were more thoroughly investigated, studies intensively addressed key questions such as the relationship between positive and negative affect, and models incorporating SWB with physical and mental health were proposed. The third phase, beginning in the 1990s, has initiated studies that consider SWB from the viewpoints of major psychological and sociological processes: cognitive functions such as judgment and memory, emotionality and mood, stress and coping, communication and social relations (Diener, 1994; Strack, Argyle, & Schwarz, 1991; Veenhoven, 1991).

The current stage of the research may give impetus to the transformation of the SWB construct *from a static attribute to a dynamic process*. Both the declarative and the differential aspects of SWB may help in this direction, as they highlight interactive effects either between the person communicating SWB and the potential audience attending to it, or among components active within the person's SWB structure. An important ingredient in the dynamic approach to SWB is the flexibility of the construct. While showing temporal stability and cross-situational consistency, SWB is also found to be sensitive to changes such as the ones occurring in life events or psychotherapy (Diener, 1994). The conception of differential types also suggests that one can simultaneously express different positions of SWB without necessarily presenting an inconsistent self, but rather an integration of "possible selves" (Markus & Nurius, 1986).

A major implication of the currently suggested typlogical model concerns *therapeutic and intervention programs* aimed at promoting SWB on either the individual or the group level. It is now evident that the manipulation of SWB can be accomplished along various lines according to the specific dimensions being tackled. Moreover, a decision to intervene through a given dimension may result in strengthening a certain type of SWB, and this choice should be considered beforehand. For example, enhancing positive affect in an unhappy person may lead to different consequences than reducing negative affect, because in the first instance, the person must also know how to handle frequently aroused and seemingly contradictory affects of both negative and positive quality, whereas in the second instance, he or she must adapt to a more relieved but emotionally shallow life of deflated affects. The individual's developmental stage along the lifespan may be an important consideration in this regard. Thus, on the basis of arguments reviewed earlier, one should decide whether it would be preferable to promote life satisfaction in an older person rather than mend his or her skewed affect balance. Another example is the need for the therapist to decide whether to focus on the present of the older client rather than foster an unfeasibly favorable future evaluation. In making these decisions, the typological model presented here could serve as a frame of reference for generating such structural changes in one's SWB configuration. The consideration of this model becomes especially relevant when the goal to move people from most undesirable (Cell 4 types in the suggested typologies) to most desirable (Cell 1 types) conditions proves so often unrealistic. Here, the incongruous types may offer more practical, albeit less than perfect, alternatives.

In any therapeutic intervention, however, caution should be exercised while implementating the proposed conceptualization. Thus, before dealing with specific types, it might be helpful to discuss with the clients the implications of their raw SWB evaluations and the related declarative functions possibly involved. For instance, self-orienting evaluations may be more tentative and negotiable than self-expressive evaluations; self-presentational and simulative evaluations may have more social repercussions than defensive evaluations. When the SWB evaluations do suggest certain differential types, it would be prudent to assess whether persons moving from congruous to incongruous types are really able to tolerate the inherent inconsistency of their condition, and even take advantage of it. A most facilitative strategy might be to reframe clients' feelings and problems in terms of the proposed model, and to consult them on their options.

SWB is still theoretically vague and largely elusive: It confusingly combines cognition and affect, personality disposition and transitory effects, self-consciousness and self-presentation. This very nature, however, might explain some of its potential contribution to professional work in mental health, because the shifting combinations make SWB a relevant starting point, perhaps a vehicle, for addressing different psychological functions and processes. By relating to the aging process in particular, SWB actually signifies the dialectical task imposed on every aging individual: sustaining the contentment of continuous growth while facing potential deterioration and loss. It appears that even if happiness becomes less and less tangible, the *pursuit* of happiness may never be over.

REFERENCES

American Psychiatric Association. (1994). *Diagnostic and statistical manual of mental disorders* (4th ed.). Washington, DC: Author.

Andrews, F. M., & Herzog, A. R. (1986). The quality of survey data as related to age of respondent. *Journal of the American Statistical Association, 81*, 403–410.

Andrews, F. M., & Inglehart, R. F. (1979). The structure of subjective well-being in nine Western societies. *Social Indicators Research, 6*, 73–90.

Andrews, F. M., & McKennell, A. C. (1980). Measures of self-reported well-being: Their affective, cognitive, and other components. *Social Indicators Research, 8*, 127–155.

Andrews, F. M., & Robinson, J. P. (1991). Measures of subjective well-being. In J. P. Robinson, P. R. Shaver, & L. S. Wrightsman (Eds.), *Measures of personality and social psychological attitudes* (Vol. 1, pp. 61–114). San Diego: Academic Press.

Andrews, F. M., & Withey, S. B. (1976). *Social indicators of well-being: Americans' perceptions of life quality.* New York: Plenum Press.

Austin, J. L. (1962). *How to do things with words.* London: Oxford University Press.

Bradburn, N. M. (1969). *The structure of psychological well-being.* Chicago: Aldine.

Brenner, B. (1975). Quality of affect and self-evaluated happiness. *Social Indicators Research, 2*, 315–331.

Brief, A. P., Butcher, A. H., George, J. M., & Link, K. E. (1993). Integrating bottom-up and top-down theories of subjective well-being: The case of health. *Journal of Personality and Social Psychology, 64*, 646–653.

Bryant, F. B., & Veroff, J. (1984). Dimensions of subjective mental health in American men and women. *Journal of Health and Social Behavior, 25*, 116–135.

Campbell, A. (1981). *The sense of well-being in America: Recent patterns and trends.* New York: McGraw-Hill.

Campbell, A., Converse, P. E., & Rodgers, W. L. (1976). *The quality of American life: Perceptions, evaluations, and satisfactions.* New York: Russel Sage.

Cantril, H. (1965). *The pattern of human concerns.* New Brunswick, NJ: Rutgers University Press.

Carp, F. M. (1989). Maximizing data quality in community studies of older people. In M. P. Lawton & A. R. Herzog (Eds.), *Special research methods for gerontology* (pp. 93–122). Amityville, NY: Baywood.

Carstensen, L. L., & Cone, J. D. (1983). Social desirability and the measurement of well-being in elderly persons. *Journal of Gerontology, 38,* 713–715.

Carstensen, L. L., Gross, J. J., & Fung, H. H. (1997). The social context of emotional experience. *Annual Review of Gerontology and Geriatrics, 17,* 325–352.

Chamberlain, K. (1988). On the structure of subjective well-being. *Social Indicators Research, 20,* 581–604.

Compton, W. C., Smith, M. L., Cornish, K. A., & Qualls, D. L. (1996). Factor structure of mental health measures. *Journal of Personality and Social Psychology, 76,* 406–413.

Costa, P. T., & McCrae, R. R. (1980). Influence of extroversion and neuroticism on subjective well-being: Happy and unhappy people. *Journal of Personality and Social Psychology, 38,* 668–678.

Costa, P. T., Jr., McCrae, R. R., & Zonderman, A. B. (1987a). Environmental and dispositional influences on well-being: Longitudinal follow-up of an American national sample. *British Journal of Psychology, 78,* 299–306.

Costa, P. T., Jr., Zonderman, A. B., McCrae, R. R., Cornoni-Huntley, J., Locke, B. Z., & Barbano, H. E. (1987b). Longitudinal analyses of psychological well-being in a national sample: Stability of mean levels. *Journal of Gerontology, 42,* 50–55.

deHaes, J. C. J. M., Pennink, B. J. W., & Welvaart, K. (1987). The distinction between affect and cognition. *Social Indicators Research, 19,* 367–378.

Diener, E. (1984). Subjective well-being. *Psychological Bulletin, 95,* 542–575.

Diener, E. (1994). Assessing subjective well-being: Progress and opportunities. *Social Indicators Research, 31,* 103–157.

Diener, E., & Emmons, R. A. (1984). The independence of positive and negative affect. *Journal of Personality and Social Psychology, 47,* 1105–1117.

Diener, E., Emmons, R. A., Larsen, R. J., & Griffin, S. (1985). The satisfaction with life scale. *Journal of Personality Assessment, 49,* 71–75.

Diener, E., Larsen, R. J., Levine, S., & Emmons, R. A. (1985). Intensity and frequency: Dimensions underlying positive and negative affect. *Journal of Personality and Social Psychology, 48,* 1253–1265.

Diener, E., Sandvik, E., & Larsen, R. J. (1985). Age and sex effects for emotional intensity. *Developmental Psychology, 21,* 542–546.

Diener, E., Sandvik, E., & Pavot, W. (1991). Happiness is the frequency, not the intensity, of positive versus negative affect. In F. Strack, M. Argyle, & N. Schwarz (Eds.), *Subjective well-being: An interdisciplinary perspective* (pp. 119–139). Oxford, UK: Pergamon.

Diener, E., Sandvik, E., Pavot, W., & Gallagher, D. (1991). Response artifacts in the measurement of subjective well-being. *Social Indicators Research, 24,* 35–56.

Filipp, S. H. (1996). Motivation and emotion. In J. E. Birren & K. W. Schaie (Eds.), *Handbook of the psychology of aging* (4th ed., pp. 218–235). San Diego: Academic Press.

Fujita, F., Diener, E., & Sandvik, E. (1991). Gender differences in negative affect and well-being: The case for emotional intensity. *Journal of Personality and Social Psychology, 61,* 427–434.

Gaitz, C. M., & Scott, J. (1972). Age and the measurement of mental health. *Journal of Health and Social Behavior, 13,* 55–67.

Gatz, M., & Hurwicz, M. L. (1990). Are old people more depressed? Cross-sectional data on Center for Epidemiological Studies Depression Scale factors. *Psychology and Aging, 5,* 284–290.

George, L. K. (1981). Subjective well-being: Conceptual and methodological issues. *Annual Review of Gerontology and Geriatrics, 2,* 345–382.

Green, D. P., Goldman, S. L., & Salovey, P. (1993). Measurement error masks bipolarity in affect ratings. *Journal of Personality and Social Psychology, 64,* 1029–1041.

Gurin, G., Veroff, J., & Feld, S. (1960). *Americans view their mental health*. New York: Basic Books.

Gutmann, D. (1987). *Reclaimed powers: Toward a new psychology of men and women in later life*. New York: Basic Books.

Haring, M. J., Stock, W. A., & Okun, M. A. (1984). A research synthesis of gender and social class as correlates of subjective well-being. *Human Relations, 37*, 645–657.

Headey, B., Holmstrom, E., & Wearing, A. (1985). Models of well-being and ill-being. *Social Indicators Research, 17*, 211–234.

Headey, B., Veenhoven, R., & Wearing, A. (1991). Top-down versus bottom-up theories of subjective well-being. *Social Indicators Research, 24*, 81–100.

Herzog, A. R., & Rodgers, W. L. (1981). The structure of subjective well-being in different age groups. *Journal of Gerontology, 36*, 472–479.

Herzog, A. R., & Rodgers, W. L. (1986). Satisfaction among older adults. In F. M. Andrews (Ed.), *Research on the quality of life* (pp. 235–251). Ann Arbor: University of Michigan, Institute for Social Research.

Horley, J., & Little, B. R. (1985). Affective and cognitive components of global subjective well-being measures. *Social Indicators Research, 17*, 189–197.

Hoyt, D. R., & Creech, J. C. (1983). The Life Satisfaction Index: A methodological and theoretical critique. *Journal of Gerontology, 38*, 111–116.

Huyck, M. H. (1990). Gender differences in aging. In J. E. Birren & K. W. Schaie (Eds.), *Handbook of the psychology of aging* (3rd ed., pp. 124–132). San Diego: Academic Press.

Israel Central Bureau of Statistics. (1994). *Statistical abstract of Israel* (Vol. 45). Jerusalem: Author.

Jahoda, M. (1958). *Current concepts of positive mental health*, New York: Basic Books.

Johns, G. (1981). Difference score measures of organizational behavior variables: A critique. *Organizational Behavior and Human Performance, 27*, 443–463.

Kammann, R., Farry, M., & Herbison, P. (1984). The analysis and measurement of happiness as a sense of well-being. *Social Indicators Research, 15*, 91–115.

Kastenbaum, R. (1982). Time course and time perspective in later life. *Annual Review of Gerontology and Geriatrics, 3*, 80–101.

Kozma, A., & Stones, M. J. (1987). Social desirability in measures of subjective well-being: A systematic evaluation. *Journal of Gerontology, 42*, 56–59.

Larsen, R. J., Diener, E., & Emmons, R. A. (1985). An evaluation of subjective well-being measures. *Social Indicators Research, 17*, 1–17.

Larson, R. (1978). Thirty years of research on the subjective well-being of older Americans. *Journal of Gerontology, 33*, 109–125.

Lawton, M. P. (1975). The Philadelphia Geriatric Center Morale Scale: A revision. *Journal of Gerontology, 30*, 85–89.

Lawton, M. P. (1983). The varieties of well-being. *Experimental Aging Research, 9*, 65–72.

Lawton, M. P., Kleban, M. H., Rajagopal, D., & Dean, J. (1992). Dimensions of affective experience in three age groups. *Psychology and Aging, 7*, 171–184.

Lazarus, R. S. (1991). *Emotion and adaptation*. New York: Oxford University Press.

Lewinsohn, P. M., Redner, J. E., & Seeley, J. R. (1991). The relationship between life satisfaction and psychosocial variables: New perspectives. In F. Strack, M. Argyle, & N. Schwarz (Eds.), *Subjective well-being: An interdisciplinary perspective* (pp. 141–169). Oxford, UK: Pergamon.

Liang, J. (1984). Dimensions of the Life Satisfaction Index A: A structural formulation. *Journal of Gerontology, 39*, 613–622.

Liang, J., & Bollen, K. A. (1983). The structure of the Philadelphia Geriatric Center Morale Scale: A reinterpretation. *Journal of Gerontology, 38*, 181–189.

Lomranz, J., Friedman, A., Gitter, G., Shmotkin, D., & Medini, G. (1985). The meaning of time-related concepts across the lifespan: An Israeli sample. *International Journal of Aging and Human Development, 21*, 87–107.

Lowry, J. H. (1984). Life satisfactions time components among the elderly. *Research on Aging 6*, 417–431.

Lucas, R. E., Diener, E., & Suh, E. (1996). Discriminant validity of well-being measures. *Journal of Personality and Social Psychology, 71*, 616–628.

Markus, H., & Nurius, P. (1986). Possible selves. *American Psychologist, 41*, 954–969.

McCrae, R. R. (1986). Well-being scales do not measure social desirability. *Journal of Gerontology*, *41*, 390–392.

McKennell, A. C. (1978). Cognition and affect in perceptions of well-being. *Social Indicators Research*, *5*, 389–426.

McNeil, J. K. Stones, M. J., & Kozma, A. (1986). Subjective well-being in later life: Issues concerning measurement and prediction. *Social Indicators Research*, *18*, 35–70.

Michalos, A. C. (1980). Satisfaction and happiness. *Social Indicators Research*, *8*, 385–422.

Michalos, A. C. (1985). Multiple discrepancies theory (MDT). *Social Indicators Research*, *16*, 347–414.

Michalos, A. C. (1986). An application of multiple discrepancies theory (MDT) to seniors. *Social Indicators Research*, *18*, 349–373.

Moum, T. (1988). Yea-saying and mood-of-the-day effects in self-reported quality of life. *Social Indicators Research*, *20*, 117–139.

Myers, D. G., & Diener, E. (1995). Who is happy? *Psychological Science*, *6*, 10–19.

Neugarten, B. L., Havighurst, R. J., & Tobin, S. S. (1961). The measurement of life satisfaction. *Journal of Gerontology*, *16*, 134–143.

Newmann, J. P. (1989). Aging and depression. *Psychology and Aging*, *4*, 150–165.

Okun, M. A. (1987). Life satisfaction. In G. L. Maddox (Editor-in-Chief), *The encyclopedia of aging* (pp. 399–401). New York: Springer.

Ortiz, V., & Arce, C. H. (1986). Quality of life among persons of Mexican descent. In F. M. Andrews (Ed.), *Research on the quality of life* (pp. 171–191). Ann Arbor: University of Michigan, Institute for Social Research.

Pavot, W., & Diener, E. (1993). Review of the satisfaction with life scale. *Psychological Assessment*, *5*, 164–172.

Reker, G. T., & Wong, T. P. (1985). Personal optimism, physical and mental health: The triumph of successful aging. In J. B. Birren & J. Livingston (Eds.), *Cognition, stress, and aging* (pp. 134–173). Englewood Cliffs, NJ: Prentice-Hall.

Reker, G. T., & Wong, P. T. P. (1988). Aging as an individual process: Toward a theory of personal meaning. In J. E. Birren & V. L. Bengtson (Eds.). *Emergent theories of aging* (pp. 214–246). New York: Springer.

Ryff, C. D. (1989).Happiness is everything, or is it? Explorations on the meaning of psychological well-being. *Journal of Personality and Social Psychology*, *57*, 1069–1081.

Ryff, C. D. (1991). Possible selves in adulthood and old age: A tale of shifting horizons. *Psychology and Aging*, *6*, 286–295.

Ryff, C. D., & Keyes, C. L. M. (1995). The structure of psychological well-being revisited. *Journal of Personality and Social Psychology*, *69*, 719–727.

Sauer, W. J., & Warland, R. (1982). Morale and life satisfaction. In D. J. Mangen & W. A. Peterson (Eds.), *Research instruments in social gerontology*: *Vol. 1. Clinical and social psychology* (pp. 195–240). Minneapolis: University of Minnesota Press.

Scheier, M. F., & Carver, C. S. (1992). Effects of optimism on psychological and physical well-being: Theoretical overview and empirical update. *Cognitive Therapy and Research*, *16*, 201–228.

Schulz, R. (1985). Emotion and affect. In J. E. Birren & K. W. Schaie (Eds.), *Handbook of the psychology of aging* (2nd ed., pp. 531–543). New York: Van Nostrand Reinhold.

Schwarzer, R., & Jerusalem, M. (1995). Optimistic self-beliefs as a resource factor in coping with stress. In S. E. Hobfoll & M. W. de Vries (Eds.), *Extreme stress and communities: Impact and intervention* (pp. 159–177). Dordrecht, The Netherlands: Kluwer.

Shedler, J., Mayman, M., & Manis, M. (1993). The illusion of mental health. *American Psychologist*, *48*, 1117–1131.

Shmotkin, D. (1990). Subjective well-being as a function of age and gender: A multivariate look for differentiated trends. *Social Indicators Research*, *23*, 201–230.

Shmotkin, D. (1991a). The role of time orientation in life satisfaction across the lifespan. *Journal of Gerontology: Psychological Sciences*, *46*, 243–250.

Shmotkin, D. (1991b). The structure of Life Satisfaction Index A in elderly Israeli adults. *International Journal of Aging and Human Development*, *33*, 131–150.

Shmotkin, D. (1992). The apprehensive respondent: Failing to rate future life satisfaction in older adults. *Psychology and Aging*, *7*, 484–486.

Shmotkin, D. (1996). *Behavioral declaration: Stating one's future behavior as a social affair and an issue of prediction.* Unpublished manuscript, Tel Aviv University, Tel Aviv, Israel.

Shmotkin, D., & Hadari, G. (1996). An outlook on subjective well-being in older Israeli adults: A unified formulation. *International Journal of Aging and Human Development, 42*, 271–289.

Staats, S., Partlo, C., & Stubbs, K. (1993). Future time perspective, response rates, and older persons: Another chapter in the story. *Psychology and Aging, 8*, 440–442.

Staats, S., & Skowronski, J. (1992). Perceptions of self-affect: Now and in the future. *Social Cognition, 10*, 415–431.

Stacey, C. A., & Gatz, M. (1991). Cross-sectional age differences and longitudinal change on the Bradburn Affect Balance Scale. *Journal of Gerontology: Psychological Sciences, 46*, 76–78.

Stenback, A. (1980). Depression and suicidal behavior in old age. In J. E. Birren & R. B. Sloane (Eds.), *Handbook of mental health and aging* (pp. 616–652). Englewood Cliffs, NJ: Prentice-Hall.

Stock, W. A., Okun, M. A., & Benin, M. (1986). Structure of subjective well-being among the elderly. *Psychology and Aging, 1*, 91–102.

Stones, M. J., & Kozma, A. (1985). Structural relationships among happiness scales: A second order factorial study. *Social Indicators Research, 17*, 19–28.

Strack, F., Argyle, M., & Schwarz, N. (Eds.). (1991). *Subjective well-being: An interdisciplinary perspective.* Oxford, UK: Pergamon.

Tabachnick, B. G., & Fidell, L. S. (1989). *Using multivariate statistics* (2nd ed.). New York: Harper Collins.

Taylor, S. E., & Brown, J. D. (1988). Illusion and well-being: A social psychological perspective on mental health. *Psychological Bulletin, 103*, 193–210.

Veenhoven, R. (1984). *Conditions of happiness.* Dordrecht, Holland: D. Reidel.

Veenhoven, R. (1991). Questions on happiness: Classical topics, modern answers, blind spots, In F. Strack, M. Argyle, & N. Schwarz (Eds.), *Subjective well-being: An interdisciplinary perspective* (pp. 7–26). Oxford, UK: Pergamon.

Veenhoven, R. (1994). Is happiness a trait? *Social Indicators Research, 32*, 101–160.

Veit, C. T., & Ware, J. E. (1983). The structure of psychological distress and well-being in general populations. *Journal of Consulting and Clinical Psychology, 51*, 730–742.

Waterman, A. S. (1993). Two conceptions of happiness: Contrasts of personal expressiveness (eudaimonia) and hedonic enjoyment. *Journal of Personality and Social Psychology, 64*, 678–691.

Weinberger, D. A. (1990). The construct validity of the repressive coping style. In J. L. Singer (Ed.), *Repression and dissociation: Implications for personality, theory, psychopathology, and health* (pp. 337–386). Chicago: University of Chicago Press.

World Health Organization. (1996). *Basic documents* (41st ed.). Geneva, Switzerland: Author.

CHAPTER 2

Control
Cognitive and Motivational Implications

LAWRENCE C. PERLMUTER AND ANGELA S. EADS

With the exception of the pioneering interventional studies of Langer and Rodin (1976; Rodin & Langer, 1977; Rodin, Timko, & Harris, 1985), most of the research that has investigated the relationship between perceptions of control and aging have utilized self-reports to determine the extent to which advancing age is associated with changes in perceived control (Blanchard-Fields & Robinson, 1987). Although the self-report procedure is sound in itself, it may have peculiar limitations with respect to assessing age-related changes in perceived control; that is, when individuals are asked to respond to specific questions or scenarios that depict control, older individuals may respond differently than younger individuals to these inquiries, not because their perception of control has changed, but rather because the particular scenario or question may be lacking in appropriateness for either group. Thus, the requisite standardization procedures involved in test construction (i.e., presenting the respondent with a topic for judgment) may limit test validity. In other words, if young and old respondents answer a given question differently, is it because they perceive more or less control, or is the stem of the test item differentially appropriate to young or old individuals? As a result of the potential limitations surrounding exclusive reliance on self-reports, we primarily utilize experimental paradigms that examine how choice and control affect motivation and performance in younger and older individuals. We examine laboratory as well as field studies and propose some principles that may be useful in enhancing the perception of control in the elderly. In constructing our experiments, be they in the laboratory or in the field, we operate always under the limitation that imposes a compromise be-

LAWRENCE C. PERLMUTER AND ANGELA S. EADS • Department of Psychology, Finch University of Health Sciences/The Chicago Medical School, North Chicago, Illinois 60064.

Handbook of Aging and Mental Health: An Integrative Approach, edited by Jacob Lomranz. Plenum Press, New York, 1998.

tween the reality that we have created for our participants and the existing analytic technologies (Mostofsky, Chapter 23, this volume).

INTRODUCTION

Definitional Considerations

In this chapter we examine how perceived control can be deployed to increase motivation, performance, and quality of life in the aged. For most theorists, the perception of control has the important function of improving the quality of life by increasing the sense of preparedness through belief in a predictable environment. Despite some commonality in the definition of perceived control, emphases vary among theorists. For example, Adler (1929) viewed control as "an intrinsic necessity of life," whereas White (1959) viewed control as a basic need, analogous to a biological necessity. Baron and Rodin (1978) discussed control as the ability to regulate or influence intended outcomes through selective responding. Langer (1975) has suggested a vital distinction between actual control and illusory control, whereas others have distinguished primary control from secondary control (Heckhausen & Schulz, 1995). Secondary control has a strong adaptive flavor, because it suggests the possibility of discovering control even within a highly controlling environment. Savage, Perlmuter, and Monty (1979) have adopted the illusory feature of control depicted in Robert Frost's description, "freedom is being easy in the harness."

Almost all of these definitions are characterized by a strong, personal evaluative focus that is intrinsic to control; that is, through perceptual interpretive processes, individuals are presumed to view a situation according to their needs, past, present, and future. Such perceptions, in turn, are analogous to a mechanism for coping proposed by Lazarus and Folkman (1984).

Whether the perception of control is best described as the belief in the power that one has to effect an outcome or the ability to discover personal control within a highly controlling environment, the common element throughout these definitions relates to the primary role of the self and its sense of efficacy. In turn, the sense of self-efficacy is reciprocally changed through the self-appraisal of behavioral outcomes. Hence, Bandura's notion (1977) of reciprocal causality plays a vital role in this conceptualization. Kegan (Chapter 9, this volume) provides a more comprehensive description of how perceptions of the ability to complete the work of life may change with time. Kegan's description gives consideration to the significance that the role of personal efficacy plays relative to the socialization process characteristic of Western society.

Control is of special significance for the elderly because physical, emotional, as well as psychosocial changes may result in decreased opportunities for actual control (Aldwin, 1991). However, despite changes in physical reality, the illusory aspect of control can persist unabated. Thus, we examine control in its many facets in order to better understand how it can be exploited to enhance the quality of life for those individuals who may perceive that control is no longer effective, as in earlier days.

Attributions and Control

Psychologists and other observers of behavior are wont to proffer that, irrespective of the nature of the events that befall an individual, the specific outcome of the event cannot be predicted or adequately understood without regard to the way in which the individual *perceives* the event (Schmidt, 1985). Such perceptions often develop in conjunction with attributions that individuals generate regarding the reason for, or the meaning of, the event. Attributions, along with their related perceptions, jointly determine cognitive and affective outcomes that, in turn, have a variety of consequences, ranging from changes in simple, overt behaviors to physiological stress reactions, to actual shortening of life itself.

Weiner (1974) had earlier suggested that attributions simplify the world psychologically, presumably by enabling the observer to make sense of events. As attributions enhance perceptions of predictability and orderliness in the universe, they thereby enhance perceived control and motivation. There are a number of studies that broadly support this conjecture. Rakowski and Hickey (1992) showed that mortality rates were significantly lower in older individuals who attributed difficulties with their health status to a disease or specific problem, rather than to old age. Presumably, individuals who lived longer attributed their problems to a more controllable event, namely, their disease, rather than to the ineluctable process of advancing age.

Although these speculations regarding perceptions and attributions appear post hoc and tautological, we show how these processes can be studied prospectively. In addition, we discuss an intervention that, sui generis, *affects* attributions for behavior and that, in turn, can increase motivation and strengthen the degree to which individuals attribute behavior to their own efforts.

The exercise of choice and enhancement of control is so powerful that it has positive effects despite the intrinsic liking or disliking for the setting in which control is exercised. Specifically, whether veridical or illusory, opportunities for exercising choice can strengthen attributions and increase individuals' sense of involvement with a task, irrespective of its intrinsic interest for the participants. In other words, by enhancing the perception of control, it is possible to strengthen the *linkage* or connection between individuals' self-initiated efforts and the outcome of their behavior.

Control can have beneficial effects even if behavior is ineffective in producing the desired change. Individuals with diabetes mellitus are burdened by a variety of risk factors and complications that are largely a consequence of the level of glucose in the blood (Rand et al., 1985). It is widely recognized that the incidence of retinopathy increases as glucose levels increase (Nathan, Singer, Godine, Harrington, & Perlmuter, 1986). To help reduce glucose levels, individuals are instructed and encouraged to monitor regularly their blood sugars. Such monitoring procedures are demanding; thus, adherence rates are low (Orne & Binik, 1989). Results showed that the frequency with which individuals monitored their glucose levels had little impact in reducing blood glucose levels, and from this perspective, the monitoring procedure was ineffective. However, more frequent monitoring was associated with significant reductions in the incidence of retinopathy (Rand et al., 1985). Presumably, the *choice* to monitor their blood glucose levels provided individuals with a sense of control that motivated healthful practices that, in turn, reduced susceptibility to this serious and disabling complication.

Choice, Control, and Performance

In this section, we examine how choice and control can be used to increase motivation, thereby enhancing cognitive performance in young and elderly individuals. Since some of these studies have been reviewed (Perlmuter & Monty, 1989), we describe the basic paradigm and provide only a brief overview of the results.

The present research grew out of an attempt to integrate opposing views of the role of the participant in the learning situation, namely, one that views the individual as a passive recipient of stimulation and another that views the individual as an active participant (Kimble & Perlmuter, 1970). Basically, in the present studies, we sought to determine whether performance could be improved by forcing subjects' active participation in the learning task. To this end, subjects made choices over some of the materials to be learned. It was reasoned that the opportunity to exercise choice would strengthen the subject's perception of control and responsibility for performance and thereby increase motivation. Hobfoll and Wells (Chapter 5, this volume) proposed a similar hypothesis that suggests that cognitive resources (such as choice) play a positive role in an elderly person's ability to adjust and adapt to the losses associated with growing old.

Choice Facilitates New Learning in Young and Old Subjects

In many of these studies, we used a paired associates task in which individuals attempted to learn associations between stimuli and respective response terms. Participants were assigned randomly to experimental conditions.

To evaluate the motivational effectiveness of choice with minimal bias or confounding, we selected tasks that had little intrinsic interest to individuals. In addition, we selected tasks in which changes in performance could be assessed objectively. In the *Choice* condition, individuals were presented with stimuli, each accompanied by two or more potential response terms. Subjects chose one response to be learned to each stimulus and thus, a paired associates list was uniquely fashioned by each subject. In the comparison, or *Force*, condition,

individuals were exposed to identical materials, but response terms were assigned, based on the selections of yoked Choice subjects. Except where otherwise stated, verbal materials had moderate to low levels of scaled meaningfulness and thus were generally difficult to learn. In the present study (Perlmuter,
Monty, & Chan, 1986), participants were middle-aged and older males who
had sought assistance from a memory clinic for their self-diagnosed memory
problems.

The results showed (Figure 2–1) that Choice subjects not only learned to a

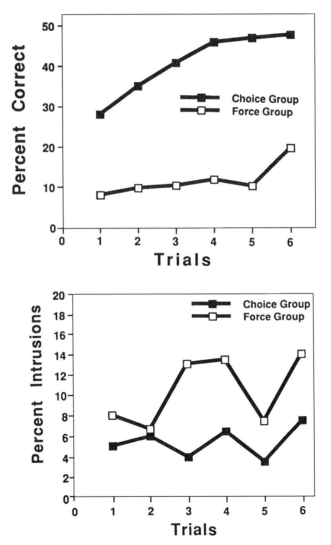

Figure 2–1. Mean percent correct responses and mean percent intrusions across trials in
Choice and Force subjects.

higher level, but they also committed fewer intrusion errors across the paired associate trials. Apparently, even for individuals who evaluated their memory skills as poor, the opportunity to choose response words was sufficiently salient to increase control and motivation, and thereby to improve performance.

Choosing from Similar Undesirable Options

In another paired associate study (Monty & Perlmuter, 1972) with college-aged participants, the stimuli were common words, whereas the response terms were paralogs and thus quite difficult to learn. Because paralogs are by definition relatively unfamiliar (e.g., zobel) they would constitute pairs of nondesirable or meaningless options from which to choose. When performance on the paired associate learning task was compared for Choice and Force subjects, as predicted, there were no beneficial effects of choice on the learning of the paired associates. In a study with Japanese students, Takahashi (1992) used Japanese characters to construct either words or nonwords, and the results fully replicated those reported here.

Choice from Highly Dissimilar Options

In another paired associate study (Monty, Geller, Savage, & Perlmuter, 1979), each pair of response options was constructed of one meaningful word and one paralog. Although the meaningful response term constitutes a reasonable option for selection, one element is missing from this scenario, namely, the opportunity to *reject* a possible alternative; that is, on the initial appraisal of the materials, the paralog is likely to be discounted, a priori, as an option, and thus it might not undergo the necessary scrutiny by which choice and rejection develop.

The majority of Choice subjects (approximately 70%) selected the *meaningful* word in each pair. The meaningful word in each pair was assigned to the Force subjects. As predicted, there were no benefits accruing to choice. There was even a tendency for Choice subjects to perform somewhat poorer than Force subjects.

Next, we examined the 30% of the subjects in the Choice condition who selected one or more paralogs as response words. A yoked Force group was enlisted that learned materials that were identical to those selected by the Choice subjects, namely, primarily words and a few paralogs as responses. In this comparison, the Choice subjects displayed the typical positive effects of choice. Apparently, for these "maverick" Choice subjects who, through selection of the paralogs, were able to *discover* choice, the process of rejection was satisfied, and thus performance was enhanced.

This study provides a clear indication that the act of choosing per se does *not* enhance the perception of control. Thus, to be beneficial, choice requires, at a minimum, two viable alternatives, both of which must receive consideration, and one of these must undergo the process of rejection. That is, objectively undesirable alternatives are unlikely to receive adequate consideration a priori, and the criteria for an *autonomous* choice are unlikely to have been satisfied (Steiner, 1979). These results indicate that choice and rejection may be separable processes, and unless rejection is a constituent part of choosing, the enhancement of perceived control is thereby nullified or preempted.

The Explicit Role of Rejection

In the next study, rejection and choice constituted overt behaviors so that their effects could be evaluated separately (Perlmuter & Monty, 1982). The task assessed recognition memory. Specifically, subjects were presented with a series of lines of (meaningful) words containing either two or four words per line. The task was to remember one (target) word on each line. The subjects were of college age and were assigned at random to one of three conditions.

In the Rejection condition, subjects proceeded down the page, crossing out the word or words on each line that they wanted *not* to learn, leaving only one remaining target word on each line. In the Choice condition, subjects underlined the target word on each line that they wanted to learn, while in the Force condition, the target word had been underlined previously and subjects reunderlined and studied it.

On a recognition test, individuals indicated whether the word was "old" or "new" (i.e., had been previously exposed or had not been previously exposed, respectively). Results showed that the poorest recognition was evident in the Force condition, and the best recognition was evident in the Rejection condition, with the Choice condition intermediate. Apparently, in enhancing performance, rejection produced even stronger positive effects than those resulting from choice.

Does Choice Enhance Motivation?

While we have proposed that choice increases motivation, to this point, the only evidence for this account is that the learning of chosen items was superior to the learning of assigned items. To assess the effectiveness of choice in increasing motivation, we required subjects to perform a simple (motor) reaction time task concurrent with the learning of their paired associates (Perlmuter, Scharff, Karsh, & Monty, 1980). Choice subjects not only learned paired associates better than their Force counterparts, but also reaction times were significantly faster for Choice than for Force subjects (Figure 2–2).

In a second study, the reaction time task was presented after subjects had chosen their desired materials, but before the opportunity to formally learn these. Again, reaction times were significantly faster for Choice subjects. Thus, choice has positive effects extending beyond the specific task in which it was exercised.

The opportunity to choose not only enhances motivation, but it also changes

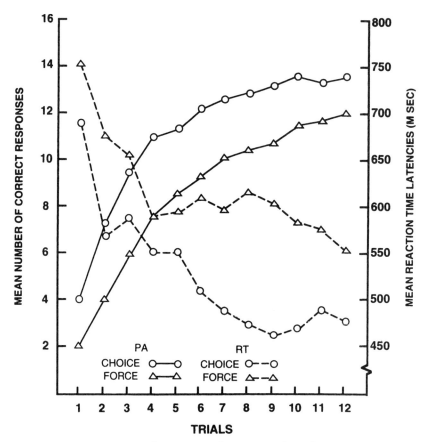

Figure 2–2. Mean reaction time latencies and mean number of correct responses on the paired associates task across trials for Choice and Force subjects.

the perception of a task in a positive direction. In this study, subjects were able to choose only a portion (25%) of their responses for a paired associate task, whereas the remainder were assigned (Monty, Rosenberger, & Perlmuter, 1973). Still another group chose 25% of the responses, but this was in the concluding portion of the task. Those individuals who chose early in the task learned the chosen *and* assigned materials significantly better than those who were assigned all or a portion of the materials to be learned. These results were replicated in young children with a reading comprehension test in which individuals who were permitted to choose one story at the start of the procedure had significantly higher reading comprehension scores than those for whom all of the stories had been assigned (Perlmuter & Monty, 1977). Thus, the benefits of choice extend beyond the specific materials that have been chosen, and the effects of choice are compatible with a general motivation explanation as proposed by Hull (1943).

In the next section, we briefly identify a few principles regulating the effectiveness of choice and then examine some field studies that have utilized choice and control.

Choice and the Enhancement of Perceived Control: Some Principles

The previously cited studies illustrate some elemental determinants of the relationship between choice and motivation. A first principle is that despite its semblance to freedom, choice is effective only in the presence of specific constraints. Specific criteria must be met for choice to be effective. These include consideration of the options presented for choosing, namely, they must differ from each other to a moderate degree, and they must also be potentially desirable (Harvey & Johnston, 1973). For most individuals, paralogs satisfied neither criterion; thus, choice was ineffective.

Second, as a moderator, choice is very robust; that is, while in a later section we offer some caveats to this generalization, irrespective of the age of the participant, and even in a task of low intrinsic interest, the opportunity to exercise choice enhances cognitive performance. In addition to improving performance, choice reduces distractibility; that is, choice not only increased motivation, but it also decreased interference among materials, as evidenced by the relatively low percentage of intrusions (mistaken responses) on the paired associates task (Figure 2–1). The effectiveness of choice in reducing intrusions is an important feature because, for older individuals, susceptibility to interference from contextual or background stimuli constitutes one of the primary indices of age-related cognitive decline (Kleigl & Lindenberger, 1978). We have proposed (Perlmuter, 1991) that among the benefits of enhanced control is the more effective *differentiation* between to-be-learned (target) materials and potentially interfering contextual stimuli. To the extent that such effects of choice reflect a more generalized process, enhanced differentiation consequent to choice can have a variety of benefits, including a reduction in the magnitude of reactions to stressful stimuli (Stotland & Blumenthal, 1964); that is, by increasing the distinctiveness of the target, choice reduces its confusability with the background. If the target has aversive qualities, these would less likely generalize to the background or to contextual material, thereby reducing the overall level of aversiveness.

Third, these studies have shown that the process of rejection is not only implicitly a part of the process of choosing but also may be the more important element that contributes to the effectiveness of choice and control.

Choice and the Perception of Control in Clinical Settings

To illustrate the benefits and limitations of choice and control in clinical settings, we turn next to some pioneering experimental studies reviewed by Wallston (1989). In the first study, an attempt was made to reduce stress associated with an unpleasant medical procedure, namely, bowel cleaning, using a barium enema. Individuals were assigned randomly to one of three conditions. In advance of the delivery of the enema, one group chose one of three alternative regimens. To enhance predictability and control, a second group received detailed descriptions of the anticipated experiences associated with one barium procedure, while a third group received the standard barium procedure. There were no differential effects associated with these interventions, as reflected by self-reports of control and helplessness.

In a second experiment (Wallston, 1989), oncology patients were recruited. One group received a choice of one of three antiemetic agents, whereas the control group was informed only of the anticipated experiences associated with the treatment. For ethical reasons, the experimental protocol was restricted to these two conditions. Patients in the Choice condition used fewer helpless descriptors to depict their state, while revealing no difference in self-reports of perceived control from the predictability group.

Finally, in a third study (Wallston, 1989), some postsurgical patients were assigned to a predictability condition in which the discomfort and debilitations to be expected following surgery were described. In a second condition, postsurgical patients were provided choices over various behavioral options, such as sleep and bathing schedules. The comparison or no-treatment group received neither choice nor predictability. During the postsurgical period, perceptions of control in both experimental groups were similar to those in the no-treatment group. However, in the Choice group, increasing amounts of perceived control were correlated with the number of options that participants had explicitly *rejected*.

What do these results reveal about the effectiveness of choice in enhancing control with medical patients? First, they show that there is no ineluctable or automatic linkage between the act of choosing and perceived control. In both the barium enema study and the cancer study, subjects were presented with options, none of which were pleasant. Thus, whether choice failed to enhance the perception of control because of the absence of pleasing or desirable options, or because the options were similar on the dimension of unpleasantness, cannot be differentiated. In any case, to paraphrase William Shakespeare, *there is no choice in rotten apples*.

In other clinical settings, choice plays a more positive role. For example, choosing between psychological health and the personal degradation that can be associated with an addiction may provide a meaningful choice, and clinicians are beginning to utilize the construct of choice and motivation as an integral component of psychotherapy (Miller & Rollnick, 1991). Their approach to therapy posits that clients with addictions are most likely to have successful treatment outcomes when they independently come to a realization about the need for behavior change, namely, the availability of options for change. This approach is contrasted with more traditional treatment methods, such as confrontation and required admissions of powerlessness over one's addiction. Rather, Miller and Rollnick suggest that techniques that maximize clients' perceptions of control over their treatment are most effective at enhancing feelings of efficacy in coming to terms with their addiction. Inherent in this approach is the notion that by the act of *rejecting* the desire to continue using their preferred substance, clients gain a sense of empowerment. Given the relatively high rate of success with this technique (Rollnick & Morgan, 1995), it appears that a therapeutic environment that encourages personal involvement in the decision to change also enhances the sense of self, thereby increasing motivation to act. Likewise, Gutmann (Chapter 12, this volume) provides another application of the role of self as a moderator in the adjustment to adversity observed in clients presenting with the onset of psychopathology during old age.

The concordance between the laboratory studies and the field studies is comforting because it shows that the laboratory provides a valid analog for the explication of choice. More importantly, the laboratory provides a valid proving ground that can be used to protect patients with serious diseases from being exposed to interventions of unproved effectiveness.

The studies reported earlier identify some of the benefits and limitations in the usefulness of control in medical settings. However, a large body of evidence supports the notion that environments and interventions that enhance autonomy and control can motivate and increase adherence to medical regimen and improve the health status of elderly nursing home residents (for a review, see Williams, Deci, & Ryan, 1995).

Individual Differences and the Effectiveness of Choice

It is taken as axiomatic that to be maximally effective, an intervention should be compatible with specific needs or characteristics of the individual (Shute, 1993). Anderson (1995) matched participants' internality orientation (rated by teachers) and competence (IQ) with a choice manipulation. The assumption was that individuals who scored highest on these variables would benefit maximally from the opportunity to exercise choice. Subjects were kindergarten children (aged 5–6½ years old) who, because of their age, could be expected to have less well-formed experiences with the effects of choice and control. Because of subjects' inability to read, a face–name paired associates procedure was used, in which five faces, unfamiliar to the subjects, were presented individually, each accompanied by two names. The names were read to the participants.

In the Choice condition, subjects chose the name that they wanted to associate with the respective face; in the Force condition, names were assigned as described previously. Since internality scores and IQ were highly correlated, subjects were divided into three groups based on their IQ score, thus comprising a $3 \times 2 \times 5$ mixed design (IQ score, three levels; Choice/Force; trials, five). Results showed that the learning of the face–name associations improved across trials (Figure 2–3). Neither IQ nor choice was significant as main effects, but the interaction (IQ $\times$ Choice $\times$ Trials) was highly significant. Specifically, choice was maximally effective only for those individuals with a high competence orientation, as reflected in elevated IQ levels. Although not significant, when groups with the lowest competence scores were compared, there was a trend

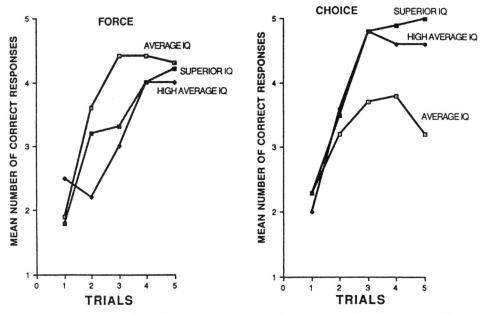

Figure 2–3. Mean number of correct responses in the Average, High Average, and Superior IQ groups in the Force (left panel) and Choice (right panel) groups.

for choice to have an adverse effect on performance relative to that exhibited by Force subjects.

In summary, absent the appropriate levels of individual-difference variables, performance was not benefitted by choice. On the other hand, when choice was compatible with individual characteristics, its positive effects were highly significant.

Choice and Cognitive Function in a Low Autonomy Sample

To continue the theme of examining choice in special populations, we recruited members of a Veterans Administration Day Treatment Center (Eads, 1996, Study 2). Subjects were assigned at random either to a Choice or a Force group, and their task was to learn a list of paired associates. Subjects ranged in age from 62 to 81 years old. Choice subjects selected their response words from available pairs, whereas responses were assigned for Force subjects. The number of correct responses increased significantly across trials, and more importantly, the *Force* group performed significantly better than the Choice group (Figure 2–4). Moreover, the percentage of intrusive responses was significantly greater in the Choice group.

These results appear *inconsistent* with those reported by Perlmuter et al. (1986). It had been shown (Figure 2–1) that subjects who were motivated to seek treatment (control) for their self-diagnosed memory problems benefitted from

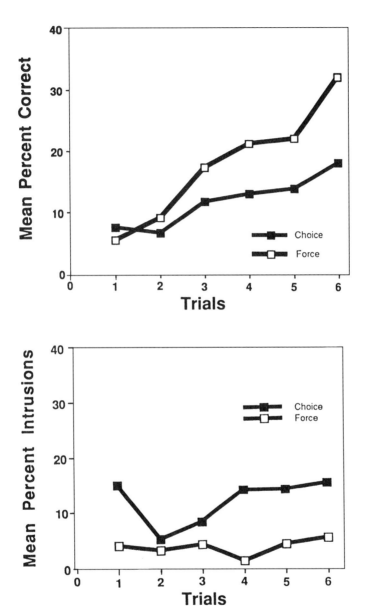

Figure 2–4. Mean percent correct responses and mean percent intrusions across trials for Choice and Force subjects.

choice. Conversely, the subjects in the present study (Eads, 1996, Study 2) were besought with a variety of psychosocial and medical problems that likely increased their dependency on social services, thereby decreasing their autonomy. Apparently, the day center members were burdened by the *opportunity* to choose, whereas the subjects recruited from the memory clinic were motivated by the opportunity to choose.

In summary, as in the Anderson study (1995) (Figure 2–3) with kindergarten children, the necessary *coincidence* between individual differences and the opportunity to experience control determines whether choice is a benefit, a burden, or simply irrelevant. Overall, these results show that treatment effectiveness is increased by matching the features of the intervention with the characteristics of the subject. Parenthetically, the issue of matching patients to treatments has even broader research implications (Brewin & Bradley, 1989); that is, the hallowed procedure of randomization may not provide the appropriate experimental strategy if individuals in the treatment group and in the control group are each required to engage in specific behaviors.

Choosing, Age, Educational Attainment, and Cognitive Performance

The purpose of the next study (Eads, 1996, Study 1) in this sequence was to examine the effects of choice in enhancing cognitive performance in young (Mean = 21 years) and older adults (Mean = 71 years). Young and older subjects were assigned at random either to a Choice group or a Force group. Thus, choice/force and age (young/old) were crossed in this factorial design.

The paradigm utilized a learning task in which lines of (meaningful) words with two or four words per line were presented. Subjects examined these materials, and then in the Choice group, individuals selected a *target* word on each line to be learned; in the Force group, the target word was assigned. Recognition testing occurred 1 week later. The test involved a presentation of one word from each line, either the target word or one of the nonchosen (background) word(s). Specifically, on the test trial, participants were shown an old word (previously presented) along with a new word (not previously presented); that is, in each pair, there was one old word (target or background) and one new word. Subjects indicated which word was "old." Subjects had been informed that each pair would contain a previously exposed word; thus, guessing would produce a correct score, on average, 50% of the time.

The basic results showed that recognition accuracy was significantly poorer in the elderly than in the young. Moreover, the benefits of choice were evident in the young, whereas in the elderly, recognition accuracy of chosen materials was indistinguishable from that of assigned materials. Overall, age appeared to have attenuated the typical improvements in performance that result from choosing.

To examine further the age-attenuated effects of choice, we classified the old participants into one of two groups based on years of formal educational attainment. For individuals with greater than a high school education, the opportunity to choose significantly improved target recognition accuracy. In other words, for the more competent elderly individuals, choice produced a pattern of performance that was highly similar to that observed in the young subjects. In a sense, choice motivated and rejuvenated performance. Such effects are consistent with the notion proposed by Gatz (Chapter 4, this volume) that increased education levels may provide a cognitive reserve that may increase the sense of self-efficacy, thereby enabling individuals to benefit from choosing. An alternative account is that higher levels of education may predispose to a class of behaviors that are qualitatively different from those that individuals with less education are wont to pursue. Thus, higher education may provide individuals with more behavioral options that, in turn, promote decision making, choice, and control.

By comparison, participants with only a high school education or less exhibited similar recognition accuracy, irrespective of their membership in the Choice or Force condition. Furthermore, in the low education group, the exercise of choice resulted in significantly better recognition of background (contextual) words as compared to target words. Apparently, as with kindergarten-aged children, when competence is relatively low, choice can degrade performance.

In this same study, we examined how individuals allocated their attentional resources to target and background stimuli. To this end, we categorized subjects into one of two groupings, namely, those with target recognition scores *greater* than background recognition scores (Target Learners), and those with target recognition scores *less* or equal to background recognition scores (Background Learners). More elderly than young participants were Background Learners; however, the opportunity to choose did improve the allocation of attentional resources (Table 2–1). Apparently, under specifiable conditions, choice not only enhances motivation, thereby improving performance, but it also facilitates the more effective allocation of attention, a provision that is especially salient for the elderly.

Table 2–1. Chi-Square Tables for Young and Old Subjects with Choice/Force by Target/Background Learner Variables

	Choice group	Force group
Young subjects		
Target learners	24	16
Background learners	6	14
$\chi^2(1) = 4.80$; $p \leqslant .01$		
Old subjects		
Target learners	22	10
Background learners	17	26
$\chi^2(1) = 6.27$; $p = .01$		

Choice and Attributions for Performance

In addition to enhancing motivation, we explored the idea that choice enhances performance by increasing the strength of attributions and sense of self-involvement with a task. To examine self-attributions, we return to the study utilizing elderly day-care participants (Eads, 1996, Study 2). Immediately following the paired associates learning trials, a brief questionnaire was presented, instructing individuals to rate on a 7-point scale the amount of choice and control they perceived over the task. Subjects also rated the extent to which luck, skill, and effort influenced their performance. Finally, subjects were asked to rate their ability to improve their performance in the future. These data were treated in two ways. First, attributions were examined as dependent variables by comparing Choice and Force groups. It was expected that attributions to choice, control, and skill would be enhanced by the opportunity to choose, whereas attributions to luck and chance would be reduced.

Results showed that on a 7-point scale, subjects in the Choice group (mean = 4.8 ± 1.9) tended to report higher *perceptions of choice* relative to the Force group (mean = 3.1 ± 1.9), $p = .07$. Furthermore, Choice subjects (mean = 6.0 ± 1.0) made significantly stronger attributions to *skill* than Force subjects (mean = 4.5 ± 1.5), $p = .03$. Although all other attributions were in the predicted direction, none differed significantly between groups. Thus, despite the significant degradation in paired associates learning occasioned by choice, the opportunity to choose tended to generate stronger, positive, self-directed attributions.

Next, we evaluated the relationship or linkage between attributions and task performance. In examining these analyses, it is important to note that participants had not been provided with any information about their performance, nor were they asked to rate their performance. Zero-order correlations between paired associates learning scores and attributions for performance showed different patterns in the Choice and Force groups (Table 2–2). The correlations between attributions reflecting control and skill are positively related to perfor-

Table 2–2. Zero-Order Correlations between Paired Associates Learning and Self-Attributions in the Choice (*N* = 10) and Force Groups (*N* = 9) (Higher Attributions Indicate Stronger Belief)

Attributions	Choice group	Force group
Perceived control	.77*	.34
Reported skilfullness	.69*	−.31
Ability to improve	−.77**	.30
Perceived luck	−.42	.00
Expended effort	.54	.17

$*p \leq .05$
$**p \leq .01$

mance and are relatively strong in the Choice group. Furthermore, the negative correlation between performance and the ability to improve suggests that Choice subjects may have perceived their effort as more maximal, with less opportunity for future improvement. This pattern was not evident for Force subjects, who tended to report less effort expenditure. Because of the relatively small sample size, tests for differences in the strength of correlations revealed no significant differences.

In summary, even in a task of low intrinsic interest, the opportunity to choose tended to effect greater task involvement as well as more positive self-attributions, despite poorer performance occasioned by choice.

The next set of analyses provided a replication for the relationship between attributions and performance (Eads, 1996, Study 1). It will be recalled that recognition accuracy was evaluated in young versus old individuals who learned under either Choice or Force conditions. We now report attributions for performance in these groups using a 2 × 2 analysis of variance with young/old as one variable and choice/force as the second variable. Elderly individuals expressed weaker attributions with respect to perceptions of choice and control, task satisfaction, and skill (Table 2–3). Furthermore, a number of attributions were strengthened by the opportunity to choose. However, Choice subjects expressed weaker attributions to skill, a finding that replicates the results of Burger (1989).

To examine the linkage between self-attributions, experimental conditions, and performance, multiple regression models were developed with target recognition as the dependent variable (Table 2–4). Age also served as a predictor. Attributions to control and luck were not only significant predictors of recognition performance, but also these variables interacted with choice, as predicted; that is, this linkage between the attributions and performance was *different* in the Choice and the Force group. Subsequent analyses revealed that two attributions (control and luck) had a significant association with performance only in the Choice group.

Table 2–3. Mean Attributions and Standard Deviations for Young and Old Subjects in the Choice and Force Groups

	Young subjects		Old subjects		
	Choice	Force	Choice	Force	p value
Perceived choice	5.07 ± 1.2	3.53 ± 1.6	3.97 ± 1.8	3.42 ± 1.9	a*,b**
Perceived control	5.40 ± .89	5.00 ± 1.3	4.33 ± 1.5	4.47 ± 1.8	a***
Satisfaction with performance	4.67 ± 1.1	5.03 ± .89	3.00 ± 1.5	2.92 ± 1.2	a***
Perceived luck	2.47 ± 1.4	2.21 ± 1.2	3.03 ± 1.4	3.23 ± 1.6	a**
Perceived skill	5.74 ± 1.5	5.95 ± 1.4	3.60 ± 2.0	4.88 ± 2.0	a***,b**

a = difference between age groups
b = difference between choice/force groups
*$p \leq .05$
**$p \leq .01$
***$p \leq .001$.

Table 2–4. Regression Models with Age,
Choice/Force, and Selected Attributions
as Predictors of Performance

DEPENDENT VARIABLE: Target Learning

Predictor	Beta	R^2 change
Model 1		
Age group (young/old)	−.34	.11***
Choice/force	−.27	.07***
Perceived control	.18	.03**
Choice/force × Control	−.73	.02*
Model 2		
Age group (young/old)	−.34	.11***
Choice/force	−.20	.04*
Perceived luck	−.21	.04**
Choice/force × Luck	.79	.04**
Model 3		
Age group (young/old)	−.34	.11***
Choice/force	−.20	.04*
Perceived skill	.17	.02
Choice/force × Skill	−.60	.01

*$p \leq .05$
**$p \leq .01$
***$p \leq .001$.

Thus, in summary, choice not only increased the strength of some personal attributions, but more importantly, it strengthened the linkage between attributions and performance, an especially important benefit for older individuals who may begin to perceive that their personal ability to effect outcomes has diminished. Additionally, Gatz (Chapter 4, this volume) has proposed that an enhanced sense of personal agency provides individuals with a source of optimism. In turn, increased optimism may strengthen the sense of well-being, thereby enhancing motivation. To the extent that individuals learn from their performance, the opportunity to choose generates a feed-forward loop that provides a continued source of motivation.

Enhancing the Perception of Control through Behavioral Monitoring

A molecular view of behavior would permit the description of an action as being composed of a sequence of movements that, in turn, would derive from choices being made at each juncture in the sequence (Perlmuter & Langer, 1982). Although such a description might be applicable to novel or recently learned behaviors, routinely performed behaviors become devoid of the sense of choice and control. Thus, a skillfully executed action, such as tying the laces in one's shoes, provides little sense of competence or control to the performer, that is, until an injury, such as a cerebral accident, deprives the individual of the facility to perform this routine behavior and it must be relearned.

Because routine behaviors are generally not performed deliberately, their performance fails to enhance the performer's perception of control. This lost opportunity to experience control can be especially costly to many elderly individuals whose living conditions and daily activities may provide relatively few novel challenges that require deliberate action. However, if encouraged to discover choice in routinely performed behaviors, individuals may become more generally attentive, and they may also experience a rejuvenated sense of competence and control.

To implement these ideas, we developed a behavioral monitoring task that encouraged individuals to discover choices within their routine behaviors (Perlmuter & Langer, 1982). In a pilot study, experimentally naive individuals were recruited from an adult day center. All participants maintained a diary for three successive weeks, requiring daily entries. Participants were assigned at random to one of three groups. In the *repeat monitoring* group, subjects responded in writing to three questions each day. For example, they indicated their choice of the first beverage of the day, how much they drank, their enjoyment of the beverage. A second group, *varied monitoring*, monitored a different behavior daily (e.g., color of shirt selected, snack chosen, etc.) and answered three questions, similar to those already described. In the third group, the *rejection* group, the same behaviors were targeted as in the second (varied choice) group. However, instead of focusing on that which was chosen, subjects indicated three alternatives that might have been chosen but were not. Following the 3-week intervention, the rejection group reported the strongest perceptions of control and motivation, but because the sample size was small, these results remain suggestive.

To provide a conceptual replication of this intervention, we recruited 40 learning-disabled children, ranging in age from 10–13 years (Turner, 1994). This population was selected because members often report diminished feelings of behavioral control. Participants were assigned at random to a behavioral monitoring group, in which they monitored a behavior each day and reported what a particular choice had been and whether they enjoyed it, similar to the first group described above (Perlmuter & Langer, 1982). Another group received the rejection intervention, as described earlier. Subjects indicated a chosen activity or option and then generated three alternatives that might have been chosen but were not. For both groups, entries were made into a diary for 5 days each week over 3 weeks. The study used a double-blind procedure.

The pre–post study design assessed performance prior to the intervention and within a week of its conclusion. To measure distractibility, numbers and letters were presented auditorially at one per second, and individuals were required to tally either one of these while ignoring the other. The groups performed similarly prior to treatment, but the improvement in performance following treatment was significantly greater in the rejection condition than in the monitoring condition. Apparently, the rejection intervention fostered increased attentional control while decreasing distractibility—one of the characteristics of individuals with this disorder.

On a second task, problem solving was required. Generally, highly impulsive individuals with low control perform poorly on this test. Problem-solving abilities were similar between groups prior to treatment, but following the intervention, the rejection group exhibited a significantly greater improvement in the number and quality of solutions than the comparison group. Apparently, as a result of the discovery of alternatives and choice, the rejection intervention brought about a more deliberate pattern of behavior that strengthened the sense of control.

Can the Opportunity to Choose Be Harmful?

Despite its many benefits, the exercise of choice can also increase the probability as well as the intensity of a failure experience (Schultz & Heckhausen, 1996). Complications following choice include experiences that could inhibit successful execution of control, such as having to choose one career path over another, physical impairment resulting from behavioral choices, and random negative events, such as being laid off from a chosen job. In these instances, *actual* opportunities for control may be limited, and such experiences are likely to decrease perceptions of control, at least temporarily. Several authors have offered explanations of the manner by which individuals may compensate for these potentially damaging experiences. Goal pursuits may be altered to better fit the conditions of one's environment (Lachman & Leff, 1989); attributions may be made to explain the circumstances that decrease one's control (Weiner, 1974); individuals may engage in "downward comparison" of the self to other, less fortunate persons (Taylor & Lobel, 1990), and Kuhl (1986) has suggested that elderly persons with decreased opportunities for control may derive a sense of control by choosing passivity, a choice in itself. Therefore, although having control may increase the possibility of failure, it appears that the development of the perception of control may allow individuals to retain the belief in their own efficacy.

CONCLUSION

The extent to which the quality of life depends upon motivation, behavior, and the perception of control is becoming increasingly clear. Less well appreciated is how routine behaviors provide opportunities for maintaining the perception of control throughout life, but most especially in the elderly, for whom the number of options available for control are likely to have been diminished.

Because they are so elemental and common, societal values have come to trivialize the significance of routine behaviors. However, our studies have shown that through behavioral monitoring, it is possible to enhance the perception of control by enabling individuals to discover choice within the performance of these most elemental behaviors.

As a result of its paradoxical nature, as illustrated by its phenomenological and illusory qualities, control cannot merely be awarded directly to an individual. Such an award would reduce the potential effectiveness of control by reinforcing its external source as well as its illusory quality. To generate a veridical perception of control, various criteria must be satisfied. Perhaps the most important consideration is that personal effort, such as through making choices, is required to enhance the perception of control.

Since choice and control increase the likelihood of positive outcomes as well as the risk for some untoward results, it should first be determined whether individuals will benefit from such interventions. For some groups of individuals, choice may produce positive or null effects, but for others, it may produce negative consequences. Thus, an intervention designed to increase control must be executed with full consideration of the possible range of sequelae.

Through various mechanisms, choice and control can guide an effective intervention. For example, the opportunity to exercise choice can contribute to the strengthening of the sense of self. By enabling individuals to exercise choice, motivation and the perception of control can be enhanced. Other personal attributions for performance, such as skill and effort, may also be increased. Irrespective of its effects upon performance, choice appears to increase the linkage between positive attributions and performance, thereby providing the individual with a strengthened sense of self.

Finally, in addition to improving the quality of life, it is important to encourage behavior change through increased control, because it is now recognized that nearly half of all deaths in America are both premature and attributable to destructive behavior (Williams et al., 1995). Thus, the accrual of the recognition of control over one's behaviors may prevent the untimely loss of well-being and life itself.

ACKNOWLEDGMENTS.   We want to express our thanks to Hadassa Kubat, who assisted with data collection and analyses. We also express our appreciation to Brian Hitsman and Samantha Faber, who assisted with data collection, and to Daniel Swichkow, who facilitated recruitment of a portion of these subjects.

REFERENCES

Adler, A. (1929). *The science of living.* New York: Greenburg.

Aldwin, C. M. (1991). Does age affect the stress and coping process? Implications of age differences in perceived control. *Journal of Gerontology: Psychological Sciences, 46,* 174–180.

Anderson, K. S. (1995). *Individual differences moderate the effects of choice in performance of kindergarten children.* Unpublished master's thesis, Finch University of Health Sciences/The Chicago Medical School, Chicago, IL.

Bandura, A. (1977). Self efficacy: Towards a unifying theory of behavior change. *Psychological Review, 84,* 191–215.

Baron, R., & Rodin, J. (1978). Perceived control and crowding stress. In A. Baum, J. E. Singer, & S. Valins (Eds.), *Advances in environmental psychology* (pp. 145–190). Hillsdale, NJ: Erlbaum.

Blanchard-Fields, F., & Robinson, S. L. (1987). Age differences in the relationship between controllability and coping. *Journal of Gerontology, 52,* 497–501.

Brewin, C. R., & Bradley, C. (1989). Patient preferences and randomized clinical trials. *British Medical Journal, 299,* 313–315.

Burger, J. M. (1989). Negative reactions to increases in perceived personal control. *Journal of Personality and Social Psychology, 56*, 246–256.

Eads, A. S. (1996). *The effects of choice on performance and motivation in elderly individuals.* Unpublished master's thesis, Finch University of Health Sciences/The Chicago Medical School, Chicago, IL.

Harvey, J. H., & Johnston, S. (1973). Determinants of the perception of control. *Journal of Experimental Social Psychology, 9*, 164–179.

Heckhausen, J., & Schulz, R. (1995). A life-span theory of control. *Psychological Review, 102*, 284–304.

Hull, C. L. (1943). *Principles of behavior.* New York: Appleton-Century-Crofts.

Kimble, G. A., & Perlmuter, L. C. (1970). The problem of volition. *Psychological Review, 77*, 361–384.

Kleigl, R., & Lindenberger, U. (1978). Age differences in processing relevant versus irrelevant stimuli in multiple item recognition learning. *Journal of Gerontology, 33*, 87–93.

Kuhl, J. (1986). Aging and models of control: The hidden costs of wisdom. In M. M. Baltes & P. B. Baltes (Eds.), *The psychology of control and aging* (pp. 1–34). Hillsdale, NJ: Erlbaum.

Lachman, M. E., & Leff, R. (1989). Perceived control and intellectual functioning in the elderly: A five year longitudinal study. *Developmental Psychology, 25*, 722–728.

Langer, E. J. (1975). The illusion of control. *Journal of Personality and Social Psychology, 32*, 311–328.

Langer, E. J., & Rodin, J. (1976). The effects of choice and enhanced personal responsibility for the aged: A field experiment in an institutional setting. *Journal of Personality and Social Psychology, 34*, 191–198.

Lazarus, R. S., & Folkman, S. (1984). *Stress, appraisal and coping.* New York: Springer.

Miller, W. R., & Rollnick, S. (1991). *Motivational interviewing: Preparing people to change addictive behavior.* New York: Guilford.

Monty, R. A., Geller, E. S., Savage, R. E., & Perlmuter, L. C. (1979). The freedom to choose is not always so choice. *Journal of Experimental Psychology: Human Learning and Memory, 5*, 170–178.

Monty, R. A., & Perlmuter, L. C. (1972). The role of choice in learning as a function of meaning and between and within subject designs. *Journal of Experimental Psychology, 94*, 235–238.

Monty, R. A., Rosenberger, M. A., & Perlmuter, L. C. (1973). Amount and locus of choice as sources of motivation in paired associates learning. *Journal of Experimental Psychology, 97*, 16–21.

Nathan, D. M., Singer, D. E., Godine, J. E., Harrington, C., & Perlmuter, L. C. (1986). Retinopathy in older type II diabetics: Association with glucose control. *Diabetes, 35*, 797–801.

Orne, C. M., & Binik, Y. M. (1989). Consistency in adherence across diabetic regimen demands. *Health Psychology, 8*, 27–43.

Perlmuter, L. C. (1991). Choice enhances performance in non-insulin-dependent diabetics and controls. *Journal of Gerontology: Psychological Sciences, 46*, 218–223.

Perlmuter, L. C., & Langer, E. J. (1982). The effects of behavioral monitoring on the perception of control. *Clinical Gerontologist, 1*, 37–43.

Perlmuter, L. C., & Monty, R. A. (1977). The importance of perceived control: Fact or fantasy? *American Scientist, 65*, 759–765.

Perlmuter, L. C., & Monty, R. A. (1982). Contextual effects on learning and memory. *Bulletin of the Psychonomic Society, 20*, 290–292.

Perlmuter, L. C., & Monty, R. A. (1989). Motivation and aging. In L. W. Poon, D. C. Rubin, & B. S. Wilson (Eds.), *Everyday cognition in adulthood and late life* (pp. 373–393). New York: Cambridge University Press.

Perlmuter, L. C., Monty, R. A., & Chan, F. (1986). Choice, control, and cognitive functioning. In M. M. Baltes & P. B. Baltes (Eds.), *The psychology of control and aging* (pp. 91–118). Hillsdale, NJ: Erlbaum.

Perlmuter, L. C., Scharff, K., Karsh, R., & Monty, R. A. (1980). Perceived control: A generalized state of motivation. *Motivation and Emotion, 4*, 35–44.

Rakowski, W., & Hickey, T. (1992). Mortality and the attribution of health problems to aging among older adults. *American Journal of Public Health, 82*, 1139–1141.

Rand, L. I., Krolewski, A. S., Aiello, L. M., Warram, J. H., Baker, R. S., & Maki, T. (1985). Multiple factors in the prediction of risk of proliferative diabetic retinopathy. *New England Journal of Medicine, 313*, 1433–1438.

Rodin, J., & Langer, E. J. (1977). Long-term effects of a control relevant intervention with the institutionalized aged. *Journal of Personality and Social Psychology, 35,* 897–902.

Rodin, J., Timko, S., & Harris, S. (1985). The construct of control: Biological and psychological correlates. *Annual Review of Gerontology, 5,* 3–55.

Rollnick, M., & Morgan, M. (1995). *Motivational interviewing—increasing readiness for change.* New York: Guilford.

Savage, R. E., Perlmuter, L. C., & Monty, R. A. (1979). Effect of reduction in the amount of choice and the perception of control on learning. In L. C. Perlmuter & R. A. Monty (Eds.), *Choice and perceived control* (pp. 91–106). Hillsdale, NJ: Erlbaum.

Schmidt, A. J. M. (1985). Cognitive factors in the performance level of chronic low back pain patients. *Journal of Psychosomatic Research, 29,* 183–189.

Schultz, R., & Heckhausen, J. (1996). A life span theory of successful aging. *American Psychologist, 51,* 702–714.

Shute, V. J. (1993). A macroadaptive approach to tutoring. *Journal of Artificial Intelligence in Education, 4,* 61–93.

Steiner, I. D. (1979). Three kinds of reported choice. In L. C. Perlmuter & R. A. Monty (Eds.), *Choice and perceived control* (pp. 21–22). Hillsdale, NJ: Erlbaum.

Stotland, E., & Blumenthal, A. (1964). The reduction of anxiety as a result of the expectation of making a choice. *Canadian Journal of Psychology, 18,* 139–145.

Takahashi, M. (1992). Memorial consequences of choosing nonwords: Implications for interpretations of the self-choice effect. *Japanese Psychological Research, 34,* 35–38.

Taylor, S., & Loebl, M. (1990). Social comparison activity under threat: Downward evaluation and upward contacts. *Psychological Review, 96,* 569–575.

Turner, M. L. (1994). *Increasing the perception of control and its effects on performance in learning disabled children.* Unpublished doctoral dissertation, Finch University of Health Sciences/ The Chicago Medical School, Chicago, IL.

Wallston, K. A. (1989). Assessment of control in health care settings. In A. Steptoe & A. Appels (Eds.), *Stress, personal care, and health* (pp. 85–105). Brussels, Belgium: Wiley.

Weiner, B. (1974). *Achievement, motivation, and attribution theory.* Morristown, NJ: Gerald Learning Press.

White, R. W. (1959). Motivation reconsidered: The concept of competence. *Psychological Review, 66,* 297– 333.

Williams, G. C., Deci, E. L., & Ryan, R. M. (1995). *Building partnerships by supporting autonomy: Promoting maintained behavior change and positive health outcomes.* Unpublished manuscript, University of Rochester, Rochester, NY.

CHAPTER 3

Resilience in Adulthood and Later Life

Defining Features and Dynamic Processes

CAROL D. RYFF, BURTON SINGER,
GAYLE DIENBERG LOVE, AND MARILYN J. ESSEX

INTRODUCTION

The study of mental health in old age, as throughout the life course, has addressed primarily the nature of mental illness, disorders, and difficulties. Health
in this framework is essentially the "absence of illness"—to the extent that one
does not suffer from various forms of mental problems, one is deemed mentally
healthy. Such a negative approach, which prevails in the assessment of physical
health as well, fails to address individuals' capacities to thrive and flourish, that
is, go beyond the absence of illness, or neutrality, into the presence of wellness
(Ryff, 1995; Ryff & Singer, 1996; 1998). In this chapter, we examine the relevance
of positive psychological well-being for understanding mental health in adulthood and later life. Such a focus on the positive underscores, we believe, the
unique strengths *and* vulnerabilities of the current elderly population.

Elevating the side of strengths, we propose a conceptualization of *resilience*,
which speaks to the capacities of some aging persons to stay well, recover, or
even improve, in the face of cumulating challenge. Growing old for many is a
time of life when life stresses accumulate; as such, it provides a compelling
period in the life course for the study of resilience and how it comes about. We
distinguish between resilience as a set of outcome criteria, and resilience as a

CAROL D. RYFF, GAYLE DIENBERG LOVE, AND MARILYN J. ESSEX • Institute on Aging, University of
Wisconsin–Madison, Madison Wisconsin 53706.   BURTON SINGER • Office of Population Research, Princeton University, Princeton, New Jersey 08544.

Handbook of Aging and Mental Health: An Integrative Approach, edited by Jacob Lomranz. Plenum
Press, New York, 1998.

dynamic process. Our formulation is illustrated with recent empirical findings from two longitudinal studies, one involving life histories of individuals in late midlife, and the other involving a specific transition of old age (community relocation). In both, we examine protective factors that appear to account for resilience in the face of adversity. We approach such factors from a multidisciplinary standpoint that incorporates an array of sociodemographic, psychosocial, and biological resources.

The first section of our chapter provides a brief review of prior literatures on resilience, giving emphasis to the conceptualizations, empirical findings, and age focus that characterize previous studies. We then summarize our own approach to the phenomenon of resilience and illustrate select parts of it with ongoing studies. A final section reviews future research directions to advance understanding of later life resilience as well as interventive directions to promote resilience in the elderly.

PRIOR STUDIES OF RESILIENCE

Resilience has various meanings in prior research. In some investigations, the construct has been used to refer to how one functions in the face of adversity; that is, *outcome profiles* associated with life difficulties are the focus of interest. Three key areas of investigation illustrate this approach, commencing with Rutter's 10-year study of children of parents diagnosed as mentally ill. Because many of these offspring did not become mentally ill themselves or exhibit maladaptive behavior (Rutter, 1985, 1987; Rutter, Maughan, Mortimore, & Ouston, 1979), Rutter subsequently defined resilience as the positive pole of an individual's response to stress and adversity (Rutter, 1990). Most of the key dependent variables in this research (e.g., adverse temperament, conduct disorders, affective disorders, depression) are not, however, positive. In another longitudinal investigation, Garmezy and colleagues (Garmezy, 1991, 1993; Garmezy, Masten, & Tellegen, 1984) followed children from low socioeconomic status (SES) backgrounds with negative family environments and found that although some showed less competence and more disruptive profiles, other disadvantaged children were competent (judged by teachers, peers, school records) and did not display behavior problems. In this work, resilience was defined as the capacity for recovery and maintaining adaptive functioning following incapacity (Garmezy, 1991), or the positive side of adaptation after extenuating circumstances (Masten, 1989).

In a third pioneering investigation, Werner and colleagues (Werner, 1993, 1995; Werner & Smith, 1977) followed a cohort of children born in Kauai for over three decades, one-third of whom were designated as high risk because they were born into poverty and lived in troubled environments (parental psychopathology, family discord, poor child-rearing conditions). Of these high-risk children, one-third grew up to be competent, confident, and caring adults. Werner's conception of resilience emphasized sustained competence under stress (Werner, 1995; Werner & Smith, 1992).

With the growing evidence of such resilience came further lines of inquiry that focused on the *protective factors* that could explain these positive responses to stress or adversity (Masten & Garmezy, 1985; Rutter, 1985). Werner (1995) referred to such factors as the "mechanisms that moderate (ameliorate) a person's reaction to a stressful situation or chronic adversity" so that adaptation is more successful than if protective factors were absent (p. 81). The aim thus was to show *how* children exposed to chronic poverty, parental psychopathology, parental divorce, serious caregiving deficits, or the horrors of war did *not* show psychological or health dysfunction. Prior candidates to account for stress resistance in children have included temperament and personality attributes, family cohesion and warmth, and external social supports (Garmezy, 1993) as well as high IQ, problem-solving abilities, quality parenting, stable families, and high SES (Garmezy et al., 1984). Werner (1995) distinguished among protective factors *within the individual* (e.g., affectionate and good-natured in infancy and early childhood; outgoing, active, autonomous, bright, and possessing positive self-concepts in middle childhood and adolescence); those *in the family* (close bonds with at least one nurturing, competent, emotionally stable parent); and those *in the community* (support and counsel from peers and elders in the community). Analytically, these protective factors have variously been construed as compensatory factors that have direct, independent effects on outcomes (Garmezy et al., 1984; Masten, 1989), or as interactive influences that moderate the effects of exposure to risk (Rutter, 1985, 1987; Zimmerman & Arunkumar, 1994).

A separate line of resilience research emerged, not from the study of children growing up under adverse circumstance, but from longitudinal studies of *personality*. The typological work of Jack Block (1971; Block & Block, 1980) pointed to the "ego-resilients" among adolescents and young adults as those who were well adjusted and interpersonally effective. Klohnen (1996) recently rekindled interest in ego-resiliency, defining it as a "personality resource that allows individuals to modify their characteristic level and habitual mode of expression of ego-control so as to most adaptively encounter, function in, and shape their immediate and long-term environmental contexts" (p. 1067). Klohnen finds strong relationships between ego-resiliency and effective functioning in diverse areas of life (e.g., global adjustment, work and social adjustment, physical and psychological health). Other recent work (Robins et al., 1996) extends the personality–typological approach to resilience in a mixed ethnic sample of adolescent boys, exploring implications for developmental problems and outcomes. Outside of the research realm, but also targeted on adulthood, are recent clinical accounts of extreme cases of abuse and successful recovery from them via critical psychosocial factors (Higgins, 1994).

As these prior studies indicate, resilience has been primarily the domain of developmental researchers dealing with early childhood and adolescence. Only recently, perhaps with the aging of the aforementioned longitudinal samples, has the focus shifted to early and middle adulthood. The study of resilience in later life remains largely uncharted territory, which is unfortunate, given that aging is characterized by incrementing profiles of physical, social, and psychological challenge. As such, it is a particularly promising period in the life course to investigate mechanisms of resilience and vulnerability. Moreover, with longitudinal aging studies, it is possible to track the long-term reach of early life adversities and early established profiles of resilience.

Among researchers who explicitly address the life course significance of resilience, Staudinger, Marsiske, and Baltes (1995) have proposed connections between the developmental psychopathological approach to resilience, as evident in the aforementioned child-focused studies, and ideas of "reserve capacity," a construct from lifespan developmental theory, referring to an individual's potential for change, especially continued growth. This work underscores distinctions between resilience as recovery from trauma, and resilience as maintenance of development despite the presence of threat or risk. Extensive prior research in multiple aging domains (i.e., cognition, self, social transactions) is reviewed, although few of the reported studies include explicit measures of developmental reserve/continued growth linked with particular risks or threats.

To these many prior investigations, we bring three observations. First, we note that most conceptions of resilience, whether focused on the *capacity to withstand adversity* or *capacity for recovery* of adaptive functioning following adversity, are operationalized according the absence-of-illness conceptions of health; that is, one maintains functioning, or recovers, to the extent that he or she is *not ill*, mentally or physically. This limited conception of resilience ignores the capacity of the organism to thrive and flourish after challenge, qualities central to understanding positive human health (Ryff & Singer, 1998). Looking for the *presence of wellness* following adversity comprises a more demanding and rigorous conception of resilience than the avoidance of psychopathology or negative behavioral outcomes, the usual gold standards. More fundamentally, this observation calls for greater attention to the outcome criteria that define resilience. As the preceding literature illustrates, the question of outcome has typically been overshadowed by efforts to formulate the risk factors that create vulnerability, or the protective factors that enable adaptive functioning.

Second, we note that extant research has given limited attention to the exact nature of the stressors confronting children of poverty or parental psychopathology, or resilient adults. In most cases, stress is inferred from troubled situations rather than empirically delineated, both in terms of objective events/experiences and their reactions to them. Furthermore, as Werner (1995) reminds, the majority of stresses (e.g., parental neglect) *and* protective factors (e.g., child personality) have consisted of psychosocial factors, thereby neglecting biological insults as stressors as well as physiological mechanisms involved in protective resources.

At the other end of the life course, we acknowledge the literature on *successful aging* (Baltes & Baltes, 1990; Berkman, Seeman, Albert et al., 1993; Bond, Cutler, & Grams, 1995; Rowe & Kahn, 1987; Schulz & Heckhausen, 1996) that has delineated high levels of physical, cognitive, and personal functioning in later life and explored their correlates (sociodemographic, behavioral, physiological). This research neglects, however, how such profiles of success intersect with the actual challenges or stresses of later life, and how they are effectively engaged. Without consideration of such challenges, it is impossible to map the dynamic processes through which successful aging is achieved or maintained.

A third, and related, observation is to underscore the need to study resilience as a longitudinal process. Paradoxically, although much of the early work on resilience has been conducted with longitudinal studies, the identification of factors to account for stress resistance has been largely post hoc (i.e., protective factors are identified *after* resilience has been established). Such an approach makes it difficult to determine which factors are necessary, and which may be peripheral, in explaining resilient outcomes. Prospective longitudinal studies that include a priori prediction and testing of hypothesized risk or protective factors have little presence in extant literature. Later life is an auspicious time to implement such prospective studies, because life challenges are then accumulating, and individual differences in health and well-being becoming more pronounced.

RESILIENCE AS WELL-BEING
IN THE FACE OF CHALLENGE

In this section, we elaborate a conceptualization of resilience, both as an outcome and as a process. The discussion of outcome criteria begins with a brief summary of prior research on psychological well-being across the adult life course. First, multiple dimensions of well-being provide empirical indicators of the positive aspects of psychological functioning that are central to a formulation of resilience as the capacity to flourish, and not just avoid dysfunction or illness, vis-à-vis challenge. These components of wellness, we argue, also have significance for physical health via the "physiological substrates of flourishing" (Ryff & Singer, 1998). Second, we present our dynamic conception of the resilience process and discuss a multidisciplinary array of protective factors hypothesized to account for resilience. Many of these are established areas of inquiry in the social sciences, although explicit connection of them with the maintenance of well-being in the face of challenge (i.e., resilience) has not been addressed. Adding to the usual psychosocial buffering factors, we describe three specific avenues for tracking protective mechanisms at the biological level.

Psychological Well-Being: Defining Dimensions and Life-Course Trajectories

Numerous prior publications (Ryff, 1989, 1991, 1995, 1996; Ryff & Keyes, 1995; Ryff & Singer, 1996) have summarized empirical findings for six theory-guided dimensions of psychological well-being. These include autonomy, environmental mastery, personal growth, positive relations with others, purpose in life, and self-acceptance. Such dimensions were derived from points of convergence of prior accounts of positive psychological functioning, including life-span developmental theory (Buhler & Massarik, 1968; Erikson, 1959; Jung, 1933;

Neugarten, 1973), clinical psychology (Allport, 1961; Maslow, 1968; Rogers, 1961), and mental health literatures (Birren & Renner, 1980; Jahoda, 1958). Collectively, these dimensions encompass a breadth of wellness that includes positive evaluations of one's self and one's life, a sense of continued growth and development, the belief that life is purposeful and meaningful, the possession of quality relations with others, the capacity to manage effectively one's life and surrounding world, and a sense of self-determination. In essence, numerous components of human flourishing are included.

The dimensions are operationalized with structured self-report instruments. Data from multiple groups, including mixed-age local probability samples, national survey samples, and focused longitudinal studies, have thus far been collected. Cross-sectional studies have shown diverse, but replicable, patterns of age trajectories of well-being (Ryff, 1989, 1991; Ryff & Keyes, 1995; Ryff & Singer, 1996). Environmental mastery, for example, consistently shows incremental patterns with age; purpose in life and personal growth consistently show declining profiles from young adulthood to midlife and old age; self-acceptance repeatedly has shown no significant age differences. For autonomy and positive relations with others, findings have varied between showing incremental age profiles or no age differences. Women consistently score higher than men on positive relations and in some samples (including cross-cultural comparisons) have also scored higher on personal growth. The remaining aspects of well-being show few gender differences.

Viewed in concert, these studies suggest possible strengths *and* vulnerabilities in psychological functioning over the life course. In the absence of longitudinal data spanning multiple decades of adult life, it is impossible to know whether the findings represent aging, maturational processes, enduring cohort differences, or some combination of both. Whatever the interpretation, the outcomes underscore previously unrecognized vulnerabilities among current samples of older persons—to wit, the replicative consistency of downward age trends for purpose in life and personal growth, even among samples of healthy, well-educated, economically comfortable older adults. These patterns may speak to the claim that current social institutions lag behind the added years of life that many persons now experience (Riley, Kahn, & Foner, 1994). "Structural lag," that is, may heighten the challenges faced by contemporary older adults.

Resilience as an Outcome: Toward Mind–Body Integration

Drawing on the previous studies of psychological well-being, we define resilience as the *maintenance, recovery, or improvement in mental or physical health following challenge*. Such a formulation goes beyond prior conceptions that have focused on "absence of illness" indicators of resilience (e.g., not becoming depressed, anxious, or physically ill in the face of adversity). Our definition also brings physical health into the conception of resilience, thereby underscoring a joint emphasis on the mind and the body in understanding positive functioning. Positive physical health, like mental health, includes not only the absence of illness (e.g., avoidance of disease, chronic conditions, health symptoms, physical limitations) but also the presence of the positive (e.g., functional abilities, aerobic capacities, healthy behaviors—diet, exercise, sleep).

Life challenge is also fundamental to our conception of resilience. Thus, the model is not about lives of smooth sailing, where all goes well and one manages to evade adversity, but rather is about successful *engagement* with life challenges. The later years are replete with such challenges, making old age a particularly valuable period for understanding how such challenges are successfully negotiated. A central feature of our research program is tracking naturally occurring challenges and their cumulation over time. How individuals remain healthy and well in the face of these challenges is a fundamental route to understanding resilience as a dynamic process.

Resilience as a Dynamic Process: Delineating Key Protective Factors

Following a multidisciplinary approach, we propose that the phenomenon of resilience results from the inner workings of multiple protective factors. At the *sociological, social structural level* are sociodemographic resources such as education, income, and occupational status. Prior literature on class and health (Adler et al., 1994; Dohrenwend, Levav, & Shrout, 1992; Kessler & Cleary, 1980; Marmot, Ryff, Bumpass, Shipley, & Marks, 1997) has documented an extensive array of health benefits associated with higher status positions as well as the vulnerabilities linked with lower SES standing. Much of this research has, however, focused on accounting for differential profiles of psychological disorders, physical morbidity, or mortality. Our emphasis, in contrast, is on the role of these sociodemographic variables in accounting for positive health (mental and physical) outcomes as well as contributing to positive profiles of other psychological, social, and biological protective factors.

At the *psychological level* is another array of factors that have been investigated as possible mediators or moderators of stressful life experience. These include how individuals interpret, cope with, or react to their life events (e.g., Aldwin, 1991; Carver, Scheier, & Weintraub, 1989; Kling, Seltzer, & Ryff, 1997; Lazarus & Folkman, 1984; Pearlin, 1991; Ryff & Essex, 1992; Thoits, 1994, 1995) as well as the ways in which their enduring personality characteristics influence how everyday problems are handled (Bolger & Schilling, 1991; Heady & Wearing, 1989; Ormel, Stewart, & Sanderman, 1989). These individual-level factors may well influence the adaptive ways in which life stresses and challenges are encountered, although, again, the bulk of prior knowledge has elaborated the negative, dysfunctional aspects of such factors (e.g., neuroticism, emotion-focused coping). A positive characterization of protective factors converges with efforts to portray the individual as a psychological activist, capable of proactive and effective problem solving, rather than being passively buffeted about by external forces (Thoits, 1994).

At the *social–relational level* is the voluminous literature on social supports and their ameliorative effects on response to stressful life events (Adler & Matthews, 1994; Cohen, 1988; House, Landis, & Umberson, 1988; McLeod & Kessler, 1990; Seeman, 1996; Thoits, 1995). Thus, for diverse life problems, researchers have examined the buffering effects of social integration, social network properties, and perceived support. Moreover, a recent review of 81 studies revealed that social support was reliably related to multiple aspects of physiology, including the cardiovascular, endocrine, and immune systems (Uchino, Cacioppo, & Kiecolt-Glaser, 1996). Family relationships and family life have also been extensively studied for their health consequences, although the focus has been on the negatives (e.g., divorce, widowhood, caregiving) and how they compromise health, with much less attention given to the ways in which family life contributes to human flourishing (see Ryff & Seltzer, 1996; Ryff & Singer, 1998).

Sociodemographic, psychological, and social–interactional protective factors are not, in and of themselves, innovative directions for the study of resilience. On the contrary, the extensive prior literature cited earlier speaks to the prominence of these areas in identifying the prevalence of, or the buffering of the impact of, stress. Our intent is to channel what is known about these factors to the specific task of understanding *who remains well, regains their wellness, or improves in the face of cumulating adversity*. What is thus new is the effort to *integrate* these factors to explain resilience, conceptualized as the presence of the positive in mental and physical health. In addition, our aim is to establish connections between these social-psychological protective factors and those that are biological. The biological side of resilience is largely an undeveloped subject, primarily because stress research has focused almost exclusively on *failures* in the adaptation process. Thus, little is known about optimal biological functioning under challenge. We propose three specific avenues to explicate protective mechanisms at the *biological level*: optimal allostasis, immune competence, and cerebral activation asymmetry. These, we have argued elsewhere (Ryff & Singer, 1998), provide empirical inroads to the "physiological substrates of flourishing"; that is, they delineate different aspects of autonomic, neuroendocrine, and immune function linked with quality living.

Optimal Allostasis. Allostasis, meaning "stability through change" (Sterling & Eyer, 1988, p. 638), is a concept that emphasizes that healthy functioning requires continual adjustments and alterations of the internal physiological milieu; that is, in responding and adapting to environmental demands, normally functioning physiological systems exhibit fluctuating levels of activity. Alternatively, "allostatic load" refers to the strain on multiple organs and tissues (McEwen & Stellar, 1993) that accumulates via the wear and tear associated with *acute shifts* in physiological reactivity in response to negative stimuli and via *chronic elevations* in physiological activity.

Seeman et al. (1997) operationalized allostatic load with numerous indicators of physiological system impairment: high systolic and diastolic blood pressure as indices of cardiovascular activity; waist–hip ratio as an index of metabolism and adipose tissue disposition; serum high density lipoproteins (HDL) and total cholesterol as indices of atherosclerotic risk; blood plasma levels of gly-cosylated hemoglobin indicate glucose metabolism; 12-hour integrated urinary cortisol excretion as an indicator of hypothalamic-pituitary-adrenal (HPA) axis activity; and urinary epinephrine and norepinephrine excretion levels as in-dices of sympathetic nervous system (SNS) activity. A study of elderly persons showed that those with higher allostatic load and no reported cardiovascular disease (myocardial infarction, stroke, diabetes, high blood pressure) at baseline had higher incidence of declining cognitive function (particularly memory decline) and declining physical performance (Seeman et al., 1994) 2.5 years later. Not surprisingly, they also had high incidence of cardiovascular disease. Thus, elevated allostatic load predicted multiple types of organ system breakdown.

"Optimal allostasis," in contrast, addresses *successful* physiological adap-tation to the challenges and stresses of life. In this context, it is *maintenance in normal operating ranges* of the multiple components of cardiovascular activ-ity, metabolism, atherosclerotic risk, HPA-axis activity, and SNS activity that operationalizes "effective warding off of stress."[*] In addition to adaptive re-sponses to stress, optimal allostasis is promoted by experiences with the positive in life (e.g., fulfilling life purposes, quality relationships) via their ameliorative physiological effects. Here, measurement of selected brain opioids, such as B-endorphins and leucine and methionine enkephalins, is relevant. These en-dorphins have powerful effects in counteracting negative emotions and promot-ing positive ones (Panksepp, 1981, 1993; Solomon et al., 1987). Dopamine from the catecholamine systems is also pertinent, as positive human emotionality has been related to heightened dopamine activity (Depue & Iacono, 1989; Depue, Luciana, Arbisi, Collins, & Leon, 1994). Central nervous system (CNS) opioid peptides, activated by prolonged physical exercise, are also relevant for their promotion of both physical and mental well-being (Hoffmann, 1997; Morgan, 1997). Finally, oxytocin (OXY), an instigator of maternal behavior, nurturant feelings of acceptance, and social bonding (Insel, 1992; Panksepp, 1993; Uvnäs-Moberg, 1997), and a facilitator of sexual gratification via facilitation of male and female sexual responses (Pederson, Caldwell & Brooks, 1990; Insel, 1992; Pank-sepp, 1992), may be a further relevant marker of optimal allostasis.

The essential idea embodied by these lines of inquiry is that an organism remains healthy and well through (1) effective warding off of stress and its physiological sequelae, and (2) via encounters with the positives in life and their physiological substrates. These avenues of optimal allostasis, we propose, are part of understanding the mechanisms of human resilience.

Immune Competence. Substantial evidence exists that stress and nega-tive psychological and social factors influence both cellular and humoral indica-tors of immune status and function (Cohen & Herbert, 1996; Kiecolt-Glaser,

---

[*]A related model of the positive response to stress is Dienstbier's (1989) formulation of "physiologi-cal toughness," which refers to a pattern of arousal (i.e., low SNS arousal base rates combined with strong, responsive challenge-induced SNS–adrenal–medullary arousal, with resistance to brain catecholamine depletion and suppression of pituitary adrenal–cortical responses) that works in interaction with effective psychological coping to comprise positive physiological reactivity.

Malarkey, Cucioppo, & Glaser, 1994; Maier, Watkins, & Fleshner, 1994). Suppression of immune function has been found across numerous forms of life adversity (e.g., taking examinations; caring for relatives with chronic disease; suffering marital discord; experiencing high levels of unpleasant daily events, chronic stress, and negative moods). In the case of infectious disease, consistent evidence also links stress and negative affect with disease onset and progression (Cohen, 1996; Stone et al., 1992).

On the positive side, we underscore the importance of considering how healthy mental states, such as possessing a strong sense of meaning and purpose in life, or supportive love relationships, contribute to resistance to, or recovery from, threats to the immune system (Ryff & Singer, 1998). Melnechuk (1988) summarizes literature relating positive feelings, religious beliefs, expression of goals, and hopes to regression of cancers and other autoimmune disorders. Persons with positive life outlooks also showed differences in wound healing and tissue repair. Quality relationships have also been implicated in survival time following breast cancer diagnosis (Spiegel, Kraemer, Bloom, & Gottheil, 1989).

How do these positive experiences and states of mental well-being serve *protective* roles? We propose that deeply experienced aspects of well-being provide a bedrock of psychological strengths that contributes to optimal operating ranges for multiple physiological systems, and these, in turn, modulate immune function (operationalized with an array of indicators, such as antibody titers, natural killer (NK) cells, T suppressor/cytotoxic lymphocytes). Explication of these *positive pathways* has been neglected in scientific studies of human health, despite suggestive autobiographical accounts, such as Victor Frankl's (1959/1992) life in the concentration camps, or Mark Mathabane's (1986; see also Singer & Ryff, 1998) childhood under apartheid in South Africa, both of which speak poignantly to the power of meaningful life pursuits, belief in one's own potentialities, and supportive love relationships in fostering health and well-being in the face of enormous adversity. One critical aspect of health in both life stories was remarkable immune competence.

Cerebral Activation Asymmetry. Extensive prior research shows that the two cerebral hemispheres play an asymmetrical role in the experience of positive versus negative effect (Davidson, 1992a, 1992b). Decreased activation in the left prefrontal region is associated with increased vulnerability to depression, while increased activation is associated with dispositional positive affect (Tomarken, Davidson, Wheeler, & Doss, 1992) and with coping styles found to be protective against depressive symptomatology (Tomarken & Davidson, 1994). Similarly, individual differences in anterior asymmetry associated with emotional responding are seen as vulnerabilities, which in combination with negative environmental events, produce depressive symptomatology (Davidson, 1993). Thus, given the same negative life event, an individual with baseline left anterior hypoactivation is hypothesized to show more intense depressive symptoms compared with one showing left anterior hyperactivation.

These neurophysiological substrates of emotional reactivity are also implicated in immune function. A comparison of extreme and stable patterns of left- and right-sided prefrontal activation patterns showed that right frontal subjects had significantly lower NK cell activity in contrast to left-frontal subjects (Kang, Davidson, Coe et al., 1991). Emerging evidence also links hemispheric asymmetries to cortisol secretion in emotionally threatening or aversive situations. Wittling and Pfluger (1992) manipulated viewing of an emotional film with lateralized projection of visual stimuli to the left or right hemisphere and found that the right-hemispheric group showed marked cortisol elevation in response to the aversive film compared to those in the same group who saw a neutral film, or those in the left-hemispheric group who saw either film. Davidson (1995) further demonstrated that subjects with increased right-sided prefrontal activation have higher cortisol levels and slower recovery to baseline following presentation of negative stimuli.

From the perspective of positive brain function, we propose that individuals with high profiles of psychological well-being are those who possess capacities to activate positive affective processes in the face of negative environmental stressors. Such capabilities likely reflect enduring differences in dispositional mood *and* established patterns of emotional reactivity. Emerging connections between cerebral asymmetry, immune function, and cortisol secretion further elaborate the interweaving of physiological avenues through which the possession of positive mental health contributes to physical health.

In summary, optimal allostasis, immune competence, and cerebral activation asymmetry comprise promising routes to explore the separate and interactive physiological substrates of flourishing, and thereby, how individuals maintain optimal health in the face of life adversity. Our formulation underscores continual exchange and feedback between these different physiological systems as well as how they affect, and are affected by, other psychological and social protective factors. Explicating the bidirectional pathways through which these biological and psychosocial factors are linked with mental and physical health outcomes is the essence of the larger resilience research agenda.

ILLUSTRATIVE STUDIES

We describe select parts of ongoing studies in this section to illustrate how the previous formulation guides our program of empirical research. A first study involves a longitudinal investigation of a large random sample of high school graduates who have been followed for more than 35 years. In this work, we are primarily interested in compiling life-history data to understand profiles of health and well-being in midlife. A second study involves a short-term longitudinal investigation that has followed a sample of aging women through a major life transition. Along the way, these women have also experienced numerous other life challenges. Thus, in both investigations, we emphasize the *cumulation of adversity* in respondents' lives, as well as the impact of key protective factors, in trying to understand resilience. Both studies also involve a typological approach, where the objective is to work in the neglected space that exists between traditional variable-focused, nomothetic analyses and single, case-study analyses (see Singer, Ryff, Carr, & Magee, in press).

Life Histories and Resilience in Midlife

How diverse events and experiences across multiple life domains comprise life histories, and how such histories are linked with psychological resilience are questions we have explored with the Wisconsin Longitudinal Study (WLS). This study was begun in 1957 with a random sample of over 9,000 Wisconsin high school graduates. Data were initially collected on respondents' family background, starting resources, academic abilities, youthful aspirations and, in subsequent waves (1970, 1975, 1992–1993), on educational and occupational achievements, work events and conditions, family events, social support and relationships, social comparisons, and physical and mental health. This comprehensive, multidomain, across-time information provides the data from which we have constructed life histories.

Guiding Principles.   We follow various guiding principles to organize the expansive array of life-history information (see Singer et al., in press). First, we emphasize the *cumulation of adversity* in respondents' lives. The idea that negative life events and difficult conditions compromise health has long-standing presence in social science research (e.g., Harris, Brown, & Bifulco, 1990; Kessler & Magee, 1993; McLeod & Kessler, 1990; Turner & Lloyd, 1995; Wheaton, 1990). The life-history approach calls for tracking of negative events in multiple life domains, thereby capturing patterns of "pile up." Cumulation can also refer to the enduring, persistent features of life strains (chronic problems), which may have important links to physiological substrates.

For some individuals, cumulative adversity may, however, be offset by an analogous *cumulation of advantage.* These may come in multiple forms: starting resources (e.g., growing up in an intact family, high parental SES), personal capabilities and abilities (e.g., IQ), realization of desired life transitions (e.g., job promotions, marriage, parenthood), and positive evaluations of different aspects of life (e.g., job or marital satisfaction). The idea of cumulative advantage is also not new, although, in prior work, it has been invoked to explain inequalities in scientific productivity (Cole & Singer, 1991; Merton, 1968), or health advantages of higher educational attainment (Ross & Wu, 1996). We seek to broaden the applicability of the idea to encompass multiple domains of life. Cumulative advantage, we hypothesize, has ameliorative, protective benefits that may be central to understanding human resilience.

Our life history research also emphasizes the importance of how people *react* to their experiences of adversity (or advantage). This interest converges with the extensive prior research on coping (Lazarus & Folkman, 1984; Menaghan, 1983; Pearlin, 1991, Pearlin & Schooler, 1978; Thoits, 1995), which constitute key protective factors on the psychological level (as we noted earlier).

However, because our life histories include not only unexpected life events, but also chronic conditions, normative life transitions, and general life evaluations, we broaden the scope of what is typically examined as reactive responses.

At the social level, we have emphasized the importance of quality relationships with significant others, thereby converging with the extensive social support literature (Cohen & Wills, 1985; House et al., 1988; Wethington & Kessler, 1986). Beyond considering how meaningful relationships buffer the effects of stress, we also seek to illuminate the role of significant others in contributing to one's sense of positive self-regard, esteem, and worth.

A further feature of the social world that may afford protective influence is one's position in the social hierarchy. Social hierarchies are ubiquitous features of human and animal life. We adopt a broad view of hierarchy that includes not only traditional SES classifications (e.g., education, income, occupational status), but also considers ability hierarchies, positions of influence in the family and community, degree of autonomy and authority in the workplace, and subjective social comparisons with others. We suggest that high social standing in some stable hierarchy (and its cumulation over time) has positive health consequences.

We have drawn on these guiding principles, which converge with protective factors discussed earlier, to address how different life histories are linked with particular mental health profiles (e.g., depressed, resilient, vulnerable, healthy) in the midlife WLS respondents. For present purposes, we describe findings for one subgroup of respondents: *resilient women*. Our classification of resilience in this study reflects the *recovery* conception; to be classified as resilient, respondents had to have reported a prior episode (or episodes) of major depression (assessed with a subset of items from the Composite International Diagnostic Interview, CIDI), but at the time of the 1992–1993 data collection, reported high psychological well-being (using the previously described six dimensions). The sample included 168 women who fit this description.

Multiple Pathways to Resilience.   Our methodological procedures for analyzing the life histories of these women are summarized elsewhere (Singer, Ryff, Carr, & Magee, in press). Briefly, we began with the writing of randomly selected individual biographies, which included extensive numbers of variables. The biographies were then reviewed for commonalities and subsequently thinned to more generic descriptions, organized according to the guiding principles. We then test the distinguishability of the life histories in one mental health group (i.e., the resilient) with individuals in other groups (i.e., depressed, vulnerable, healthy). Such procedures illustrate our intent to work in the middle ground between strictly idiographic and nomothetic approaches.

Our analyses distinguished four primary life-history pathways to resilience among these midlife women. The first pathway (subgroup H_1) was comprised of women with generally positive beginnings (e.g., high starting abilities, no alcoholism in childhood home) who subsequently experienced upward job mobility. They also perceived that their achievements in life compared favorably with their parents and siblings. Despite these advantages, all of these women had experienced the death of one parent, most had participated in caregiving for an ill person, and approximately half had two or more chronic conditions. Thus, their lives involved multiple difficulties of particular acute or chronic adversities that were offset by positive work experiences, good beginnings, and favorable self-evaluations.

The second subgroup, H_2, was comprised of women for whom the primarily early life adversity was growing up with alcohol problems in the childhood home. All women in the subgroup met this condition. In addition, many (65%) of these women had experienced three or more major acute events (e.g., death of parent, child, spouse; divorce; job loss). However, the women had important advantages involving social relationships and social participation, early employment with stable or upward occupational status, and positive social comparisons. The latter pluses are presumably part of why the women reported high psychological well-being despite their early and later life adversities.

The third subgroup, H_3, showed primarily advantage in early life: All had parents who were both high school graduates, no alcohol problems existed in the childhood home, and the women had high starting abilities (high school grades, IQ). Later, however, they confronted various forms of adversity (e.g., poor social relationships, downward occupational mobility, job loss, divorce, single parenthood, caregiving). Thus, their lives were characterized by various forms of family adversity occurring largely in adulthood, but they began their journeys with important early strengths that likely facilitated their recovery from adverse experiences.

The final subgroup, H_4, were women whose early lives showed mixed advantages (intact families, no alcoholism) and disadvantage (all had one parent with less than a high school diploma). As life unfolded, the women confronted an array of adversities: job loss, downward mobility, living with alcohol problems in the home, divorce/single parenthood, high profiles of major acute events. This array of negatives, combined with their less than uniformly positive beginnings, makes difficult the explanation for their resilience. As such, this subgroup underscores the need for additional information pertaining, for example, to their reactions to different life challenges or the quality of their significant social relationships.

Overall, the analyses underscore the diversity in what was bad and good in these women's lives: difficulties occurred across multiple life domains; some were chronic and enduring, others acute; some occurred early in life, others in adulthood. Their advantages and resources also varied across the life domains in which they occurred. From this variety emerged *differing tales* of why the women may have succumbed to depression and what were their routes out of it. Thus, rather than present a uniform characterization of the life histories of all 168 resilient women, our analysis clarified *diverse pathways* through adversity to high psychological well-being. The protective roles of positive experiences of advantage (e.g., good starting resources), quality social relationships, advancements in work hierarchies, and favorable reactions (e.g., positive social comparisons) are central to the overall resilience story.

Links to Biology. Currently, we are collecting comprehensive biological data on a subset of WLS respondents to incorporate the previously discussed protective factors of optimal allostasis, immune competence, and cerebral activation asymmetry. The basic objective is to evaluate the extent to which the cumulation of adversity (or advantage), along with profiles on the other psychosocial protective factors, can be used to *predict* these aspects of midlife physiological functioning. In this investigation, we focus on resilience as the ability to *withstand adversity*, that is, the capacity to maintain high psychological well-being, despite an extensive accumulation of negative life events and difficult enduring conditions. The fundamental hypothesis is that resilience for these individuals stems from strong positive profiles on optimal allostasis, immune competence, and cerebral activation asymmetry, as well as psychological, social, and sociodemographic protective factors. Consistent with prior analyses, we expect these protective factors to combine in different ways for different subgroups of respondents. Because the respondents are entering their sixties decade, the profiles of resilience and vulnerability will also serve as important predictive markers for how the later years are traversed. The aim is to track the unfolding mental and physical health of respondents as a function of cumulative prior challenges and multidisciplinary profiles of protective resources.

Later Life and the Cumulation of Challenge

To document our claim that later life is a period in which life challenges rapidly accumulate, we summarize data from the Wisconsin Study of Community Relocation. This short-term longitudinal investigation is following over 300 older women (average age = 70) through a major life transition of high prevalence among older women: relocation from one's prior home to an apartment or retirement community (moves to nursing homes are *not* included). We obtained extensive demographic, psychosocial, and health assessments prior to these moves, as well as three times following the move (i.e., 1–2 months, 7–8 months, and 13–15 months later).

Although the specific focus was on relocation, at each wave of data collection, the women were asked about other types of life events (e.g., changes in marital status, household composition, or income; deaths of family or friends; illnesses or injuries of self or significant others; moves; job changes) that had happened recently or since we last interviewed them. The respondents were also given the opportunity to identify other significant events in an open-ended framework.

Central to the idea of *cumulative challenge* is the question of how many such events occurred in the lives of our sample respondents over a slightly less than 2-year period (average time interval from T_1 to T_4 was 21 months). We counted the cross-time distribution of events for a subsample of 189 women who had completed all four waves of the study (data collection is still underway). Collectively, the respondents reported a total number of *1,485 events*, which were collapsed into three general categories: positive (e.g., births, promotions,

Table 3–1. Distribution of Cumulative Events

		Number of Positive Events			
		0-1	2-3	4+	
Number of Negative Events	0-2	30 (15.8%)	25 (13.2%)	13 (6.8%)	68 (35.9%)
	3-5	34 (17.9%)	27 (14.2%)	17 (8.9%)	78 (41.2%)
	6+	17 (8.9%)	15 (7.9%)	11 (5.8%)	43 (22.7%)
		81 (42.8%)	67 (35.4%)	41 (21.6%)	189

celebrations), negative (e.g., deaths, health events, difficulties in relationships) or neutral (e.g., starting–stopping a job; someone moving in–out of respondent's home). Of the total events reported, 61% (909) were negative, 33% (483) were positive, and about 6% (93) were neutral.

Table 3–1 summarizes the distribution of cumulative events for the 189 respondents, cross-classifying positive and negative events. Entries in the cells of the table are numbers of persons who had experienced a particular numerical combination of positive and negative events. The number of total events reported over this period for a single person was 25, with respondents on average reporting 9 events. The maximal number of negative events reported per person over the data-collection period was 20, with the mean being 5 negative events. Approximately 23% of respondents reported 6 or more negative events, while a comparable 22% reported 4 or more positive events. Alternatively, few (about 16%) reported a low incidence of positive *and* negative events. What we draw attention to in this table are (1) the generally high profile of events occurring over this relatively brief time period, thereby underscoring our claim that later life is a time when life *challenges cumulate*; (2) the overall *variability* in the distribution of the magnitude of these events, thereby pointing to the utility of such cumulation indices in explicating differential profiles of health and well-being and intervening resilience processes; and (3) the evidence that for many respondents, life is replete with *both* positive and negative occurrences. Because the positives may play an important role in *offsetting* the impact of negative events, we consider it particularly important to track cumulation of them as well. As described in the WLS study, the cumulation of adversity *and* advantage are requisite to understanding resilience.

Our data collection for these idiographically reported events also included assessments of respondents' *emotional reactions* to these experiences and their view of the events' overall impact. Respondents were able to select their own words to describe their reactions, thereby providing powerful assessments of a key guiding principle described in the WLS research, namely, how the event is interpreted by the respondent. Whether such events are perceived as threats or nonthreats is fundamental to mapping the physiology of the stress response, and more specifically, allostatic load or optimal allostasis. Analyses of these reaction data and their ties to subsequent health outcomes are currently underway.

Resilient Outcomes in Later Life

In addition to documenting the cumulation of life challenges, the relocation study also provides an opportunity to assess the prevalence of individuals who, in fact, demonstrate resilient outcomes, that is, show maintenance, recovery of, or improvement in health and well-being over time in the face of challenge. Our multiple-wave data thus permit the tracking of *dynamic mental and physical health trajectories.* To illustrate such dynamics, we classified respondents according to their mental and physical health stability or change over the prior waves of data collection.

Dynamic mental health trajectories are based on respondents' composite profiles on six scales of psychological well-being (Ryff, 1989, 1995; Ryff & Keyes, 1995; Ryff & Singer, 1996) described earlier. We first distinguished between different levels of overall well-being: *High well-being* is defined as moderately or strongly agreeing with 11 of 14 items (80%) on any 4 of the 6 well-being scales; *low well-being* is defined as disagreeing (strongly, moderately, slightly) or slightly agreeing with 9 of 14 items on any 4 of the 6 well-being scales. Those not meeting criteria for high or low well-being are defined as having *medium well-being.* Following these definitions, approximately 50% of respondents were classified as having medium levels of well-being across the four waves of prior data, about 35% were classified as having high well-being, and about 15% were classified as having low well-being. Consistent with prior findings, these definitional criteria and distributions reflect the skewed distributions of well-being (i.e., people tend to rate themselves positively on the measures).

Moving to *dynamic trajectories,* we further distinguished between respondents who show *stability* in overall well-being across the prior waves (i.e., they maintained statuses of high, medium, or low well-being), from those who showed *improved* well-being (i.e., those who went up from low or medium to medium or high at any subsequent wave), from those who showed *declining* well-being (i.e., those who went down from high or medium to medium or low at

Table 3-2. Mental Health × Physical Health Histories

Physical Health (T_1 - T_4)

Mental Health (T_1 - T_4)	Improving	Stable-High	Stable-Med/Low	Fluctuating	Declining	
Improving	12	15	22		8	57
Stable-High	12	6	10		8	36
Stable-Med/Low	13	7	20		7	47
Fluctuating	5	3	3		2	13
Declining	5	6	16		9	36
	47	37	71		34	189

Resilient   80/189 = .423

Mixed   48/189 = .254

Vulnerable   61/189 = .323

any subsequent wave). These designations are represented in Table 3–2 (note the combining of stable medium and low, due to the low prevalence of low well-being). Also included were respondents who showed *fluctuating* (i.e., going up and down over time) profiles of well-being.

Similar procedures were followed to characterize respondents' physical health profiles across the four waves of prior assessment. Three key indicators were used: chronic conditions, physical symptoms, and recent falls. (These, we acknowledge, address only negative aspects of physical health; further analyses that incorporate positive indicators, such as high functional abilities, positive subjective health, and positive health behaviors, are in progress). About 40% of our respondents reported having at least one chronic condition that interfered

with their activities either moderately or a great deal. Thus, we created a dichotomous variable for *interfering chronic conditions*. Similarly, about 47% of respondents reported having at least one symptom that interfered with their
activities moderately or a great deal. Thus, we created a dichotomous variable
for *interfering symptoms*. At the Time 1 interview, approximately 25% of respondents reported falling at least once in the preceding year. A final dichotomous variable was created for assessing *recent falls*. These three indicators
were then combined into a general trichotomous variable, which was defined as
having low (having all three negative criteria), medium (having one or two
negative criteria), or high (having no negative criteria) physical health status.

The dynamic physical health trajectory is based on patterns of stability or
change from the first and last waves of data collection (data for all indicators
were not available at all four waves). Following the mental health classification,
we distinguished those who showed physical health *stability* (i.e., maintained
high or medium–low status), from those who *improved* (i.e., went up from low or
medium to medium or high), and those who *declined* (i.e., went down from high
or medium to medium or low). Because we were using only two times of
measurement for physical health, fluctuating profiles could not be ascertained.

Table 3–2 summarizes the results of this cross-classification of dynamic
mental and physical health trajectories. We note that these analyses are based on
189 women for whom complete longitudinal data were available (i.e., four
waves). Consistent with our prior formulation, we define as *Resilient* those respondents who have *maintained* high levels of mental or physical health across
time, or have shown *improvement* or *recovery* in either mental or physical
health, or both. We labeled as *Vulnerable* those respondents who showed *decline*
on either mental or physical health through time. A third category of *Mixed*
respondents referred to those who showed either fluctuating mental health
profiles or medium–low stability profiles on either mental or physical health.

Following this classification scheme, approximately 42% of the sample was
classified as Resilient, about 32% as Vulnerable, and 25% as Mixed. These
preliminary analyses thus bespeak the prevalence of positive, improving, or
recovering profiles of health and well-being in a sample of older women confronted with a significant life transition (community relocation) as well as
numerous other co-occurring challenges. Table 3–3 provides the combined data
on dynamic health trajectories with the preceding life event distributions. Specifically, for each cell of the event distribution table, we indicate the number
of respondents who were classified as Resilient, Vulnerable, or Mixed. These
data reveal that all three health groups are present in all cells of the event
distributions, and with frequencies to challenge a solely event-based explanation of positive health and well-being (i.e., the healthy are those with high
prevalence of positive events and low prevalence of negative events). Similarly,
vulnerability is not characterized by high levels of negative events and low levels
of positive events. Positive and negative event distributions do not, in short,
provide explanation for who shows health resilience or vulnerability. To understand how these outcomes come about, it is necessary to look elsewhere. This is

Table 3-3. Distribution of Health Catergories × Cumulative Events

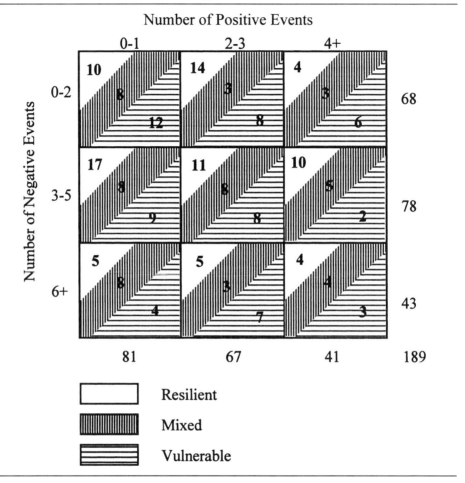

where we turn to the previously described protective factors (sociodemographic, psychological, social, biological) to account for resilience and vulnerability. We next provide a brief summary of the empirical findings compiled thus far on one particular category of protective factors, namely, psychological resources.

Later Life Protective Factors: Interpretive Mechanisms and Coping

Prior publications from the relocation study have documented the influence of particular psychological resources in accounting for improved profiles of well-being over the course of this life transition. Central among these have been *interpretive mechanisms*, which refer to multiple psychosocial processes (e.g., social comparisons, reflected appraisals, behavioral self-perceptions, psychological centrality) through which individuals interpret and give meaning to their life experiences (Ryff & Essex, 1992). These mechanisms were derived from the self-concept literature, and our relocation findings as well as other related studies (Heidrich & Ryff, 1993a, 1993b, 1996) have demonstrated their significance in mediating or moderating the impact of life challenges on psychological well-being.

Focusing on *change* in the premove to postmove period (T_1 to T_2), Kling, Ryff, and Essex (1997) investigated the hypothesis that psychological well-being would be *enhanced* by increasing the importance (centrality) of life domains where respondents saw themselves improving, and, concomitantly, decreasing the importance of domains where they saw themselves declining. Such change would illustrate adaptive shifts in the self-concept. Supportive evidence was obtained in two life domains (health, friends), where gains in psychological well-being were linked with the aforementioned patterns. Other life domains (e.g., economics, family) showed reverse patterns where gains in well-being were associated with giving more importance to areas of perceived decline, possibly reflective of a proactive, problem-focused coping orientation (i.e., giving more attention to areas of difficulty).

Smider, Essex, and Ryff (1996) investigated emotional adaptation to relocation as a function of baseline resources (e.g., premove levels of environmental mastery, autonomy, and personal growth) and contextual aspects of the move itself (e.g., whether the move was voluntary, stressful of the move, experiencing unexpected gains in the move). This study showed that women with greater premove resources were more emotionally resilient (i.e., showed greater happiness and less anger and sadness) in the face of negative contextual factors. However, the emotional "boost" of unexpected gains was greatest for women with lower premove resources.

The impact of coping orientations on changes in psychological well-being was examined in a study (Kling et al., 1997) that contrasted the experience of community relocation with a separate, less normative later life challenge (i.e., caregiving for an adult child with mental retardation). The guiding hypothesis was that women experiencing community relocation,the more normative challenge, would report higher psychological well-being *and* use problem-focused coping more frequently than women with long-term-care responsibilities. As predicted, more positive *changes* in well-being across time were reported by the relocation sample, which also showed more problem-focused coping. Caregiving respondents, however, showed stronger links between coping and well-being, underscoring possible gains in expertise that accompany challenges of lengthy duration.

Other work, currently underway, explores other psychological (e.g., personality traits) as well as sociodemographic (e.g., education levels) and social–relational (e.g., social supports, confidante) resources in illuminating who in the relocation transition is able to maintain high levels of well-being, or even surpass prior levels. The intersection of these protective factors with the previously described biological protective factors (i.e., optimal allostasis, immune competence, cerebral activation asymmetry) in accounting for the respondents' future profiles of health and well-being is the target of future research.

SUMMARY AND FUTURE DIRECTIONS

The purpose of this chapter has been to elevate the place of positive psychological functioning in understanding mental health in later life. We put forth the construct of resilience to illuminate, theoretically and empirically, how some individuals are able to maintain, recover, or improve their health and well-being in the face of cumulative life challenges. Our formulation draws distinctions between resilience as an outcome, and resilience as a process. Central to the latter is a multidisciplinary formulation of protective factors, operative at the sociodemographic, psychological, social, and biological levels, that are believed to explain how resilience comes about. Selective findings from two longitudinal studies, one involving life-history data from high school to midlife, and the other involving a multiwave later life transition, were reviewed to illustrate various features of our formulation of resilience. Much additional work remains to be done to test the separate and interactive influences of the various protective factors in accounting for mental and physical vitality in later life.

We close our chapter with a brief consideration of intervention programs, which we see as a particularly compelling route to advance knowledge of life-course resilience. Of particular interest are those interventions designed to foster key components of psychological well-being (e.g., purpose in life, commitment to goals and pursuits). Examples of such already-occurring interventions include the work of Steven Danish, who conducts a Skills Training Program with adolescents (Danish, 1997; Danish et al., 1992). Known as Going for the Goal (GOAL), this is a school-based program taught by high school students to middle-junior high school students in interactive classroom sessions. Adolescents learn how to (1) identify positive life goals; (2) focus on the process (not the outcome) of goal attainment; (3) use a general problem-solving model; (4) identify health-promoting behaviors that can facilitate goal attainment; (5) identify health-compromising behaviors that can impede goal attainment; (6) seek and create social support; and (7) transfer these skills from one life context to another. Since it was developed in 1987, it has been taught to approximately 15,000 students in over 20 cities nationwide.

At the other end of the life course, old age, where our earlier evidence points to declines in purpose in life and personal growth among the elderly, the need for programs and interventions is perhaps even greater. Here, we point to two naturally occurring interventions that address these exact problems in old age. First, the Center for Creative Retirement in North Carolina (Brown, 1990) illustrates a new approach to fulfillment in later life that revolves around community volunteer work and educational pursuits, both of which are explicit routes toward engendering purpose and continued growth. Second, in the Israeli *kibbutzim*, older individuals maintain a place of importance and purpose in community life and communal responsibility (Leviathan, 1989). Both examples illustrate social initiatives that sustain these vital ingredients to health and well-being into old age.

As such, these interventions constitute powerful contexts within which to track the proposed mechanisms and processes involved in positive mind–body spirals. What, for example, is the profile of allostatic load, immune competence, and cerebral activation asymmetry for individuals participating in such programs? How are these indicators, in turn, linked with physical and mental health outcomes down the road? Pursuit of these questions illustrates what we see as "activist science," that is, the synthesis of health-promoting interventions with scientific investigations designed to track underlying mechanisms as well as distal health outcomes. The central feature of such an enterprise is that questions about physiological substrates of flourishing are framed in the context of specific intervention programs that are designed to enhance aspects of positive mental health.

Seeking to advance health-promoting interventions, we are mindful that they would ultimately be applied to mere mortals who will, at some point, show signs of decline, deterioration, and, finally, die. We are not, therefore, promoting a *Dorian Gray* (Wilde, 1891/1962) model of aging in which the ultimate goal is to maintain vitality, if not youthfulness, at all costs. Rather, the objective is to look carefully at those who, as they age, experience notable quality of life vis-à-vis the problems that come their way. These individuals have much to teach us about the mysteries of positive human health.

ACKNOWLEDGMENTS.   This research was supported by the John D. and Catherine T. MacArthur Foundation Research Network on Successful Midlife Development (Ryff), the Socioeconomic Status and Health Network (Singer), and grants from the National Institute on Aging (R01AG08979, Ryff and Essex; R01AG013613, Ryff and Singer) and National Institute of Health Center for Research Resources to the University of Wisconsin Medical School (M01 RR03186).

REFERENCES

Adler, N. E., Boyce, T., Chesney, M. A., Cohen, S., Folkman, S., Kahn, R .L., & Syme, S. L. (1994). Socioeconomic status and health: The challenge of the gradient. *American Psychologist, 49,* 15–24.

Adler, N. E., & Matthews, K. (1994). Health psychology: Why do some people get sick and some stay well? *Annual Review of Psychology, 45,* 229–259.

Aldwin, C. M. (1991). Does age affect the stress and coping process? Implications of age differences in perceived control. *Journal of Gerontology, 46,* 174–180.

Allport, G. W. (1961). *Pattern and growth in personality.* New York: Holt, Rinehart & Winston.

Baltes, P. B., & Baltes, M. M. (Eds.). (1990). *Successful aging: Perspectives from the behavioral sciences.* New York: Cambridge University Press.

Berkman, L. F., Seeman, T. E., Albert, M. et al. (1993). High, usual and impaired functioning in community-dwelling older men and women: Findings from the MacArthur Foundation Research Network on Successful Aging. *Journal of Clinical Epidemiology, 46,* 1129–1140.

Birren, J. E., & Renner, V. J. (1980). Concepts and issues of mental health and aging. In J. E. Birren &

R. B. Sloane (Eds.), *Handbook of mental health and aging* (pp. 3–33). Englewood Cliffs, NJ: Prentice-Hall.

Block, J. H. (1971). *Lives through time*. Berkeley, CA: Bancroft Books.

Block, J. H., & Block, J. (1980). The role of ego-control and ego-resiliency in the organization of behavior. In W. A. Collins (Ed.), *Development of cognition, affect, and social relations: The Minnesota Symposium on Child Psychology*, (Vol. 13, pp. 39–101). Hillsdale, NJ: Erlbaum.

Bolger, N., & Schilling, E. A. (1991). Personality and the problems of everyday life: The role of neuroticism in exposure and reactivity to daily stressors. *Journal of Personality*, *59*, 355–386.

Bond, L. A., Cutler, S. J., & Grams, A. (Eds.). (1995). *Promoting successful and productive aging*. Thousand Oaks, CA: Sage.

Brown, P. L. (1990, November 29). For some, "retired" is an inaccurate label. *New York Times*, pp. B1–B2.

Buhler, C., & Massarik, F. (Eds.). (1968). *The course of human life*. New York: Springer.

Carver, C. S., Scheier, M. F., & Weintraub, J. K. (1989). Assessing coping strategies: A theoretically based approach. *Journal of Personality and Social Psychology*, *56*, 267–283.

Cohen, S. (1988). Psychosocial models of social support in the etiology of physical disease. *Health Psychology*, *7*, 269–297.

Cohen, S. (1996). Psychological stress, immunity, and upper respiratory infections. *Current Directions in Psychological Science*, *5*, 86–89.

Cohen, S., & Herbert, T. B. (1996). Health psychology: Psychological factors and physical disease from the perspective of human psychoneuroimmunology. *Annual Review of Psychology*, *47*, 113–142.

Cohen, S., & Wills, T. A. (1985). Stress, social support, and the buffering hypothesis. *Psychological Bulletin*, *2*, 310–357.

Cole, J. R., & Singer, B. (1991). A theory of limited differences: Explaining the productivity puzzle in science. In H. Zuckerman, J. R. Cole, & J. T. Bruer (Eds.), *The outer circle: Women in the scientific community* (pp. 277–340). New York: Norton.

Danish, S. J. (1997). Going for the Goal: A life skills program for adolescents. In G. Albeee & T. Gullotta (Eds.), *Prevention works* (pp. 291–312). Newbury Park, CA: Sage.

Danish, S. J., Mash, J. M., Howard, C. W., Curl, S. J., Meyer, A. L., Owens, S., & Kendall, K. (1992). *Going for the Goal Leader Manual*, Department of Psychology, Virginia Commonwealth University, Richmond, VA.

Davidson, R. J. (1992a). Anterior cerebral asymmetry and the nature of emotion. *Brain and Cognition*, *20*, 125–151.

Davidson, R. J. (1992b). Emotion and affective style: Hemispheric substrates. *Psychological Science*, *3*, 39–43.

Davidson, R. J. (1993). Cerebral asymmetry and emotion: Conceptual and methodological conundrums. *Cognition and Emotion*, *7*, 115–138.

Davidson, R. J. (1995). Cerebral asymmetry, emotion and affective style. In R. J. Davidson & K. Hugdahl (Eds.), *Brain asymmetry* (pp. 000–000). Cambridge, MA: MIT Press.

Depue, R. A., & Iacono, W. G. (1989). Neurobehavioral aspects of affective disorders. *Annual Review of Psychology*, *40*, 457–492.

Depue, R. A., Luciana, M., Arbisi, P., Collins, P., & Leon, A. (1994). Dopamine and the structure of personality: Relation of agonist-induced dopamine activity and positive emotionality. *Journal of Personality and Social Psychology*, *67*, 485–498.

Dienstbier, R. A. (1989). Arousal and physiological toughness: Implications for mental and physical health. *Psychological Review*, *96*, 84–100.

Dohrenwend, B. P., Levav, I., & Shrout, P. E. (1992) Socioeconomic status and psychiatric disorders: The causation–selection issue. *Science*, *255*, 946–951.

Erikson, E. (1959). Identity and the life cycle. *Psychological Issues*, *1*, 18–164.

Frankl, V. E. (1992). *Man's search for meaning: An introduction to logotherapy*. Boston, MA: Beacon Press. (Original published 1959)

Garmezy, N. (1991). Resiliency and vulnerability of adverse developmental outcomes associated with poverty. *American Behavioral Scientist*, *34*, 416–430.

Garmezy, N. (1993). Vulnerability and resistance. In D. C. Funder, R. D. Parke, C. Tomlinson-Keasey, & K. Widaman (Eds.), *Studying lives through time: Personality and development* (pp. 377–398). Washington, DC: American Psychological Association.

Garmezy, N., Masten, A. S., & Tellegen, A. (1984). The study of stress and competence in children: A building block for development. *Child Development, 55,* 97–111.

Harris, T., Brown, G. W., & Bifulco, A. (1990). Loss of parent in childhood and adult psychiatric disorder: A tentative overall model. *Development and Psychopathology, 2,* 311–328.

Heady, B., & Wearing, A. (1989). Personality life events, and subjective well-being: Toward a dynamic equilibrium model. *Journal of Personality and Social Psychology, 57,* 731–739.

Heidrich, S. M., & Ryff, C. D. (1993a). The role of social comparison processes in the psychological adaptation of elderly adults. *Journal of Gerontology, 48,* P127–P136.

Heidrich, S. M., & Ryff, C. D. (1993b). Physical and mental health in later life: The self-system as mediator. *Psychology and Aging, 8,* 327–338.

Heidrich, S. M., & Ryff, C. D. (1996). The self in later years of life: Changing perspectives on psychological well-being. In L. Sperry & H. Prosen (Eds.), *Aging in the twenty-first century: A developmental perspective* (pp. 73–102). New York: Garland.

Higgins, G. O. (1994). *Resilient adults: Overcoming a cruel past.* San Francisco: Jossey-Bass.

Hoffmann, P. (1997). The endorphin hypothesis: In W. P. Morgan (Ed.), *Physical activity and mental health* (pp. 163–177). Washington, DC: Taylor & Francis.

Holmes, K. F. (1994). Human ecology and behavior and sexually transmitted bacterial infections. *Proceedings of the National Academy of Sciences, 91,* 2448–2455.

House, J. S., Landis, K. R., & Umberson, D. (1988). Social relationships and health. *Science, 241,* 540–545.

Insel, T. R. (1992). Oxytocin: A neuropeptide for affiliation—evidence from behavioral, receptor autoradiographic, and comparative studies. *Psychoneuroendocrinology, 17,* 3–35.

Jahoda, M. (1958). *Current concepts of positive mental health.* New York: Basic Books.

Jung, C. G. (1933). *Modern man in search of a soul.* New York: Harcourt, Brace & World.

Kang, D. H., Davidson, R. J., Coe, C. I. et al. (1991). Frontal brain asymmetry and immune function. *Behavioral Neuroscience, 105,* 860–869.

Kessler, R. C., & Cleary, P. (1980). Social class and psychological distress. *American Sociological Review, 45,* 463–478.

Kessler, R. C., & Magee, W. J. (1993). Childhood adversities and adult depression: Basic patterns of association in a U.S. national survey. *Psychological Medicine, 23,* 679–690.

Kiecolt-Glaser, J. K., Malarkey, W. B., Cacioppo, J. T., & Glaser, R. (1994). Stressful personal relationships: Immune and endocrine function. In R. Glaser & J. K Kiecolt-Glaser (Eds.), *Handbook of human stress and immunity* (pp. 321–340). San Diego: Academic Press.

Kling, K. C., Ryff, C. D., & Essex, M. J. (1997). Adaptive changes in the self-concept during a life transition. *Personality and Social Psychology Bulletin, 23,* 989–998.

Kling, K. C., Seltzer, M. M., & Ryff, C. D. (1997). Distinctive late life challenges: Implications for coping and well-being. *Psychology and Aging, 12,* 288–295.

Klohnen, E. C. (1996). Conceptual analysis and measurement of the construct of ego-resiliency. *Journal of Personality and Social Psychology, 70,* 1067–1079.

Lazarus, R. S., & Folkman, S. (1984). *Stress, appraisal, and coping.* New York: Springer.

Leviathan, U. (1989). Successful aging: The kibbutz experience. *Journal of Aging and Judaism, 42,* 71–92.

Maier, S. F., Watkins, L. R., & Fleshner, M. (1994). Psychoneuroimmunology: The interface between behavior, brain, and immunity. *American Psychologist, 49,* 1004–1017.

Marmot, M., Ryff, C. D., Bumpass, L. L., Shipley, M., & Marks, N. F. (1997). Social inequalities in health: Converging evidence and next questions. *Social Science and Medicine, 44,* 901–910.

Maslow, A. (1968). *Toward a psychology of being* (2nd ed.). New York: Van Nostrand.

Masten, A. S. (1989). Resilience in development: Implications of the study of successful adaptation for developmental psychopathology. In D. Cicchetti (Ed.), *The emergence of a discipline: Rochester Symposium on Developmental Psychopathology* (Vol. 1, pp. 261–294). Hillsdale, NJ: Erlbaum.

Masten, A. S., & Garmezy, N. (1985). Risk, vulnerability, and protective factors in developmental psychopathology. In B. B. Lahey & A. E. Kazdin (Eds.), *Advances in clinical child psychology* (Vol. 8, pp. 1–52). New York: Plenum Press.

Mathabane, M. (1986). *Kaffir boy*. New York: Penguin.

McEwen, B. S., & Stellar, E. (1993). Stress and the individual. *Archives of Internal Medicine, 153,* 2093–2101.

McLeod, J. D., & Kessler, R. C. (1990). Socioeconomic status differences in vulnerability to undesirable life events. *Journal of Health and Social Behavior, 31,* 162–172.

Melnechuk, T. (1988). Emotions, brain, immunity, and health: A review. In M. Clynes & J. Panksepp (Eds.), *Emotions and psychopathology* (pp. 181–247). New York: Plenum Press.

Menaghan, E. D. (1983). Individual coping efforts: Moderators of the relationship between life stress and mental health outcomes. In H. B. Kaplan (Ed.), *Psychosocial stress: Trends in theory and research* (pp. 157–191). New York: Academic Press.

Merton, R. K. (1968). The Matthew Effect in science. *Science, 159,* 59–63.

Morgan, W. P. (Ed.). (1997). *Physical activity and mental health* (Series in Health Psychology and Behavioral Medicine). Washington, DC: Taylor & Francis.

Neugarten, B. L. (1973). Personality change in late life: A developmental perspective. In C. Eisdorfer & M. P. Lawton (Eds.), *The psychology of adult development and aging*. Washington, DC: American Psychological Association.

Ormel, J., Stewart, R., & Sanderman, R. (1989). Personality as modifier of the life change–distress relationship. *Social Psychiatry and Psychiatric Epidemiology, 24,* 187–195.

Panksepp, J. (1981). Brain opiods—a neurochemical substrate for narcotic and social dependence. In S. Cooper (Ed.), *Theory in psychopharmacology* (pp. 149–175). New York: Academic Press.

Panksepp, J. (1992). Oxytocin effects on emotional processes: Separation distress, social bonding, and relationships to psychiatric disorders. *Annals of the New York Academy of Sciences, 652,* 243–252.

Panksepp, J. (1993). Neurochemical control of moods and emotions: Amino acids to neuropeptides. In M. Lewis & J. M. Haviland (Eds.), *Handbook of emotions* (pp. 87–106). New York: Guildford.

Pearlin, L. I. (1991). The study of coping: An overview of problems and directions. In J. Eckenrode (Ed.), *The social context of coping* (pp. 261–276). New York: Plenum Press.

Pearlin, L. I., & Schooler, C. (1978). The structure of coping. *Journal of Health and Social Behavior, 19,* 2–21.

Pederson, C. A., Caldwell, J. D., & Brooks, P. J. (1990). Neuropeptide control of parental and reproductive behavior. In D. Ganten & D. Pfaff (Eds.), *Current topics in neuroendocrinology: Vol. 10. Behavioral aspects of neuroendocrinology* (pp. 81–113). New York: Springer-Verlag.

Riley, M. W., Kahn, R. L., & Foner, A. (1994). *Age and structural lag*. New York: Wiley.

Robins, R. W., John, O. P., Caspi, A., Moffitt, T. E., & Stouthamer-Loeber, M. (1996). Resilient, overcontrolled, and undercontrolled boys: Three replicable personality types. *Journal of Personality and Social Psychology, 70,* 157–171.

Rogers, C. R. (1961). *On becoming a person*. Boston: Houghton Mifflin.

Ross, C. E., & Wu, C. L. (1996). Education, age, and the cumulative advantage in health. *Journal of Health and Social Behavior, 37,* 104–120.

Rowe, J. W., & Kahn, R. L. (1987). Human aging: Usual and successful. *Science, 237,* 143–149.

Russell, B. (1958). *The conquest of happiness*. New York: Liveright. (Original published 1930)

Rutter, M. (1985). Resilience in the face of adversity: Protective factors and resistance to psychiatric disorder. *British Journal of Psychiatry, 147,* 598–611.

Rutter, M. (1987). Psychosocial resilience and protective mechanisms. *American Journal of Orthopsychiatry, 22,* 323–356.

Rutter, M. (1990). Psychosocial resilience and protective mechanisms. In J. Rolf, A. S. Masten, D. Cicchetti, K. H. Neuchterlein, & S. Weintraub (Eds.), *Risk and protective factors in the development of psychopathology* (pp. 181–214). New York: Cambridge University Press.

Rutter, M., Maughan, N., Mortimore, P., & Ouston, J. (1979). *Fifteen thousand hours: Secondary schools and their effects on children*. Cambridge, MA: Harvard University Press.

Ryff, C. D. (1989). Happiness is everything, or is it? Explorations on the meaning of psychological well-being. *Journal of Personality and Social Psychology, 57,* 1069–1081.

Ryff, C. D. (1991). Possible selves in adulthood and old age: A tale of shifting horizons. *Psychology and Aging, 6,* 386–295.

Ryff, C. D. (1995). Psychological well-being in adult life. *Current Directions in Psychological Science, 4,* 99–104.

Ryff, C. D. (1996). Psychological well-being. In J. E. Birren (Ed.), *Encyclopedia of gerontology: Age, aging, and the aged* (pp. 365–369). San Diego: Academic Press.

Ryff, C. D., & Essex, M. J. (1992). The interpretation of life experience and well-being: The sample case of relocation. *Psychology and Aging, 7,* 507–517.

Ryff, C. D., & Keyes, C. L. M (1995). The structure of psychological well-being revisited. *Journal of Personality and Social Psychology, 69,* 719–727.

Ryff, C. D., & Seltzer, M. M. (Eds.) (1900). *The parental experience in midlife.* Chicago: University of Chicago Press.

Ryff, C. D., & Singer, B. H. (1996). Psychological well-being: Meaning, measurement, and implications for psychotherapy research. *Psychotherapy and Psychosomatics, 65,* 14–23.

Ryff, C. D., & Singer, B. H. (1998). The contours of positive human health. *Psychological Inquiry, 8,* 1–28.

Schulz, R., & Heckhausen, J. (1996). A life span model of successful aging. *American Psychologist, 51,* 702–714.

Seeman, T. E. (1996). Social ties and health: The benefits of social integration. *Annals of Epidemiology, 6,* 442–451.

Seeman, T., Charpentier, P., Berkman, L., Tinetti, M., Guralnik, J., Albert, M., Blazer, D., & Rowe, J. (1994). Predicting changes in physical performance in a high-functioning elderly cohort: Mac-Arthur Studies of Successful Aging. *Journal of Gerontology, 49,* M97–M108.

Seeman, T. E., Singer, B. H., Rowe, J. W., Horwitz, R. I., & McEwen, B. S. (1997). The price of adaptation: Allostatic load and its health consequences: MacArthur Studies of Successful Aging. *Archives of Internal Medicine, 157,* 2259–2268. pSinger, B. H., & Ryff, C. D. (1997). Racial and ethnic inequalities in health: Environmental, psychosocial, and physiological pathways. In B. Devlin, S. E. Feinberg, D. Resnick, & K. Roeder, (Eds.), *Intelligence, genes, and success. Scientists respond to the Bell Curve* (pp. 89–122). New York: Springer-Verlag.

Singer, B. H., Ryff, C. D., & Magee, N. J. (in press). Linking life histories and mental health: A person-centered strategy. In A. Raferty (Ed.), *Sociological methodology.*

Smider, N. A., Essex, M. J., & Ryff, C. D. (1996). Adaptation to community relocation: The interactive influence of psychological researches and contextual factors. *Psychology and Aging, 11,* 362–371.

Solomon, G. F., Fiatarone, M. A., Benton, D., Morley, J. E., Bloom, E., & Makinodan, T. (1987). Psychoimmunologic and endorphin function in the aged. *Annals of the New York Academy of Sciences, 54,* 143–158.

Spiegel, D., Kraemer, H. C., Bloom, T. R., & Gottheil, E. (1989). Effect of psychosocial treatment on survival of patients with metastatic breast cancer. *Lancet, ii,* 888–891.

Staudinger, U. M., Marsiske, M., & Baltes, P. B. (1995). Resilience and reserve capacity in later adulthood: Potentials and limits of development across the life span. In D. Cicchitti & D. J. Cohen (Eds.), *Developmental psychopathology: Vol. 2. Risk, disorder, and adaptation* (pp. 801–847). New York: Wiley.

Sterling, P., & Eyer, J. (1988). Allostasis: A new paradigm to explain arousal pathology. In J. Fisher & J. Reason (Eds.), *Handbook of life stress, cognition, and health* (pp. 629–649). New York: Wiley.

Stone, A. A., Bovbjerg, D. H., Neale, J. M., Napoli, A., Valdimarsdottir, H. et al. (1992). Development of common cold symptoms following experimental rhinovirus infection is related to prior stressful life events. *Behavioral Medicine, 8,* 115–120.

Thoits, P. A. (1994). Stressors and problem-solving: The individual as psychological activist. *Journal of Health and Social Behavior, 35,* 143–159.

Thoits, P. A. (1995). Stress, coping, and social support processes: Where are we? What next? *Journal of Health and Social Behavior,* (Extra Issue), 53–79.

Tomarken, A. J., Davidson, R. J., Wheeler, R. I., & Doss, R. C. (1992). Individual differences in anterior brain asymmetry and fundamental dimensions of emotion. *Journal of Personality and Social Psychology, 62*, 676–687.

Tomarken, A. J., & Davidson, R. J. (1994). Frontal brain activation in repressors and non-repressors. *Journal of Abnormal Psychology, 103*, 339–349.

Turner, R. J., & Lloyd, D. A. (1995). Lifetime traumas and mental health: The significance of cumulative adversity. *Journal of Health and Social Behavior, 36*, 360–376.

Uchino, B. N., Cacioppo, J. T., & Kiecolt-Glaser, J. K. (1996). The relationship between social support and physiological processes: A review with emphasis on underlying mechanisms and implications for health. *Psychological Bulletin, 119*, 488–531.

Uvnäs-Moberg, K. (1997). Physiological and endocrine effects of social contact. *Annals of the New York Academy of Sciences, 287*, 146–163.

Werner, E. E. (1993). Risk, resilience, and recovery: Perspectives from the Kauai Longitudinal Study. *Development and Psychopathology, 5*, 503–515.

Werner, E. E. (1995). Resilience in development. *Current Directions in Psychological Science, 4*, 81–85.

Werner, E. E., & Smith, R. S. (1977). *Kauai's children come of age.* Honolulu University of Hawaii Press.

Werner, E. E., & Smith, R. S. (1992). *Overcoming the odds: High risk children from birth to adulthood.* Ithaca, NY: Cornell University Press.

Wethington, E., & Kessler, R. C. (1986). Perceived support, received support, and adjustment to stressful life events. *Journal of Health and Social Behavior, 27*, 78–89.

Wheaton, B. (1990). Life transitions, role histories and mental health. *American Sociological Review, 55*, 209–223.

Wilde, O. (1962). *The picture of Dorian Gray.* New York: Signet Classics. (Original published 1891)

Wittling, W., & Pfluger, M. (1992). Neuroendocrine hemisphere asymmetries: Salivary cortisol secretion during lateralized viewing of emotion-related and neutral films. In C. Kirschbaum, G. F. Read, & D. H. Hellhammer (Eds.), *Assessment of hormones and drugs in saliva in biobehavioral research* (pp. 129–146). Toronto: Hogrefe & Huber.

Zimmerman, M. A., & Arunkumar, R. (1994). Resiliency research: Implications for schools and policy. *Social Policy Report (Society for Research in Child Development), 8*, 1–17.

PART II

Stress, Coping, and Mental Health

In light of the accumulated research on stress in the various domains of life, the time is ripe to integrate such knowledge in order to comprehend its impact on mental health, aging, and life-course processes (Elder, George, & Shanahan, 1996; Pearlin & Skaff, 1996) so that further research in this area can be carried out under unifying models. Part II proposes conceptualizations covering a broad spectrum of coping with various levels of stress. While all the chapters in this section relate to stress and eventual pathology, they also present the possibilities of constructive coping; hence, they are more like "maturity models" than "loss-deficit models" (Knight, 1992). Gatz (Chapter 4) presents a theory-building scheme anchored in a lifespan developmental perspective and based on three encompassing images of old age, as well as on her elaboration of four propositions essential for a model of aging and mental disorders in the elderly. Psychopathology is viewed as the product of diathesis, constitutional vulnerability, and stress. This model integrates previous models (e.g., the vulnerability–stress model) and constructs (e.g., person–environment fit), sheds light on the concept of depression (see Chapters 21 and 23 by Katz and Mostofsky, respectively) and the age of onset of pathology (see Gutmann, Chapter 12) as well as on the concepts of reserve capacity and optimism in old age (see Chapters 1 and 3 by Shmotkin and Ryff et al., respectively). Gatz's developmental diathesis–stress model incorporates biological vulnerability, stressful life events, and psychological diathesis. This innovative conceptualization integrates research and provides guidance for treatment and prevention.

The promotion of theory in gerontology could benefit from the "gerontolization" of other relevant models, presently not part of the discipline of gerontology. This is the approach adopted by Hobfoll and Wells (Chapter 5) in applying "conservation of resources" (COR) theory to an understanding of stress and coping in later life and integrating COR theory with a developmental multidimensional conceptualization of adaptation to long-term stress (Lomranz, 1990). COR theory tries to predict how both gains and losses will affect older adults. It emphasizes the primacy of resource loss, suggesting that the loss of an object or condition is more potent than its seemingly equivalent gain, since loss threatens survival, and gain only brings pleasure. In elaborating the development of "resources caravans" in later life, the authors emphasize the integrative impact of trajectories of stress. The model helps us to better understand the joint impact of development, stress, and the social–historical context on coping and adjustment, as well the changes that may occur in the nature of the resources themselves along a lifetime (see Ryff et al. and Gatz, Chapters 1 and 3, respectively). It also provides a further understanding of the impact of social support, family resources, developmental transitions and tasks, and the journey of resource caravans.

The number of elderly victims of extreme stress is, unfortunately, increasing. Our century has witnessed the greatest of world wars; moreover, large-scale traumatic events and threats to life, property, or security continue to occur in communities throughout the world. Thus, it becomes important to view the elderly in a community perspective, as part of a community that has experienced severe stress (Hobfoll & de Vries, 1995), and to endeavor to comprehend reactions to stress and the long-term impact of stress on aging. Furthermore, while approaches that purported to "understand the healthy through understanding the sick" have come under much criticism, we should avoid throwing the baby out with the bath water and bear in mind the merits of studying the implications of pathology on health. It is with these in mind that we approach the last two chapters in this section.

Solomon and Ginzburg (Chapter 6) shed light on the relationship between trauma and aging. On the basis of the Israeli experience, they demonstrate how aging affects adjustment to current trauma, as well as how trauma experienced in earlier developmental stages affects adjustment to aging (Hobfoll & Wells, Chapter 5). They reveal that when the elderly find themselves under stress that affects the entire community (e.g., missiles falling during the Gulf War), they function adequately and do not differ in affect or coping strategies, unlike the situations in which they are characterized as a group of "aged," while their younger counterparts play an active role in the war (e.g., fighting at the front). As for the millions who suffer from trauma in their youth and encounter it again in their old age, it seems they are more vulnerable, respond with higher distress, and experience a reawakening of the earlier traumas.

Relating lifelong stressors to physical and mental well-being and adaptation to old age, while highlighting the importance of negative life events and trauma at various stages on the life course, Kahana and Kahana (Chapter 7) integrate some of the cogent issues in stress research as they present their temporal–spatial model of cumulative life stress. The model recognizes both the impact of temporal (e.g., timing of onset, duration of impact, age specificity) and spatial dimensions of stressors (e.g., type of stress, protective resources, magnitude of impact) on late life well-being. Their work takes into account cumulative life stress (see Chapter 5 by Hobfoll & Wells) as well as recent life events; it spans community-based general populations as well as those who have endured extreme trauma (see Chapter 6 by Solomon & Ginzburg). Their model promotes our understanding of this area by integrating cogent themes in gerontology with stress research.

REFERENCES

Elder, G., George, L., & Shanahan, M. (1996). Psychological stress over the life course. In H. Kaplan (Ed.), *Psychological stress* (pp. 247–292). New York: Academic Press.

Hobfoll, S., & de Vries, M. (1995). *Extreme stress and communities: Impact and intervention.* Boston: Kluwer Academic.

Knight, B. (1992). *Older adults in psychotherapy: Case histories.* Newbury Park, CA: Sage.

Lomranz, J. (1990). Long-term adaptation to traumatic stress in light of adult development and aging perspectives. In M. P. Stephens, J. Crowther, S. H. Hobfoll, & D. Tennenbaum (Eds.), *Stress and coping in later-life families* (pp. 99– 121). Washington, DC: Hemisphere.

Pearlin, L., & Skaff, M. (1996). Stress and the life course. *Gerontologist, 36*(2), 239–247.

CHAPTER 4

Toward a Developmentally Informed Theory of Mental Disorder in Older Adults

Margaret Gatz

BACKGROUND AND CONTEXT

> A theory is an attempt to explain.... Explicit theory-building is crucial to research, and especially to intervention.
>
> Bengtson (1995)

This chapter represents an exercise in theory building, setting out propositions that are essential for a model of mental disorder in older adults. The intent is to provide a framework that will be useful to research and practice through implications for etiology, course, treatment, and prevention.

The initial elements required for any theory in clinical psychology are a model of person and a model of change. These are derived from a lifespan perspective on development. A lifespan developmental perspective has been the dominant theoretical force within psychology for describing adult development and aging, from Baltes and Schaie (1973) and Riegel (1976) to Baltes and Baltes (1990) and Baltes (1993). The major features of a lifespan developmental perspective are summarized in this chapter.

There have been some past attempts to infer from lifespan developmental concepts to prevention and treatment (e.g., Baltes & Danish, 1979; Nolen-Hoeksema, 1988; Smyer, 1987; Staudinger, Marsiske, & Baltes, 1995). However, there has not been systematic extension in the form of explicit propositions

Margaret Gatz • Department of Psychology, University of Southern California, Los Angeles, California 90089-1061.

Handbook of Aging and Mental Health: An Integrative Approach, edited by Jacob Lomranz. Plenum Press, New York, 1998.

about aging and psychopathology. This chapter presents a beginning effort in this respect.

In addition to a lifespan developmental perspective, this undertaking reflects the widely held view that psychopathology is a product of both diathesis (or constitutional vulnerability) and stress (Davison & Neale, 1996). This diathesis–stress viewpoint has much in common with quantitative genetics, which holds that behavior is the product of both genes and environment (Plomin, DeFries, & McClearn, 1990), and with biosocial models of deviance (e.g., Raine, Brennan, & Farrington, 1997).

A diathesis–stress viewpoint has rarely been extended developmentally, although some researchers have begun to argue for a developmental approach to psychopathology (e.g., Asarnow & Goldstein, 1986; Cicchetti, 1993; Kazdin & Kagan, 1994, whose focus is children and adolescents; Gatz, Kasl-Godley, & Karel, 1996, whose focus is older adults).

Several further points are germane to the propositions about mental disorder and aging offered in this chapter. In this theory-building exercise, influences on developmental outcomes are themselves regarded developmentally; that is, vulnerabilities and stressors each have their own developmental trajectories. Additionally, physical illness and chronic conditions—customarily subsumed by gerontologists among other losses and stressful life events that occur in old age—are taken to represent age-related change in physiological function.

The theoretical framework offered in this chapter blends three images of old age and mental health that are evident in everyday thinking on this topic. One image could be called "genetic legacy." The key element in this picture is that in old age, whatever one has inherited from one's parents reveals itself. Indeed, many people express the fear of ending up with precisely those diseases that they witnessed in their parents, from colon cancer to Alzheimer's disease.

A second image might be called "environmental insults." Here, the diseases of old age are seen as the net result of accumulated stress and abuse of a lifetime, as the manifestation of unique insults associated with old age, or perhaps as both of these. A traditional gerontological joke goes, "If I'd known I was going to live this long, I'd have taken better care of myself." The other version of the environmental insults image is captured by the belief that, what with all the ailments, losses, and other indignities inflicted on an older person, depression is virtually inevitable.

A third, everyday image might be called "maturity." Here, the governing opinion is that wisdom and a sense of balance accrue over one's lifetime. Hence, with aging, one might actually become better able to weather the vicissitudes dealt by life. Traces of these images are apparent in the sections that follow.

LIFESPAN DEVELOPMENTAL PERSPECTIVE

Five concepts are essential to a lifespan developmental perspective. These draw chiefly on Baltes (1987); they also reflect the influence of other theorists, including Riegel (1976) and Neugarten (1977), but are not directly adopted from any one source (see Gatz, 1989; Gatz, Harris, & Turk-Charles, 1995; Gatz, Pearson, & Fuentes, 1984).

1. *Identity*. It is the same person who passes through the lifespan, exhibiting intraindividual change, moving to different life stages, and maintaining a sense of continuity. Indeed, it is common for gerontologists to comment that, as people age, they become more and more like themselves.

2. *Cohort*. One is born, matures, and ages within a given historical period or generation. Age and cohort are inextricably linked; thus, it is difficult to isolate what aspects of a person are traceable to age per se, and what to the historical and cultural cohort into which the person was born. This concept increases in complexity for those who move from one culture to another, each with its distinct sociopolitical and historical context, or for ethnic minorities who live in two cultures—majority and minority. These people may rightly be regarded as having multiple cohorts.*

3. *Multiple interaction*. There are multiple interrelated sources of influence on change, including normative influences, both biological and social, and nonnormative influences (Baltes, Reese, & Lipsitt, 1980). Development is multidirectional, consisting of both gains and losses. Finally, development is multidimensional, and there can be intraindividual differences across dimensions as well as over time.

4. *Diversity*. Older adults are heterogeneous, and variability in development is observed between individuals. The fact that there are interindividual differences within age groups means that performance distributions for different age groups overlap considerably. What is true on average about differences between young and old may not be true for a particular older adult compared to a particular younger adult, nor may it correctly represent a particular older adult's performance now compared to him- or herself at a younger age.

5. *Agency*. It is fundamental to the model of person that the individual is viewed as having an active role in his or her own development, managing various changes, making choices, and creating meaning. The person is not simply the passive recipient of events and influences.

More recently, Baltes has proposed a framework of seven propositions to describe the nature of human aging (Baltes, 1991, 1993; Baltes & Baltes, 1990; Staudinger et al., 1995). These build on his previous writings about the lifespan developmental perspective (e.g., Baltes, 1987; Baltes & Danish, 1979).

The first proposition asserts the concept of heterogeneity, specifically, that the course of aging shows a great deal of interindividual variability. The second proposition indicates the need to distinguish among normal, optimal, and pathological aging. The third proposition is key, propounding the view that in old age, there is considerable developmental reserve capacity. The emphasis is on the extent to which older adults are capable of new learning, called plasticity. Developmental reserve capacity can be thought of as the upper and lower limits of development. In general, range of plasticity decreases with age. Reserve capacity is discussed elsewhere in gerontology as representing homeostatic reserves on which the individual may draw at times of stress in order to bring the

---

*The author thanks Jacob Lomranz for urging consideration of multiple historical contexts.

system back into equilibrium. Furthermore, physically or cognitively frail individuals, that is, those with reduced reserves, may temporarily or permanently be pushed across a threshold into functional impairment under conditions of physiological or psychological stress (Fries, 1989; Mortimer, 1994). Similarly, Baltes and Baltes (1990) opine that losses become visible under demanding performance conditions when the demand meets or exceeds the available reserve.

The fourth and fifth propositions describe those areas of cognitive functioning that show decline with aging, namely, "fluid mechanics" (i.e., intellectual abilities that relate to processing information, such as speed and memory strategies), and those areas that do not, namely, "knowledge and cognitive pragmatics." The latter can therefore be used to offset losses in the former. The sixth proposition indicates that with aging, the tradeoff between gains and losses becomes less favorable.

Finally, the seventh proposition asserts the resiliency of the individual in confronting these changes. Resilience refers to the processes by which the individual adapts when confronted by losses, decrements, and other stressful circumstances. Baltes and Baltes (1990) describe those processes in terms of *selective optimization with compensation*. Older adults whose capacity to cope is taxed or exceeded by the demands of the environmental context can elect to reduce the number of domains to be managed, selecting those where they feel most competent, or to adjust their expectations through comparing themselves with others. Coping effectively entails compensation, such as writing things down to reduce reliance on one's memory, or using social support to make up for aging-related losses (Dixon, 1995; Staudinger et al., 1995). In the interpersonal domain, Carstensen (1992) has described a process similar to selective optimization, whereby older adults reduce the number of relationships to be maintained, focusing on those that are most important. Lastly, Schulz and Heckhausen (1996) have expanded the principles of managing diversity, selectivity, and compensation into a life-course model of successful development that emphasizes the role of primary and secondary control strategies.

Lifespan concepts and propositions about the nature of aging give form to a model of person and a model of change relevant to mental health. However, they are not explicit about the nature of psychopathology or possibilities for intervention in older adults. The propositions presented in the following section take these lifespan developmental principles into account in suggesting elements that are necessary for a clinical psychology of later life.

A FRAMEWORK OF PROPOSITIONS
ABOUT AGING AND MENTAL DISORDER

Four propositions are offered as an additional frame of reference for organizing central issues concerning psychopathology and aging. This propositions are not limited to older adults, but their emphases reflect points of consensus and controversy from clinicians and researchers in aging.

Developmental Diathesis–Stress Model

A variety of diatheses, stressors, and protective factors determine whether an individual will show mental disorder in later life. Each diathesis, stressor, and protective factor has a developmental trajectory. These trajectories have different forms (e.g., linear increase, linear decreases, nonlinear change).

The vulnerability–stress model, first applied to the etiology of schizophrenia (Zubin & Spring, 1977), specifies that psychopathology is a product of vulnerabilities (genetic propensities or acquired biological liabilities) and stressors (negative life events, such as loss of a parent, or chronic stressful situations, such as unemployment). Vulnerability and stress both contribute to occurrence of disorder. The model has been extended; for example, with respect to schizophrenia in adolescence and early adulthood, three central constructs have been proposed: vulnerability factors, stressful environmental stimuli, and protective factors (social support, intelligence, and healthy patterns of family interaction) (Asarnow & Goldstein, 1986). In other interpretations, diatheses extend to include attributional styles (Spangler, Simons, Monroe, & Thase, 1993) and personality modes (Coyne & Whiffen, 1995) as risks for depression. As well, expanding on the idea of person–environment fit (Lawton & Nahemow, 1973), the stress dimension can be seen as encompassing psychosocial stressors, prejudice, physical barriers, and harmful environmental exposures. Protective factors explain why someone who might otherwise be expected to be at risk for a disorder does not develop the disorder (Garmezy, 1993).

None of these dimensions are without controversy. Much current literature overinvests in biological explanations. The role of life stress in contributing to mental disorder is not straightforward. And protective factors can be problematic to measure, seemingly representing the positive pole of risk factors (e.g., high eduction is protective, whereas low education is a risk factor). However, it makes sense to organize influences in terms of these dimensions. Finally, it must be specified that diatheses, stressors, and protective factors may be interactive as well as simply additive; for example, a stressful situation may make long-standing deficits in interpersonal skills more consequential, or protective factors may only play a role under conditions of vulnerability.

As already noted, there are also obvious parallels between a vulnerability–stress model and a quantitative genetic model that seeks to learn the relative contribution of genetic influences and environmental influences on the appearance of a disorder, and that considers the possibility of gene–environment correlations and interactions (see also Rende & Plomin, 1992). Making this connection compels broadening the idea of stress to encompass a wide range of environmental factors, not simply life events.

Gatz et al. (1996) suggested extending these notions to a lifespan developmental diathesis–stress perspective, applicable to disorders including depression, anxiety disorders, schizophrenia and paranoid disorders, personality disorders, and dementia. Nolen-Hoeksema (1988) proffered that a lifespan perspective, if applied to depression, would lead to three questions: (1) whether the causes of depression are similar from one age group to another, (2) how differences in rates of depression between age groups should be explained, and (3) whether experiences at one stage of life affect vulnerability to depression at other stages of life.

The developmental diathesis–stress model expands on the first of these questions by suggesting that the causes of disorder can usefully be organized in terms of diatheses and stressors. With respect to answering the second question, the developmental diathesis–stress model posits that the way to account for age differences not only in rate of disorder, but also in etiology and phenomenology, is by considering age and cohort differences in diathesis, stress, and protective factors. The pivotal detail is that developmental changes across different life stages are incorporated not only for the target disorder, but also for influences on the disorder.

Examples of developmental changes in diatheses and stressors are readily available. Aging is associated with changes in neurotransmitter functioning that could be relevant to cognitive and emotional symptoms. Genetic influences can also change during development, with genes turning on or turning off at different ages (Pedersen, 1996). Several types of Alzheimer's disease associated with identified gene mutations can appear in middle to old age with no indication earlier in life.

Aging is associated with changes in the likelihood of certain stressful life events (e.g., bereavement). Considering stress developmentally, however, must go beyond cataloging frequencies of events by age. It also incorporates the developmental source of people's interpretations of transitions and events that they are undergoing (Gutmann, Chapter 12, this volume); that is, the accumulation of experiences over time shapes people's reaction to the present. Temporal context is further invoked by several observations: events themselves have a duration; events often are interpreted in terms of whether they are "on time" or "off time"; and perceptions are affected by awareness of how near one is to the probable end of one's lifespan (Neugarten & Hagestad, 1976). In these ways, replying to Nolen-Hoeksema's (1988) third question, experiences at one life stage do affect both vulnerability and resilience to disorder at later ages.

Different elements of the model may interact over time. For example, stressors earlier in the individual's development, such as loss of a parent or experiencing extreme trauma, may alter biological or psychological vulnerability to other events later in life, such that susceptibility is increased (see Lomranz, 1995).* In addition, some types of depression are characterized by co-occurrence of a hopelessness attributional style and a negative event (Spangler et al., 1993). Stated in quantitative genetic terms, diathesis and stress show gene–

---

*Hobfoll's conservation of resources theory (Hobfoll & Wells, Chapter 5, this volume) offers an integrative framework that organizes what is known about stress in later life, including interactions with attributional style and social context. This chapter will not duplicate the extensive review provided by those authors.

environment correlation. In one demonstration of interaction between vulner-abilities and stressors, data from adult twin pairs were used to determine that, while across the entire sample there was some temporary elevation in depressive symptoms after a stressful event, the effect was magnified for those with a genetic propensity (Kendler, Neale, Heath, Kessler, & Eaves, 1995). Cognitive diathesis may also have an influence on what events will actually be encountered in a person's life (Monroe & Simons, 1991). This phenomenon is further substantiated by quantitative genetic results indicating genetic influence for life events (Plomin, Lichtenstein, Pedersen, McClearn, & Nesselroade, 1990).

Diathesis–stress interactions have been reported for dementia as well. For example, relationship between smoking history and Alzheimer's disease was modified by whether or not there was an identified genetic vulnerability (either family history of dementia or presence of an ∊4 allele of the apolipoprotein E gene) (Van Duijn, Havekes, Van Broeckhoven, Knijff, & Hofman, 1995).

Protective factors that increase with age have been suggested to include ego integrity, use of more mature coping styles or defense mechanisms, and wisdom, defined as expertise in the human condition and the course of life (Baltes, 1991; Kivnik, 1993; Vaillant, 1977). Wisdom might be considered as a particular sort of cognitive pragmatics pertaining to self-knowledge (Staudinger et al., 1995). Self-knowledge includes less dependence on expectations of others, with behavior increasingly motivated by one's own attitudes and feelings (see Reifman, Klein, & Murphy, 1989). Betty Friedan (1993) quotes an 80-year old friend of hers: "I'm more and more myself. But I'm more comfortable with differences, not uptight about them. I suppose along the way I got a larger vision, somehow ... I'm not envious of anybody else and I'm not anguished about my own failures" (p. 572).*

The increase in these protective factors answers a paradox posed by Knight (1992): "As a clinician, the question I most often find myself asking about [older] clients is, 'Why aren't they more depressed?' ... With the accumulation of clinical experience, my conclusion has grown stronger over the years that older adults are, in fact, more mature than younger adults (myself included) in some significant ways" (p. 186).†

Summarizing these various ideas, a depiction of a developmental diathesis–stress model from Gatz et al. (1996) is reproduced as Figure 4–1. It illustrates for depressive symptoms how biological and psychological diatheses and stressful life events might change with age. It provides a rubric for examining sources of depressive symptoms across the lifespan and accounting for differences in rates of depression. Tentative trajectories for each influence are drawn, based on available literature. The frequency and importance of stressful life events is shown as curvilinear. Biological vulnerability is depicted as accelerating with age (primarily reflecting the association of depression with chronic illness). Psychological vulnerability is portrayed as decreasing with age as a consequence of improved wisdom and knowledge of one's own abilities and limits. Thus, protective factors are indirectly reflected through the decline in psychological

---

*Reprinted with the permission of Simon & Schuster, copyright © 1993 by Betty Friedan.
†Copyright © 1992 by Sage Publications. Reprinted by permission of Sage Publications.

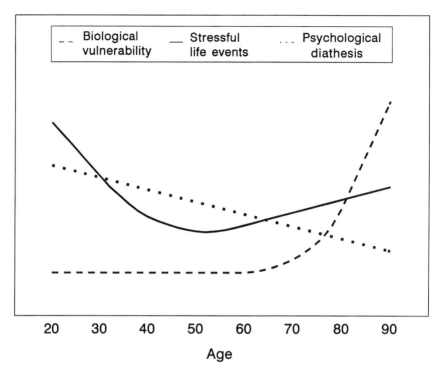

Figure 4–1. Depiction of developmental changes in the magnitude of influence on depressive symptomatology exerted by biological vulnerability (dashed line), psychological diathesis (dotted line), and stressful life events (solid line). From Gatz et al. (1996). Reprinted with the permission of Academic Press.

vulnerability. The combined area under these curves at different ages should correspond to the prevalence of depressive symptoms at those ages.

The diagram in Figure 4–1 is a schematic, with the curves intended to reflect what is currently known. There have been two empirical studies relevant to testing the model. Mirowsky and Ross (1992) tested the influence of decreased survival among the most disadvantaged individuals, increased physical dysfunction with age, erosion of personal control, and changes in social status over the life cycle (i.e., gains and losses of marital partners, employment, and income) in accounting for age group differences in symptoms of depression. Blazer, Burchett, Service, and George (1991) controlled for biological factors and stressful life events that are correlated with age: chronic illness, physical disability, reduced income, and loss of close relatives. Both groups found that the covariates could largely explain cross-sectional age differences in depressive symptoms. In addition, Mirowsky and Ross (1992) inferred an underlying benefit of increased maturity to explain why average levels of depression were not more responsive to accelerating declines and losses. Next, the developmental diathesis–stress model needs to be expanded beyond depression, with further operationalization and empirical testing of diatheses, stressors, and protective factors.

Age of Onset

The etiology of disorder will differ according to age of onset. To a large extent, there will be continuities such that disorders in old age will have a history from younger ages, while disorders seemingly occurring first in old age will often have an identifiable physiological element in their etiology.

A critical consideration, emphasized by Kahn (1977), is the distinction between mental disorder that occurs for the first time in old age and mental disorder that had its first onset in younger adulthood and has continued as a chronic or episodically recurring mental illness into old age. Kahn referred to the former as true geriatric mental illness. Even before Kahn, Abraham (1919/1953) urged that the age of the patient not be confused with the duration and history of the problem, suggesting that the latter was more informative in determining treatment and prognosis. Gatz et al. (1996) recommended expanding Kahn's two types into three categories: (1) those who had the disorder earlier in life and experience a continuation or reappearance; (2) those with some difficulty earlier in life, such as dysfunctional ways of coping with stress, that only becomes sufficiently problematic later in life to result in mental disorder; and (3) those who experience disorder for the first time in old age. An example of the second category would be someone with mild borderline characteristics who presents him- or herself for treatment for the first time at age 60, complaining of depression. From the point of view of completeness, note that there can also be older adults who had a disorder earlier in life but do not show evidence of any disturbance in old age, and that many people never exhibit disorder at any age.

Along with other writers in gerontology, Baltes and Baltes (1980) distinguish normal, optimal (or successful), and pathological aging. Subsequent interest lies chiefly in identifying the features of successful aging (e.g., Schulz & Heckhausen, 1996). Implicit to the propositions in this chapter is the applicability of the same concepts across the spectrum of aging individuals, although recognizing that different factors may have different weights when accounting for pathological aging. Especially in the instance of true geriatric mental illness, it is relevant to bear in mind that the individual had successfully developed through earlier life stages, including acquisition of abilities of selection and compensation.

New disorder in older life is most prototypically exemplified by dementia of the Alzheimer's type, which is exceedingly rare at younger ages. For other disorders, rates are lower in older adults than in younger adults, suggesting both that there may be a secular trend toward more disorder among those adults who are now younger than 65, and that there is no upsurge of mental disorder upon reaching old age (Regier et al., 1988).

Furthermore, there is some evidence to imply that those who show schizophrenia or depression in old age, with no prior history of disorder, often have a neurobiological explanation for disease onset. For example, Kinzie, Lewinsohn, Maricle, and Teri (1986) determined that only 8% of depressed older adults had no contribution from physical illness or medication. Steingart and Herrmann (1991) obtained support for the hypothesis that depression occurring for the first time in old age more often was apparently associated with occult neurological impairment or brain atrophy.

In exploring genetic and environmental influences on symptoms of depression in a sample of twins, we (Gatz, Pedersen, Plomin, Nesselroade, & McClearn, 1992) found that heritability was greatest for somatic symptoms and psychomotor retardation, and that these effects were most pronounced for the older half of the sample (aged 62 and above). The influence of shared rearing environment was substantially larger than is usually found in quantitative genetic studies of personality traits and temperament, and was stronger in young than in old, with its most marked influence on depressed mood. This result is consistent with the suggestion that traumatic events shared by children (such as divorce of their parents) may influence depression in adult life, or—more likely—that parents may inadvertently or deliberately teach offspring ways of interpreting the world that make their offspring more or less vulnerable to depression later in life. Nonshared influences, in other words, nonnormative influences or stressful life events, were the most important component of all in accounting for individual differences in depressive symptoms.

The findings for somatic symptoms and psychomotor retardation lead to a hypothesis that in older adults, genetic influences, conceivably represented by a latent variable such as "fatigue," account for the depressive symptoms and explain the correlation between depressive symptoms and medical illness.

Reserve Capacity

The appearance of disorder depends in part on reserve capacity. Individuals with greater reserve can suffer greater loss without showing disorder, while individuals whose daily life is closer to the limits of their reserve are in greater jeopardy of being stressed beyond that threshold.

The notion of reserve capacity comes from the idea that essentially all organs show an age-related decline in maximum performance, with ability to maintain homeostasis becoming diminished as the reserve capacity decreases. Sufficient depletion of reserve will result in the appearance of chronic disease (Fries, 1983). Similarly, as the brain ages, there is normally occurring neuron loss that may result in the depletion of reserve capacity or alterations in neurotransmitter availability.

Mortimer (1995) describes how this perspective gives new insight into the etiology of dementia, arguing that dementia is the net result of a lifetime of growth and degeneration of the brain—that the sum of brain development during childhood and damage resulting from a variety of insults over the life course determines whether and when a critical threshold of functioning brain tissue is reached at which an individual is no longer capable of normal intellectual performance and fulfills criteria for the diagnosis of dementia. (pp. 132–133)*

People start life with different degrees of brain reserve capacity. Decline can be gradual or abrupt (e.g., stroke), and a clinical brain disease such as Alzheimer's disease can accelerate neuronal loss.

For Baltes (1993) and associates, reserve capacity also is predominantly a cognitive concept, although the knowledge systems encompass not only intelligence but also everyday competence and social problem solving, expert knowledge (typing, music, sports, clinical psychology, law), and self-knowledge. The focus of much of the research from this group has been the use of training to activate the reserves. While baseline reserve capacity gradually decreases with age, developmental reserve capacity—assessed by a "testing the limits" procedure—can be increased with training. Additionally, their findings confirm the greater magnitude of cognitive reserve for cognitively normal older adults in contrast to those with dementia (Baltes, Kühl, & Sowarka, 1992).

The concept of reserve capacity may also be applicable to affect. Regulation of emotions can be considered as a kind of pragmatics or expert knowledge. Given biological decrements and social losses, this emotional expertise serves as a protective factor (Staudinger et al., 1995).

On this basis, for purposes of setting out a theory of mental disorder in older adults, the concept of affective reserve is proposed, analogous to the better established but still hypothetical construct of cognitive reserve. Affective reserve, like cognitive reserve, would be characterized by considerable plasticity, conferred by various protective factors. Conversely, depletion of affective reserve such that an individual is brought near a critical threshold would provide an explanation for depression.

An important feature of depression in older adults is that it is closely related to physical health. Katz (Chapter 21, this volume) emphasizes that medical illness and disease-related changes in the brain are implicated in the pathogenesis of late-onset depression, and, in turn, that depressive disorder can have an amplifying effect on medical conditions. It is well established that prevalence rates of depressive disorder are notably elevated for older adults in medical settings (e.g., Reifler, 1994). Katz (Chapter 21, this volume) summarizes the evidence demonstrating that this elevation is more than just a reaction to the stress of illness, and that the fatigability and related symptoms are part of a comorbid reverberating process.

The concept of affective reserve capacity provides a construct to mark the common process that is involved. A quantitative genetic model reflecting this hypothesis is shown in Figure 4–2. This is a bivariate model, where the questions of interest are the extent to which the correlation between depressive

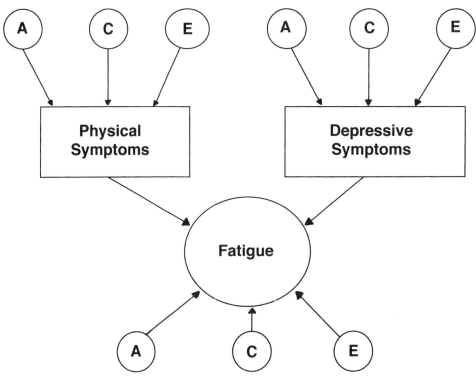

Figure 4–2. Quantitative genetic model indicating how fatigue may serve as affective reserve. *Note*: A = variance attributable to additive genetic effects; C = variance attributable to shared [correlated] environmental influences; E = variance attributable to nonshared environmental, or nonnormative, influences.

symptoms and medical illness reflects a common genetic or environmental etiology, and whether the effects of these genetic and environmental factors are mediated through a common underlying phenotype (Eaves, Eysenck, & Martin, 1989). Here, the common underlying phenotype is hypothesized to be fatigue. Fatigue denotes lowered affective reserve, which both manifests itself in depressive symptoms and explains the correlations between depressive symptoms and medical illness. By extension, affective reserve offers a way to understand depressive side effects often documented to follow from certain illnesses or medications, for instance, hypertensive medication. Specifically, the medication may reduce affective reserve rather than acting directly to cause depression.* The conceptualization portrayed in the figure now requires empirical refinement and evaluation.

*The author thanks Ira Katz for this example.

Optimism

Subjective attributions about one's psychological well-being may be either pessimistic or optimistic. Optimism is the more adaptive attribution.

Clinical observation suggests that very old individuals not infrequently are characterized by an unusual degree of optimism, almost to the extent of seeming naive. This clinical observation has an empirical basis in the relationship between optimism and physical health. Specifically, optimism is related to immune functioning (data summarized by Seligman, 1991), and optimists tend to have superior health habits (Scheier & Carver, 1992).

Psychology research groups that have concerned themselves with optimism have not been particularly interested in aging. Nonetheless, their definitions and conclusions converge on a number of key points that bear on the place of optimism in a series of propositions concerning mental health and aging. Here, optimism is regarded as a protective factor.

Scheier and Carver (1992) define optimism as a positive orientation to life, in which one generally believes that one will experience good outcomes. Optimists and pessimists have characteristic coping styles, with optimists using active, planful, problem-focused strategies as well as positive reinterpretation (i.e., making the best of a rotten situation), and pessimists using denial or disengagement from goals. A sense of personal agency ("When I make plans, I can make them work") is one source of optimism, in combination with a trusting attitude (perceiving that one's environment is not hostile and that there are people available who can and will provide help if needed). Optimism is similar to, but not the same as, self-esteem, sense of personal mastery, or positive affectivity, while pessimism is distinguished from depression, neuroticism, or negative affectivity.

In Seligman's (1991) view, optimism is the belief that one's actions will matter. Optimism is an explanatory style that (1) sees the causes of good events as permanent (e.g., due to traits or abilities) but the causes of bad events as temporary, (2) generalizes from good events but not from bad, and (3) "blames" the self for good events but not for bad. In contrast, depressives see negative events as due to stable and global causes. In both definitions, optimism emphasizes choice. Longitudinally, there is a high correlation in individuals over time for their explanatory style for negative events. However, there is relatively little consistency in explanatory style for positive events (Burns & Seligman, 1989).

Pessimism is a risk factor for depression. Optimism may actually represent something of a cognitive distortion, although clearly one with beneficial consequences. Compared to nondepressed optimists, depressed people are more accurate judges of their own social skills and better at admitting to both their failures and their successes (Lewinsohn, Mischel, Chaplin, & Barton, 1980).

Considerable literature in aging has concerned itself with self-rated health and with other subjective judgments such as age identification. In gerontology, paralleling the aforementioned findings with respect to optimism, it appears that both judging one's health to be "excellent" or "good" rather than "fair" or "poor," and judging one's age to be "middle-aged" rather than "old" are predictive of more positive psychological and physical outcomes (see Mossey, 1995). Particularly intriguing is that self-rated health is strongly predictive of longevity. The mechanism is not fully understood; however, it seems possible that those people who report more optimistic self-ratings of their health may be responding on the basis of self-knowledge that is not completely accessible to others, or that positive feelings are protective through a psychoneuroimmunological pathway (Leedham, Meyerowitz, Muirhead, & Frist, 1995).

Thus, optimism appears to represent a key dimension of adaptation for older adults, as for adults of other ages. Heidrich and Ryff (1993) have demonstrated that social comparison processes are an important means by which the self-system works to help older individuals maintain positive psychological well-being despite having poor physical health status. Social comparison entails both deriving inspiration from those perceived as better off than oneself and finding comfort in realizing that others are worse off than oneself.

An enduring issue in gerontological literature is combating myths about old age, for example, that old age equates with loss of memory, sexlessness, non-productivity, and powerlessness (Butler, 1985). At the same time, a great deal of gerontological research does concern cognitive decline or diseases of old age. The danger of negative stereotypes is that they can become internalized and lead to lowered self-esteem and aspirations (Kuypers & Bengtson, 1973). Yet, as Baltes and Baltes (1990) have emphasized, aging is comprised of both negative and positive changes, with the balance between gains and losses becoming less positive with age. Thus, overidealized stereotypes, or "countermyths" signified by advertisements of presumably elderly persons with gray hair but unlined faces and unnaturally lean and athletic bodies, may be no more factual than the myths (Gatz et al., 1984).

Optimism provides a means to reconcile myth and countermyth. Research on optimism and self-rated health would argue that countermyth is generally the better choice. As Heidrich and Ryff (1993) note, the outcome of social comparison is what is important. Therefore, if the countermyth provides inspiration and positive role models, then it will serve self-esteem. Only if the countermyth results in unfavorable social comparisons will it work against psychological well-being. Indeed, myths might often be equated with depressive realism.

Myth and countermyth have parallels in overestimation and underestimation of mental disorder. Overestimation leads to pathologizing normal responses to common difficulties of everyday life. Underestimation means that a disorder may be misconstrued as normal rather than as pathological. In the area of dementia, Adelman (1995) has described the "Alzheimerization of aging." A campaign against this disease, including overestimation in the form of characterizing Alzheimer's disease as an epidemic (Robertson, 1990), has brought more funding. The tradeoff is that other aspects of normal aging may receive less research attention. At the individual level, overestimation is manifested in the tendency to assume that any mental lapse in an older person is diagnostic of Alzheimer's disease.

Underestimation and overestimation pertain as well to controversies about the frequency of depression in later life. Warnings about the problem of under-diagnosis (e.g., Friedhoff, 1994) are far more common than warnings about overdiagnosis. Underdiagnosis is customarily inferred from the discrepancy between community surveys showing high rates of depressive symptoms among older adults in contrast to low rates of depression according to diagnostic criteria. Not meeting diagnostic criteria has been explained by older adults' special reluctance to endorse symptoms of sadness or loss of interest or pleasure in things (e.g., Gallo, Anthony, & Muthén, 1994; Nolen-Hoeksema, 1988), which are the filter questions in the diagnostic interview schedule. However, the phenomenon of scoring above the cutoff on a self-report depression scale, while not meeting diagnostic criteria for major depressive disorder, is also highly characteristic of adolescents (Gotlib, Lewinsohn, & Seeley, 1995), making the argument somewhat less persuasive.

Although speculative, findings about positive bias in subjective judgments could be extended to depression. From this point of view, understating symp-toms of depression represents an optimistic subjective self-rating. These older adults may exemplify an optimistic explanatory style, for example, recognizing impediments in their lives, but viewing the causes as temporary, not pervasive, and not their fault. Perhaps it would be more realistic to be depressed, but it is more adaptive not to be.

Binstock (1994) has further highlighted the problem of overdiagnosis, or at least of overmedicalization, by pointing out how much easier it is for the society to prescribe pills for an older person who is understandably discouraged due to his or her life circumstances than to help that person obtain relevant supports. Notice that medication tacitly confirms that the cause is permanent and internal, and that the cure is external; in contrast, focusing on situational factors and practical solutions conveys that the cause is temporary and external. Drugs reinforce a depressive explanatory style; changing the environment urges a more optimistic explanatory style.

The value of an optimistic explanatory style for older adults in the face of life stress holds parallels to the shift from primary to secondary control proposed by Schulz and Heckhausen (1996) as occurring in conjunction with an increas-ingly unfavorable tradeoff between gains and losses. Primary control empha-sizes changing one's environment, whereas secondary control entails changing cognitions, such as valuing what is attainable rather than what is not, and making causal attributions that protect the self. Schulz and Heckhausen see the balancing of primary and secondary control as instantiating selection and com-pensation.*

CONCLUSION AND SIGNIFICANCE

This exercise in theory building has suggested four propositions that pro-vide a framework for mental health in later life. These propositions (summarized

*See also Perlmuter and Eads, Chapter 2, this volume.

Table 4-1. Psychopathology and Aging: Four Propositions

1. There are a variety of diatheses, stressors, and protective factors that determine whether an individual will show mental disorder in later life. Each diathesis, stressor, and protective factor has a developmental trajectory. These trajectories have different forms (e.g., linear increase, linear decrease, nonlinear change).
2. The etiology of disorder will differ according to age of onset. To a large extent, there will be continuities such that disorders in old age will have a history from younger ages, while disorders seemingly occurring first in old age will often have an identifiable physiological element in their etiology.
3. The appearance of disorder depends in part on reserve capacity. Individuals with greater reserve can suffer greater loss without showing disorder, while individuals whose daily lives are closer to the limits of their reserves are in greater jeopardy of being stressed beyond that threshold.
4. Subjective attributions about one's psychological well-being may be either overpessimistic or overoptimistic. Optimism is the more adaptive.

in Table 4–1), and the conceptual scheme in which they are embedded, provide guidance with respect to prevention, treatment, and maintenance.

A lifespan developmental perspective contributes the model of person and model of change. Especially relevant is the notion of resilience, in particular, the process of selective optimization with compensation. This concept can be applied in preventive intervention and in psychotherapy. To date, implications for intervention based on selective optimization with compensation have been tested chiefly for cognition (e.g., Baltes, 1991). However, extension to other domains and to psychotherapeutic intervention are suggested by Carstensen's (1992) socioemotional selectivity theory. Thus, a therapist might encourage clients toward less rather than more activity, selecting those commitments that are most central or most enjoyable, and focusing on them (Knight, 1992).

The lifespan perspective is complemented by diathesis–stress theories of psychopathology and analytic models from quantitative genetics. The lead proposition argues for considering the developmental trajectory of each influence in order to understand the developmental course of mental disorder. A developmental perspective makes evident ways in which early intervention has the possibility to prevent later disorder. In addition, the different dimensions—biological and psychological vulnerability factors, psychosocial and environmental stressors, and protective factors—denote different possible points for intervention. These include teaching an optimistic attributional style, supplying environmental aids to enable more independent functioning, and using life experiences—pragmatics—to confront present stressors.

Knight (1992) has contrasted a "loss–deficit model" and a "maturity model" for psychotherapy with older adults. The loss–deficit model, which has been the dominant approach in the psychotherapeutic literature, emphasizes helping the older client adjust to and grieve for the losses that accompany aging. In the maturity model, the focus of treatment is using the life experiences and maturity of older adults to cope with present problems and prepare for those in the future.

Another lifespan developmental construct, reserve capacity, has important preventive implications. Preventing depletion of cognitive reserve, or enhancing reserve earlier in life, can delay or prevent an individual from reaching a critical threshold of cognitive decline (Mortimer, 1995). Just as cognitive reserve helps to explain the etiology of dementia, a construct such as affective reserve would help to account for depression and associated phenomena.

Despite an underlying loss of reserve with age, much reserve can remain latent (Baltes, 1991). Additionally, whether one is aging normally, optimally, or pathologically, it seems likely that optimism is a factor in allowing maximal use of reserve capacity, in that optimism includes a belief in personal agency and the possibility of change (see Seligman, 1991).

In summary, these propositions about aging and mental health, and the conceptual scheme in which they are embedded, direct attention to (1) a developmental perspective on diathesis, stress, and protective factors, including their interactions and correlations over time; (2) the importance of age of onset for etiology and treatment; (3) affective reserve, as a construct parallel to cognitive reserve, to describe both an older individual's latent potential and the fragility of functioning near a critical threshold; and (4) the adaptive qualities of optimism.

ACKNOWLEDGMENTS.   The author thanks Beth Meyerowitz for comments on an earlier draft of this chapter, as well as the participants in the Herczeg Institute First International Forum at Kibbutz Shefayim. Their critique during the discussion of this chapter is reflected in the postconference revision. Finally, the assistance of the Computing Support Center at State University of New York, Plattsburgh, is greatly appreciated.

REFERENCES

Abraham, K. (1953). The applicability of psychoanalytic treatment to patients at an advanced age. In S. Steury & M. L. Blank (Eds.), *Readings in psychotherapy with older people* (pp. 18–20). Washington, DC: U.S. Department of Health, Education, and Welfare. (Original published 1919).

Adelman, R. C. (1995). The Alzheimerization of aging. *Gerontologist, 35,* 526–532.

Asarnow, J. R., & Goldstein, M. J. (1986). Schizophrenia during adolescence and early adulthood: A developmental perspective on risk research. *Clinical Psychology Review, 6,* 211–235.

Baltes, M. M., Kühl, K.-P., & Sowarka, D. (1992). Testing for limits of cognitive reserve capacity: A promising strategy for early diagnosis of dementia? *Journal of Gerontology: Psychological Sciences, 47,* P165–P167.

Baltes, P. B. (1987). Theoretical propositions of life-span developmental psychology: On the dynamics between growth and decline. *Developmental Psychology, 23,* 611–623.

Baltes, P. B. (1991). The many faces of human aging: Toward a psychological culture of old age. *Psychological Medicine, 21,* 837–854.

Baltes, P. B. (1993). The aging mind: Potential and limits. *Gerontologist, 33,* 580–594.

Baltes, P. B., & Baltes, M. M. (1990). Psychological perspectives on successful aging: The model of selective optimization with compensation. In P. B. Baltes & M. M. Baltes (Eds.), *Successful aging: Perspectives from the behavioral sciences* (pp. 1–34). New York: Cambridge University Press.

Baltes, P. B., & Danish, S. J. (1979). Intervention in life-span development and aging: Issues and concepts. In R. R. Turner & H. W. Reese (Eds.), *Life-span developmental psychology: Intervention* (pp. 44–78). New York: Academic Press.

Baltes, P. B., Reese, H. W., & Lipsitt, L. P. (1980). Life-span developmental psychology. *Annual Review of Psychology, 31*, 65–110.

Baltes, P. B., & Schaie, K. W. (1973). On life-span developmental research paradigms: Retrospects and prospects. In P. Baltes & K. W. Schaie (Eds.), *Lifespan developmental psychology: Personality and socialization* (pp. 366–395). New York: Academic Press.

Bengtson, V. L. (1995, September). *Theories and models in social gerontology.* Talk delivered as part of the Multidisciplinary Colloquium Series in Gerontology, Andrus Gerontology Center, University of Southern California, Los Angeles.

Binstock, R. H. (1994). Depression, biomedical ethics and health policy. *Gerontologist, 34* [Special Issue], 291.

Burns, M., & Seligman, M. E. P. (1989). Explanatory style across the life-span: Evidence for stability over 52 years. *Journal of Personality and Social Psychology, 56*, 471–477.

Butler, R. N. (1985). Health, productivity, and aging: An overview. In R. N. Butler & H. P. Gleason (Eds.), *Productive aging: Enhancing vitality in later life* (pp. 1–13). New York: Springer.

Carstensen, L. L. (1992). Social and emotional patterns in adulthood: Support for socioemotional selectivity theory. *Psychology and Aging, 7*, 331–338.

Cicchetti, D. (1993). Developmental psychopathology: Reactions, reflections, projections. *Developmental Review, 13*, 471–502.

Coyne, J. C., & Whiffen, V. E. (1995). Issues in personality as diatheses for depression: The case for sociotropy–dependency and autonomy–self-criticism. *Psychological Bulletin, 118*, 358–378.

Davison, G. C., & Neale, J. M. (1996). *Abnormal psychology* (6th ed.). New York: Wiley.

Dixon, R. A. (1995). Promoting competence through compensation. In L. A. Bond, S. J. Cutler, & A. Grams (Eds.), *Promoting successful and productive aging* (pp. 220–238). Newbury Park, CA: Sage.

Eaves, L. J., Eysenck, H. J., & Martin, N. G. (1989). *Genes, culture, and personality: An empirical approach.* London: Academic Press.

Friedan, B. (1993). *The fountain of age.* New York: Simon & Schuster.

Friedhoff, A. J. (1994). Consensus development conference statement: Diagnosis and treatment of depression in late life. In L. S. Schneider, C. F. Reynolds, III, B. C. Lebowitz, & A. J. Friedhoff (Eds.), *Diagnosis and treatment of depression in late life* (pp. 493–511). Washington, DC: American Psychiatric Press.

Fries, J. F. (1983). The compression of morbidity. *Milbank Quarterly, 61*, 397–419.

Fries, J. F. (1989). The compression of morbidity: Near or far? *Milbank Quarterly, 67*, 208–232.

Gallo, J. J., Anthony, J. C., & Muthén, B. O. (1994). Age differences in the symptoms of depression: A latent trait analysis. *Journal of Gerontology: Psychological Sciences, 49*, P251–P264.

Garmezy, N. (1995). Children in poverty: Resilience despite risk. *Psychiatry: Interpersonal and Biological Processes, 56*, 127–136.

Gatz, M. (1989). Clinical psychology and aging. In M. Storandt & G. R. VandenBos (Eds.), *The adult years: Continuity and change* (pp. 79–114). Washington, DC: American Psychological Association.

Gatz, M., Harris, J., & Turk-Charles, S. (1995). Older women and health. In A. L. Stanton & S. J. Gallant (Eds.), *Psychology of women's health: Progress and challenges in research and application* (pp. 491–529). Washington, DC: American Psychological Association.

Gatz, M., Kasl-Godley, J. E., & Karel, M. J. (1996). Aging and mental disorders. In J. E. Birren & K. W. Schaie (Eds.), *Handbook of the psychology of aging* (4th ed., pp. 367–382). San Diego: Academic Press.

Gatz, M., Pearson, C., & Fuentes, M. (1984). Older women and mental health. In A. U. Rickel, M. Gerrard, & I. Iscoe (Eds.), *Social and psychological problems of women: Prevention and crisis intervention* (pp. 273–299). New York: Hemisphere/McGraw-Hill.

Gatz, M., Pedersen, N. L., Plomin, R., Nesselroade, J. R., & McClearn, G. E. (1992). The importance of shared genes and shared environments for symptoms of depression in older adults. *Journal of Abnormal Psychology, 101*, 701–708.

Gotlib, I. H., Lewinsohn, P. M., & Seeley, J. R. (1995). Symptoms versus a diagnosis of depression: Differences in psychosocial functioning. *Journal of Consulting and Clinical Psychology, 63*, 90–100.

Heidrich, S. M., & Ryff, C. D. (1993). Physical and mental health in later life: The self-system as mediator. *Psychology and Aging*, *8*, 327–338.

Kahn, R. L. (1977). Perspectives in the evaluation of psychological mental health problems for the aged. In W. D. Gentry (Ed.), *Geropsychology: A model of training and clinical service* (pp. 9–19). Cambridge, MA: Ballinger.

Kazdin, A. E., & Kagan, J. (1994). Models of dysfunction in developmental psychopathology. *Clinical Psychology: Science and Practice*, *1*, 35–52.

Kendler, K. S., Neale, M. C., Heath, A. C., Kessler, R. C., & Eaves, L. J. (1995, June). *Studies of major depression and anxiety disorders in female twins from the Virginia Twin Registry*. In K. S. Kendler (Chair), Psychiatric Genetics, symposium conducted at the meeting of the 8th International Congress on Twin Studies, Richmond, VA.

Kinzie, J. D., Lewinsohn, P., Maricle, R., & Teri, L. (1986). The relationship of depression to medical illness in an older community population. *Comprehensive Psychiatry*, *27*, 241–246.

Kivnik, H. Q. (1993). Everyday mental health: A guide to assessing life strengths. *Generations*, *17*, 13–20.

Knight, B. G. (1992). *Older adults in psychotherapy: Case histories*. Newbury Park, CA: Sage.

Kuypers, J. A., & Bengtson, V. L. (1973). Social breakdown and competence. *Human Development*, *16*, 181–201.

Lawton, M. P., & Nahemow, L. (1973). Ecology and the aging process. In C. Eisdorfer & M. P. Lawton (Eds.), *The psychology of adult development and aging* (pp. 619–674). Washington, DC: American Psychological Association.

Leedham, B., Meyerowitz, B. E., Muirhead, J., & Frist, W. H. (1995). Positive expectations predict health after heart transplantation. *Health Psychology*, *14*, 74–79.

Lewinsohn, P., Mischel, W., Chaplin, W., & Barton, R. (1980). Social competence and depression: The role of illusory self-perceptions. *Journal of Abnormal Psychology*, *89*, 203–212.

Lomranz, J. (1995). Endurance and living: Long-term effects of the Holocaust. In S. E. Hobfoll & M. W. deVries (Eds.), *Extreme stress and communities: Impact and intervention* (pp. 325–352). Dordrecht, The Netherlands: Kluwer.

Mirowsky, J., & Ross, C. E. (1992). Age and depression. *Journal of Health and Social Behavior*, *33*, 187–205.

Monroe, S. M., & Simons, A. D. (1991). Diathesis–stress theories in the context of life stress research: Implications for depressive disorders. *Psychological Bulletin*, *110*, 406–425.

Mortimer, J. A. (1994). What are the risk factors for dementia? In F. Huppert, C. Brayne, & D. O'Connor (Eds.), *Dementia and normal aging* (pp. 208–229). Cambridge, UK: Cambridge University Press.

Mortimer, J. A. (1995). Prospects for prevention of dementia and associated impairments. In L. A. Bond, S. J. Cutler, & A. Grams (Eds.), *Promoting successful and productive aging* (pp. 131–147). Newbury Park, CA: Sage.

Mossey, J. M. (1995). Importance of self-perceptions for health status among older persons. In M. Gatz (Ed.), *Emerging issues in mental health and aging* (pp. 124–162). Washington, DC: American Psychological Association.

Neugarten, B. L. (1977). Personality and aging. In J. E. Birren & K. W. Schaie (Eds.), *Handbook of the psychology of aging* (pp. 626–649). New York: Van Nostrand Reinhold.

Neugarten, B. L., & Hagestad, G. O. (1976). Age and the life course. In R. H. Binstock & E. Shanas (Eds.), *Handbook of aging and the social sciences* (pp. 35–55). New York: Van Nostrand Reinhold.

Nolen-Hoeksema, S. (1988). Life-span views on depression. In P. B. Baltes, D. L. Featherman, & R. M. Herner (Eds.), *Lifespan development and behavior* (Vol. 9, pp. 203–241). Hillsdale, NJ: Erlbaum.

Pedersen, N. L. (1996). Gerontological behavior genetics. In J. E. Birren & K. W. Schaie (Eds.), *Handbook of the psychology of aging* (4th ed., pp. 59–77). San Diego: Academic Press.

Plomin, R., DeFries, J., & McClearn, J. (1990). *Behavioral genetics: A primer*. San Francisco: W. H. Freeman.

Plomin, R., Lichtenstein, P., Pedersen, N. L., McClearn, G. E., & Nesselroade, J. R. (1990). Genetic influence on life events during the last half of the life span. *Psychology and Aging*, *5*, 25–30.

Raine, A., Brennan, P., & Farrington, D. (1997). Biosocial bases of violence: Conceptual and theoretical issues. In A. Raine, P. Brennan, D. P. Farrington, & S. A. Mednick (Eds.), *Biosocial bases of violence* (pp. 1–20). New York: Plenum Press.

Regier, D. A., Boyd, J. H., Burke, J. D., Rae, D. S., Myers, J. K., Kramer, M., Robins, L. N., George, L. K., Karno, M., & Locke, B. Z. (1988). One-month prevalence of mental disorders in the United States. *Archives of General Psychiatry, 45,* 977–986.

Reifler, B. V. (1994). Depression: Diagnosis and comorbidity. In L. S. Schneider, C. F. Reynolds, III, B. D. Lebowitz, & A. J. Friedhoff (Eds.), *Diagnosis and treatment of depression in late life* (pp. 55–59). Washington, DC: American Psychiatric Press.

Reifman, A., Klein, J. G., & Murphy, S. T. (1989). Self-monitoring and age. *Psychology and Aging, 4,* 245–246.

Rende, R., & Plomin, R. (1992). Diathesis–stress models of psychopathology: A quantitative genetic perspective. *Applied and Preventive Psychology, 1,* 177–182.

Riegel, K. F. (1976). The dialectics of human development. *American Psychologist, 31,* 688–700.

Robertson, A. (1990). The politics of Alzheimer's disease: A case study in apocalyptic demography. *International Journal of Health Services, 20,* 429–442.

Scheier, M. F., & Carver, C. S. (1992). Effects of optimism on psychological and physical well-being: Theoretical overview and empirical update. *Cognitive Therapy and Research, 16,* 201–228.

Schulz, R., & Heckhausen, J. (1996). A life span model of successful aging. *American Psychologist, 51,* 702–714.

Seligman, M. E. P. (1991). *Learned optimism.* New York: Knopf.

Smyer, M. A. (1987). Life transitions and aging: Implications for counseling older adults. *Counseling Psychologist, 12,* 17–28.

Spangler, D. L., Simons, A. D., Monroe, S. M., & Thase, M. E. (1993). Evaluating the hopelessness model of depression: Diathesis–stress and symptom components. *Journal of Abnormal Psychology, 102,* 592–600.

Staudinger, U. M., Marsiske, M., & Baltes, P. B. (1995). Resilience and reserve capacity in later adulthood: Potentials and limits of development across the life span. In D. Cicchetti & D. J. Cohen (Eds.), *Developmental Psychopathology: Vol. 2. Risk, disorder, and adaptation* (pp. 801–847). New York: Wiley.

Steingart, A., & Herrmann, N. (1991). Major depressive disorder in the elderly: The relationship between age of onset and cognitive impairment. *International Journal of Geriatric Psychiatry, 6,* 593–598.

Vaillant, G. E. (1977). *Adaptation to life.* Boston: Little, Brown.

van Duijn, C. M., Havekes, L. M., Van Broeckhoven, C., de Knijff, P., & Hofman, A. (1995). Apolipoprotein E genotype and association between smoking and early onset Alzheimer's disease. *British Medical Journal, 310,* 627–631.

Zubin, J., & Spring, B. (1977). Vulnerability: A new view of schizophrenia. *Journal of Abnormal Psychology, 86,* 103–126.

CHAPTER 5

Conservation of Resources, Stress, and Aging

Why Do Some Slide and Some Spring?

STEVAN E. HOBFOLL AND JENNIFER D. WELLS

Conceptions of later adulthood have often portrayed a picture of the frail elderly, spiraling toward loneliness and loss (Lerner & Gignac, 1992). Furthermore, later life has generally been conceptualized as separate from earlier adult life in some qualitative manner, such that once you were young then you became middle aged, and then one day you were old, the proverbial riddle of the Sphinx. This chapter suggests that rather than a distinct developmental phase, later life is influenced by the caravan of resources that the person has obtained, protected, or lost throughout earlier life. This caravan is shaped by the lifetime experiences of the individual, the context of the family, and the framework of society for older adults. Who among us looks back at our earlier life and says, "That was a different person?" Rather, we see ourselves as having continuity with that earlier self. Our change is incremental. Yet, at the same time, we must acknowledge that changes do occur, and that these cumulatively affect us. So too, at any age, illness and death profoundly affect us and those around us, and as these changes are more prevalent with age, the caravan may move faster in our later years.

When examining stress in later life, typically, the changes associated with this stage are conceived of as a series of losses (Labouvie-Vief, 1985; Rosow, 1974). Health and cognitive abilities deteriorate, loved ones pass on or move away, and our social roles dwindle as we lose our roles at work and within the now grown families, whose members are the new heads of their own families. This viewpoint ignores the potential gains in resources that come with later life. Economic freedom and increased leisure time, allowing people to explore new

STEVAN E. HOBFOLL AND JENNIFER D. WELLS • Applied Psychology Center, Department of Psychology, Kent State University, Kent, Ohio 44242.

Handbook of Aging and Mental Health: An Integrative Approach, edited by Jacob Lomranz. Plenum Press, New York, 1998.

part-time careers or volunteer in areas that have long interested them, are also frequent occurrences in later life. Medical advances have translated to good health for older individuals and allow for an enjoyment of these gains. Many older adults travel extensively and are socially more active than at any earlier time in their lives. In addition, freedom from child rearing and from the structured 8-hour workday that characterized midlife may also translate to a release from some of the most stressful roles in life (Harris, 1990).

The increased longevity in Western nations, coupled with a large portion of the population now in their forties and fifties, presages a change in attitudes toward the elderly both in terms of how older adults are regarded, and how positively they regard themselves. At the turn of this century, only 40% of individuals could expect to live beyond 65 years of age, whereas today, greater than 70% of individuals live beyond this age. Furthermore, the number of old old (85 and older) in America has increased by 50% in each decade since 1940 (Rosenwaike, 1985). With greater numbers comes greater voice in politics, larger influence as consumers, and a more integrated role within families that continue to depend on parents for economic support. These changes may, in turn, result in an increased sense of power and agency. One wonders if the elderly will achieve the esteemed status afforded to them in some non-Western cultures (e.g., filial piety in East Asian cultures; see Sung, 1995), but meaningful changes in this regard are already occurring and will, we think, accelerate.

This chapter focuses on how conservation of resources theory (COR) might aid our prediction of how both gains and losses will affect older adults. Stress is inevitable in life, and late adulthood certainly has many special attributes that involve the stress experience. We will analyze people's resource caravan on both the individual and broader societal levels and suggest possible avenues for future research, theory, and social policy formation.

CONSERVATION OF RESOURCES (COR) THEORY

Basic Concepts

Conservation of resources (COR) theory (Hobfoll, 1988, 1989, 1998) is a general stress theory that may have special implications for an understanding of stress and coping in later life. In this section, we explicate COR theory in order to show how it might inform conceptualizations of stress as people age.

COR theory begins with the assumption that *individuals strive to obtain, retain, and protect that which they value.* This basic assumption is depicted as transcending culture, age, and environment; that is, it is seen as a universal human motivation (Hobfoll & Lilly, 1993; Hobfoll, Lilly, & Jackson, 1991). These things that individuals value are termed resources. In one sense, there is an endless list of resources people value, but we have concentrated on what we might call primary, shared resources. These are the resources that tend to hold wide acceptance as being important to people (Hobfoll, 1998).

There are a number of ways to divide resources, and one method that we have found helpful is to categorize them into four groups: (1) objects, (2) conditions, (3) personal characteristics, and (4) energies. Among these, we have resources that are valued for themselves, such as health, and other resources that are only valued as a means of obtaining intrinsically valued resources, such as health insurance.

Object resources are physical in nature. Objects are resources to the extent they aid in survival (e.g., shelter, transportation) or have acquired value due to a combination of demand and scarcity (e.g., diamonds). As Maslow (1968) theorized, meeting survival needs is a basic step in building well-being. Although more superficial, enormous energy is also expended toward acquiring objects that have no such utility, other than the prestige or pleasure factor in owning them. Our investigations to date suggest that people strongly rate necessity resources higher than luxury resources (Hobfoll et al., 1991). However, although more highly rated, once necessity resources are acquired, inordinate and even ultimately harmful emphasis is often placed on acquiring luxury resources. An example of this is working to the point of ignoring family to pay for a luxury home or car. People's ratings of resources and their behavior appears to be highly incongruent in such cases, but their behavior indicates the emphasis that is often placed on acquiring objects.

Conditions provide access to other elements of survival and can influence opportunities for obtaining love, status, and object resources. Conditions are resources to the extent that they confer status or make other resources available. Conditions include a good marriage, a valued role at work, and tenure. In later life, the circumstances of retirement, which include having health insurance, whether one's spouse is alive and healthy, and the status of the family (e.g., intact, dispersed) are important condition resources. Unlike other resources, we have noted that condition resources are usually acquired over the long term, but may, on the other hand, be quickly lost. For example, it may take decades to acquire a certain job status, with no quicker route available, but layoffs may end that status in the time it takes to write and receive a company memorandum. How condition resources are shaped to match the changing demands of pre and postretirement life may be a critical area for study (Riley, Kahn, & Foner, 1994).

Personal resources include personal attributes (e.g., mastery, self-esteem) and skills (e.g., having a profession or trade). Personal resources shape how people frame their experiences. This framing has been seen almost solely in a cognitive light, but COR theory suggests that those high in personal resources can cognitively frame their experiences positively, because of the actual utility of their resources. Their optimism, for example, is based on the abilities and skills that contributed to their very sense of mastery and optimism. Indeed, optimism, where these underlying actual skills and attributes are lacking, is likely to lead to failure and a plummeting of resources.

Energy resources are resources to the extent they provide access to other resources and, as such, they have no intrinsic value. Included in this category are knowledge, money, credit, and insurance. For older individuals, some energy resources may lose their value with people's changing roles. For example, child-care knowledge may have little utility after children leave the nest. For a person given a role as grandparent, in contrast, such a resource may have continued value and be a principal source of self-esteem. The role structure of the older adult's life will determine the extent to which such resources have continued value. Other resources, such as money and credit, will have ongoing value, but often change in terms of their replaceability following retirement.

Psychological stress is depicted within COR theory as occurring when resources in any of these categories are (1) lost, (2) threatened, or (3) invested without consequent, expected resource gain in turn. Acute stress conditions tend to create a more immediate and rapid threat or loss of resources. Chronic stressors, even of moderate intensity, chip away at people's resource reservoirs. All of us are at risk of these challenges to our resources. However, the elderly may have more difficulty replenishing resources (see Baltes, 1987, 1997). For example, as life goes on, many social resources are lost to death and social mobility such that the potential cadre of long-term relationships inevitably dwindles as people's own parents, old friends, and older relatives die or become infirm. Older individuals, however, have also gained valuable experience in the effective use of resources, and they may be able to apply this knowledge to limit resource loss and enhance resource gains.

In order to obtain, retain, and protect resources, COR theory suggests that other resources are put into service. Sometimes the same resource is used to preserve itself. For instance, individuals may call on social support to help preserve threat to their social ties, or they may rely on self-esteem to bolster themselves when their self-esteem is threatened, say, with retirement. At other times, one resource is used to bolster another resource. For example, individuals may call on social support to bolster self-esteem, in an instance when self-esteem is threatened.

Schönpflug (1985) instructs us to be mindful that resource investment itself results in threat or loss of resources. We cannot combat stress without incurring the costs of arming our defense (see also Baltes, 1987, 1997). For example, finances may need to be used and favors may need to be called in. In other situations, resources are not necessarily lost in combating stress, but they are risked. For example, a widow may place her sense of mastery on the line when having to take over family finances. A failure at this task may indeed result in loss of some of that sense of mastery, but success may also bolster mastery.

Schönpflug's insights are critical on two counts. First, they emphasize that people with greater resource reservoirs are more likely to be able to invest or risk their resources. A good example of this is provided by Lieberman (Chapter 16, this volume). Citing findings from his research program, he suggests that "healthy" families caring for an older adult with Alzheimer's disease are more likely than unhealthy families to rely on their own resource base rather than external resources (e.g., outside services). Second, Schönpflug's proposition indicates that people may be cautious in their attempts to manage stress because they fear that the very acts of coping may have more dire loss consequences than the stress challenge. Accepting that an elderly parent needs extensive nursing care may result in a decision no longer to struggle with the daily challenges of home caregiving, which required ongoing taxing of their resources. Hence, even though placing their parent in a nursing home is very stressful, it may require less ongoing resource loss in service of coping with home care (Aneshensel, Pearlin, & Schuler, 1993).

Distinguishing COR Theory from Other Stress Theories. It is instructive at this juncture to compare COR theory with other stress theories. First, although COR theory contains a cognitive component, idiographic appraisal is less emphasized in COR theory than in other stress theories (Lazarus & Folkman, 1984). COR theory posits that individuals do evaluate their resources, losses, and gain, but this personal evaluation is viewed as a product of more or less objective factors. Even the very resources that we have studied have been found to be reducible to a list of some 74 resources that hold shared value across people and cultures (Hobfoll, Lilly, & Jackson, 1991). Second, COR theory suggests that people act to obtain, retain, and protect their resources even when current stress is low. This places the stress and coping process in the realm of everyday life. When we purchase insurance, we pay a premium for its value in that it may offset future financial or health crises. When we invest in relationships, we do so not only for their intrinsic value, but also because we do not wish to someday be alone and unloved.

The objective nature of resource challenges is particularly poignant in an understanding of aging. There is little evidence that cognitive changes are responsible for the changing nature of stress in people's later life. Dementia, if it does occur, tends to occur very late in life and does not characterize the lives of most older adults. Instead, it is the more common changes that occur such as retirement, children growing and leaving the nest, economic security or insecurity, health status of self and loved ones, and increasingly, caring for an extreme aged parent (age 85 and over) that affect the conditions of people's lives at this stage (Thorson, 1995).

The Primacy of Resource Loss

COR theory also suggests that loss and gain are not equivalent. Loss of the same object or condition is more potent than its seemingly equivalent gain. Research by Tversky and Kahneman (1981) suggests that this bias may be a basic cognitive framework. We have argued that its basis lies in the fact that loss is more likely to threaten survival. In an evolutionary sense, people were often at the edge of survival, such that loss was intolerable. Gain, in contrast, is valued to the extent that it prevents or offsets loss, or to the extent that it brings pleasure. Pleasure, however, has no survival value. From this perspective, gain takes on meaning in the context of loss, and we have found that gains actually increase under loss conditions as resources are mobilized to combat stress (Hobfoll & Lilly, 1993). For older adults, this may be a critical point, because their survival is more easily threatened due to health, economic, and social threats. Also, if older adults enter a more generative, prosocial developmental phase (Aldwin,

1990), they can develop increased concerns for risk of resource loss to their children and grandchildren, not just to themselves.

Because (1) resource loss is more potent than gain, (2) stress follows from resource loss, and (3) people must utilize resources to cope with resource loss or threat of loss, people's resource reservoirs become depleted after a period of loss or threat. With their resources more depleted, those experiencing stress are increasingly likely to encounter loss cycles (Baltes, 1987, 1997). At each turn of the cycle, they are less likely to have either a strong resource or the appropriate resource to offset the next demand (Baltes, 1997; Diener & Fujita, 1995; Thoits, 1995). This results in loss cycles of increasing momentum and potency. Gatz (Chapter 4, this volume) discusses the concept of "reserve capacity" as it relates to mental disorder in the elderly. Consistent with COR predictions, she suggests that persons high in reserve can withstand greater loss without demonstrating disorder compared to persons with depleted reserve, who will more likely show disorder at an earlier juncture in the coping process.

Of course, gain cycles will also occur. When individuals gain in resources, they are more likely to have additional resources to invest in further resource gain. However, because loss is more potent than gain, gain cycles are likely to have less momentum or potency than loss cycles.

For example, following death of his spouse, a man loses an array of resources including love, a source of esteem, help with tasks, and a source of emotional support. When the next stressor occurs, perhaps a health problem, it may not be possible to recuperate at home. Entering into a nursing home might accelerate feelings of aging and alienation years before they might have occurred. The nursing home might also deplete financial resources. Now, with fewer health, emotional, task, esteem, and financial resources, he would be even more vulnerable when confronting the financial problems that emerge.

There are a number of reasons why a gain in the form of finding a new partner might not have the equivalent positive effect. One principal reason is that other gains are less likely to be part of the resource caravan that accompanies this change. Also, as we have argued, we have a cognitive bias that favors loss and makes us more sensitive to the loss process. Hence, Wortman and Silver (1987) have shown how people are deeply influenced by loss of a loved one over a decade later, but there is no sign of an equivalent positive effect for remarriage. This is not to say that remarriage cannot have profound positive influences, only that it is not equivalent to the comparable loss.

Development of the Resource Caravan in Later Life

At this juncture, we would like to integrate COR theory with Lomranz's (1990) multidimensional theory of adaptation to long-term stress. We feel that this integration helps illuminate our central thesis as to why some resources spring and some slide in later life. An initial attempt along these lines has already been formulated by Lomranz, and we would like to further elucidate the implications of such an integration.

Lomranz's (1990, 1995) model depicts three trajectories that influence the stress process. These include (1) the normal developmental sequence (e.g., schooling, leaving home, retirement), (2) a trauma timeline (e.g., impact of a major trauma as it vibrates across time and one's lifespan), and (3) the historical backdrop of stressful events during people's lives (e.g., World War II, the emergence of Israeli statehood, the Great Depression). He suggests that these three timelines crate potential stressors that contribute to people's stress experience. In turn, Lomranz argues that personal, social, and environmental resources, as depicted in COR theory, are employed to combat these stressors. He makes the critical point that people are influenced along a continuous developmental process. Thus, at any stage, the prior stages influence the current stress experience. A further, key insight of his thinking is that individuals' personal histories should not be separated from the social context in which they live their lives. People are instead seen as both shaped by and actively shaping their world. For example, he illustrates how the Holocaust experience not only influenced its survivors, but also, more surprisingly, how these survivors contributed to creating and shaping Israeli society.

We propose a further integration of these two theories. Not only do people use their resources to counteract the losses and threats that are a product of their personal, traumatic, and historical timelines, but these timelines are the very things that create the context for the growth or diminishment of their resource reservoirs. Moreover, the societal context also determines the nature to which people's resources will have good fit with demands. Let us take these two points separately.

Developmental, Trauma, and Historical Sequelae Produce Resources.
Many authors (e.g., Hobfoll, 1988; Sarason, Pierce, & Sarason, 1990) have argued that research on resources, such as mastery, optimism, and social support, has been introduced in such a way as to suggest that these resources are static, and as if they were just bestowed on people pell-mell. Lomranz's model suggests instead that resources may either develop or diminish because of the nature of the developmental, trauma, and historical sequences of individuals' lives. Family stability, love, and support during ongoing development will, for example, contribute to enduring self-esteem and sense of coherence (Antonovsky, 1979). Exposure to personal or societal traumatic stress in the form of rape or the Holocaust experience might, in contrast, challenge self-esteem and sense of coherence. As many Holocaust survivors lost major segments of their families, it is also clear how traumatic stress can deeply alter social resources.

The social-historical context also influences the resource caravan. Holocaust survivors who came to Israel met great prejudice and were often blamed for "going like lambs to slaughter." This led many rather than seeing themselves as heroic survivors to feel out of touch with their new homeland. General economic difficulties in Israel further challenged their ability to obtain and protect their resources. However, as Israelis learned more about their Holocaust experience, Israeli society came to view survivors in a different light. Solomon (1995) suggests that the historical and developmental sequences also interact. In her recent work, she finds that descendants of Holocaust survivors in Israeli remain differentially affected by combat experiences.

Historical Sequelae and the Fit of Resources.   We would further suggest that the fit of resources is also influenced by the historical timeline. For example, elderly Asians in Toronto may have the appropriate resources for their culture of origin, but not for their current culture. Immigration alters the historical back-drop because people move into a new society that is shaped and fashioned by a different history. Perhaps there is no more striking example of this as when Holocaust survivors attempted to return to their homelands in Poland and other countries, and found that their historical place had been essentially erased. As Jews, they no longer had a historical foothold in the society.

This is not to say that people passively either have or lack fit of their resources to a historical or social context. In earlier work, we have suggested that resources do not simply "fit" a context. Rather, people act to fit their resources to their contexts. Those high in mastery, for example, shape their social support in a way that it meets their demands and perhaps even avoid the use of social support when it is less appropriate to situational demands (Hobfoll, Shoham, & Ritter, 1991). COR theory further posits that the extent this fitting process is successful is, in part, dependent on the array of resources people have and the flexibility of the social structure in which they are embedded.

Older adults may have a rich array of resources and the flexibility to fit their resources to demands. Baltes and Baltes's (1990) model of selective optimization with compensation describes such adaptation in later life. In the model, selection refers to the process by which older persons choose and focus on meaningful life experiences in the face of losses associated with aging. For example, Lang and Carstensen (1994) found that older adults engage in proactive selection strategies to ensure that the number of close relationships remains the same as when they were younger—despite decreases in their social networks. Optimization refers to strategies employed to enrich and maintain individual's resources at the highest possible level during periods of loss. For example, an older adult may choose to remain near close friends and family rather than relocating. Finally, compensation involves reliance on elderly persons' own or outside resources in order to lessen the effect of losses (e.g., using escort services when no longer able to drive).

Societal structures prevent older adults from applying their resources (Riley et al., 1994). One of the clearest examples of this is forced retirement, whereby people who are fully capable are demobilized from the workforce. Their ability to support themselves and to contribute economically to their society is derailed. Some individuals who have very rich resource reserves can find a way to go around this obstacle, for example, if they can be their own boss or have an independent profession. Others, however, are prevented from fitting their resources to their demands.

Again, we must not fall into the trap of viewing later adult life as necessarily being characterized by loss cycles. Indeed, a more accurate portrayal of the aging process may be that suggested by Shmotkin (Chapter 1, this volume). He describes all aging individuals as facing the subjective well-being challenge of continued gains and personal development in spite of possible loss and deterioration. However, even if, as we suggest, loss cycles are more potent than gain cycles, there are a number of reasons why gain cycles have special relevance in later life. Many people are able to develop substantial savings and pensions for later life. This may allow them to enjoy life in ways that were not possible earlier. Personal resources are also likely to be enhanced with age, including increased wisdom (Baltes, Staudinger, Maercker, & Smith, 1995), control (Perlmuter, Goldfinger, Sizer, & Monty, 1989), and higher cognitive development (Souvaine, Lahey, & Kegan, 1990). Grandchildren may bring special joy, and this often comes without the responsibility of having to endure the burdening aspects of child rearing. Free time may also increase opportunities for interaction with loved ones and friends—opportunities that the hustle of earlier life may have curtailed. With the swelling of the older population in society, attractive retirement villages have sprouted, and there is finally time for prolonged games of golf. Nevertheless, we should not confuse these gain opportunities as being available to too wide a segment of society. The increasing division between rich and poor in many countries may be especially difficult for older adults who have fewer opportunities to replenish resources, and for whom inflation may detract from their purchasing and even their survival power.

Lomranz's multidimensional framework for adaptation aids understanding of this process and encourages investigation of the special effects that trauma have on the stress and coping process. COR theory suggests that traumatic events may deeply impact stress because they result in large, usually unanticipated losses, and because loss may be so deep as to prevent resource rebound. Where the trauma influences a society or appreciable segment of the population, such as the case of war or major, natural disaster, the societal support structure is also often disrupted as well. Giel (1990) suggests that when this occurs, resource replenishment on the individual level may be sacrificed for societal demands of resource replenishment. An example provided by Giel is of a village that was devastated by a landslide. Following the disaster, increased prejudice between the rich and poor limited opportunities for poorer residents to regain a foothold in the rebuilding of their resources. A similar pattern can be noted in the United States after World War I, when antiblack demonstrations, riots, and even lynchings occurred across many areas of the United States at a time paralleling the postwar recession (Tuttle, 1970). This limited the advancement of many African Americans who had made headway during the expanded war economy and migration from rural to urban areas.

A number of researchers have examined the extent and longevity of the impact of the Holocaust on survivors (e.g., Eitenger & Major, 1993; Nadler & Ben-Shushan, 1989). Other traumatic events, in contrast, have not been well researched in terms of the length and possible fading of their long-term impact. There is a paucity of information on the influence of either individual trauma events, such as rape, or communal traumatic events, such as being disaster victims, or being exposed to war, either when they occur in later life or when they have occurred much earlier. Hobfoll and Lomranz, along with their colleagues

(Hobfoll, Lomranz, Eyal, Bridges, & Tzemach, 1989; Lomranz, Hobfoll, Johnson, Eyal, & Tzemach, 1994), found that during war, the elderly may actually be at less risk than middle-aged individuals. Likewise, Thompson, Norris, and Hanacek (1993) found older adults to be less distressed than middle-aged and young people following Hurricane Hugo. Still, this aspect of the integration of COR and the multidimensional framework for adaptation awaits further investigation.

Based on an integration of these two models, we hypothesize that traumatic events will have a general negative impact that will be long-term. We also recognize that a small percentage of those affected may actually become stronger from such experiences. However, we would add that members of the latter group would only have positive outcomes if they are able to recreate a strong resource base. In other words, health and well-being require an accumulated base of resources. If the individual has experienced extreme resource loss, recovery will necessarily be long term, and larger social systems (e.g., the family, the state) will be needed to help in the process of rebuilding resources. This is not to romanticize this process, however, as we feel that COR theory and the evidence to date suggest that the major effect will not be positive. As an example, see Solomon and Ginsburg's discussion of Holocaust survivors' poor adaptation to the Gulf War (Chapter 6, this volume).

Implications of COR Theory for Family Coping

COR theory suggests that social support acts as a link between people's personal resources and the resources of the larger social system (Hobfoll & Freedy, 1990; Hobfoll & Vaux, 1993; Norris & Kasniasty, 1992). Seen this way, social support acts as a conduit for resource transfer. Through social support, people receive emotional aid, support on tasks, information, and a sense of group membership (Hobfoll, 1998).

The first line of social support lies within the family (Hobfoll, 1986) and, indeed, families develop a mutual obligation to confer aid upon each other. Clearly, nonprofessional caregivers for the infirm elderly are overwhelmingly family members (Stone, Cafferata, & Sangl, 1987; Stull, Kosloski, & Kercher, 1994), and, as Lieberman and Fisher (1995) point out, in such situations, all members of the family are affected—not just the primary caregiver. Families often mobilize to help in times of crisis, and their help has been found to have a generally positive effect. Indeed, the presence versus the absence of such support may be pivotal in separating those with the ability to withstand major stress challenges from those who cannot (Brown & Harris, 1978).

However, both COR theory and the integrative framework for adaptation also caution about another possibility. Specifically, Lomranz's developmental sequence particularly stresses family interaction—processes such as marriage, entry into parenthood, launching children from the nest, and widowhood. These developmental transitions can either strengthen or weaken families. COR theory suggests that there will be a cumulative trend across these events. This does not mean that those who have a poor marriage will necessarily have a troubled launching of their children, but that the transitions do rely upon common resources. As such, poor outcomes at the juncture of one transition will increase the probability of poor outcomes at the next developmental stage. This follows because the poor outcome will likely have stemmed from a very resource-demanding situation, a lack of resources, or both. All three of these eventualities are likely to lead to further resource depletion. This resource depletion, in turn, reduces the chances of success at the next transitional stage.

It is difficult to see how the transition from school in late adolescence is linked to the transition to retirement in later life. However, if we examine transitions that overlap, such as retirement and health concerns, then the link is clearer. Adding to this formula, the fact that later life is a period of multiple transitions, in a way mirroring late adolescence in terms of number of new, major transitions, it becomes clearer how this linking evolves. When adding the condition that resources receive demands from multiple sources, it becomes more apparent how the spring versus the slide alternatives emerge.

Finally, COR theory suggest that we must also remember that families share resource burdens. Although we have discussed the positive side of this coin, it should also be emphasized that this means that stress contagion (Riley & Eckenrode, 1986) and pressure-cooker effects (Hobfoll & London, 1986) are also likely. Stress contagion occurs when people who are emotionally linked share stressors across these social linkages. By so doing, they not only experience their own stress, but also are exposed to the stress of their loved ones. The pressure-cooker effect suggests that rather than being linear, this sharing of stress may especially overburden those with more intimate social support. In particular, the hubs of support linkages are at risk. In many cases, older adults are these hubs, because they are deeply emotionally linked to their children and what occurs in their children's lives. It is striking that we know relatively little about the social support that grandparents and older parents provide their families. Some insights are emerging along these lines from research within the African American and Hispanic communities in the United States, where grandparents are often the primary caregiver for their children's children (Chase-Lansdale, Brooks-Gunn, & Zamsky, 1994; Garcia, 1993; Wilson, 1986). However, we will have much to learn about this phenomenon and, in particular, how it may burden the older adult.

FUTURE DIRECTIONS

When stress research failed to find a strong link between stress and mental and physical health (Rabkin & Streuning, 1976), investigators searched for possible moderating effects of resources (Dohrenwend & Dohrenwend, 1974; Hobfoll, 1988). However, initial research in this area also failed to find particularly strong moderating effects of individual resources such as self-esteem, mastery, and social support. What we believe researchers have missed is the fact that resources emerge in caravans, that is, linked systems along the lifespan.

When resources are evaluated more globally, evidence strongly suggests that resources have a major influence on physical and psychological outcomes (Hobfoll, 1988, 1989; Hobfoll & Lilly, 1993). Recent researchers (Diener & Fujita, 1995; Turner & Marino, 1994; Thoits, 1995) are studying this phenomenon and confirming that when seen in aggregate, people's resources are the fountainhead of their psychological and physical health (Hobfoll, 1998).

Research on older adults has special importance in uncovering the phenomenon of resource caravans for three reasons. First, by virtue of their being older, the long-term effects of resource accumulation and depletion can be studied. Second, because later life is often accompanied by multiple transitions, processes that are overlapping may be studied in a way that is rare during the lifespan. Third, we know that significant resource losses are likely in later life in the areas of health, loss of loved ones, and employment roles. This means that later life is a special laboratory for the study of stress that may shed light on this process throughout the lifespan.

Finally, insight into the life journey of resource caravans may aid our understanding of how to help older adults cope with the inevitable stressors that accompany later life. By viewing later life as linked in this way to a lifelong process, we also gain an attachment with older individuals, whatever our age, and by so doing will be less likely to see older individuals as anything but ourselves in another metamorphosis.

REFERENCES

Aldwin, C. M. (1990). The elders life stress inventory: Egocentric and nonegocentric stress. In M. A. P. Stephens, J. H. Crowther, S. E. Hobfoll, & D. L. Tennenbaum (Eds.), *Stress and coping in later-life families* (pp. 44–69). New York: Hemisphere.

Aneshensel, C. S., Pearlin, L. I., & Schuler, R. H. (1993). Stress, role captivity, and the cessation of caregiving. *Journal of Health and Social Behavior, 34*, 54–70.

Antonovsky, A. (1979). *Health, stress, and coping.* San Francisco: Jossey-Bass.

Baltes, P. B. (1987). Theoretical propositions of lifespan developmental psychology: On the dynamics between growth and decline. *Developmental Psychology, 23*, 611–623.

Baltes, P. B. (1997). On the incomplete architecture of human ontogeny: Selection, optimization, and compensation as foundations of developmental psychology. *American Psychologist, 52*, 366–380.

Baltes, P. B., & Baltes, M. M. (1990). Psychological perspectives on successful aging: The model of selective optimization with compensation. In P. B. Baltes & M. M. Baltes (Eds.), *Successful aging: Perspectives from the behavioral sciences* (pp. 1–34). Cambridge, UK: Cambridge University Press.

Baltes, P. B., Staudinger, U. M., Maercker, A., & Smith, J. (1995). People nominated as wise: A comparative study of wisdom-related knowledge. *Psychology and Aging, 10*, 155–166.

Brown, G. W., & Harris, T. (1978). *The social origins of depression: The study of psychiatric disorder in women.* New York: Free Press.

Chase-Lansdale, P. L., Brooks-Gunn, J., & Zamsky, E. (1994). Young African-American multigenerational families in poverty: Quality of mothering and grandmothering. *Child Development, 65*, 373–393.

Diener, E., & Fujita, F. (1995). Resources, personal strivings, and subjective well-being: A homothetic and idiographic approach. *Journal of Personality and Social Psychology, 68*, 926–935.

Dohrenwend, B. S., & Dohrenwend, B. P. (Eds.). (1974). *Stressful life events: Their nature and effects.* New York: Wiley.

Eitinger, L., & Major, E. F. (1993). Stress of the Holocaust. In L. Goldberger & S. Breznitz (Eds.), *Handbook of stress: Theoretical and clinical aspects* (2nd ed., pp. 617–640). New York: Free Press.

Garcia, C. (1993). What do we mean by extended family? A closer look at Hispanic multigenerational families. *Journal of Cross Cultural Gerontology, 8*, 137–146.

Giel, R. (1990). Psychosocial processes in disasters. *International Journal of Mental Health, 19*, 7–20.

Harris, D. K. (1990). *The sociology of aging* (2nd ed.). New York: Harper & Row.

Hobfoll, S. E. (1986). Social support: Research, theory, and applications from research on women. In S. E. Hobfoll (Ed.), *Stress, social support, and women* (pp. 239–256). New York: Hemisphere.

Hobfoll, S. E. (1988). *The ecology of stress.* New York: Hemisphere.

Hobfoll, S. E. (1989). Conservation of resources: A new attempt at conceptualizing stress. *American Psychologist, 44*, 513–524.

Hobfoll, S. E. (1998). *Stress, culture, and community: The psychology and philosophy of stress.* New York: Plenum Press.

Hobfoll, S. E., & Freedy, J. R. (1990). The availability and effective use of social support [Special issue: Social support and clinical psychology.] *Journal of Social and Clinical Psychology, 9*, 91–103.

Hobfoll, S. E., & Lilly, R. S. (1993). Resource conservation as a strategy for community psychology. *Journal of Community Psychology, 21*, 128–148.

Hobfoll, S. E., Lilly, R. S., & Jackson, A. P. (1991). Conservation of social resources and the self. In H. O. F. Veiel & U. Baumann (Eds.), *The meaning and measurement of social support: Taking stock of 20 years of research* (pp. 125–141). Washington, DC: Hemisphere.

Hobfoll, S. E., Lomranz, J., Eyal, N., Bridges, A., & Tzemach, M. (1989). Pulse of a nation: Depression mood reactions of Israel to Israel–Lebanon War. *Journal of Personality and Social Psychology, 56*, 1002–1012.

Hobfoll, S. E., & London, P. (1986). The relationship of self-concept and social support to emotional distress among women during war. *Journal of Social and Clinical Psychology, 12*, 87–100.

Hobfoll, S. E., Shoham, S. B., & Ritter, C. (1991). Women's satisfaction with social support and their receipt of aid. *Journal of Personality and Social Psychology, 61*, 332–341.

Hobfoll, S. E., & Vaux, A. (1993). Social support: Resources and context. in L. Goldberger & S. Breznitz (Eds.), *Handbook of stress: Theoretical and clinical aspects* (2nd ed., pp. 685–705). New York: Free Press.

Labouvie-Vief, G. (1985). Intelligence and cognition. In J. E. Birren & K. W. Schaie (Eds.), *Handbook of the psychology of aging* (2nd ed., pp. 500–530). New York: Van Nostrand Reinhold.

Lang, F. R., & Carstensen, L. L. (1994). Close emotional relationships in late life: Further support for proactive aging in the social domain. *Psychology and Aging, 9*, 315–324.

Lazarus, R. S., & Folkman, S. (1984). *Stress, appraisal, and coping.* New York: Springer.

Lerner, M. J., & Gignac, M. A. M. (1992). Is it coping or is it growth? A cognitive–affective model of contentment in the elderly. In L. Montada, S. H. Fillip, & M. J. Lerner (Eds.), *Life crises and experiences of loss in adulthood* (pp. 321–337). Hillsdale, NJ: Erlbaum.

Lieberman, M. A., & Fisher, L. (1995). The impact of chronic illness on the health and well-being of family members. *Gerontologist, 35*, 94–102.

Lomranz, J. (1990). Long-term adaptation to traumatic stress in light of adult development and aging perspectives. In M. P. Stephens, J. Crowther, S. E. Hobfoll, & D. Tennenbaum (Eds.), *Stress and coping in later-life families* (pp. 99–121). Washington, DC: Hemisphere.

Lomranz, J. (1995). Endurance and living: Long-term effects of the Holocaust. In S. E. Hobfoll & M. W. deVries (Eds.), *Extreme stress and communities: Impact and intervention* (pp. 325–352). Dordrecht, The Netherlands: Kluwer Academic.

Lomranz, J., Hobfoll, S. E., Johnson, R., Eyal, N., & Tzemach, M. (1994). A nation's response to attack: Israelis' depressive reactions to the Gulf War. *Journal of Traumatic Stress, 7*, 55–69.

Maslow, A. H. (1968). *Toward a psychology of being.* New York: Van Nostrand Reinhold.

Nadler, A., & Ben-Shushan, D. (1989). Forty years later: Long-term consequences of massive traumatization as manifested by Holocaust survivors from the city and the kibbutz. *Journal of Consulting and Clinical Psychology, 57*, 287–293.

Norris, F., & Kaniasty, K. (1992, August). *Disasters deplete social support: Implications for practice.* Paper presented at the meetings of the American Psychological Association, Washington, DC.

Perlmuter, L. C., Goldfinger, S. H., Sizer, N. R., & Monty, R. A. (1989). Choosing to improve performance. In P. S. Fry (Ed.), *Psychological perspectives of helplessness and control in the elderly* (pp. 395–411). Amsterdam, The Netherlands: North-Holland.

Rabkin, J. G., & Streuning, E. L. (1976). Life events, stress, and illness. *Science, 194*, 1013–1020.

Riley, D., & Eckenrode, J. (1986). Social ties: Subgroup differences in costs and benefits. *Journal of Personality and Social Psychology, 51*, 770–778.

Riley, M. W., Kahn, R., & Foner, A. (Eds.). (1994). *Age and structural lag.* New York: Wiley.

Rosenwaike, I. (1985). *The extreme aged in America: Portrait of an expanding population.* Westport, CT: Greenwood.

Rosow, I. (1974). *Socialization to old age.* Berkeley: University of California Press.

Sarason, B. R., Pierce, G. R., & Sarason, I. G. (1990). Social support: The sense of acceptance and the role of relationships. In B. R. Sarason, I. G. Sarason, & G. R. Pierce (Eds.), *Social support: An interactional view* (pp. 97–128). New York: Wiley.

Schönpflug, W. (1985). Goal directed behavior as a source of stress: Psychological origins and consequences of inefficiency. In M. Frese & J. Sabini (Eds.), *The concept of action in psychology* (pp. 172–199). Hillsdale, NJ: Erlbaum.

Solomon, Z. (1995). The pathogenic effects of war stress: The Israeli experience. In S. E. Hobfoll & M. W. deVries (Eds.), *Extreme stress and communities: Impact and intervention* (pp. 229–246). Dordrecht, The Netherlands: Kluwer Academic.

Souvaine, E., Lahey, L. L., & Kegan, R. (1990). Life after formal operations: Implications for a psychology of the self. In C. N. Alexander & E. J. Langer (Eds.), *Higher stages of human development: Perspectives on adult growth* (pp. 229–257). New York: Oxford University Press.

Stone, R. I., Cafferata, G. L., & Sangl, J. (1987). Caregivers of the frail elderly: A national profile. *Gerontologist, 27*, 616–626.

Stull, D. E., Kosloski, K., & Kercher, K. (1994). Caregiver burden and generic well-being: Opposite sides of the same coin? *Gerontologist, 34*, 88–94.

Sung, K. T. (1995). Measures and dimensions of filial piety in Korea. *Gerontologist, 35*, 240–247.

Thoits, P. A. (1995). Identity-relevant events and psychological symptoms: A cautionary tale. *Journal of Health and Social Behavior, 36*, 72–82.

Thompson, M. P., Norris, F. H., & Hanacek, B. (1993). Age differences in the psychological consequences of Hurricane Hugo. *Psychology and Aging, 8*, 606–616.

Thorson, J. A. (1995). *Aging in a changing society.* New York: Wadsworth.

Turner, R. J., & Marino, F. (1994). Social support and social structure: A descriptive epidemiology. *Journal of Health and Social Behavior, 35*, 193–212.

Tuttle, W. M., Jr. (1970). *Race riot: Chicago in the Red Summer of 1919.* New York: Atheneum.

Tversky, A., & Rabneman, D. (1981). The framing of decisions and psychological voice. *Science, 24*, 453–458.

Wilson, M. N. (1986). Perceived parental activity of mothers, fathers and grandmothers in three generational black families. *Journal of Black Psychology, 12*, 43–60.

Wortman, C. B., & Silver, R. C. (1987). Coping with irrevocable loss. In G. R. VandenBos & B. K. Bryant (Eds.), *Cataclysms, crises, and catastrophes: Psychology in action* (pp. 189–235). Washington, DC: American Psychological Association.

Chapter 6

War Trauma and the Aged

An Israeli Perspective

ZAHAVA SOLOMON AND KARNI GINZBURG

INTRODUCTION

Posttraumatic Stress Disorder

The pathogenic effects of traumatic events have been consistently documented over a large range of populations and occurrences (Wilson & Raphael, 1993). At the same time, considerable variability in human response to trauma has been documented (e.g., Solomon, Mikulincer, & Waysman, 1991). Although many survivors are able to put the trauma behind them and resume their lives, others are detrimentally affected. They may suffer a deterioration of health and social functioning, along with a large variety of psychological disturbances, including anxiety, depression, somatization (Solomon, 1993), and posttraumatic stress disorder (PTSD), which is the most common and conspicuous psychological sequela of trauma (American Psychiatric Association, 1994).

PTSD is characterized by intrusive recollections of the traumatic event, psychic numbing, and symptoms of autonomic nervous system arousal. The syndrome may occur in an acute form, with its characteristic clinical symptoms appearing within 6 months of the traumatic event. Alternatively, its onset may be delayed or its emergence reactivated (American Psychiatric Association, 1994). Delayed PTSD is diagnosed when the symptoms appear for the first time and with no apparent warning only 6 or more months after the traumatic event. It emerges either spontaneously or following some trigger (Solomon, 1993). Reactivation is the emergence of a full-blown syndrome in individuals previously asymptomatic. It is usually precipitated by exposure to another stressful or

ZAHAVA SOLOMON AND KARNI GINZBURG • The Bob Shapell School of Social Work, Tel Aviv University, Tel Aviv 69978, Israel.

Handbook of Aging and Mental Health: An Integrative Approach, edited by Jacob Lomranz. Plenum Press, New York, 1998.

traumatic stimulus that is reminiscent of the original traumatic event (Solomon, 1993). Either acute or delayed PTSD may become chronic. Chronic PTSD is diagnosed when the symptoms persist for longer than 6 months (American Psychiatric Association, 1994). In many cases, in fact, PTSD does tend to be chronic, with recurring remissions and relapses. These relapses may take the form of an exacerbation of the subclinical symptoms that had persisted throughout the period of remission or the form of reactivation of prior trauma. Its chronic nature means that it can either be alleviated or intensified with the passage of time.

Reciprocal Relations between Trauma and Old Age

Current trauma literature recognizes that both features of both the traumatic event and the victim may mediate the trauma's immediate and long-term psychological effects. These features include the length and severity of the traumatic event (e.g., Rutledge, Hunter, & Dahl, 1979), the gender (e.g., Solomon, 1995) and socioeconomic status of the victim (e.g., Green, Grace, Lindy, & Leonard, 1990), and the social support available to the victim (e.g., Solomon, 1993). With the exception of trauma experienced in childhood, however, relatively little attention has been paid to the interplay of the traumatic event and the survivor's developmental stage. The prevailing trend is to treat adults as a single, unified population (Lomranz, 1994). The tendency may stem from the fact that much of the theory and study of trauma is rooted in prevailing psychoanalytic theories, which postulate that personality is by and large determined in childhood, and that human development virtually terminates in adolescence. The outcome of this assumption is that the trauma literature does not adequately take into account our present understanding that people continue to develop throughout the life cycle, and that every stage has its particular resources and concerns, which may affect how individuals respond to the trauma.

This chapter looks at the reciprocal relations between trauma and aging. The first part of the chapter explores the effect of this developmental stage on adjustment to current trauma, asking whether the elderly cope with and adjust to such trauma differently from younger adults. The second part explores whether prior experiences, including earlier exposure to trauma, affects persons' adjustment to aging, that is, whether the aging process of trauma victims differs from that of persons who had the good fortune to have been spared earlier trauma.

THE IMPACT OF CURRENT TRAUMA
ON OLD AGE

Perspectives on the Impact of Traumatic Experiences in Old Age

The literature offers three distinct views, each supported by empirical evidence, of the impact of traumatic events on the psychosocial adjustment of the elderly.

One view claims that the aged are largely a weak and vulnerable group, have fewer resources than younger persons to cope with traumatic stress, and are at particularly high risk for adjustment difficulties following traumatic events. It further maintains that the aged are rigid in their responses and use regressive and nonadaptive defense mechanisms. In accordance with this view, Friedsman (1961) and Bolin and Klenow (1982–1983) reported that older victims tend to react with a greater sense of deprivation than younger victims to roughly equivalent losses, while others reported that they have specific, age-related problems and needs following a disaster. These include difficulty in coping with the heavy physical work of cleanup and repair (Huerta & Horton, 1978); the need for selected support services, such as transportation and shopping, to help them extend their life space beyond the home (Poulshock & Cohen, 1975); and, frequently, the need for more help than younger persons in dealing with the financial, legal, and tax issues that arise following a disaster (Huerta & Horton, 1978). The "vulnerability perspective" is further supported by studies showing high levels of depression (McNaughton, Smith, Patterson, & Grant, 1990) among elderly victims of stressful experiences, a low level of perceived quality of life (Melick & Logue, 1985–1986), increased use of sedatives and tranquilizers (Melick & Logue, 1985–1986), and poorer immune function (McNaughton et al., 1990).

A second view regards the aged as a resilient population that can adjust better than younger victims to traumatic experiences. The "resilience perspective" is supported by studies showing that elderly persons adjust better than their juniors in the aftermath of trauma. Elderly victims have reported better recovery than younger victims following a major tornado (Bolin & Klenow, 1988). They have been found to express less fear, worry, and despair than younger survivors in the aftermath of a natural disaster, and more positive emotions, such as security, cheerfulness, and contentment (Bell, 1978; Huerta & Horton, 1978). Studies show less family and emotional disruption among elderly disaster victims (Bolin & Klenow, 1982–1983), as well as lower alcohol consumption (Miller, Turner, & Kimball, 1981). Following an earthquake, elderly victims reported less intrusion of the experience into their lives in the form of unsolicited recollections, thoughts, and dreams of the event than their juniors, though the PTSD rates were much the same (Goenjian et al., 1994).

These salutary findings can be attributed to a number of possible factors. One is that the aged usually experience less disruption of their daily routine and work following disaster than do younger victims (Bolin & Klenow, 1982–1983). They would thus perceive the disaster as less stressful than younger victims, who are subject to more secondary stressors (such as financial loss derived from disruption of work). A related factor might be that, being more restricted to their homes, more occupied with themselves, and less involved in the external world, including in the rescue efforts in the aftermath of a disaster, than younger victims, the aged are less exposed to the full brunt of the trauma. Their exposure is more confined to their own losses and they are relatively shielded from the suffering of others. This, too, could lead them to experience the situation as less stressful. Finally, some professionals have argued that their more extensive life experience, including prior exposure to trauma, might make the aged more resilient to traumatic stress. Various scholars hold that life events serve as an "immunizer," claiming that multiple stressful experiences contribute to the development of useful coping styles and thereby facilitate adaptation (Epstein, 1983; Meichenbaum, 1985).

A third view holds that vulnerability and resilience to stress are not age-dependent, and that the elderly do not differ from others in their emotional reaction to trauma. This view is supported by studies showing that there were no age-related differences in the levels of worry, anxiety, depression, avoidance, sleep disturbances, nightmares, intrusiveness, forgetfulness, and lack of confidence experienced after a disaster (Hagstrom, 1995; Miller et al., 1981; Ollendick & Hoffmann, 1982). It is also supported by the finding that the same percentage—33%—of elderly and younger victims of a disaster reported positive changes in their lives or emotional functioning as result of the events related to the disaster (Ollendick & Hoffmann, 1982).

In short, the literature is highly inconsistent on the impact of trauma on the elderly. At least part of the problem may derive from the methodological shortcomings of many of the studies. Many studies fail to report on either or both the sampling procedure (e.g., Bolin & Klenow, 1982–1983; McNaughton et al., 1990) and response rate (e.g., Bell, 1978; Gray & Calsyn, 1989; Kilijanek & Drabek, 1979; Poulshock & Cohen, 1975). Some do not use a control group (e.g., McNaughton et al., 1990; Melick & Logue, 1985–1986), and some are based on data gathered by nonstandardized interviews or from impressions (e.g., Friedsman, 1961; Goenjian et al., 1994). All of these flaws would make a consistent picture quite unlikely.

Another difficulty is that a very large range of events is involved, from robbery through accidents, from natural disasters through wars. Some of the events are natural and others are man-made; some affect individuals, whereas others affect whole communities, while the victims themselves may experience varying degrees of exposure and destruction. All and any one of these variables, as well as many others, can affect the psychological outcome. Compounding the problem of obtaining a clear picture is that catastrophes often occur without warning and without pattern. They are thus not the sort of thing that a researcher can approach with a preplanned study design. Moreover, they happen to very different types of populations. Aged urbanites may be quite different from aged rural folk or villagers. At the least, the two groups would be likely to have different social, family, and economic structures, as well as different personal resources, such as education and income, which may also affect the psychological outcome. Given all of these variables, it is hardly surprising that the literature does not provide an unequivocal answer as to whether or how the age at which a person is exposed to trauma affects its psychological impact.

The Elderly Trauma Victim: The Israeli Perspective

Israel is a small country that events have, unfortunately, made a natural laboratory for the study of stress. Few people reach old age without experiencing stressful life events, such as serious illness, the death of a loved one, and so forth. But the life experiences of most elderly Israelis include not only these personal crises, but also major communal disasters. The great majority of elderly Israelis are immigrants, most of them refugees, who came to Israel shortly after its founding, when it was a poor and struggling State, uncertain that it would survive the enmity of its neighbors. Those from Africa and the Middle East fled their countries or snuck out, often following severe persecution or pogroms and braving many dangers to reach the country. Those from Europe had survived the Nazi Holocaust in hiding or in concentration or prison camps, and had lost the better part of their families. Both groups arrived with little in the way of personal possessions; both had to make substantial adjustments in their way of life. Moreover, both they and the "old-timers" who had arrived before the State was founded lived through at least several of the seven full-fledged wars and countless terrorist attacks that the country has suffered in its short years of existence. These experiences may have affected the coping of Israeli elderly with current adversities.

Here, we take a look at four studies that examined the coping of elderly Israelis in comparison to that of their younger counterparts during two wars: the 1982 Lebanon War and the 1991 Gulf War.

The Lebanon War was a relatively contained military operation that lasted for several months over the summer of 1982. It took place on Lebanese soil, and although Israeli soldiers were at danger at the fire line, the civilian population, including the elderly, were not exposed to direct danger. While there was considerable television and newspaper coverage of the war, with daily casualty counts and funerals, the day-to-day routine of most Israelis was not directly affected.

In a prospective nationwide study, Hobfoll, Lomranz, Eyal, Bridges, and Tzemach (1989) assessed the depressive mood of the Israeli population before, during, and after the Lebanon War. They found a marked elevation in depressive mood at the onset of the war, followed by a decrease in depression during the intensive period of the war, suggesting adaptation to the stressful situation. Dividing the sample into four age groups (young adults aged 18–22; midadults aged 23–40; midlifers aged 41–60; and older adults aged 61 and over), they found that while the older adults exhibited the same pattern of increased depression and subsequent habituation as the young adults, their depressive mood had intensified more, indicating stronger reaction to war stress.

The Gulf War, 10 years later, was quite different from the Lebanon War. In this war, the entire population, again, including the elderly, was on firing line. Thirty-nine missiles struck Israel, most of them landing in densely populated neighborhoods in and around Tel Aviv. The missiles damaged or destroyed a considerable number of homes and caused a certain amount of bodily injury and even loss of life. Even where there was no direct damage, the threat of gas and biological attack, with unknown but terrifying consequences, hung over people's heads.

The Gulf War was stressful for most Israelis, but it posed particular problems for Israel's elderly, who made up over 10% of the country's population at the time and happened to be highly concentrated in the targeted and stricken areas. While essential services were kept running, many "nonessential" services were radically curtailed. Among other things, the senior citizens' centers to which many elderly went for everything from company to instrumental services were shut. Since the missile danger tended to keep people indoors, close to gas-sealed rooms, the closure of the centers made the elderly even more housebound than they usually were and greatly augmented the isolation to which they were subject at the best of times.

The emergency procedures that were adopted during the war also posed special problems for the elderly. Many older persons lacked the manual dexterity needed to fit the gas masks; some had trouble hearing the air-raid sirens; yet others found it difficult to understand the emergency instructions broadcast over the radio and television. On the whole, they had more difficulty than their juniors in settling into their sealed room in the short time that was available between the air-raid alarm and missile strikes. Some dealt with the problem by sealing up their entire apartment, which meant that they spent long hours in sunless, airless confinement. For those with impaired vision or hearing, seclusion in the sealed room further aggravated their sense of isolation.

How they fared was examined by a comprehensive longitudinal survey conducted by the Israeli Defense Force's Department of Behavioral Sciences (Carmeli et al., 1992). The study investigated the attitudes, behavior, coping, and morale of the elderly. It found that the elderly did not differ significantly from the rest of the population in their knowledge of the protective procedures, their satisfaction with the amount and clarity of the media information on the subject, or in actually carrying out the emergency instructions; that is, about the same proportion of elderly obeyed instructions to seal rooms and wear gas masks as the rest of the population, and about the same proportions did and did not hoard food and supplies. As the researchers explain it, Israel's elderly are well versed in wars and did not need a great deal of prompting to do what was required under the circumstances.

However, the study also revealed that, in some ways, the aged did differ from the rest of the adult population. One is that they found the war less disruptive of their daily routine and work, and less damaging economically than their juniors. Only 16% of the aged reported that the disruption of their routine bothered them a great deal, in contrast to 35% of the younger subjects. Similarly, the impact on family relations was less salient among the elderly. Seventy percent of them reported that their family relations were not affected, in comparison to 50% of the younger subjects.

On the other hand, throughout most of the war, the elderly felt that they managed less well than their juniors. Figure 6–1 shows the coping reported by the two populations at various points of the war. At the start of the war, the aged, according to their self-reports, coped only slightly less well than the rest of the population. However, while the rest of the population reported that they coped better as the war progressed, throughout much of that period, the aged reported that they coped worse. It was only toward the very end of the war, when the missile strikes were few and far between and tended to be off-target, that their coping improved and reached the level of that of the rest of the population.

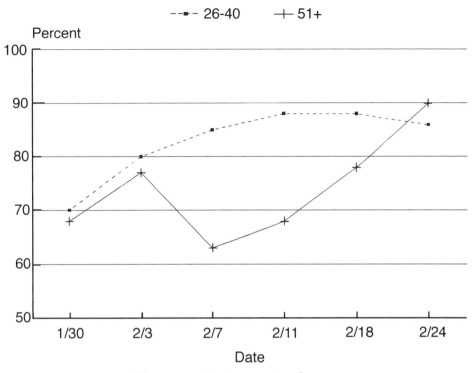

Figure 6–1. Coping over time by age.

In other words, the study suggests that while, on a practical level, the aged continued to function adequately during the war, obeying the emergency instructions and going on with their lives, emotionally they found it harder to cope with the missile strikes and suffered greater distress than their juniors.

In another study conducted during the Gulf War, my colleagues and I (Prager & Solomon, 1995a, 1995b) examined the relation between age and distress level, measured by two indices: "affective distress"—defined as a temporary, perceivable change in mood or feeling likely to be disturbing to the individual—and "social interaction distress"—a temporary, perceivable change in patterns of behavior toward and in interaction with the social and physical environment. The study was conducted on 164 persons between 50 and 91 years of age, divided into a "younger" group (age range 50–69; $M = 64.8$) and an "older" group (age range 70–91; $M = 77.0$). Findings showed almost no difference in the mean stress scores of the two age groups on both measures of distress. Nor did the two age groups differ in their perceived control of the situation or attribution of meaning to events and their outcomes.

The last study that we discuss in this connection was carried out by Lomranz and Ayal (1994). This was a longitudinal study of the Gulf War, similar to one the authors had undertaken of the Lebanon War. It examined depressive mood in four age groups at four points of time: before the threat of war was on the horizon, under the threat of impending war, during the war, and after the end of the war. The findings indicate that during the war, depressive mood rose in all the age groups, but while a significant age difference was found at the two points of time preceding the fighting, none was found during or after. Before the threat of war was in the air, the base depression rate of the aged and middle-aged was higher than of the young age group; then, when war was impending, the level of depression among the aged rose strikingly, only to even out with that of the rest of the population during the war. In other words, while the aged were particularly disturbed by the anticipation of war, they felt much the same as younger Israelis during the war itself.

The findings of the four studies can be summarized as follows: During the Lebanon War, in which younger persons played an active role in the war effort but the rest of the population was not directly threatened, the elderly responded more strongly to the stress, with a sharper rise in depressive mood, than their juniors. During the Gulf War, however, when most of the population was exposed to the threat in similar measure, the elderly did not differ from the rest of the population in either depressive mood or distress and used similar cognitive coping strategies. Moreover, for all practical purposes, they handled the emergency orders and used the protective measures as well as their younger counterparts and reported being less bothered than their juniors by the disruption of their daily routine. The only notable difference was in their perceptions of their coping: The elderly perceived their coping as poorer than the rest of the population. This may be related to the generally lower sense of self-efficacy among the aged.

THE IMPACT OF EARLIER TRAUMA
ON COPING WITH CURRENT TRAUMAS
IN OLD AGE

The Reawakening of Earlier Traumas in the Aging Process

Millions of today's elderly all over the world have suffered traumatic events in their youth. The combatants, refugees, and prisoners of war of World War II, along with the survivors of the Nazi Holocaust and atomic bomb, who are today in their seventies, eighties, or nineties, are some of many examples.

The literature suggests that many of them have been deeply scarred. Empirical studies conducted about 40 years after the World War II, when the victims were well into their sixties, have shown that former prisoners of war had high rates of PTSD, hovering between about 50% and 85% (Goldstein, Van Kammen, Shelly, Miller, & Van Kammen, 1987; White, 1983), as well as high levels of depression (Page, Engdahl, & Eberly, 1991) and anxiety (Goldstein et al., 1987). Similarly, studies of Holocaust survivors point to posttraumatic residues. For example, studies report that 30–60% of the survivors show considerable emotional distress (Carmil & Carel, 1986; Levav & Abramson, 1984), manifested mainly in PTSD (Kuch & Cox, 1992), and especially in sleep disturbances (Rosen, Reynolds, Yaeger, Houck, & Horowitz, 1991). Although a number of studies have found recovery (Kluznik, Speed, Van Valkenburg, & Magraw, 1986; Sperr, Sperr, Craft, & Boudewyns, 1990), the evidence thus far seems to point to lasting damage among a good proportion of trauma victims.

The chronic nature of PTSD renders trauma survivors vulnerable for the rest of their lives. Moreover, some of the features of old age make it a particularly high-risk period for either delayed-onset or reactivated PTSD.

Aging generally entails a reduction of activity and a shift from planning to reminiscing, and from occupation with current events to the review and rethinking of one's life. In the course of this shift, the aging individual may be brought face-to-face with his or her past, often forgotten or ignored till then. Indeed, trauma survivors try hard to put their past behind them. They put great effort into building new lives and invest considerable energy in their work and family. Often, with the complicity of the surrounding society, they suppress their traumatic memories or force them into the background of their lives. The altered perspective of old age may force them up to the foreground again (Hertz, 1990).

The process can be seen among the Holocaust survivors in Israel. While the physical needs of the survivors who immigrated to Israel were met with remarkable generosity, their emotional needs were met with what became known as a "conspiracy of silence." Veteran Israelis were unwilling to listen to what the survivors had undergone in the Holocaust. The survivors were encouraged to make new lives for themselves and to participate actively in the building of the young State. They were discouraged from "dwelling on the past" and working through their experiences. As they aged, their attention shifted back to the past, while social and cultural changes in the country have led to greater interest on the part of other Israelis. In fact, Israeli society now encourages the Holocaust survivors to bear witness to the events, bringing to the surface repressed traumatic memories. While the acknowledgment of the Holocaust sufferings is to be seen as a positive development, the awakening of dormant memories among people who have not had a chance to work them through can be highly distressing.

In addition, aging inevitably entails many losses and exit events, from retirement through the death of spouse, relatives, and friends. Painful in themselves, such losses may be particularly distressing for previously traumatized individuals, whom they often remind of the losses in the traumatic event. Several case reports demonstrated the exacerbation of repressed memories and triggering of delayed PTSD following such events (e.g., Hermann & Eryavec, 1994).

Retirement may be a source of dread for elderly Holocaust survivors. Not only does it entail a loss of the structure, routine, self-esteem, status, and social interaction that are vital to all of us, but it brings down one of the major protective shields that trauma survivors have against being flooded by memories. The fact that inability to work resulted in almost certain death in the concentration camps can only increase the survivors' anxiety about retiring.

The deterioration of health is also a feature of the aging process that may lead to the onset of delayed or reactivated PTSD. Findings show that as they age, both Holocaust survivors and prisoners of war tend to become more ill, and more frequently so, than comparable individuals with no such traumatic past. The deterioration of health has been documented to trigger the outbreak of delayed PTSD (Hamner, 1994). The situation is complicated when elderly survivors are hospitalized or placed in nursing homes. Observations of Holocaust survivors suggest that many of them find hospitalization extremely traumatic, since it echoes and revives their former ordeal (Danieli, 1994; Hirschfield, 1977). They are again separated from their loved ones, confined, and sometimes required to share quarters with strangers; they are exposed to bodily smells and noises that remind them of their persecution, placed in a position of helplessness, and told what to do by authorities they had learned to mistrust. Clinical evidence (Hirshfeld, 1977) indicates that in more than a few cases, hospitalization brings about psychotic-like delusions of being back in the concentration camp, with the confined survivors accusing the doctors and nurses of Nazi-like experimentation.

The Reawakening of Earlier Trauma through Symbolic Association

Various studies have shown that PTSD and other trauma residuals can be provoked by events, even seemingly trivial ones, that bear for the survivor symbolic association with his or her earlier trauma. For example, two studies have shown that movie and television coverage of military violence can reactivate dormant PTSD in veterans (Brockway, 1988; Jones & Lovell, 1987). Similarly, Long, Chamberlain, and Vincent (1994) demonstrated that media coverage of the warfare in the Gulf revived memories of earlier combat among Vietnam veterans who had never presented combat-related psychological problems, resulting in increased PTSD rates.

Similar evidence of reactivation following exposure to minor stressors was found among Holocaust survivors. Eaton, Sigal, and Weinfeld (1982) observed elevated levels of distress among Jewish Holocaust survivors when the Jewish community in Montreal was under strain due to local political issues. They concluded that the political stress awakened dormant feelings of insecurity among the survivors. Kahana, Harel, and Kahana (1989), who studied Holocaust survivors and comparable controls living in Israel, found that the survivors showed more constant concern for the future and lower morale than the others.

In the same vein, empirical evidence suggest that when faced with a major stressor, Holocaust survivors exhibited more distress than others; that is, cancer patients with a Holocaust background manifested more psychological distress (Baider, Peretz, & De-Nour, 1992) and displayed a lower level of coping potential (Baider & Sarell, 1984) than comparable cancer patients. It seems that the past trauma left them vulnerable, and when faced with new major trauma, their vulnerability was unmasked and they were not able to mobilize the adaptive coping.

Aged Holocaust Survivors in the Gulf War

As noted earlier, the Gulf War imposed special stresses on Israel's elderly population as a whole. In addition to these, it created even further stresses for Holocaust survivors, for it bore a disturbing resemblance to aspects of their Holocaust experience. These included the often repeated threat of gas attack, the machinations of a megalomaniacal tyrant, and the targeting of unarmed civilians, coupled with the government policy of restriction, leaving them totally passive, all of which had the power to evoke troublesome memories.

Although there is a great deal of evidence to the effect that Holocaust survivors, and especially aged Holocaust survivors, are a vulnerable group, the literature leaves open the question whether their Holocaust experience impairs or facilitates their coping with adversity. The literature on coping offers two contradictory views: the inoculation perspective and the vulnerability perspective.

The inoculation perspective holds that stress contributes to the development of useful coping strategies, that each similar hardship increases familiarity, leading to a decrease in the amount of perceived stress and enabling more successful adaptation in future stressful situations (Epstein, 1983; Janis, 1971; Keinan, 1979). Eysenck (1983) refines this view somewhat by proposing the utility of both similar and dissimilar stressors. A stressor, he states, can promote either "direct tolerance" or similar stressors in the future and/or "indirect tolerance" of dissimilar stressors.

Applied to Holocaust survivors, the inoculation perspective would predict them to weather the Gulf War either with greater equanimity than their agemates, if the direct tolerance model is advanced, or with the same equanimity, if the indirect cross-tolerance model is the basis for prediction.

The vulnerability perspective considers repeated exposure to stressful events a risk factor. It holds that every stressful life event depletes available coping resources and thereby increases vulnerability to subsequent stress (Coleman, Butcher, & Carson, 1980; McGrath, 1970; Selye, 1956; Vinokur & Selzer, 1975).

Numerous studies of posttrauma point to the pathogenic effect of recurrent exposure. Silver and Wortman (1980) found that people who had experienced extreme stress in the past were more vulnerable to the aftereffects of a subsequent stressor. Similarly, Solomon, Mikulincer, and Jacob (1987) found, in a younger population, that the accumulated stress of multiple wars had a largely detrimental impact on the ability of soldiers to retain their emotional equilibrium in battle; soldiers who had stress reactions in their first war were more likely to break down in the second. Other studies suggest that exposure to traumatic events leaves the victims more vulnerable in general. Solomon, Oppenheimer, Elitzur, and Waysman (1990a) found that after a soldier was traumatized in war, he did not return to his prewar level of control, even if he coped successfully with a subsequent war. Titchner (1986; Titchner & Ross, 1974) has argued strongly that exposure to a traumatic event may issue in a process of posttraumatic decline and leave permanent psychological effects, especially proneness to anxiety reactions.

Applied to Holocaust survivors, the vulnerability perspective would predict them to fare much worse than other elderly Israelis during the Gulf War,
whether they perceived that war as a similar stress or as a symbolic reminder of
the first.

My colleagues and I (Hantman, Solomon, & Prager, 1994; Solomon & Prager,
1992) addressed the question of whether Holocaust survivors responded differently to the Gulf War than their non-Holocaust age-mates and, if so, how. Did
they respond with more anxiety or less? Or was there no substantial difference?
To put it differently, did the trials they endured during the Holocaust help them
cope with the difficulties of the Gulf War or evoke old anxieties that impaired
their ability to manage?

To answer these questions, we surveyed 192 senior citizens during the Gulf
War. Sixty-one (31.8%) of the sample were Holocaust survivors (Mean age = 68.3;
$SD = 7.2$); 131 (68.2%) were not (Mean age = 72.9; $SD = 7.5$). Most of them (88%)
lived in their own homes; the rest were residents of an urban community home
for the aged. Utilizing standardized questionnaires, we measured perceptions of
danger (level of personal safety during the war, e.g., "To what degree you feel that
your life is in danger?", "To what degree you assess that the country of Israel is in
danger of being annihilated?"), wartime psychological distress (stress symptoms; e.g., nightmares, startle response), and state–trait anxiety.

The findings show that elderly Holocaust survivors responded to the Gulf
War with greater distress than elderly nonsurvivors (see Table 6–1).

Holocaust survivors viewed the war as more dangerous, rating their own
danger, the danger of Israel's being annihilated, and the danger of the war to
their families higher than their nonsurvivor age-mates. They displayed both
greater state anxiety and greater trait anxiety than nonsurvivors. And significantly more survivors than nonsurvivors reported more specific, war-related
distress in the form of sleep disturbances (68.9% vs. 51.5%), concentration
difficulties or memory impairment (54.1% vs. 36.6%), apprehension and tension
(80.3% vs. 64%), nightmares (41% vs. 23.7%), loss of interest in significant

Table 6–1. Psychological Ratings during the Gulf War
for Elderly Israeli Survivors of the Holocaust and Other
Elderly Subjects[a]

	Holocaust survivors (N = 61)		Other subjects (N = 131)		
	Mean	SD	Mean	SD	F(1100)
Peceptions of danger	−0.2	0.9	0.5	1.1	2.29
Psychological distress	42.9	11.9	33.0	10.1	6.20
State anxiety	47.4	13.2	36.5	13.0	6.27
Trait anxiety	50.3	10.4	41.5	7.4	7.53[b]

[a]A multivariate analysis of covariance was performed with age, sex, education, religiosity, health, and proximity to bomb sites as covariates. Overall F
= 2.43, $df = 4,97$, $p < .05$.
[b]$p < .005$, with Bonferroni correction (Miller, 1981) for multiple comparisons.

activities (59% vs. 40.8%), sense of detachment from others (28.8% vs. 10.4%), as well as stronger feelings of panic and fear (37.7% vs. 16.9%), irritability (72% vs. 46.2%), excitability (65.6% vs. 48.1%), and feelings of hopelessness (42.6% vs. 11.6%).

In short, on all four of the measures, Holocaust survivors showed greater vulnerability than nonsurvivors. Moreover, with the exception of the sense of danger, the differences remained significant when the background factors that might bias the findings, including the differences in mean age and gender in the two groups, were controlled for.

We also assessed the impact of other prior stressful experiences on the responses of the elderly to the Gulf War (Hantman et al., 1994). These included both "objective" experiences of losing a child and earlier exposure to war and to war-related events, and the "subjective" sense of having previously experienced an event similar to the Gulf War. The nature of the "similar" event was neither defined nor queried, since the aim of this question was to investigate the role of symbolic associations in the response to stress. Surprisingly, none of the "objective" life events had any impact on how either the survivor or nonsurvivor group coped. But the "subjective" sense of having previously undergone a similar stressful experience had a significant impact on the coping of the survivors, though not on that of the nonsurvivors. Holocaust survivors who reported having had a prior experience similar to the Gulf War were even more vulnerable than other survivors. They reported a significantly greater sense of danger, lower sense of self-efficacy, and a higher level of trait, though not of state, anxiety. Among non-Holocaust survivors, no such differences were found. Neither their sense of danger, their self-efficacy, or their level of anxiety was affected by whether they had a prior experience similar to the Gulf War.

The findings of this study clearly show that Holocaust survivors were more vulnerable during the Gulf War than nonsurvivors. The findings to the effect that the survivors felt more danger, had higher state anxiety, and reported more symptoms of war-related stress than nonsurvivors show the residue of stress left by the Holocaust in the survivors' lives. So does the finding that they have higher trait anxiety than nonsurvivors. Together, these findings suggest that the survivors retain from their Holocaust experience both a generalized sensitivity to stress and a more specific sensitivity to the stress of war.

The findings are consistent both with the abundance of evidence that points to the pervasive, long-lasting damage of exposure to traumatic events and with the evidence cited earlier to the effect that survivors suffer from psychological difficulties that can be traced back to their Holocaust ordeal (e.g., Eitinger, 1980; Neiderland, 1968). They are also consistent with findings that the survivors are particularly susceptible to the resurgence of Holocaust-related memories, anxieties, and stresses in old age (Dasberg, 1987; Lomranz, 1990; Nadler, 1983). They are consistent, too, with studies of Holocaust survivors (Shanan & Shahar, 1983) that demonstrate their elevated sensitivity to issues of safety and security.

It seems that for many survivors, the Gulf War exacerbated or reactivated the trauma of the Holocaust. Similar exacerbation or reactivation was found by Christenson, Walker, Ross, and Maltbie (1981) among aging World War II veterans. Presenting a case of a reactivation "precipitated by an event that simulated the original trauma," they went on to suggest that "losses associated with involutional age, including parental loss, children leaving home, pending retirement and increasing medical disability all serve as stressors that may reactivate a latent traumatic stress disorder" (p. 985).

Like the studies reported here, studies of reactivation of traumas in the civilian sphere have also shown that reactivation can occur after many years of dormancy, and can be triggered by events only remotely reminiscent of the original trauma. For example, it has been shown that reactivation of unresolved grief reactions, in which the bereaved are suddenly reemerged in the mourning process—with all its attendant feelings of sadness, pining, and depression—can be triggered by a large range of events from deliberate recall through incidental reminders of the death (Lindeman, 1944). Similarly, Burgess and Halmstrom (1974) and Notman and Nadelson (1976) report the unresolved feelings of rape victims emerging many years after the assault and giving rise to acute depression, anxiety, and phobic behaviors, much like those commonly experienced in the period immediately following a rape. These findings suggest that it was indeed the associations of the Gulf War with the Holocaust (however remote the actual resemblance may have been), and their power to exacerbate or trigger reactivations of the survivors' Holocaust trauma, that made that war such a potent stressor.

The current findings are the reverse of the only other systematic study that assessed the effects of recurrent exposure among the elderly. Norris and Murrel (1988) found that elderly flood victims who had experienced prior floods fared emotionally better than those who had not. The Holocaust experience of the elderly survivors in our study did not similarly help them cope with the Gulf War. The discrepancy may be accounted for by two explanations.

One is that Israel's Holocaust survivors had probably experienced far more prior traumatic stress in their lives than either Norris and Morrel's flood victims or their nonsurvivor Israeli age-mates, who, as noted earlier, had been exposed to more potentially traumatic hardship than elderly people in less war-ridden parts of the world. Our findings suggest that even if life's "ordinary" stressors and natural disasters may strengthen a person's ability to cope, a massive catastrophe such as the Holocaust by and large depletes it.

The other explanation is that manmade disasters wreak a great deal more emotional damage than natural ones (Beigel & Berren, 1985; Frederick, 1980). Navon (1992) attributes the difference to the tendency of people to perceive the victims of human violence, as opposed to the victims of natural catastrophes, as at least partly responsible for their plight and to the aspersion that follows upon that perception. This explanation is supported by the cool reception that Holocaust survivors received when they first arrived in Israel, when they were blamed for everything from going to their deaths like sheep to the slaughter, to using unscrupulous means to survive. At the same time, it has been frequently pointed out that traumatic events undermine victims' basic trust and their belief in the goodness and continuity of the world (Janoff-Bulman, 1989). It might be argued that since survivors of man-made disasters experience not only of the unreliability of nature but also the cruelty and treachery of people, the damage to their trust is that much more extensive.

The finding that survivors who reported having had an earlier experience similar to the Gulf War showed more distress than those who did not points to the ability of a similar, earlier stressor—even if that similarity is purely subjective—to intensify the later stress it resembles. This finding is consistent with the results of a series of studies conducted on Israeli soldiers in the Lebanon War who had had acute or posttraumatic reactions to previous conflicts (Solomon, 1993). These studies indicated that the more the soldier's Lebanon encounter reminded him of his earlier traumatic experience, the more likely it was to exacerbate residual symptoms or to trigger a reactivation of his previous stress reaction. Like the Gulf War, the later stressor did not have to be as intense as the first or even of objectively major dimensions; it was enough that, in the soldier's mind, it resembled the first and evoked memories and associations.

Moreover, previous studies with war-induced stress casualties suggest that reactivation of prior trauma leaves the casualty even more vulnerable than before, suffering from more severe psychopathology and poorer psychosocial functioning (Solomon, Oppenheimer, Elitzur, and Waysman, 1990b). It seems that when exposed to the second trauma, the victims' resources were quite depleted, as their "reserved" resources had been used up in coping with the after-effects of the first experience.

The finding in the same study that none of the objective stresses queried—neither participation in other wars, nor the loss of loved ones—affected the survivors' coping with the Gulf War brings home the importance of the subjective meaning of an event in the reactivation of earlier traumas. Although it is common to speak of survivors as a group, individual survivors undoubtedly differ in how well they worked through their experience. Their subjective feelings during and about the Gulf War may be one index of that working through. This interpretation suggests that it was the survivors who sustained the most serious and long-lasting psychological injuries in the Holocaust who reported both previous experiences similar to the Gulf War and the strongest distress during it.

In summary, the study of the responses of Israel's Holocaust survivors to the Gulf War indicates that they continue to suffer from the detrimental results of their experience, even into old age. If the Gulf War can be taken as a reliable indicator, their Holocaust experience does not immunize them to subsequent stresses. On the contrary, it seems to have made it more difficult for them to endure the hardships. Or, in the words of the psychologist, Emanuel Berman, "Trauma does not heal trauma. Trauma only adds to trauma. Trauma deepens trauma" (cited in Solomon, 1993, p. 209).

REFERENCES

American Psychiatric Association. (1994). *Diagnostic and statistical manual of mental disorders* (4th ed.). Washington, DC: Author.

Baider, L., Peretz, T., & Kaplan De-Nour, A. (1992). Effect of the Holocaust on coping with cancer. *Social Science and Medicine, 34*, 11–15.

Baider, L., & Sarell, M. (1984). Coping with cancer among Holocaust survivors in Israel: An exploratory study. *Journal of Human Stress, 10*, 121–127.

Beigel, A., & Berren, M. R. (1985). Human induced disasters. *Psychiatric Annals, 15*, 143–150.

Bell, B. D. (1978). Disaster impact and response: Overcoming the thousand natural shocks. *Geron-tologist, 18*, 531–540.

Bolin, R., & Klenow, D. J. (1982–1983). Response of the elderly to disaster: An age-stratified analysis. *International Journal of Aging and Human Development, 16*, 283–296.

Bolin, R., & Klenow, D. J. (1988). Older people in disaster: A comparison of black and white victims. *International Journal of Aging and Human Development, 26*, 29–43.

Brockway, S. (1988). Case report: Flashback as a posttraumatic stress disorder (PTSD) symptom in a WWII veteran. *Military Medicine, 153*, 372–373.

Burgess, A. W., & Halmstrom, C. C. (1974). Rape trauma syndrome. *American Journal of Psychiatry, 131*, 981–986.

Carmeli, A., Mevorach, L., Leiberman, N., Taubman, A., Kahanovitz, S., & Navon, D. (1992). *The Gulf War: Home front in a test of crisis, final report.* Department of Behavioral Sciences, Israel Defense Force. [Hebrew]

Carmil, D., & Carel, R. S. (1986). Emotional distress and satisfaction in life among Holocaust survivors: A community study of survivors and controls. *Psychological Medicine, 16*, 141–149.

Christenson, R. M., Walker, J. L., Ross, D. R., & Maltbie, A. A. (1981). Reactivation of traumatic conflicts. *American Journal of Psychiatry, 138*, 984–985.

Coleman, Y. C., Butcher, Y. N., & Carson, R. C. (1980). *Abnormal psychology and modern life.* Glenview, IL: Scott, Foresman.

Danieli, Y. (1994). As survivors age: Part I. *Clinical Quarterly, 4*, 1–7.

Dasberg, H. (1987). Psychological distress of Holocaust survivors and their offspring in Israel, forty years later: A review. *Israel Journal of Psychiatry and Related Sciences, 24*, 243–256.

Eaton, W. W., Sigal, J. J., & Weinfeld, M. (1982). Impairment in Holocaust survivors after 33 years: Data from an unbiased community sample. *American Journal of Psychiatry, 139*, 773–777.

Eitinger, L. (1980). The Concentration Camp Syndrome and its late sequelae. In J. Dimsdale (Ed.), *Survivors, victims and perpetrators* (pp. 127–161). Washington, DC: Hemisphere.

Epstein, S. (1983). Natural healing processes of the mind: Graded stress inoculation as an inherent coping mechanism. In D. Michenbaum & M. Yarenko (Eds.), *Stress reduction and prevention* (pp. 39–66). New York: Plenum Press.

Eysenck, H. J. (1983). Personality as a fundamental concept in scientific psychology. *Austrian Journal of Psychology, 35*, 289–304.

Frederick, C. J. (1980). Effects of natural vs. human-induced violence. *Evaluation and Change* [Special Issue], 71–75.

Friedsman, H. J. (1961). Reactions of older persons to disaster-caused losses: An hypothesis of relative deprivation. *Gerontologist, 1*, 34–37.

Goenjian, A. K., Majarian, L. M., Pynoos, R. S., Steinberg, A. M., Manoukian, G., Tavosian, A., & Fairbanks, L. A. (1994). Posttraumatic stress disorder in elderly and younger adults after the 1988 earthquake in Armenia. *American Journal of Psychiatry, 151*, 895–901.

Goldstein, G., Van Kammen, W., Shelly, C., Miller, D., & Van Kammen, D. (1987). Survivors of imprisonment in the Pacific theatre during World War II. *American Journal of Psychiatry, 144*, 1210–1213.

Gray, D., & Calsyn, R. J. (1989). The relationship of stress and social support to life satisfaction: Age effects. *Journal of Community Psychology, 17*, 214–219.

Green, B. L., Grace, M. C., Lindy, J. D., & Leonard, A. C. (1990). Race differences in response to com-bat stress. *Journal of Traumatic Stress, 3*, 379–393.

Hagstrom, R. (1995). The acute psychological impact on survivors following a train accident. *Journal of Traumatic Stress, 8*, 391–402.

Hamner, M. B. (1994). Exacerbation of posttraumatic stress disorder symptoms with medical ill-ness. *General Hospital Psychiatry, 16*, 135–137.

Hantman, S., Solomon, Z., & Prager, E. (1994). The effect of previous exposure to traumatic stress on the responses of elderly people to the Gulf War. In J. Lomranz & G. Naveh (Eds.), *Trauma and old age: Coping with the stress of the Gulf War* (pp. 59–72). Jerusalem: JDC. [Hebrew]

Hermann, M. D., & Eryavec, G. (1994). Delayed onset post traumatic stress disorder in World War II veterans. *Canadian Journal of Psychiatry, 39*, 439–441.

Hertz, D. G. (1990). Trauma and nostalgia: New aspects on the coping of aging Holocaust survivors. *Israel Journal of Psychiatry and Related Sciences, 27*, 189–198.

Hirschfield, M. J. (1977). Care of the aging Holocaust survivors. *American Journal of Nursing, 20,* 1187–1189.

Hobfoll, S., Lomranz, J., Eyal, N., Bridges, A., & Tzemach, M. (1989). Pulse of a nation: Depressive mood reactions of Israelis to the Israel–Lebanon War. *Journal of Personality and Social Psychology, 56,* 1002–1012.

Huerta, F., & Horton, R. (1978). Coping behavior of elderly flood victims. *Gerontologist, 18,* 541–546.

Janis, I. L. (1971). *Stress and frustration.* New York: Harcourt Brace Jovanovich.

Janoff-Bulman, R. (1989). Assumptive worlds and the stress of traumatic events: Applications of the schema construct. *Social Cognition, 7,* 113–136.

Jones, G. H., & Lovell, J. W. T. (1987). Delayed psychiatric sequelae among Folkland War veterans. *Journal of the Royal College of General Practitioners, 37,* 34–35.

Kahana, B., Harel, Z., & Kahana, E. (1989). Clinical and gerontological issues facing survivors of the Nazi Holocaust. In P. Marcus & A. Rosenberg (Eds.). *Healing their wounds* (pp. 197–211). New York: Praeger.

Keinan, G. (1979). *The effects of personality and training variables on the experiences, stress and quality of performance in situations where physical integrity is threatened.* Unpublished doctoral thesis, Tel-Aviv University, Tel Aviv, Israel.

Kilijanek, T. S., & Drabek, T. E. (1979). Assessing long-term impacts of a natural disaster: A focus on the elderly. *Gerontologist, 19,* 555–566.

Kluznik, J. C., Speed, N. H., Van Valkenburg, C., & Magraw, R. (1986). Forty-year follow-up of United States prisoners of war. *American Journal of Psychiatry, 143,* 1443–1446.

Krause, N. (1987). Exploring the impact of a natural disaster on the health and psychological well-being of older adults. *Journal of Human Stress, 13,* 61–69.

Kuch, K., & Cox, B. J. (1992). Symptoms of PTSD in 124 survivors of the Holocaust. *American Journal of Psychiatry, 149,* 337–340.

Levav, I., & Abramson, J. H. (1984). Emotional distress among concentration camp survivors: A community study in Jerusalem. *Psychological Medicine, 14,* 215–218.

Lindemann, E. (1944). Symptomatology and management of acute grief. *American Journal of Psychiatry, 101,* 141–148.

Lomranz, J. (1990). Long-term adaptation to traumatic stress in light of adult development and aging perspectives. In M. A. Stephens, S. Crowther, S. Hobfoll, & D. L. Tennebaum (Eds.), *Stress and coping in later life families* (pp. 99–121). Washington, DC: Hemisphere.

Lomranz, J. (1994). Preface: Stress, trauma, and old age during the Gulf War. In J. Lomranz & G. Naveh (Eds.), *Trauma and old age: Coping with the stress of the Gulf War* (pp. 1–11). Jerusalem: JDC. [Hebrew]

Lomranz, J., & Eyal, N. (1994). A longitudinal study of depressive moods of men and women in several age groups during the Gulf War. In J. Lomranz & G. Naveh (Eds.), *Trauma and old age: Coping with the stress of the Gulf War* (pp. 13–29). Jerusalem: JDC. [Hebrew]

Long, N., Chamberlain, K., & Vincent, C. (1994). Effect of the Gulf War on reactivation of adverse combat-related memories in Vietnam veterans. *Journal of Clinical Psychology, 50,* 138–144.

McGrath, J. E. (1970). Setting measures and theses: An integrative review of some research of social and psychological factors in stress. In J. E. McGrath (Ed.), *Social and psychological factors in stress* (pp. 558–596). New York: Holt, Rinehart & Winston.

McNaughton, M. E., Smith, L. W., Patterson, T. L., & Grant, I. (1990). Stress, social support, coping resources, and immune status in elderly women. *Journal of Nervous and Mental Disease, 178,* 460–461.

Meichenbaum, D. (1985). *Stress inoculation training.* New York: Pergamon Press.

Melick, M. E., & Logue, J. N. (1985–1986). The effect of disaster on the health and well-being of older women. *International Journal of Aging and Human Development, 21,* 27–38.

Miller, J. A., Turner, J. G., & Kimball, E. (1981). Big Thompson Flood victims: One year later. *Family Relations, 30,* 111–116.

Miller, R. G. (1981). *Simultaneous statistical influence.* New York: Springer.

Nadler, A. (1983). Social psychology and social issues: Research and theory on help seeking and help receiving in applied settings. In A. Nadler & J. D. Fisher (Eds.), *New directions in helping* (Vol. 3). New York: Academic Press.

Navon, D. (1992, August). Appendix: Public fear legitimization. In A. Carmeli, L. Mevorach, N. Leiberman, A. Taubman, S. Kahanovitz, & D. Navon (Eds.), *The Gulf War: The home front in a test of crisis.* IDF, Department of Behavioral Sciences.

Neiderland, W. G. (1968). The problem of the survivor. In H. Krystal (Ed.). *Massive psychic trauma* (pp. 8–23). New York: International Universities Press.

Norris, F. H., & Murrel, S. A. (1988). Prior experience as a moderator of disaster impact on anxiety symptoms in older adults. *American Journal of Community Psychology, 16,* 665–683.

Notman, M., & Nadelson, C. (1976). The rape victim: Psychodynamic consideration. *American Journal of Psychiatry, 133,* 408–412.

Ollendick, D. G., & Hoffmann, M. (1982). Assessment of psychological reactions in disaster victims. *Journal of Community Psychology, 10,* 157–167.

Page, W. F., Engdahl, B. E., & Eberly, R. E. (1991). Prevalence and correlates of depressive symptoms among former prisoners of war. *Journal of Nervous and Mental Disease, 179,* 670–677.

Poulshock, S. W., & Cohen, E. S. (1975). The elderly in the aftermath of a disaster. *Gerontologist, 15,* 357–361.

Prager, E., & Solomon, Z. (1995a). Cognitive control as a buffer of war-induced stress in a middle-aged and older Israeli sample. *Aging and Society, 15,* 355–374.

Prager, E., & Solomon, Z. (1995b). Correlates of war-induced stress responses among late middle-aged and elderly Israelis. *International Journal of Aging and Human Development, 41,* 203–220.

Rosen, J., Reynolds, C. F., Yaeger, A. L., Houck, P. R., & Horowitz, L. F. (1991). Sleep disturbances in survivors of the Nazi Holocaust. *American Journal of Psychiatry, 148,* 62–66.

Rutledge, H. E., Hunter, E. J., & Dahl, B. B. (1979). Human values and the prisoner of war. *Environment and Behavior, 11,* 227–244.

Selye, H. (1956). *The stress of life.* New York: McGraw-Hill.

Shanan, J., & Shahar, O. (1983). Cognitive and personality functioning of Jewish Holocaust survivors during midlife transition in Israel. *Archives of Psychology, 135,* 275–294.

Silver, R. L., & Wortman, C. B. (1980). Coping with undesirable life events. In J. Garber & M. E. P. Seligman (Eds.), *Human helplessness* (pp. 279–340). New York: Academic Press.

Solomon, Z. (1993). *Combat stress reaction: The enduring toll of war.* New York: Plenum Press.

Solomon, Z. (1995). *Coping with war-induced stress: The Gulf War and the Israeli response.* New York: Plenum Press.

Solomon, Z., Mikulincer, M., & Jacob, B. R. (1987). Exposure to recurrent combat stress: Combat stress reaction among Israeli soldiers in the 1982 Lebanon War. *Psychological Medicine, 17,* 433–440.

Solomon, Z., Mikulincer, M., & Waysman, M. (1991). Delayed and immediate onset posttraumatic stress disorder: The role of life events and social resources. *Journal of Community Psychology, 19,* 231–236.

Solomon, Z., Oppenheimer, B., Elizur, Y., & Waysman, M. (1990a). Exposure to recurrent combat stress: Can successful coping in a second war heal combat-related PTSD from the past? *Journal of Anxiety Disorders, 4,* 141–145.

Solomon, Z., Oppenheimer, B., Elizur, Y., & Waysman, M. (1990b). Trauma deepens trauma: The consequences of recurrent combat stress reaction. *Israel Journal of Psychiatry and Related Sciences, 27,* 233–241.

Solomon, Z., & Prager, E. (1992). Elderly Israeli Holocaust survivors during the Persian Gulf War: A study of psychological distress. *American Journal of Psychiatry, 149,* 1707–1710.

Sperr, E. V., Sperr, S. J., Craft, R. S., & Boudewyns, P. A. (1990). MMPI profiles and posttraumatic symptomatology in former prisoners of war. *Journal of Traumatic Stress, 3,* 369–378.

Titchner, J. L. (1986). Post-traumatic decline: A consequence of unresolved destructive drives. In C. R. Figley (Ed.), *Trauma and its wake: Vol. 2. Traumatic stress, theory, research and intervention* (pp. 5–20). New York: Brunner/Mazel.

Titchner, J. L., & Ross, W. O. (1974). Acute or chronic stress as determinants of behavior, character, and neuroses. In S. Arieti & E. B. Brody (Eds.), *American handbook of psychiatry* (2nd Ed., pp. 39–60). New York: Basic Books.

Vinokur, A., & Selzer, M. (1975). Desirable versus undesirable life events: Their relationship to stress and mental distress. *Journal of Personality and Social Psychology, 32,* 329–337.

White, N. S. (1983). Post-traumatic stress disorder [Letter to the editor]. *Hospital and Community Psychiatry, 34,* 1061–1062.

Wilson, J. P., & Raphael, B. (1993). *International handbook of traumatic stress syndromes.* New York: Plenum Press.

CHAPTER 7

Toward a Temporal–Spatial Model of Cumulative Life Stress

Placing Late-Life Stress Effects in a Life-Course Perspective

BOAZ KAHANA AND EVA KAHANA

INTRODUCTION AND BACKGROUND

This chapter provides a conceptual framework for integrating the life-course research paradigm (Elder, George, & Shanahan, 1996) with the study of late-life stress effects. We discuss and integrate a series of studies, conducted by the authors and associates, that consider diverse ways in which lifelong stressors and trauma may impact on psychological well-being in later life and on adaptation to old age. The conceptual framework we propose recognizes both temporal and spatial dimensions of stressors and of their impact on late-life well-being. We also explore temporal and spatial dimensions of resistance resources and of stress impact as we propose a life-course-relevant stress paradigm.

This chapter complements the efforts of Gatz's work (Chapter 4, this volume), which attempts to build a theoretical framework for linking principles of life-course development to psychopathology. Gatz's framework, consistent with formulations of Zubin and Burdock (1965) is based on a focus of constitutional vulnerability (termed *diathesis*) and on stress as two elements that might contribute to late-life psychopathology. Our focus relates to a better understanding of the texture and timing of stress effects across the life course, focusing on the

BOAZ KAHANA • Department of Psychology, Cleveland State University, Cleveland, Ohio 44115. EVA KAHANA • Department of Sociology, Case Western Reserve University, Cleveland, Ohio 44106.

Handbook of Aging and Mental Health: An Integrative Approach, edited by Jacob Lomranz. Plenum Press, New York, 1998.

normal range of responses to stress among older individuals who manage, for the most part, to remain free of psychopathology in spite of stressful and even traumatic life circumstances. Thus, we attempt to understand the normal range of human responses to problematic life situations. This approach allows for a better understanding of the effects of stress throughout the life course, unencumbered by further complexities of constitutional vulnerabilities that may accompany the aging process and are indeed relevant to the emergence of major psychopathology in later life. Ultimately, a more detailed cumulative life-course framework for stress may incorporate stress–diatheses models of psychopathology. A major contribution of our analysis relates to the specification of both temporal and spatial dimensions of the stress process in relation to issues of life-course development. We term the framework and model we present the temporal–spatial model of cumulative life stress.

As the area of stress research has matured, there has been increasing recognition that a broad array of events and life situations place people at risk for developing negative outcomes (Wheaton, 1996). It is also recognized now that the timing of events throughout the life course may determine their differential influence on the individual (Elder et al., 1996). There has been little attention, however, paid to the potential of earlier events, as well as more recent life events, for having a cumulative influence on mental health in later life. This chapter discusses and integrates a series of studies conducted by the authors and their associates that consider diverse ways in which lifelong stressors and trauma impact on psychological well-being in later life. Data are presented to address the impact of negative life events and crises occurring early in life, throughout adult life, and in late life on mental health of the elderly. Our research spans general populations of community-based elders, as well as older individuals who have endured extreme trauma. Our studies include racially diverse, urban aged (Kahana, Oakes, Slotterback, Kercher, & Kahana, 1996a; Kahana et al., 1995; Nauta, Brooks, Johnson, Kahana, & Kahana, 1995), elderly living in Florida retirement communities (Kahana & Kahana, 1996; Kahana, Namazi, Kahana, & Brown, 1996b), and survivors of the Nazi Holocaust living in the United States and in Israel (Harel, Kahana & Kahana, 1988; Kahana, Harel, & Kahana, 1988, 1989; Kahana et al., 1997; Kahana, Kahana, Harel, & Rosner, 1988). This chapter will thus contribute to an understanding of potential and actual influences of a broad array of major life events and chronic stressors, which occur throughout life, on mental health during later life. Our conceptual discussion relates to the value of considering long-term consequences of events that occur throughout the lifespan in both a spatial and temporal perspective.

The life-course paradigm has only recently been superimposed on the study of stress. The paradigm (Elder et al., 1996) emphasizes the importance of early life transitions for shaping later life experiences and outcomes. In this framework, it is understood that a full life history of stressful events and life situations defines the experience and appraisal of later life for the individual. The importance of key historical events, such as the Great Depression, have been recognized as shaping late-life adaptation of a whole generation of individuals (Clausen, 1991).

Elder et al. (1996), call attention to four themes relevant to the stress process within the life-course-based research paradigm. These include (1) placement of human lives in a historical context, (2) recognition of both "human agency" and "social constraints" in shaping behavior, (3) consideration of the temporal framework of lives both in terms of timetables and event sequences, and (4) the view of individual lives as interdependent and linked to those of significant others. In the ensuing discussion, we attempt to address these issues as they relate to the study of late-life effects of both lifelong and recent stress. We also consider the usefulness of alternative conceptualizations and measures of stress for predicting psychological distress in late life (Kahana et al., 1995, 1996a, 1996b).

Gerontological stress research has had rich and diverse traditions, and relevant empirical work derives from approaches of general stress research and traumatic stress studies. An extensive literature has documented negative sequelae of recent stressful life events on both physical and mental health of older adults (E. Kahana, 1992). The focus of research in this field has generally been on singular, specific, recent life events such as widowhood or retirement (Chiriboga, 1992), or on the cumulative impact of diverse recent stressors, as measured by life event inventories (Dohrenwend & Dohrenwend, 1974; Kahana, Fairchild, & Kahana, 1982). The time frame considered in these studies is usually 6 months to 3 years, with the expectation that stressors have their greatest impact soon after they occur, and that stress effects have a limited duration (Norris & Murrell, 1987). Furthermore, based on their reduced social and physiological resources, the aged are thought to be particularly sensitive to health consequences of recent life stressors (Steptoe, Moses, & Edwards, 1990). With increasing sophistication of research in this area, attention has been directed to a broad array of stressors, including hassles (Lazarus & Folkman, 1984), chronic stressors (Pearlin, 1980), and acute positive (Teri & Lewinsohn, 1982) and negative events (Chiriboga, 1992). In spite of theoretical suggestions about the importance of cumulative life crises in contributing to adverse health outcomes, gerontological research has not explored the potential impact of lifelong stress exposure on late-life adaptation (Kahana, 1992b).

There is an alternative, growing research tradition that considers the enduring and long-term impact of traumatic life experiences (Wilson & Raphael, 1993). Studies focusing on trauma from the distant past have frequently dealt with wartime experiences. Researchers who have investigated the effects of war experiences among aging veterans have documented the health problems associated with combat trauma or being a prisoner of war (Blake, Cook, & Keane, 1992; Solomon, Mikulincer, & Kotler, 1987; Wilson, Harel, & Kahana, 1989). Similarly, studies of Holocaust survivors have demonstrated the negative effects of traumatic experiences endured during the Holocaust on later-life health and psychological well-being of survivors (Harel et al., 1988; Kahana et al., 1989).

Additional areas of traumatic stress research include early bereavement and other forms of victimization, such as child abuse and being the victim of a crime. Negative health and mental health sequelae have also been found in individuals who have suffered parental loss in childhood (Breier et al., 1988; Harris, 1991) or loss of a partner in adulthood (Stroebe & Stroebe, 1996). Increased general health complaints and somatic concerns have been shown in parents after the death of an adult child (Shanfield & Swain, 1984), and childhood abuse has been associated with a variety of adult health and mental health problems (Arnold & Rogers, 1990; Breier & Runtz, 1988). Indications exist that even decades after the occurrence of significant loss events, the survivors continue to ruminate about these events and search for meaning related to them (Tait & Silver, 1989). Although singular traumas associated with the distant past have been shown to influence health and mental health in later life, it remains to be clarified which types of trauma are most harmful.

The impact of early life stress has generally been studied in clinical populations and among groups exposed to specific traumatic events. The focus of these studies has been on a singular, albeit overwhelming trauma, whereas the relative impact of a lifetime experience of diverse crises has seldom been investigated. There has been little research attention directed at more chronic life crises such as poverty, unemployment, and interpersonal crises, which are prevalent features of the life histories of substantial numbers of elderly people. There is now research evidence suggesting that when lifetime experiences of cumulative trauma are considered rather than the occurrence of a single traumatic life event, there is a major increase in prevalence rates of mental health problems (Turner, Wheaton, & Lloyd, 1995). There may be much to be learned from considering accumulated lifetime trauma comprised of both chronic and acute events (Kahana, et al., 1995).

EMPIRICAL PERSPECTIVES

We now turn to our empirical work exploring the impact of both recent life events and cumulative life crises on late-life psychological well-being. All of the research we review considers late-life mental health consequences of cumulative life stress. In addition, our studies are relevant to life-course-related issues of social timing, historical time and place, linked lives, and social constraints and opportunities. Our recent studies and a conceptual framework we developed for understanding successful aging (Kahana & Kahana, 1996) introduce issues of human agency as relevant to our temporal–spatial model of cumulative life stress. Where study findings have been previously published, we provide only narrative summaries. Where findings are presented in print for the first time, more statistical detail is provided.

STUDY 1: LIFE CRISES AS RELATED
TO MENTAL HEALTH IN LATE LIFE

Our research focusing on cumulative life crises and their sequelae among urban elders sought to assess both the aggregate and individual impacts of significant negative life events or life crises that older individuals experienced throughout their lives (Kahana, Oakes, Slotterback, Kercher, & Kahana, 1996). We hypothesized that major traumatic events in aggregate, as well as individually, may impact on older adults' psychological distress. Focus on cumulative life crises was viewed as a promising approach to understanding stress–mental health linkages. Since stress is likely to translate into psychological reactions over a long period of time, we anticipated that focusing on stressors over a longer time span would maximize observations of adverse effects. Consideration of major, early life stressors also diminishes concerns about direction of causal order between stressors and their health and well-being outcomes. We focused on mental health as the major dependent variable to permit specification of the impact of both aggregate and individual stressors on alternative health and well-being outcomes. In our Study 1, mental health, the dependent variable, was defined in terms of varying degrees of psychological distress (Langner, 1962).

Study Participants

The respondents were 309 subscribers to the Health Alliance Plan, a health maintenance organization in a large Midwestern metropolitan area. They were aged 65 or older, and were living in the community at the time of the interview. Gender composition of the sample was 50.4% male and 49.6% female. The respondents were almost evenly divided between black and white racial groups. Furthermore, the two racial groups were of similar socioeconomic background. All study participants were either retired from the auto industry or spouses of retired auto workers, with a median income of $12,500. Respondents were interviewed individually in their homes by professional interviewers.

Measures

Psychological distress was measured using a modification of Langner's (1962) psychiatric symptom screening measure, which has been successfully used in prior research on psychological distress among older adults (Haug, Breslau, & Folmar, 1989) and in other studies. Recent and past life crises were assessed using the Antonovsky Life Crisis Inventory (Antonovsky, 1979). This instrument inquires about the occurrences of 19 major life stressors over the person's lifetime. The inventory was designed to assess life stress associated with employment instability and financial hardships, the death of loved ones, major interpersonal problems, life-threatening illnesses, and wartime experiences. The items cover the full lifespan, ranging from experiences in childhood up to the recent past.

Results

The two most frequently occurring events were "ever divorced or widowed," experienced by 72.5% of respondents, and "friend or person close having died in past three years," experienced by 72.2%. It is also noteworthy that 47% experienced a life-threatening illness, 45% had been unable to find work, and approximately 40% lost a parent, due to divorce or widowhood, before the age of 15. Furthermore, approximately 35% of the respondents had a sibling who died in childhood or adolescence, and 30% had a child who died. Thus, this cohort of older persons has experienced a considerable share of life crises and trauma. All of the life crises identified by Antonovsky were endorsed by substantial proportions of the sample. Even the least frequently noted event ("betrayal of another person by respondent") was endorsed by almost 8% of the sample.

Regression analyses were conducted to assess the ability of diverse life events to singularly and cumulatively predict mental health outcomes. The life crises in aggregate proved to be predictive of psychological distress ($R^2 = .22$; $p < .01$).

Psychological Distress.   Seven out of 19 individual life crises were found to be significant predictors of psychological distress. Reporting prior experiences of the following life crises was associated with reporting more psychological distress symptoms: (1) being so ill that one's life was in danger (Beta = .14, $p < .05$); (2) being divorced or widowed (Beta = .13, $p < .05$); (3) not having had enough to eat for several months (Beta = .15, $p < .05$); (4) quarreling badly with someone close to you (Beta = .13, $p < .05$); (5) very bad home conditions (Beta = .19, $p < .05$); (6) being denied a deserved promotion (Beta = .12, $p < .05$); (7) family ever in financial debt (Beta = .15, $p < .05$).

Discussion

Data from this study confirm the role of major stressors, occurring throughout life, in contributing to mental health problems during later life. As one of the initial studies considering the contribution of life crises occurring throughout life to later-life well-being, our study used a major existing scale for the assessment of life crises, which was developed by Antonovsky (1979). This scale moves beyond the general approach of linking assessment of overall stress to recently occurring events. It also encompasses specific, discrete events, along with long-term, chronic life crises. It is noteworthy that both chronic and acute stressors, and diverse types of stress ranging from interpersonal to social and financial difficulties, all contributed to late-life psychological distress. The Antonovsky Life Crisis Inventory stops short of dating the occurrences of life crises. It specifies stages during the life course when crises occurred only for some of the items included. In future studies, it would be useful to identify both timing and duration of all events considered. Such an approach will permit the identification of points during the life course when specific crises are most likely to occur and relate timing of crises to occurrence of long-term adverse outcomes.

STUDY 2: CONSIDERING THE CUMULATIVE IMPACT OF LIFE CRISES AND RECENT LIFE EVENTS

Research on stress has given increasing attention to past traumatic events extending as far back as childhood and their effects on elderly persons' psychological well-being. Another component of research has focused on recent negative life events (e.g., personal and family illness or death, marital breakdowns, financial problems) as contributing to depression and dysphoria (for a review, see Kahana, 1992b). However, the combined impact of lifelong trauma and recent life events on quality of life has not been fully explored. The purpose of our second study (Kahana, Namazi, Kercher, Kahana, & Brown, 1996) was to investigate how individual items reflecting lifelong trauma based on life crises noted in Antonovsky's and Norris's Life Crisis Inventories and items reflecting recent stressors as measured by the Elderly Care Research Center Recent Life Events Inventory (Kahana et al., 1982) affect psychological well-being in old-old persons.

Study Participants

Data for this study were derived from the third annual wave of an 8-year longitudinal study of healthy residents in three Florida retirement communities. Face-to-face interviews were conducted among the elderly, who were at least 72 years old and residents of Florida for a minimum of 9 months out of the year. The randomly selected sample consisted of 787 elderly participants. The sample was comprised mostly of women (65.6%), with an average of 13.45 years of education, a median income of $20,000–24,999, and an average age of 81 years.

Measures

The domain of psychological well-being was measured in this study by five scales: (1) Center for Epidemiological Studies Depression Scale (CES-D; Radloff, 1977), (2) Positive and Negative Affect Scales (PANAS) (Watson, Clark, & Tellegen, 1988), (3) Cognitive Life Satisfaction Scale (Diener, Emmons, Larsen, & Griffin, 1985), (4) Symptom Checklist Distress Scale (Derogatis, Lipman, & Covi, 1973), and (5) Rosenberg Self-Esteem Scales (Rosenberg, 1979).

Recent stresses were measured using the Recent Life Events Inventory (Kahana et al., 1982). This scale measures the occurrence of 11 events that have been reported with high frequency by the aged and provide evaluation of each event as a problem event.

Life crises were assessed using items from the Antonovsky Life Crisis Inventory (Antonovsky, 1979) and the Norris Life Events Inventory (Norris & Murrell, 1987). These instruments inquire about the occurrences of major life stressors over the life course. The addition of the Norris Inventory, with its inclusion of natural disasters, abuse, and criminal victimization, increased the scope of the life crises previously assessed by the Antonovsky Inventory. The items cover the full lifespan, ranging from experiences in childhood up to the recent past. This 10-item scale is referred to in this chapter as the Antonovsky–Norris Inventory.

Results

This primarily middle-class old-old population participating in the study reported far lower rates of specific life crises than did the working-class urban, elderly population considered in Study 1. The effects of early and recent life events on subjective well-being were assessed by regressing each outcome variable on individual items of the Antonovsky–Norris Inventory and Recent Life Events Inventory. Separate regression procedures indicated that individual items in both inventories accounted for some negative outcomes.

Among Antonovsky–Norris Life Crisis items, life-threatening illness, and other events were significant predictors of reduced psychological well-being. Overall, life-threatening illness was strongly linked with feelings of depression and symptom distress. In addition, experience of life-threatening illness was associated with self-esteem, life satisfaction, and negative affect. The category "other events" was strongly associated with depression, symptom distress, life satisfaction, self-esteem, and negative affect.

Several items from the Recent Life Events Inventory were also found to be significant predictors of reduced psychological well-being. The strongest relationships involved conflict with others that predicted the following: negative affect, depression, symptom distress, self-esteem, and life satisfaction. The next strongest associations occurred between financial difficulty and outcome variables of life satisfaction, as well as symptom distress, depression, self-esteem, and negative affect. Significant associations of similar strength were also found between neighbor problems and symptom distress, life satisfaction, and negative affect. Finally, family illness/injury and negative affect were strongly associated.

These findings point to the value of considering the cumulative effects of stress throughout the life course by aggregating early life crises with recent life events in stress research. These data portray small but consistent adverse effects of negative events throughout life on multiple indicators of psychological well-being. Our data support the value of considering both recent and long-term stressors and trauma in contributing to adverse effects on mental health and physical health in later life. Furthermore, both Studies 1 and 2 point to the heuristic value of in-depth exploration of wartime stress and stress related to historical events in seeking a life-course-relevant understanding of cumulative stress.

STUDY 3: FOCUS ON LINKED LIVES AND LATE-LIFE IMPACT OF EVENTS OCCURRING TO SIGNIFICANT OTHERS

The concept of linked lives in relation to stress may be addressed in considering the relative importance of self-relevant versus significant other-relevant negative life events as they contribute to late-life well-being. In a recent study (Nauta, Brooks, Johnson, Kahana, & Kahana, 1995), we explored this issue in relation to recent life events.

It has been argued that as adults age and become more "generative," using Erikson's (1963) developmental framework, events happening to significant family members may hold greater risk for negative outcomes than those happening to the self. Aldwin (1990) has termed such events as nonegocentric events and suggests that for elderly who are more focused on the next generation than on their own selves, these events assume increasing salience. In our research, we used both cross-sectional and longitudinal data to explore the relative importance of self-relevant and other-relevant events in late life. We hypothesized that there would be a positive relationship between age and the reporting of life changes attributed to nonegocentric or other-relevant events. We also hypothesized that, as older people become increasingly concerned with the welfare of others, they might suffer more adverse consequences due to significant other-relevant versus self-relevant events.

In this study, we conducted longitudinal analyses based on the urban study population described in the first study discussed in this chapter (Kahana et al., 1996a). Data were collected from 397 elderly persons enrolled in a Detroit-area health maintenance organization as part of a two-wave panel study concerned with life stress and illness. Study 3 used data collected during both waves of the study with retests involving a 1-year interval.

Egocentric and nonegocentric stressors were measured using the Geriatric Scale of Recent Life Events (Kiyak, Liang, & Kahana, 1976). Respondents were asked to indicate which events they had experienced in the year prior to the interview, and the amount of change they experienced as a consequence of the event. An individual's score on the Life Events Scale was calculated as the sum of the amount of change reported for those events the respondent had experienced.

Assignment of life events to egocentric or nonegocentric categories was done according to the scheme described by Aldwin (1990). Egocentric items are those representing circumstances that impact directly upon the individual, while those impacting on family members are described as nonegocentric. Two measures of psychological well-being were used in this study, one measuring symptoms of psychological distress, herein referred to as mental health, and one measuring morale. The mental health measure is an additive scale, consisting of 14 items from Langner's Twenty-Two Item Scale (1962). Nine of the 22 items from the Philadelphia Geriatric Center Morale Scale (Lawton, Moss, Fulcomer, & Kleban, 1982) comprised our morale measure.

Cross-sectional data reveal that both self-relevant (egocentric) and other-relevant (nonegocentric) events had significant negative effects on mental health when they were considered in separate analyses. When both types of events were entered in analyses together, only the nonegocentric events retained their negative relationship with the Langner Mental Health Scale (1962). In the longitudinal analyses, neither egocentric nor nonegocentric events were found to have a significant relationship to changes in psychological well-being over a 1-year period.

These data, based on cross-sectional analyses, provide support for the importance of other-relevant as well as self-relevant events in late life. Such effects are not observed when short-term changes in mental health over time are considered. Nevertheless, this research encourages further inquiry into the consideration of stress in the context of linked lives.

STUDY 4: STRESS VULNERABILITY BASED ON DEMOGRAPHIC CHARACTERISTICS AND STRESS APPRAISALS

In another recent paper, we explored in greater detail the role of structural constraints, reflected in sociodemographic characteristics, as well as personal appraisals along with diverse indicators of lifelong stress, recent life events, and chronic stressors (Kahana, Redmond, Hill, Kercher, Kahana, Johnson, & Young, 1995). This more comprehensive approach reflected an acknowledgment that social constraints may exacerbate the impact of diverse stressors on the elderly. At the same time, we sought to understand the processes whereby stressful life events are most likely to exert their influence on the elderly by focusing on the role of domain-specific satisfactions as potential mediators in the stress paradigm. We based our expectations in this area on prior research (Krause, 1991) that suggests that older adults are likely to assess the impact of stress by evaluating their satisfaction with specific domains in their lives such as health, family, and finances. We then synthesized these specific assessments into a general appraisal of psychological well-being. Accordingly, specific stressors may get translated into frustrations related to specific life domains, which may in turn generalize as distress.

Specific stressful experiences of the distant and recent past, as well as chronic stressors in aggregate, may translate into appraisals of the present as unsatisfying. These appraisals may lead to more global psychological distress, manifesting in symptoms of depression or anxiety. We termed this conceptual orientation a transactional stress model, predicated on appraisal-based mediators (Kahana et al., 1995).

Data we obtained as part of our study of 397 urban elders are described in Studies 1 and 3. Our findings lend support to expectations that demographic factors may pose both constraints and opportunities in relation to the stress process. Consideration of gender, marital status, race, income, and education in relation to effects of diverse stressors presented evidence of complex processes whereby social constraints shape the stress experience.

Our research documented that social structure, translated through demographic factors, may impinge on every element of the stress paradigm. On the one hand, social disadvantages may result in greater stress exposure; on the other hand, they may create lower expectations and hence diminish incongruence between aspirations and reality, thereby limiting frustrations. Our findings revealed significant positive effects of education, income, and race in relation to mental health outcomes. Interestingly, African Americans, who were of comparable socioeconomic status to whites, reported higher morale and better psychological well-being in this study. Gender effects proved to be complex, with women reporting greater satisfaction in terms of both health and activity domains, but also reporting greater psychological distress when the positive affects of domain-specific satisfaction and well-being outcomes are controlled.

Our data in this study provided partial support for an appraisal-based model of stressor effects on psychological well-being. Strongest support for the model was observed in the area of health. The significant impact of objective indicators of functional health on psychological well-being was found to be largely determined by health appraisals. The focus of this research on social constraints and opportunities is considered within a life-course framework. This study also moves our research program from primary interest in the impact of diverse stressors on outcomes to a recognition of mediators and/or moderators in the stress process.

STUDY 5: FOCUS ON LATE-LIFE EFFECTS OF EXTREME TRAUMA BASED ON SURVIVORS OF THE NAZI HOLOCAUST

The long-term impact of extreme trauma experienced in earlier life on psychological well-being, social adaptation, and physical health was examined in our major studies of elderly Holocaust survivors living in the United States and Israel (Harel, Kahana, & Kahana, 1988; Kahana, Harel, & Kahana, 1988, 1989, 1997; Kahana, Kahana, Harel, & Rosner, 1989). This study made an important contribution toward understanding long-term sequelae of major trauma. Our research was predicated on the recognition that trauma may be anchored in historical time and place. The defining feature of the stress studied was the very experience of a historical event of traumatic proportions. In studying the impact of trauma, we considered not only mental health, but also social outcomes. Furthermore, we explored whether the effects of trauma were attenuated or exacerbated by aging. We also considered personal agency in terms of coping with both immediate and long-term effects of the trauma.

The spectrum of life crises and chronic stressors that were cumulatively experienced by elderly survivors of the Holocaust have been placed in a historical and life-course perspective in our research (see Table 7–1). We argue that the trauma of the Holocaust involved a constellation of environmental assaults that, in turn, created further endurance of chronic stresses. Chronic stressors that resulted from earlier trauma of the Holocaust include intrusive memories of trauma, living with fear and mistrust, social and psychological isolation, and living with stigma (Kahana et al., 1997). The adaptive tasks confronting survivors in late life include achieving some measure of psychological well-being and maintaining physical health and social function in the face of these chronic stressors, as well as the initial trauma that set chronic stressors into motion.

Study Participants

Respondents in this research included a survivor group and a comparison group in each of two countries: the United States and Israel. Participants included Holocaust survivors who immigrated to Israel or to the United States between the end of World War II and 1965, and groups of Jewish immigrants who arrived in the United States or Israel several years prior to World War II. The total

Table 7–1. A Temporal–Spatial Framework for Cumulative Life Stress: Dimensions of Stressors

I. Dimensions of stressors	II. Salient variables or processes	III. Life-course relevance	IV. Empirical findings
1. Spatial			
a. Magnitude	Hassles		—
	Life events		Kahana, Namazi, Kahana, & Brown, 1996b
	Life crises		Kahana, Oakes, Slotterback, Kercher, & Kahana, 1996a
	Trauma		Kahana, Kahana, Harel, Kelly, Monaghan, & Holland, 1997
b. Incidence	Normative/nonnormative		Kahana, Namazi, Kahana, & Brown, 1996b
	Common/rare		Nauta, Brooks, Johnson, Kahana, & Kahana, 1995
c. Type	Health		All citations
	Financial		All citations
	Interpersonal		All citations
	Environmental		All citations
	Other		
d. Locus	Self-related/other-related	Linked lives	Nauta, Brooks, Johnson, Kahana, & Kahana, 1995
	Individual–dyadic–systemic		—
e. Desirability	Positive–negative		All citations
2. Temporal			
a. Life stage	Early life, midlife, late life		Kahana, Oakes, Slotterback, Kercher, & Kahana, 1996a
b. Historical time and place	On-time/off-time	Historical time and place	—
c. Social timing	Holocaust	Social timing	Kahana, Kahana, Harel, Kelly, Monaghan, & Holland, 1997
d. Recency	Long-term stressors		Kahana, Oakes, Slotterback, Kercher, & Kahana, 1996a
	Recent life stressors		Kahana, Namazi, Kahana, & Brown, 1996b
e. Duration	Brief vs. enduring stressors		Kahana, Oakes, Slotterback, Kercher, & Kahana, 1996a
f. Sequencing	Primary and secondary stressors		Kahana, Kahana, Harel, Kelly, Monaghan, & Holland, 1997

sample of 663 comprised 168 Holocaust survivors and 155 immigrants who settled in the United States, and 180 Holocaust survivors and 160 immigrants who settled in Israel. Respondents in both groups were from countries that were under the occupation of Nazi Germany during World War II. All respondents were individually interviewed in their own homes by trained interviewers. At the time of the study, respondents ranged in age from 45–90, with the survivors' ages being somewhat younger than respondents in the comparison groups. Women (55%) outnumbered men slightly, and a somewhat higher percentage of survivors were married relative to the comparison group (82% vs. 69%). The highest percentage of respondents originated from Poland (57%), followed by lower percentages from Czechoslovakia (13%), Germany (9%), and Hungary (8%), plus other countires (13%).

Results and Discussion

In examining Holocaust survivors living in the United States compared to those in the nontraumatized comparison group (U.S. sample) on symptoms of psychological distress (SCL-90), we found that survivors obtain significantly higher scores on all of these scales. Clinicians are thus correct in stating that trauma survivors, as a group, portray psychological symptomatology. However, this is counterbalanced by the fact that the vast majority of survivors obtain low symptomatology scores (compared to medium or high scores) on the SCL-90. Having experienced the prolonged and repeated traumas of the Holocaust, it is noteworthy that high percentages of survivors portray relatively good mental health on this measure. We note here the strong resiliency and hardiness of survivors, as a group.

An important life-course-relevant hypothesis explored in this research is that survivors would find the aging process and the elderly years particularly difficult to confront. The rationale offered by clinicians for such expectations is that Holocaust survivors do not have role models for aging, since their parents were killed before they became aged. Furthermore, the stresses of the Holocaust would render survivors more vulnerable to the normal stresses of aging (vulnerability hypothesis as opposed to inoculation hypothesis). Our research findings provide illuminating data on this question. Thus, 45% of our survivors stated that the Holocaust made it more difficult for them to cope with aging. In contrast, 29% said it made no difference, and surprisingly, 26% said that their Holocaust experience made it easier for them to cope with the aging process (e.g., "Once you survive the Holocaust, you can survive normal aging"). Our data regarding late-life events reveal that Holocaust survivors cope with the positive and negative events in their daily lives quite similarly to the comparison group in spite of their earlier traumatic life experiences.

These findings confirm expectations regarding the adverse effects of the Holocaust on survivors, but with some major modifications that support remarkable resilience. Our data do not provide evidence that Holocaust survivors as a group experience more difficulty with psychological aspects of aging than comparison groups. We have seen from our research that elderly survivors have an often unheralded potential to find meaning in adversity and to share this meaning with others.

A TEMPORAL–SPATIAL FRAMEWORK
OF LATE-LIFE STRESS EFFECTS

Based on the conceptual and empirical perspectives we reviewed, we propose a life-course-relevant conceptual framework for considering late-life sequelae of lifelong stress. This framework builds on prior classification systems in the literature (Gatz & Smyer, 1983; Pearlin, Lieberman, Menaghan, & Mullan, 1981) but introduces greater specificity and organization by simultaneously considering both *spatial* and *temporal* dimensions of stressors and addressing their relevance to the life-course paradigm (Table 7–1). By distinguishing temporal from spatial aspects of stress in our model, we introduce both life-course relevance and greater specificity to guide conceptualization and research. In addition, we also make some initial steps toward consideration of resistance resources (Table 7–2) and stress impact (Table 7–3) in a temporal–spatial framework.

As shown in the first column of Tables 7–1 to 7–3, we propose consideration of both temporal and spatial dimensions of stressors, protective resources, and outcomes in the stress model. Column I specifies components of spatial and temporal classifications used in prior research. Column II details the salient variables or processes for understanding each component of stressors, protective resources, and outcomes. Column III notes relevance to elements of the life-course paradigm and column IV provides examples based on our empirical findings, which were described earlier.

Stressors: Spatial Dimensions

Spatial dimensions of stressors refer to traditional classification systems that are relevant to the magnitude, incidence, type, locus, or desirability of the stressful event (Table 7–1). Regarding *magnitude* of stressors, in our prior research, we have been concerned primarily with events of greater magnitude, such as recent life events, life crises, and trauma. Research on the late-life impact of stressors has not generally focused on more minor stressors such as hassles. Since hassles are not generally expected to have a great impact on health and well-being in late life, studies reviewed in this chapter did not specifically deal with hassles. Regarding *incidence* of stressful events, the gerontological literature has usefully distinguished between commonly occurring or normative, and rare, nonnormative events (Kahana & Kahana, 1996). Normative events of late life include ill health and losses, and lack of person–environment fit (Kahana & Kahana, 1996). Nonnormative events such as criminal victimization or natural disasters are generally studied in the framework of traumatic stress research (Wilson & Raphael, 1993).

Table 7–2. A Temporal–Spatial Framework for Cumulative Life Stress: Dimensions of Protective Resources

I. Dimensions of protective resources	II. Salient variables or processes	III. Life-course relevance	IV. Empirical findings
1. Spatial			
Type of Resource			
a. Individual	Dispositions		
	Hopefulness/optimism		Kahana, Kahana, Harel, Kelly, Monaghan, & Holland, 1997
	Self-esteem		
	Coping stratgies	Agency	Kahana & Kahana, 1996
	Behavior		
	Preventive adaptation		
	Corrective adaptation		Kahana & Kahana, 1996
b. Environmental	Social supports		
	Financial resources		
c. Societal	Demographic background: gender, race, education	Social constraints Opportunities	Kahana, Redmond, Hill, Kercher, Kahana, Johnson, & Young, 1995; Kahana & Kahana, 1996
2. Temporal			
a. Stability of personal resources	Change vs. stability in dispositions		Kahana & Kahana, 1996
b. Timing of environmental resources	Social supports: Intermittent vs. continuous Short-term vs. long-term		Kahana, Kahana, Harel, Kelly, Monaghan, & Holland, 1997
c. Life stage specificity of resources	Childhood, adulthood, old age		—
d. Social changes affecting resources	Historical changes in opportunity structures		Kahana, Redmond, Hill, Kercher, Kahana, Johnson, & Young, 1995

Table 7–3. A Temporal–Spatial Framework for Cumulative Life Stress: Dimensions of Stress Impact and Outcomes

I. Dimensions of stress impact and outcomes	II. Salient variables or processes	III. Life-course relevance	IV. Empirical findings

1. Spatial
  a. Type of impact
	Mental health
	  Clinical problems
	    PTSD
	    Psychopathology
	    Psychological distress
	    Low morale
			Kahana, Redmond, Hill, Kercher, Kahana, Johnson, & Young, 1995
			
			All citations

	Physical health
	  Self-diagnosed illnesses
	  Self-rated overall physical health
	  Functional ability
			Kahana & Kahana, 1996

	Social functioning Meaning in life		Kahana, Kahana, Harel, Kelly, Monaghan, & Holland, 1997
b. Magnitude of impact	Degree of adverse reaction		All citations
2. Temporal a. Timing of impact onset	Immediate vs. delayed		Kahana, Kahana, Harel, Kelly, Monaghan, & Holland, 1997
b. Duration of impact	Temporary vs. long-term		—
c. Age specificity of impact (onset and duration)	Critical life stage periods of greatest impact		—
	Attenuated or exacerbated by aging		Kahana, Kahana, Harel, Kelly, Monaghan, & Holland, 1997

Regarding *type* of event, classification systems allow for an almost infinite variety. The literature on older adults typically specifies health-related, financial, and interpersonal events. The literature on trauma focuses on events in the natural or social environment, distinguishing between man-made and natural disasters (Wilson & Raphael, 1993). Our research on life crises (Kahana et al., 1996a) suggests that different types of events (e.g., loss or interpersonal conflict) may result in different patterns of long-term outcomes.

Regarding *locus* of a stressful event, consideration of self- versus other-related locus of events provides a useful bridge to the life-course paradigm outlined by Elder et al. (1996). Our empirical work (Nauta et al., 1995) has addressed distinctions between self-related and other-related (egocentric and nonegocentric) events. It is noteworthy that both our prior work, reported in Study 3, and that of Aldwin (1990) each focused only on distinctions between self- versus other-related recent life events. Yet specifying locus of the event may also be useful when applied to lifelong stress. The life-course paradigm, which we propose, may facilitate future studies of stress that explicitly acknowledge events and strains occurring to significant others in the context of linked lives. Thus, a phenomenon such as caregiving, which is a seminal example of life stress in the context of linked lives, may be studied from a life-course perspective. We have previously developed a framework for such consideration of the caregiving paradigm in a life-course framework (Young & Kahana, 1994). The model we propose here acknowledges distinctions not only between self- versus other-related events, but also recognizes dyadic and systemic perspectives on stress, implied by the concept of linked lives. Thus, events that happen to adult children may be seen as other-related events, caregiving may be viewed as a dyadic event, while one's family being in poverty would be seen as a systemic crisis.

Regarding *desirability* of event, it is useful to state that the research we reviewed focused primarily on negative life events. Early research on life events suggested that both positive and negative events can result in adverse effects based on the degree of change brought about by the event and the readaptations required (Holmes & Rahe, 1967). However, focus on the full life course has clarified that positive events happening to older adults seldom involve major life change and have little likelihood of generating negative impact. Furthermore, positive events that happened early in life seldom create an enduring negative impact, even when they involve considerable life change. Thus, the stresses of becoming a new parent or the additional responsibilities of a promotion may require short-term readjustments but are unlikely to have long-term negative effects. In evaluating desirability of events, one can apply either external or objective systems of categorization, or an internal, subjective yardstick. Subjective categorizations of event desirability have also been referred to as appraisals (Lazarus & Folkman, 1984). Since appraisals involve complex perceptual and cognitive processes, they may also be considered as elements of coping and mediators in the stress paradigm. Appraisals constitute a major focus of Study 4, which we reviewed.

Stressors: Temporal Dimensions

Temporal dimensions of stressors are closely tied to life-course issues. In categorizing stressors, our temporal consideration parallels the foregoing discussion in our empirical studies. This classification system is useful, as it helps clarify the multiple and often overlapping temporal dimensions included in cumulative life crisis measures, such as the Antonovsky Life Crisis Inventory. An examination of our model reveals that the cumulative life crisis measures do indeed reflect items relevant to all life stages and include events of varying life stages, historical time, *recency*, and *duration*. It is also notable that consideration of diverse temporal domains is overlapping in the Antonovsky Life Crisis Inventory. Thus, poverty may have occurred at any time of a person's life, whereas the discrete event of loss of a sibling is seen as relevant only if it occurred in childhood. Our framework provides conceptual guidelines for considering temporal dimensions of stress in a more clearly dimensionalized manner, so that orthogonal and overlapping dimensions may be conceptually and empirically identified and distinguished in future research.

Life stage considerations draw attention to major stages in the life course and include early life, midlife, and later-life events. Antonovsky's Life Crisis Inventory, used in Studies 1 and 2, does include events relevant to childhood, adult life, and old age. It is important to note, however, that life crisis inventories do not systematically sample events from every phase of the life course. Nor are resistance resources such as social supports and coping strategies generally categorized in a life course–sensitive manner. As interest in measurement in the field of life course research is increasing, development of life course–sensitive measures in every domain of the stress paradigm has great heuristic value (Settersten & Mayer, 1997).

Historical time is a central construct within the life-course paradigm. Although life-course researchers generally combine concepts of historical time and place (Elder et al., 1996), our temporal–spatial paradigm suggests separate consideration of those interrelated elements. Our research on survivors of the Holocaust (Study 5) represents a step toward recognizing the importance of historical time (and place). This research constitutes an in-depth focus on a historically linked trauma. In the broader context of considering diverse, cumulative life crises, timing of events could assist in linking personal and historical time (Settersten & Mayer, 1997). Thus, it is desirable to obtain the year of occurrence for specific life crises noted by respondents.

Social timing is recognized as a salient dimension related to the off-time or on-time nature of events relative to the life course. Our empirical studies did not explicitly operationalize this dimension, although some elements of timing are included in Antonovsky's operationalization of life crises throughout the life course, which is the focus of Study 1. Recency, duration, and sequence of life events are also included as distinct elements of the temporal domain.

Recency of events constituted a major focus in our prior discussion. As we have noted, stress researchers have traditionally focused on recent events defined as occurring 1 to 3 years prior to outcome assessment. Focus on such a relatively brief time frame is based on the untested assumption that proximate stressors will have the greatest impact on well-being outcomes. A life-course cumulative framework makes an important contribution by expanding the temporal frame of stressors studied. Study 2 thus included both recent life events and crises occurring throughout life in examining cumulative impact of stressors.

Duration of events refers to acuity versus chronicity of life events or crises experienced. There is a great deal of ambiguity in the stress literature regarding this important dimension. Recent life events often imply event acuity, assuming that a given event either occurred or did not occur during a specified time frame, such as the past year. Acute events generally appear to be of brief duration. In contrast, life crises often include an arbitrary marker of chronicity. Thus, for example, poverty and unemployment are counted as life crises only when they are endured for a substantial length of time. In the field of traumatic stress research, there are beginning attempts to distinguish enduring from transitory trauma (Wilson & Raphael, 1993). Study 4 among our research examples specifically sought to include a list of ongoing chronic stressors along with recent life events of briefer duration.

Sequencing of stressors is a temporal dimension that has received little prior attention. One area relevant to this domain is the distinction made between primary and secondary stressors. Secondary stressors are stressors created by the very occurrence of an original traumatic event and may reflect internalized aspects of the original trauma. For example, in our Study 5, Holocaust survivors were found to continue to confront stressful internal representations, such as intrusive memories of trauma, throughout life. This realm should be distinguished from primary versus secondary appraisals proposed by Lazarus and Launier (1978).

By distinguishing temporal from spatial dimensions of stressors, we are able to note and clarify inconsistencies in the traditional terminology in the literature. The concept of recent life events encompasses both temporal and spatial dimensions. In contrast, concepts of life crises and trauma refer only to magnitude of events, without specifying a temporal frame. Nevertheless, based on conventional usage, life crises generally imply a longer time perspective. In striving for greater precision in the field, we find it useful to designate, for each stressful event considered, both magnitude and temporal characteristics (e.g., recency and duration).

Protective Resources: Spatial Dimensions

Our research which, in aggregate, served as the impetus for developing the proposed framework, focused primarily on the explication of temporal and spatial dimensions of stressors and of outcomes. Nevertheless, we also recognize that individual, environmental, and societal resources serve important protective or predisposing roles within the stress paradigm (Kahana & Kahana, 1996;

Kahana, Kahana, & Taylor, 1998). We briefly outline salient dimensions in these areas, but do so without the specific empirical referents we could provide for our analyses of temporal and spatial dimensions of stressors.

In considering spatial dimensions of traditional buffers or protective resources within the stress paradigm, we combine psychological and sociological perspectives, and include the full spectrum of individual and environmental factors that may play protective roles or place individuals at greater risk for negative outcomes (Table 7–2). We have provided a systematic discussion of these resource factors in our recent formulation of a successful aging paradigm (Kahana and Kahana, 1996). This formulation and associated program of research proposes that successful aging may be defined in terms of dispositions, proactive adaptations, and external resources activated by older adults to meet challenges of normative stresses of aging. The spatial dimension of protective resources is primarily focused on classifying different types of resources ranging from microlevel personal dispositions and behaviors to more macrolevel indications of social constraints and opportunities. They thus address two key elements in the life-course paradigm: personal agency and social constraints or opportunities (Elder et al., 1996).

Our model of successful aging (Kahana & Kahana, 1996) includes attributional styles and personal dispositions such as optimism and self-esteem, and coping strategies such as positive comparisons, which are also discussed in the framework presented by Gatz (Chapter 4, this volume). In addition, it also extends to focus on proactive behaviors that present operational definitions for consideration of human agency. Thus, we have proposed that health promotion, planning, and helping others all reflect preventive adaptations, while marshaling social support, role substitution, and environmental modifications constitute corrective adaptations that play protective roles in the stress process, particularly during late life. Preventive and corrective proactivity are expressions of human agency in the face of normative stresses of aging, and represent life-course-relevant cornerstones of our model of successful aging.

We also incorporate demographic background variables in our model to designate social constraints and opportunities experienced by individuals that predispose them to stressful life circumstances and influence their adaptation to stressors. Our research cited in Study 4 provides empirical support for the importance of sociodemographic background in relation to stress appraisals. Our study of Florida retirees (Kahana & Kahana, 1996) also illustrates gender differences in aspects of proactivity such as health promotion.

Protective Resources: Temporal Dimensions

In conceptualizing or measuring protective resources or buffers in the stress paradigm, temporal dimensions are seldom noted. Current resources typically represent the unit of analysis even when applied to cumulative indices of stress. Yet the temporal domain is clearly relevant to understanding protective resources. In fact, the well-researched field of stability versus change in personality (Costa et al., 1986) relates to temporal dimensions of personal coping resources. Although coping resources are generally considered to be stable or trait-like, there are indications that trauma can influence such dispositional characteristics. For example, our research on Holocaust survivors suggests that dispositions of trust may be undermined by traumatic experiences (Kahana et al., 1997). Thus, it may be anticipated that life crises and trauma early in life may exert their influence on well-being, at least in part, by diminishing resistance resources.

Temporal dimensions may also be usefully considered in relation to environmental and social resources. The timing of social support is likely to be influential for determining effectiveness of support. Thus, elderly persons obtaining intermittent support or family assistance only in crisis situations may be far less likely to derive benefit than those receiving long-term and continuous support. Timing of support in relation to recent life events endured may also affect consequences. When we consider a broader life-course perspective, it also becomes apparent that lack of economic resources early in life, which characterized children of the Great Depression (Clausen, 1991), may result in frugality in later life, which can prevent frail elders from hiring paid helpers as caregivers. Elderly people who are unable to marshal paid resources may suffer psychological distress as they encounter stresses of illness in late life without sufficient social supports.

We concur with Gatz (Chapter 4, this volume) that experiences at one life stage affect vulnerability and resilience of the individual to events at later life stages. Thus, for example, the Holocaust survivors whom we studied appear to differ in their evaluation of the stressfulness of old age based on their traumatic earlier life experiences (Kahana et al., 1997).

Turning to temporal dimensions relevant to societal influences and opportunity structures, it becomes apparent that although demographic background rarely changes over time, the constraints or opportunities posed by social characteristics clearly undergo changes as society evolves. Thus, for example, female gender may pose fewer constraints for individuals experiencing divorce today compared to 30 years ago, when women faced more discrimination in entering the workforce. Consequently, divorced older women may be less stigmatized and less likely to suffer adverse mental health sequelae in the 1990s than they did 30 years earlier.

This discussion suggests that consideration of both temporal and spatial dimensions of protective resources is likely to hold great heuristic value for future research in stress and aging.

Stress Outcomes: Spatial Dimensions

In considering spatial dimensions of stress impact, alternative outcomes can be distinguished (Table 7–2). Adverse effects of stress on psychological well-being are among the most prevalent outcomes studied in the literature. It is important to note, however, that the threshold for clinical levels of psychopathology is seldom established in studies of stress among the elderly. Thus, when depression is considered as an outcome of stressful life events, typically, this is measured by higher scores on the CES-D or some other depression index, rather than based on the criterion of a clinical mental health problem (e.g., a DSM-IV diagnostic criterion for depression). Thus, when we read that stress increases depression, this typically means that as stress increases, there are greater expressions of psychological distress, as measured on a depression scale developed for the general population. Development of mental health indicators salient to the elderly poses a continuing challenge in this field. The Lawton Philadelphia Geriatric Center Morale Scale (Lawton et al., 1982) is one extensively used index of psychological well-being among the elderly. Yet even when using such an age-relevant index, there is limited reference to clinical issues. We have little understanding, based on such data, about the behaviors or lived experience of older adults reporting such distress.

In assessing the full spectrum of stress outcomes relevant to lives of the aged, it is also important to assess the impact of stress exposure on other outcome variables such as physical health, social functioning, and the ability to find meaning in life. A detailed rationale for this broader view of relevant stress outcomes is provided in our prior discussion of the successful aging model that we propose (Kahana & Kahana, 1996). In our research on old-old Florida retirees, we regularly include indications of range of daily activities engaged in as outcome measures (Kahana et al., 1996b).

Magnitude of impact represents the second major criterion among spatial classifications of outcomes. This criterion is the central focus of most studies on the effects of stress. Generally, this is assessed in the framework of cross-sectional or short-term longitudinal studies, and has been addressed in all of the studies we have reviewed. It should be noted, however, that an assumption of linearity is typically made when considering effect magnitude. Nevertheless, it is possible that there are critical levels of stress beyond which added stressors may not linearly increase impact.

Stress Outcomes: Temporal Dimensions

Because of the inherent challenges of conducting longitudinal research in the field of aging and stress, it is not surprising that little attention has been focused on temporal dimensions of stress impact. Nevertheless, there has been an indication that impact of some major life stressors, such as widowhood on psychological well-being, may diminish or even disappear after a relatively brief period (Stroebe & Stroebe, 1992). Such research is relevant to the classification of event impact as *temporary versus permanent*. The timing of impact as *immediate versus delayed* is another relevant temporal consideration. In longitudinal research, this may be addressed in distinguishing lagged from contemporaneous effects. Age specificity of stress impact is a temporal dimension with particular life-course relevance. Developmental theorists (Erikson, 1963) have thus outlined critical periods in development, suggesting that certain positive or negative experiences may have a particularly strong impact when they coincide with developmental crises. The duration of stress impact also has important and as yet little explored salience for aging research. In focusing on the aging process among individuals who experienced a broad range of stressors throughout their lives, it is of great interest whether effects of earlier stressors have been exacerbated by the aging process and by normative stresses of late life. Our research on elderly survivors of the Holocaust demonstrates interesting individual differences in this regard. Some survivors reported that the early trauma they endured made their experiences with aging easier, whereas another group suggested that the experience of their aging was more difficult because of trauma they endured, and a third group stated it made no difference (Kahana et al., 1997).

CONCLUSION

In our earlier work (Kahana, Kahana, Johnson, Hammond, & Kercher, 1994), we have called attention to the complexities and ambiguities, as well as to the promise, of the stress paradigm when it is applied to understanding the experiences and well-being of older adults. The studies reviewed in this chapter, and the conceptualization proposed, reflect our efforts to work toward further refinement and explication within this paradigm.

We have focused these efforts on explicitly addressing aspects of lifelong stress that shape late-life mental health outcomes. We attempted to depart from a gerontological framework, which isolates late life, and move toward a more integrated framework, which allows late life to take its place as one late and final stage within an interconnected life course. The stress process may be productively studied as we place the spectrum of stressors and their impact in a dual spatial and temporal context. Our model, the temporal–spatial model of cumulative stress, provides guidelines for specifying dimensions of the developmental trajectory of stressors, stress impact, and protective factors in the stress paradigm.

REFERENCES

Aldwin, C. M. (1990). The elders life stress inventory: Egocentric and non-egocentric stress. In M. A. P. Stephens, J. H. Crowther, S. Hobfoll, & D. L. Tennenbaum (Eds.), *Stress in later-life families* (pp. 49–70). New York: Hemisphere.

Antonovsky, A. (1979). *Health, stress, and coping.* San Francisco: Jossey-Bass.

Arnold, R. P., & Rogers, D. (1990). Medical problems of adults who were sexually abused in childhood. *British Medical Journal, 300,* 705–708.

Blake, D. D., Cook, J. D., & Keane, T. M. (1992). Post-traumatic stress disorder. *Journal of Clinical Psychology, 48,* 695–704.

Breier, A., Kelsoe, J. R., Kirwin, P. D., Beller, S. A., Wolkowitz, O. M., & Pickar, D. (1988). Early parental loss and development of adult psychopathology. *Archive of General Psychiatry, 45,* 987–993.

Breier, J., & Runtz, M. (1988). Symptomatology associated with childhood sexual victimization. *Child Abuse and Neglect, 12,* 51–59.

Chiriboga, D. A. (1992). Paradise lost: Stress in the modern age. In M. L. Wykle, E. Kahana, & J. Kowal (Eds.), *Stress and health among the elderly* (pp. 35–72). New York: Springer.

Clausen, J. (1991). *American lives: Looking back at the children of the Great Depression.* New York: Free Press.

Costa, P. T., Jr., McCrae, R. R., Zonderman, A. B., Barbano, H. E., Lebowitz, B., & Larson, D. M. (1986). Cross-sectional studies of personality in a national sample: 2. Stability in neuroticism, extroversion, and openness. *Psychology and Aging, 1,* 144–149.

Derogatis, L. R., Lipman, R. S., & Covi, L. (1973). SCL-90: An outpatient rating scale. *Psychopharmacology Bulletin, 9,* 13–28.

Diener, E., Emmons, R. A., Larsen, R. J., & Griffin, S. (1985). The satisfaction with life scale. *Journal of Personality Assessment, 49,* 71–75.

Dohrenwend, B. S., & Dohrenwend, B. P. (Eds.). (1974). *Stressful life events: Their nature and effects.* New York: Wiley.

Dohrenwend, B. S., Dohrenwend, B. P., Dodson, M., & Shrout, P. (1984). Symptoms, hassles, social supports, and life events: Problem of confounded measures. *Journal of Abnormal Psychology, 93,* 222–230.

Elder, G. H., George, L. K., & Shanahan, M. J. (1996). Psychosocial stress over the life course. In H. B. Kaplan (Ed.), *Psychosocial stress: Perspectives on structure, theory, life-course, and methods* (pp. 247–292). San Diego: Academic Press.

Erikson, E. (1963). *Childhood and society.* New York: Norton.

Folkman, S., & Lazarus, R. (1984). *Stress, appraisal and coping.* New York: Springer.

Gatz, M., & Smyer, M. A. (1983). Mental health and aging: Programs and evaluation. Thousand Oaks, CA: Sage.

Harris, E. (1991). Adolescent bereavement following the death of a parent: An exploratory study. *Child Psychology and Human Development, 21*(4), 267–281.

Harel, Z., Kahana, B., & Kahana, E. (1988). Psychological well-being among Holocaust survivors and immigrants in Israel. *Journal of Traumatic Stress Studies, 1*(4), 413–428.

Haug, M., Breslau, N., & Folmar, S. J. (1989). Coping resources and selective survival in mental health of the elderly. *Research on Aging, 2,* 468–491.

Holmes, R. H., & Rahe, R. H. (1967). The social readjustment rating scale. *Journal of Psychosomatic Research, 11,* 213–218.

Kahana, B. (1992). Late-life adaptation in the aftermath of extreme stress. In M. Wykle, E. Kahana, & J. Kowal (Eds.), *Stress and health among the elderly* (pp. 151–171). New York: Springer.

Kahana, B., Harel, Z., & Kahana, E. (1988). Predictors of psychological well-being among survivors of the Holocaust. In J. Wilson, Z. Harel, & B. Kahana (Eds.), *Human adaptation to extreme stress: From the Holocaust to Vietnam* (pp. 305–318). New York: Plenum Press.

Kahana, B., Harel, Z., & Kahana, E. (1989). Clinical and gerontological issues facing survivors of the Nazi Holocaust. In P. Marcus & A. Rosenberg (Eds.), *Healing their wounds: Psychotherapy with Holocaust survivors and their families* (pp. 197–211). New York: Praeger.

Kahana, B., Kahana, E., Harel, Z., Kelly, K., Monaghan, P., & Holland, L. (1997). A framework for understanding the chronic stresses of post-traumatic life: Perspectives of Holocaust survivors. In M. Gottlieb (Ed.), *Chronic stress and trauma* (pp. 315–342). New York: Plenum Press.

Kahana, B., Namazi, K., Kercher, K., & Brown, J. (1996, November 17–21). *Recent and long-term traumatic events and their effect on psychological, physical, and social domains of life.* Paper presented at the Gerontological Society of America, Washington, DC.

Kahana, B., Oakes, M., Slotterback, C., Kercher, K., & Kahana, E., (1996, August 18–21). *The late life aftermath of earlier life crises.* Paper presented at the American Sociological Association Annual Meeting, New York City.

Kahana, E. (1992). Stress, research and aging: Complexities, ambiguities, paradoxes, and promise. In M. Wykle, E. Kahana, & J. Kowal (Eds.), *Stress and health among the elderly* (pp. 239–256). New York: Springer.

Kahana, E., Fairchild, T., & Kahana, B. (1982). Adaptation. In D. J. Mangen & W. Peterson (Eds.), *Research instruments of social gerontology: Clinical and social gerontology* (pp. 145–193). Minneapolis: University of Minnesota Press.

Kahana, E., & Kahana, B. (1996). Conceptual and empirical advances in understanding aging well through proactive adaptation. In V. Bengtson (Ed.), *Adulthood and aging: Research on continuities and discontinuities* (pp. 18–41). New York: Springer.

Kahana, E., Kahana, B., Harel, Z., & Rosner, T. (1988). Coping with extreme trauma. In J. Wilson, Z. Harel, & B. Kahana (Eds.), *Human adaptation to extreme stress: From the Holocaust to Vietnam* (pp. 55–79). New York: Plenum Press.

Kahana, E., Kahana, B., Johnson, J., Hammond, R., & Kercher, K. (1994). Developmental challenges and family caregiving: Bridging concepts and research. In E. Kahana, D. Biegel, & M. Wykle (Eds.), *Family caregiving across the lifespan* (pp. 3–41). Thousand Oaks, CA: Sage.

Kahana, E., Kahana, B., & Taylor, H. (1998). Innovations in institutional care from a patient-centered perspective. In D. Biegel & A. Blum (Eds.), *Innovations in practice and service delivery across the lifespan* (pp. 377–424). New York: Oxford University Press.

Kahana, E., Redmond, C., Hill, G., Kercher, K., Kahana, B., Johnson, J., & Young, R. (1995). The effects of stress, vulnerability, and appraisals on the psychological well-being of the elderly. *Research on Aging: A Quarterly of Social Gerontology, 17,* 459–489.

Krause, N. (1991). Stressful events and life satisfaction among elderly men and women. *Journal of Gerontology, 46*(2), S84–S92.

Kiyak, A., Liang, J., & Kahana, E. (1976, August). *A methodological inquiry into the schedule of recent life events.* Paper presented at the Symposium of Life Events, American Psychological Association, New York.

Langner, T. S. (1962). A twenty-two item screening score of psychiatric symptoms indicating impairment. *Journal of Health and Human Behavior, 3,* 269–276.

Lawton, M. P., Moss, M., Fulcomer, M., & Kleban, M. H. (1982). A research and service-oriented multilevel assessment instrument. *Journal of Gerontology, 37,* 91–99.

Lazarus, R. S., & Launier, R. (1978). Stress-related transactions between person and environment. In L. A. Pervin & M. Lewis (Eds.), *Perspectives in interactional psychology* (p. 325). New York: Plenum Press.

Lazarus, R. S., & Folkman, S. (1984). *Stress, appraisal and coping.* New York: Springer.

MacDonald, A. J., & Bouchier, I. A. D. (1980). Non-organic gastrointestinal illness: A medical and psychiatric study. *British Journal of Psychiatry, 136,* 276–283.

Nauta, A., Brooks, J., Johnson, J., Kahana, E., & Kahana, B. (1995). Egocentric and non-egocentric life events as predictors of late life well-being. *Journal of Clinical Geropsychology, 2,* 3–21.

Norris, F., & Murrell, S. (1987). Transitory impact of life event stress on psychological symptoms of older adults. *Journal of Health and Social Behavior, 28,* 197–211.

Pearlin, L. I. (1980). Life strains and psychological distress among adults. In N. J. Smelser & E. H. Erikson (Eds.), *Themes of work and love in adulthood.* Cambridge, MA: Harvard University Press.

Pearlin, L. I., Lieberman, M. A., Menaghan, E. G., & Mullan, J. T. (1981). The stress process. *Journal of Health and Social Behavior, 22,* 337–356.

Radloff, L. S. (1977). The CES-D scale: A self-report depression scale for research in general population. *Applied Psychological Measurement, 1,* 385–401.

Rosenberg, M. (1979). *Conceiving the self.* New York: Basic Books.

Settersen, R., & Mayer, K. (1997). The measurement of age, age structuring, and the life course. *Annual Review of Sociology, 23,* 233–261.

Shanfield, S. B., & Swain, B. J. (1984). Death of adult children in traffic accidents. *Journal of Nervous and Mental Disease, 172,* 533–538.

Solomon, Z., Mikulincer, M., & Kotler, M. (1987). A two year follow-up of somatic complaints among Israeli combat stress reaction casualties. *Journal of Psychosomatic Research, 31,* 463–469.

Steptoe, A., Moses, J., & Edwards, S. (1990). Age related differences in cardiovascular reactions to mental stress tests in women. *Health Psychology, 9,* 18–34.

Stroebe, W., & Stroebe, M. S. (1992). Bereavement and health: Processes of adjusting to the loss of a partner. In N. L. Montada, S.-H. Filipp, & M. J. Lerner (Eds.), *Life Crises and Experiences of Loss in Adulthood* (pp. 3–22). Hillsdale, NJ: Erlbaum.

Stroebe, W., & Stroebe, M. S. (1996). The role of loneliness and social support in adjustment to loss: A test of attachment versus stress theory. *Journal of Personality and Social Psychology, 70*(6), 1241–1249.

Tait, R., & Silver, R. C. (1989). Coming to terms with major negative life events. In J. S. Uleman & J. A. Bargh (Eds.), *Unintended thought* (pp. 351–382). New York: Guilford.

Tausig, M. (1982). Measuring life events. *Journal of Health and Social Behavior, 23*, 52–64.

Teri, L., & Lewinsohn, P. (1982). Modifications of the pleasant and unpleasant events schedules for use with the elderly. *Journal of Consulting and Clinical Psychology, 50*, 444–445.

Turner, R. J., Wheaton, B., & Lloyd, D. A. (1995). The epidemiology of social stress. *American Sociological Review, 60*(1), 104–125.

Watson, D., Clark, L. A., & Tellegen, A. (1988). Development and validation of brief measures of positive and negative affect: The PANAS scales. *Journal of Personality and Social Psychology, 54*, 1063–1070.

Wheaton, B. (1996). The domains and boundaries of stress concepts. In H. B. Kaplan (Ed.), *Psychosocial stress: Perspectives on structure, theory, life-course, and methods* (pp. 29–70). San Diego: Academic Press.

Wilson, J. P., Harel, Z., & Kahana, B. (1989). *Human adaptation to extreme stress: From the Holocaust to Vietnam.* New York: Plenum Press.

Wilson, J. P., & Raphael, B. (Eds.). (1993). *International handbook of traumatic stress syndromes.* New York: Plenum Press.

Wykle, M. L., Kahana, E., & Kowal, J. (1992). *Stress and health among the elderly.* New York: Springer.

Young, R., & Kahana, E. (1994). Caregiving issues after a heart attack: Perspectives on elderly patients and their families. In E. Kahana, D. Biegel, & M. Wykle (Eds.), *Family caregiving across the lifespan* (pp. 262–284). Newbury Park, CA: Sage.

Zubin, J., & Burdock, E. (1965). The revolution in psychopathology and its implications for public health. *Acta Psychiatrica Scandinavica, 41*, 348–359.

PART III

The Adult Developing Self

Gerontology, as a comprehensive interdisciplinary discipline, must include the study of the Self (Kaufman, 1986), internalized social constraints (Kastenbaum, 1980), continuity, finitude (Kastenbaum, 1975; Kastenbaum & Kastenbaum, 1993), personality development (Ruth & Coleman, 1996), language, epistemology, and philosophy. It must also consider the interwoven phenomena of individual processes of being, social change, values, moral implications, and cultural meanings (Prilleltensky, 1997). These are the contours of Part III of this volume. Most of the present "paradigmatic" research in mental health and aging is conducted according to the positivistic approach in science. This, however, may not do justice to processes of individuality, and may force nonlinear processes and phenomena into overgeneralized patterns. Many scientists are now questioning the value of positivistic approaches. Biological models of aging (Cristofalo, 1988), for instance, emphasize the astonishing diversity and variability in development and demonstrate that gene expression is a nonlinear process that can no longer always be considered an "orderly flow of events" (p. 7). Furthermore, recently, perhaps as a result of critical methodology as well as mutual influences between disciplines in gerontology, alternative perspectives on theory have emerged, or reemerged, based on postmodern interpretive approaches (Lyotard, 1984) and critical theory (Moody, 1988). Hence, one may also find support for applications of chaos theory to aging (Hendricks, 1996). All such interpretive and critical models of theorizing shift the focus away from generalized tendencies and linear patterning (Hendricks, 1996) to epistemology, construction, and deconstruction; to underlying assumptions as well as suggested themes of meaning, preferably based on freely obtained, subjective data. The chapters in Part III fit into a combined adult-developmental and postmodern framework. They transcend the Aristotelian worldview and formulate the mental capacities by which the elderly may be able to cope with the most exacting demands placed upon them in contemporary culture. These chapters, in critically examining basic accepted assumptions, also reflect the diversity of the aging experience and the salient essence of the adult Self.

Hazan (Chapter 8) provides an intriguing conceptualization of how split, constricted, and age-related languages (literal, metaphysical, and metaphorical–pragmatic, in the life course or cycle) are used for social discourse, stigmatization, and adaptive purposes. Whereas these languages are usually interwoven, in old age, they become separated. Hazan offers the student of old age two optional language-related epistemologies for a greater understanding of the aging experience. He explicates the different spoken representations of the elderly Self as they appear in social negotiations and human dialogue, particularly marked in modern or postmodern life (see Kegan, Chapter 9). He juxtaposes the situationally anchored versus the culturally bound psychological Selves and renders them mutually exclusive (Lomranz, Chapter 10). The author stresses how the spoken, self-contrived, socially determined voice of the elderly may be heard, while their self-narrated, personal, and meaning-seeking voice may be silenced, muted, depriving them of a critical communicative resource, preventing expressions of their Self, and thus hindering their adjustment and growth. The elderly may behaviorally and vocally express the twofold patterns of existence but will keep them apart. Their fusion results in dire consequences. Hazan articulates how middle-aged people use literal, pragmatic language in order to define old age in pathological terms, distancing the actual phenomenology of aging and negatively predetermining the catastrophic image of the aging Self. Hazan clarifies, via the related analysis of language, Self, and the life cycle, how the growing-old person, using his or her resources to manage late-life incongruities and stress, finds him- or herself in a no-win situation as he or she internalizes the social discourse of aging.

We endeavor to fathom how the aged confront an extremely demanding social reality as well as the phenomenon of their diverse modes of aging. While, for instance, Hobfoll and Wells (Chapter 5) focus on stress and resources to answer these questions, Kegan (Chapter 9) focuses on the mental structures by which we organize reality. In the framework of individual and cultural constructivism, Kegan elaborates a model to explain how we construct the meaning of our changing and dynamic reality, and successfully cope with it. His model includes three qualitatively different and increasingly complex epistemological systems: the socialized, self-authoring, and self-transforming minds, each system of the mind, with its mental capacities, meeting, respectively, the demands of traditionalism, modernism and postmodernism. By recognizing one's "hidden curricula," one's epistemological approach and its level of complexity, as well as through experience or training, one may achieve a construction of meaning that enables growth (see Peskin, Chapter 13). To do so, we must transcend the captivity of socialization and develop a "gerontological curriculum" to educate and assist, as constructive–developmental educators and therapists, the elderly in orchestrating an appropriate "fit" between the mental demands of modern life and their own mental capacities.

Lomranz, in Chapter 10, attempts to integrate personality, coping behavior, mental health, and social criticism through two major components: the image of man and a proposed conceptualization of aintegration. Summarizing several major developmental lifespan conceptualizations and their implications, Lomranz demonstrates how inadequate they are to deal with the existential incompatibilities (Kegan, see Chapter 9) that face the aged, owing to their underlying assumptions of human nature. He proposes an alternative image of man and the elderly (see Gatz, Chapter 4), one that reflects a person's capability for aintegration. The concept of aintegration, contraposed to the Eriksonian concept of integration, is elucidated by dwelling on its theoretical framework and root sources in psychology and human experience. Aintegration is presented as a mental process and resultant state that reflects the ability of an adult person to feel well without having necessarily integrated all the various human biopsychosocial levels or certain entities within each level, into an overriding whole. Aintegration presents dialectics and the coexistence of seemingly contradictory elements. It embodies a possible sense of inconsistency, relativism, paradox, and tolerance for contradictions. Persons, especially the elderly, may experience an ability to consciously entertain thoughts, emotions, attitudes, and behaviors that seem inconsistent in personal, value, or cultural terms, and yet be in a state of equilibrium, well-being, and mental health. The author suggests implications for research and psychotherapy. These concepts should find their place in the larger theoretical network of personality and clinical geropsychology.

REFERENCES

Cristofalo, V. (1988). An overview of the theories of biological aging. In J. Birren & V. Bengtson (Eds.), *Emergent theories of aging* (pp. 118–127). New York: Springer.

Hendricks, J. (1996). Where are the new frontiers in aging theory? *Gerontologist, 36*, 141–144.

Kastenbaum, R. (1975). Time, death and ritual in old age. In J. Fraser & N. Lawrence (Eds.), *The study of time* (pp. 99–113). New York: Springer.

Kastenbaum, R. (1980). Habituation as a partial model of human aging. *Journal of Aging and Human Development, 13*, 159–170.

Kastenbaum, R., & Kastenbaum, B. (1993). *Encyclopedia of death.* New York: Avon Books.

Kaufman, S. (1986). *The ageless self.* Madison: University of Wisconsin Press.

Lyotard, J. F. (1984). *The postmodern condition: A report on knowledge.* Manchester, UK: Manchester University Press.

Moody, R. (1988). Towards a critical gerontology: The contribution of the humanities to theories of aging. In J. Birren & V. Bengtson (Eds.), *Emergent theories of aging* (pp. 19–40). New York: Springer.

Prilleltensky, I. (1997). Values, assumptions and practices: Assessing the moral implications of psychological discourse and action. *American Psychologist, 52*(5), 517–535.

Ruth, J.-E., & Coleman, P. (1996). Personality and aging: Coping and management of the self in later life. In J. Birren & W. Schaie (Eds.), *Handbook of the psychology of aging* (pp. 308–322). New York: Van Nostrand.

CHAPTER 8

The Double Voice of the Third Age

Splitting the Speaking Self as an Adaptive Strategy in Later Life

Haim Hazan

"Have you ever spotted a self down the corridor?" sniggered an eminent anthropologist, while exhorting against the reification of a concept replacing an ethnographic substance. Still, the discourse of selfhood is not only an analytic device, but also mainly a reflection of a certain social gaze under which cultural engendered practices are expressed. Scanning social action, this gaze recognizes and identifies the presence of selves according to their culturally audible utterances. This intriguing mixed metaphor conflating the spectral and the audible renders the self a vocal function confirmed by visual means. Attempts at disentangling the two by introducing a self-sustaining audible constant into the management of the discourse of the self are increasingly prevalent. Thus, underprivileged groups, for example, often phrase their claim to power as the right to have their own voice. Confining terms of selfhood to its spoken representations suggests the possibility of a polyphonic self composed of a multiplicity of voices.

It is the ephemeral nature of sound as against the rather perennial fixated property of sight that enables the former rather than the latter to serve various functions in communicating with others and to form an effective, flexible medium for social negotiation. This quality of lability qualifies the ear rather than the eye as a vehicle of interaction and interpretation in the era of late modernity, where the fragment rather than the whole, text rather than context, and the temporary rather than the permanent, prevail. Furthermore, the changeability of

Haim Hazan • Department of Sociology and Anthropology and the Herczeg Institute on Aging, Tel Aviv University, 69978 Tel Aviv, Israel.

Handbook of Aging and Mental Health: An Integrative Approach, edited by Jacob Lomranz. Plenum Press, New York, 1998.

the speaking self and its adaptability to differing life worlds implies as Gergen (1991, p. 83) argues in his analysis of contemporary Western society that

> increasingly we emerge as the possessors of many voices. Each self contains a multiplicity of others, singing different melodies, different verses and with different rhythms. Nor do these many voices necessarily harmonize. At times they join together, at times they fail to listen one to another and at times they create a jarring discord.

Other students of the diversity of self did not attribute this equivocality to the condition of being late modern and, indeed, couched it within the very foundation of being human. Thus Ewing (1990, p. 251) states that "in all cultures people can be observed to project multiple, inconsistent self-representations that are context dependent and may shift rapidly." Douglas (1995, p. 84) goes even further in restricting the emergence of multiple selves to non-Western societies.

> In the West, in contrast to … examples so familiar to anthropologists, the embodiment of one person for their lifetime in one body is axiomatic. In other cultures the person may go from one body to another or the one body may contain two or more persons, but claims that persons can split, or flit are not taken seriously in Western philosophy.

Late modern life or postmodern living, however, seems to close a circle and be juxtaposed with respect to the composition and status of the self, to nonindustrial societies (Strathern, 1987).

It is this flitting capacity of the self in both premodern and postmodern eras that enables persons in the two cultures to express different voices, and the question that should be posited is not only how these social structures facilitate personal polyphony, but also what these voices serve and to what extent there exists a multilogical relationship between them.

I would like to maintain that the case of the elderly in contemporary Western society could illuminate these issues, and to this end, this chapter is devoted. Briefly, it is set to argue that the marginal social position of the category of the old makes only one of its voices heard, that of the spoken self, contrived and tuned by the notes produced by society, while silencing the voice of its speaking selves, echoing sources of personal meaning and texts of self-narrated identities. Paradoxically, however, it is suggested that while the first voice of supposed general exigencies speaks in culturally conditioned, fragmented language, the other voice, that of the presumed personal and idiosyncratic, resorts to terms of human universals.

TWO SELVES: TWO VOICES

Anthropological wisdom has it that effect, rather than cause, function rather than motive, constitute the subject of its inquiry. Selfhood, therefore, to the scant extent that it has been studied, is invariably construed in terms of cultural conditioning and changing circumstances (Carrithers, Collins, & Lukes, 1985). This socially relative view turns the anthropologist's gaze to performative practices and their observed contexts, sometimes to the exclusion of past formative forces. In its extreme, the self is thus accounted for within the framework of the ethnographic present inhabited by both researcher and researchees (Crapanzano, 1980).

These assumptions are gravely challenged when the discipline focuses its attention on the lifespan and on the sense that people make of their lifelong experiences. Recording personal accounts recounted by elderly people, anthropologists found it necessary to shift their theoretical thrust from the "here and now" to the "there and then." This methodical diversion required some reconsideration of epistemological underpinning, of which the most significant was the abandonment of contextual principles in favor of universal premises as to the psychological needs of humans in general and old people in particular. Concepts such as "life-career" (Myerhoff & Simic, 1978), "continuity," and the "ageless self" (Kaufman, 1986) were formulated to enable anthropologists to encompass the entirety of one's life story and to offer a theoretically cogent interpretation of its reconstruction in old age. The more momentum that trend has gathered, the more anthropologists applied themselves to such psychologically informed perspectives (Langness & Frank, 1981). The paradox generated by this vein of research in anthropological thought was only too evident. Two conceptions of self were simultaneously invoked—one that is situationally anchored and pragmatically engineered, whereas the other is culture bound and psychologically driven. The former is a self of practical reasoning and existence, whereas the latter is a self of meaning seeking and existentialism (Cohen, 1974). The decision as to which self is predominant depends largely upon conceptual references just as much as on field data.

The coexistence of these two selves presents no novelty either for psychological theory or anthropological discourse. However, rarely has it been suggested that these two modes of personhood could be completely separate from each other and, indeed, may be mutually exclusive as alternative *modus operandi*.

Empirically, this notion of irreconcilable split between practical reasoning and the quest for meaning was sparked off in the course of an anthropological fieldwork I conducted on a self-help organization of elderly people in Cambridge, England. It was among the members of the University of the Third Age that I detected a twofold behavioral pattern consisting of practical management of daily living on the one hand, and what might be termed a metaphysical expression of reality on the other. The two states were kept as worlds apart, and it was only through an undeliberate coincidence that I was able to learn about the dire consequences of their fusion. The description of that incident provides the rationale for the argument to follow.

Members of the University set up their own research committee to investigate matters of importance to the elderly residents of Cambridge. One of the topics on their agenda was the cost of funerals and the nature of the service administered by funeral directors. Having conducted a meticulously designed inquiry into all the factors involved, and having interviewed a sizable number of respondents, the committee decided to enhance their knowledge of burial arrangements by inviting a guest speaker—a Ph.D. student who had made a study of that subject. After a hair-raising presentation concerning the gruesome abuse of the dead by undertakers and about the corrupt system surrounding it, the funeral project was, as they put it, "buried." It would appear that turning the ultimate reality into a practical issue could not withstand the encroachment of death as a forbidden taboo zone. Here, the unintended merger between the two selves brought to a halt the attempt at playing brinkmanship with death. Evidently, further and more conclusive material has to be adduced to corroborate this argument, but for the purpose of this heuristic exercise, suffice it to say that the conscious endeavor by members to distance the two selves from each other to avoid any polluting overlap is a theme running throughout the entire ethnography.

Many questions could be posed with regard to that separation. I would like to confine the discussion to the sociocultural terms that structure these two selves and to their implications to the understanding of the reality of being old in postindustrial society. The assumption, controversial as it is, that guides this approach is that selves are generated, engineered, and sustained through sociocultural processes (Rose, 1990). It is maintained that the choice and employment of adaptive strategies, such as the double self (Lifton, 1986), are induced by structural conditioning no less than by the quintessential properties of the individual. With these premises in mind, the following is set to offer a sociological discourse aimed at eliciting a model of modes of articulating experience in later life as produced and constructed by the position of the category known as "growing old" or as "the third age" in late modern society. Our theoretical stance draws on schools of thought interweaving social knowledge, cultural codes, and structure of power (Foucault, 1980). It will be shown how macrosocial forces prescribing the imagery of the lifespan construct the microinteractional fabric of organizing everyday experience by the elderly occupying that symbolic space of "the third age." The management of late life's incongruities and stresses is to be explained in terms of the handling of resources and constraints embedded in that culturally predesignated age territory.

THE MUTED VOICE: AN ANALYTIC DILEMMA

Knowledge about the old is invariably produced and disseminated by the nonold. It involves all individuals who, by mere virtue of their chronological age, are discarded into the gray territory of the "last frontier" (Fontana, 1976). It is, indeed, the unavoidable but nevertheless avoided association between death and the old that endows the latter with taboo-like attributes (Hazan, 1994). The category of the old as a culturally constructed whole delineates a symbolic space where reciprocal relationships turn into dependency, and hence standards of everyday communication and information cease to apply (Hockey & James, 1993). Denied of many social resources, the old are also deprived of the means to negotiate terms with others—their voice.

Society mutes the voice of the old by applying various methods of screening, so that what is heard on the receiving end of that distorted line is inevitably selective to befit social interests and expectations. The portrayal of aged persons

as victims of crime, social abuse, poverty, family neglect, and medical maltreat-
ment articulates a common language about aging that only attests to its medical-
ization, victimization, marginalization, infantilization, and stigmatization. In
a word, aging is made into a social problem that presupposes and predestines
the image of the aging self.

Examples of the subjugating discourse of old age are abundant. Preassumptions as to the pejorative pathological nature of aging, for example, play a major
part in medicalizing almost all forms of communication about the old. Since
diagnosis of geriatrically related syndromes is not always decidedly clinched,
and hence may rest within a gray scientific area, the range of superimposed
medical labels pertaining to aging is almost infinite. It is more often than not that
a common interest of both the physician and custodians formulates the condition of the old in medically intelligible terms so that supervisory measures can
be applied. The old person is expected to comply with a set of tests purporting to
evaluate her or his cognitive capacities and designed to establish adaptive
properties. Failure to meet such standards by appropriately demonstrated aptitudes would result in the classification of the subject as incompetent and thus in
need of care and attention. In other words, the old are deemed disoriented,
maladjusted, and incoherent unless proven otherwise. Consequently, any information produced by an old person about her- or himself, unless congruous with
the construction of reality of the nonold, is liable to be discredited. Hence,
repetitious locutions uttered by elderly persons, adherence to maxims and
aphorisms, achronological accounts of life histories, inconsistent speech–acts,
profuse recourse to reminiscences or alternatively dead silence—all serve as
testimonies to "garbled talk," "disorientation," and "senility." It has been shown
that supposedly neutral speech cues, such as slow rate of speech, bad pronuncia-
tion, and other age markers, lead hearers to draw downgrading stereotypical
inferences such as "doddery," "vague," "frail," and "upset."

The reduction of the old into corporeal attributes not only restricts the
language about the aging self to physiological determinants, but also introduces a split within the Western cultural "paradigm" of the indivisibility of body
and soul (Featherstone & Hepworth, 1990). It confines the old to a category of
social treatment such as medicine or the social welfare system, where bodies are
separated from selves (Zola, 1982). It is intriguing to observe that protest against
the social abandonment of the old often invokes the "invisibility" (e.g., Myerhoff, 1982) of the elderly as an insignia of such avoidance. However, the condition of the elderly put under the social gaze is one of overvisibility, as the old in
fact exist only as long as they are seen. Indeed, it is the separation of bodies from
selves that makes the aged only too visible. The old, the patient and the dependent, all share the overvisibility of a subject objectified and a person-cum-
persona. This adaptation-oriented perspective robbed social gerontologists of
some of the most central templates of thinking about the aging self. The result is a
theoretical impasse.

Sociocultural research into the experience of aging has formulated its frustrations by contriving concepts and theories that attest to the aborted attempt to
make sense of old age in conventional socioanthropological terms. In fact, the

very phrasing of these concepts is a self-evident admission of that failure. They all revert to nomenclature and hypotheses that negate rather than explain the subject at hand. Thus, the elderly have been sociologically declared to be "roleless" (Burgess, 1950), "deculturized" (Anderson, 1972), in a state of "no exit" (Marshall, 1979), "anomie" (Fontana, 1976), "disengaged" (Cumming & Henry, 1991), and symbolically "invisible" (Myerhoff, 1978). To rectify this conceptual myopia, a multitude of alternative constructs have been proposed, none of which stem from the self-expressed world of the aged, and all draw on social models for the aged, and indeed for the nonaged. Hence activity, continuity, lifespan development, and cultural themes (Clark & Anderson, 1967; Kaufman, 1981) were enlisted as key explanatory forms. The assumption that old age is a mere sociological extension of the other ages of man reigns supreme in the various modes and models of understanding aging, while elderly people are denied the otherwise common intellectual right to present their own worldview to the middle-aged scientific community studying them.

TWO LANGUAGES

"Old age" is represented by and to middle-aged society through the so-called "mask of aging." The aging self is masked, concealed behind specular stereotypes, objectified through medical and gerontological discourses. The elderly's self-presentation is public, often made to conform to its social image, further reinforces that image. Hepworth and Featherstone's (1991) important concept of the "mask of aging" recapitulates similar conceptualizations already suggested in the sociology of aging (e.g., Gubrium, 1994; Hazan, 1994). It proposes that the image of the elderly is part of the scopic regimes of modernity whose other inmates are the sick (most recently and blatantly, the HIV/AIDS patient), the insane, the primitive, and, ultimately, the "other" in all of its embodiments. The sociology of aging, itself a powerful image maker, is part of that scopic regime, too. It is part of the ocularcentrism of contemporary society and sociology, which gives prominence to the image and privileges of sight over sound. The ocularcentric gaze of the sociology of aging, even when self-reflexive, has tended to emphasize the visual: either the hypervisibility of the "mask" of aging or its complementary opposite, namely, the elderly's social "invisibility" (e.g., Eckert, 1980; Myerhoff, 1982; Unruh, 1983).

Masking is often a repressive act. Woodward (1991), for example, argues that repression of aging is connected to the visible oppression of old people in our society. Following Germain Greer's contention, in her recent book, *The Change* (1991), that old age generates angst, Woodward proposes that aging is not only seen as a general catastrophe but is also particularly associated with women, reflecting a Western "gerontophobia" from the aging body, regarded as bad, and split off from the youthful body, regarded as good. While the image of the elderly should be deconstructed and unmasked, the attempt may prove self-defeating. Invoking both hypervisibility and invisibility as a banner against ageism may be self-subversive, as it carries the risk of inadvertently strengthening that which it seeks to criticize. Conjuring up images, even in a critical manner, already reproduces them. To avoid that double-bind, this Chapter suggests another metaphorical venue into the aging self: non (in)visibility, but (in)audibility. I make here an attempt to lend an ear to the voices of the old as a possible means of evading the tyranny of the mirror-hall of images. What then are the social languages about the aging self and of the aging self or selves?

AGE-RELATED LANGUAGES

My argument is that any constitution of self is bound up by age categorization, and hence a transition within the age set spells a redefinition of the social self (Bernardi, 1985; Kertzer & Keith, 1984). Age groups are constituted through cultural anticipations, echoed in the various metaphors related in each and every society to the "seasons of man's life" (Levinson, Darrow, Klein, Levinson, & McKee, 1978). Such a social span of control demands different discursive frames of reference for "hearing," "discussing," "explaining," and ultimately "understanding" the various age groups defined. These discourses, in turn, often become part of their subjects' repertoire, internalized into forms of articulation that characterize the symbolic exchange practiced among members of the age group and between that group and others.

"Old age," I argue, is a symbolic category defined primarily by middle age and mainly through two discursive systems, or "languages," termed here the *literal* and the *metaphysical*. These two discursive formulations of "old age" respectively imply two socially reified views of the lifespan: the "life cycle" and the "life course." These are seen here as being primarily mechanisms of normative control rather than free alternatives open for individual choice.

Literal language is the quest for a complete identification between words and things, concepts and objects, signified and signifier. Metaphysical language is the expression of the ideal, the thing in itself rather than its representation. Both literal and metaphysical languages derive from a common origin— metonymical thinking. This is a self-contained system of communication as well as a state of mind where there is no division between signified and signifier, and hence no representations are possible (Leach, 1976). Metonymical thought, such as myth and philosophy, possesses attributes of atemporality and acontextuality beyond the "here" and "now." Conversely, nonliteral language is the articulation of reality by means of interconnecting separate semantic zones. This production of meaning is symbolic by nature, practical by function, and metaphorical by aesthetic conventions. The two linguistic modes are simultaneously present in everyday life, while their relative prevalence alters from one situation or context to another. In the case of the social discourses of old age, it will be argued that the predominant mode is the metonymical, while the metaphorical, being the core language of middle age, is absent from the construction of late life. It should be noted that an important difference between the mode of articulation, one which is responsible for the discourse of infantalization of the old (Hockey & James, 1993; Meyerowitz, 1984), is that metaphorical–pragmatic language spells rationality, causality, and logic, whereas metonymic–mythical language is presumed arational, illogical, and essentially incomprehensible. This difference has far-reaching repercussions on the construction of vindicating the dependency and ineptness imputed to the old.

Let me first discuss how middle age uses literal language in order to define old age. It has already been pointed out, at the outset of this chapter, how mass media, welfare criteria, and social stereotypes provide programs of talking about the old that are further validated by selectively induced expressions uttered by elderly people. Preassumptions as to the pathological nature of aging, for example, play a major part in medicalizing almost all forms of communication by the old. The old person is further expected to comply with a set of tests purporting to question and evaluate her or his cognitive capacities and designed to establish adaptive properties and measure "life satisfaction" (Gubrium & Lynott, 1983).

Old age and Childhood are prescribed with structurally similar social positions through the use of literal language. In childhood, this is the language of socialization, which only gradually develops into nonliteral forms such as irony and metaphor (Winner, 1990; see also Astington, 1991; Trevarthen & Logotheri, 1989). Storytelling whose moral is emphasized is presumably shared by both children and elderly. As in the case of nursery rhymes, folktales, and legends, elderly's stories are viewed as 'plotted prose with an explicit moral" (Mergler & Goldstein, 1983, p. 86), which is based on common narratives, idioms, and proverbial vocabularies (Blythe, 1979; Coupland & Coupland, 1991; Koch, 1977; Myerhoff, 1978). The elderly's "deculturated" (Anderson, 1972) discourse of "life-reviewing" and "reminiscence" can be regarded as symmetrical to childhood's socializing discourse of nursery tales and "secret-sharing" (Katriel, 1991). Both share a master narrative based on literality, metonymy, self-referentiality, and myth-like qualities (see also Searle, 1979, on literal meaning). Some psycholinguists even ventured to state that this "literal talk" is a result of deficiencies in working memory and linguistic competence (Kemper, 1988). The literal, found both in childhood and in later life, thus presents itself as an extremity—as either a point of entrance, a marker of socialization, or as a point of departure, a sign of deculturation.

In contrast to youth and old age, middle age (as conceived of and constituted by its own occupants) dictates other constraints and social prescriptions. The ideal type of midlife is concerned with effectiveness and objective information, the aligning of desires and capabilities in everyday domains such as work, love, and family life (Hepworth & Featherstone, 1982). This demands a pragmatic disposition, an outward oriented, objective frame of reference, which is furthermore capable of metaphorically—that is, nonliterally—interconnecting the various life-worlds (e.g., professional, familial, consumerist, political, etc.) of middle age. Such pragmatic, metaphorical, "better-equipped" disposition, once defined, can be used to separate and distinguish middle age from both childhood and old age.

Besides the more commonly used, abovementioned practices of the literal discourse that account for both childhood and old age, as well as make both categories accountable to the social order of middle age, there is yet another language that is part of the "discourse of aging." This language is, by and large, reserved for designating old age. It is a metaphysical language that has become the interpreting framework for discussing and authorizing the so-called "aging self." "Ego integrity" (Erikson, 1982) and "the ageless self" (Kaufmann, 1986) are two such idealized, metaphysical cultural paradigms revealing more of middle age's expectations and fears than of the actual phenomenology of aging. The trope of the old is dually occupied by the literally speaking, "confused," bedridden, and housebound elderly, as well as the aging, metaphysically speaking, "blind prophet." It is dually constituted by the archetypal "scheming hag" as well as by the literal stereotype of the "dear old thing" (Cool & McCabe, 1983).

Metaphysical interpretation is often evoked by proponents of "old age style." Woodward (1980), for example, who studied the late poems of Eliot, Pound, Stevens, and Williams, argues that aging positions the poet to see "the whole of the system." In Cohen-Shalev's (1992, p. 297) account of the late style of novelists as well as artists, it is defined as "a tendency to strip down artifice." "The relative lack of distinction between fact and fantasy, autobiography and invention, prose and poetry," he claims (p. 297), "does not result in a harmonious resolution of these opposites, but rather in a coexistence that seems to transcend logical thought categories." Viewing the elderly as incorporating the ability to "see the whole system" and "to strip down (social) artifice" is part of the metaphysical discourse of marginalization, which endows aging not only with the prescriptions of liminality, but also with the powers of estrangement. It is the unavoidable but nevertheless avoided association between death and the old that credits the latter with such a metaphysical language.

THE STRUCTURAL ORIGINS
OF AGE-RELATED LANGUAGES

The three different age-related languages (literal, metaphysical, and the metaphorical–pragmatic) can now be superimposed onto one's path of life. The dominant model found in the final stage of life in effect defines it as either a course or a cycle. Life course is an image of the linear progression of the self through the lifespan, beginning with literal language of fairy tales, legends, and nonnegotiable social perceptions, continuing with metaphorical–pragmatic articulation of reality, and ending up with a generative process governed by metaphysical wisdom. The conception of the life cycle starts at the literal, proceeds to the metaphorical, and reverts to the literal in old age. That image of the "life cycle" is very similar to the one proposed by Turner (1987). It represents childhood and old age as homologous in terms of social liminality and disengagement, or what Turner calls lack of reciprocity, which is (according to him) the basis for social prestige.

Turner's narrative, therefore, belongs to the "life cycle" type, in which youth and old age are symmetrically constructed through the literal language, "because the child and the elderly share a number of common social characteristics (such as the absence of work), and they are often described in the same pejorative and stigmatizing fashion" (Turner, 1987, p. 123). Childhood and old age, socialization and deculturation, irresponsibility and disengagement, are all the outcomes of social regulation. The dominance of literal language in those two extremes of the life cycle—childhood and old age—can also be seen as such an outcome. It is more of a socially prescribed language than an inherent part of these groups. "To speak literally" can serve as a normative control mechanism in its own right, mainly as it obliterates the need to decode the speaker's idiosyncratic, nonliteral intentions. Literal language is, therefore, the key to what Hockey and James (1993) call, in a very similar manner, the discourse of infantilization:

> The cultural pervasiveness of metaphors of childhood within the discourses surrounding aging and dependency ... has become "naturalized." It is seen as somehow inevitable, as the way things are. Through this culturally constructed model of dependency, many of those in old age and others who are infantilized—the chronically sick or disabled, for example—may be made to take a conceptual position alongside children on the margins of society. (p. 13)

The metaphysical language is in purpose not different from the literal. Through it, the nomadic aging self in late modern society is masked, muted, dubbed, and ultimately defined as the metaphysical object of "pilgrimage through life." Giddens (1991) argues that the postmodern blurring of age structure is closely linked to the rejection of the predestination narrative of identity that dominated Western thought for a long time. In his words,

> Self-identity for us [in the late modern age] forms a trajectory across different institutional settings of modernity over the duree of what used to be called the "life cycle," a term which applies more accurately to non-modern contexts than to modern ones. Modernity is a post-traditional order, in which the question, "How shall I live?" has to be answered in day-to-day decisions about how to behave, what to wear and what to eat—and many other things—as well as interpreted within the temporal unfolding of self-identity. (p. 14)

Bauman (1992) distinguishes between two symbolic types of "identity seekers": the postmodernist nomads and the Protestant (modernist) "pilgrims through life." The former wanders between unconnected places, have no preset itinerary, and hence only momentary identities, "for today," until further-notice identities. Predestination has been replaced, in their case, with uncertainty. The "pilgrims" have their destination preselected (by religion, society, gender, class, origin, etc.), guide their life according to a "life-project," crystallizing a single core identity throughout this "path of life." The "nomads" can be said to move further in the lifespan, while "pilgrims" either "progress" in the "life course" or continue along the "life cycle." Western adult society, postmodernist and all, by and large still considers its elderly according to the second narrative—that of pilgrimage.

Literal and metaphysical, in the case of the elderly, are two sides of the same coin, or, in other words, a matter of interpretation. "The language of the elder is perhaps simply all language made plain," argue Mergler and Schleifer (1985), but "speaking plainly" can be both literal and metaphysical.

There is an ambiguity inherent in the aging situation of simultaneously possessing a sense of self and otherness about oneself, a situation emanating from the split between the quintessential "I" and the socially accountable "me." Furthermore, it is because of that complete split in the life-worlds of the elderly that metaphor—being a symbolic vehicle designed to connect different worlds by means of some analogy (Davidson, 1979)—becomes impossible. It is only within such a split, for example, that "habit" can be understood as both a (literal) weary repetition and a (metaphysical) crystallization in which "the past is brought to life again, the future anticipated" (de Beauvoir, 1975, p. 696). Literal or metaphysical interpretation, in the case of both childhood and old age, does not hinge on the speaker's own intention, but rather on some collective knowledge, a socially shared record of images and stereotypes. This disciplinary convention is crucial in the case of the old. Where autobiography is too idiosyncratic and relationships are built on nonreactive networks (i.e., "social worlds"; see Unruh, 1983), nonliteral personal meaning is hardly communicable. The literal and the metaphysical, therefore, befit the discourse of aging as both a social measure of normative control and a form of talk. It enables one to understand one's words without having to decipher, in the process, one's world. The old speaker's world is hence too often muffled by the discourse of aging.

CONCLUSION: THE DOUBLE VOICE
OF THE THIRD AGE

The structural comparison drawn between childhood and old age points to yet another aspect of the specific age group under study. It should be noted that the members of the University of the Third Age (U3A) distinctly referred to themselves as belonging not to the category of "old age" but to a category they called "third age." They even created an academic organization to stand as evidence to the existence of such a "third age." This category is defined as preceding "old age" but still as different from it. One member of the group reflected on the subject by saying, "I wonder whether it has occurred to anybody else here that we are a very curious group, but then, again, we are not really old. We may say that we are ante-aged."

But what is "ante-aged"? It was, in the eyes of members, a social buffer zone between past upward careers and social integration on the one hand and the prospects of disengagement and deterioration on the other. Following the "life cycle" symmetry, I argue that the age group that is symmetrical to that "third age" is, in effect, adolescence. "Third age" (or the "young-old" as Neugarten [1976] dubbed it), one might say, is the "adolescence of old age." "Ante-age" is symmetrical to "postchildhood" (note that the life-cycle symmetry is of a reverse type, which is one of the reflections of the socially prescribed character of that paradigm). Moreover, third age and adolescence share a number of social characteristics. First and foremost, they are considered as betwixt and between— already out of their former age category, but still not part of the next category. This sense of "half-baked" categories depicts them as being caught up in ambiguity and crisis. Most significantly, these characteristics lend these age categories a social license to experiment—experiment with values, norms, social conduct, and personal behavior. I believe that their (perhaps unconscious) identification with those characteristics underpinned the creation of a "third age" by the members of the U3A, and, indeed, by aging people involved in the movement all around the world. It was this sense of ambiguity and crisis, as well as the urge to experiment with new frames of mind, that undermined the whole project of "third age."

With the dissolution of the discourse of metaphorical language, the literal/ metaphysical, on the one hand, and nonliteral on the other, become totally incongruent and mutually exclusive. Whereas usually these languages are interwoven and mixed, in old age, they become differentiated.

The young elderly entering old age occupy a social territory where social self, as defined by modes of articulating experience, is still undetermined and open to experimentation. However, the leeway for maneuvering narrows down behavioral options and, as shown in the case of the funerals project, it might disappear altogether. By internalizing the social discourses of aging, elderly people are subjected to no-win situations. They either hold on to codes of pragmatic practices and expose themselves to external sanctioning such as ridicule, inconsideration, abuse, and confinement, or conversely, if succumbing to loss of power and control, they restrict their communication with others to the literal and the metaphysical. Whichever adaptive mechanism is chosen, the authentic sense of selfhood is masked behind it. The student of old age, therefore, is forced to deliberate between two optional epistemologies: accepting the idea of one, incoherent though it might be, self-disguised behind inconsistent and at times contradictory behavioral presentations; or submitting to the notion of "a homeless mind" (Berger, Berger, & Kellner, 1973), multiple selves or doubling (Lifton, 1986), which exonerates one from the assumptions of masking at the price of challenging the very concept of selfhood. The choice of a mode of interpreting the nature of adaptive stratagems correspondingly constitutes the type of communication devices employed to comprehend the old, respond to their assumed needs, and avoid the situation of the old and the nonold being divided by a supposedly common language.

REFERENCES

Anderson, B. (1972). The process of deculturation: Its dynamics among United States aged. *Anthropological Quarterly, 45*, 209–216.

Astington, J. (1991). Narrative and the child's theory of mind. In B. Britton & A. Pellegrini (Eds.), *Narrative thought and narrative language*. Hillsdale, NJ: Erlbaum.

Bauman, Z. (1992). *Mortality and immortality and other life strategies*. Cambridge, UK: Polity Press.

Berger, P., Berger, B., & Kellner, H. (1973). *The homeless mind*. New York: Vintage.

Bernardi, B. (1985). *Age class systems: Social institutions and politics based on age*. Cambridge, UK: Cambridge University Press.

Blythe, R. (1979). *The view in winter*. New York: Harcourt Brace Jovanovitch.

Burgess, E. (1950) Personal and social adjustment in old age. In M. Derber (Ed.), *The aged and society* (pp. 138–156). Champaign, IL: Industrial Relations Research Association.

Carrithers, M., Collins, S., Lukes, S. (Eds.). (1985). *The category of the person*. Cambridge, UK: Cambridge University Press.

Clark, M., & Anderson, B. G. (1967). *Culture and aging*. Springfield, IL: Charles C Thomas.

Cohen, A. (1974). *Two dimensional man*. London: Routledge & Kegan Paul.

Cohen-Shalev, A. (1992). Self and style: The development of artistic expression from youth through midlife to old age in the works of Henrik Ibsen. *Journal of Aging Studies*, 6(3), 289–301.

Cool, L., & McCabe, J. (1983). The scheming hag and the "dear old thing": The anthropology of aging women. In J. Sokolovsky (Ed.), *Growing old in different societies* (pp. 56–71). Belmont, CA: Wadsworth.

Coupland, J., & Coupland, N. (1991). Formulating age: Dimensions of age identity in elderly talk. *Discourse Processes*, 14, 87–106.

Crapanzano, V. (1980). *Tuhami: Portrait of a Moroccan*. Chicago: University of Chicago Press.

Davidson, D. (1979). On metaphor. In S. Sachs (Ed.), *On metaphor* (pp. 98–116). Chicago: University of Chicago Press.

Cumming, E., & Henry, W. (1961). *Growing old: The process of disengagement*. New York: Basic Books.

Douglas, M. (1995). The Cloud God and the Shadow Self. *Social Anthropology*, 3, 83–94.

de Beauvoir, S. (1975). *The coming of age*. New York: Warner Communications.

Eckert, J. K. (1980). *The unseen elderly*. San Diego: Campanile Press.

Erikson, E. (1959). *Identity and the life cycle*. New York: Norton.

Erikson, E. (1982). *The life cycle completed*. New York: Norton.

Ewing, K. P. (1990). The illusion of wholeness: Culture, self and the experience of inconsistency. *Ethos*, 18, 251–278.

Featherstone, M., & Hepworth, M. (1990). Images of aging. In J. Bond & P. G. Coleman (Eds.), *Aging in society: An introduction to social gerontology*. London: Sage.

Featherstone, M., & Hepworth, M. (1991). The mask of aging and the post-modern life course. In M. Featherstone, M. Hepworth, & B. Turner (Eds.), *The body: Social process and cultural theory* (pp. 370–389). London: Sage.

Fontana, A. (1976). *The last frontier*. Beverly Hills, CA: Sage.

Foucault, M. (1979). What is an author? (Kari Hanet, Trans.). *Screen* 20(1), 13–33.

Foucault, M. (1980). *Power knowledge: Selected interviews and other writings*. Brighton, UK: Harvester Press.

Gergen, K. J. (1991). *The saturated self*. New York: Basic Books.

Giddens, A. (1991). *Modernity and self-identity: Self and society in the late modern age*. Cambridge, UK: Polity Press.

Greer, G. (1991). *The change: Women, aging, and menopause*. London: Hamish Hamilton.

Gubrium, J. (1994). *Speaking of lives*. New York: Aldine de Gruyter.

Gubrium, J. F., & Lynott, R. S. (1983). Rethinking life satisfaction. *Human Organization*, 42, 30–38.

Hazan, H. (1994). *Old Age: Construction and deconstructions*. Cambridge, UK: Cambridge University Press.

Hepworth, M., & Featherstone, M. (1982). *Surviving middle age*. Oxford, UK: Blackwell.

Hockey, J., & James, A. (1993). *Growing up and growing old: Ageing and dependency in the life course*. London: Sage.

Katriel, I. (1991). Sodot: Secret sharing as a social form among Israeli children. In I. Katriel (Ed.), *Communal webs* (pp. 183–197). Albany, NY: SUNY Press.

Kaufman, S. R. (1981). Cultural components of identity in old age. *Ethos*, 9(1), 51–87.

Kaufman, S. R. (1986). *The ageless self: Sources of meaning in late life*. Madison: University of Wisconsin.

Kemper, S. (1988). Geriatric psycholinguistics: Syntactic limitations of oral and written language. In L. Light & D. Burke (Eds.). *Language, memory and aging* (pp. 58–76). Cambridge, UK: Cambridge University Press.

Kertzer, D., & Keith, J. (Eds.). (1984). *Age and anthropological theory*. Ithaca, NY: Cornell University Press.

Koch, K. (1977). *I never told anybody: Teaching poetry writing in a nursing home*. New York: Random House.

Langness, L. L., & Frank, G. (1981). *Lives: An anthropological approach to biography.* Novato, CA: Chandler & Sharp.

Leach, E. (1976). *Culture and communication.* Cambridge, UK: Cambridge University Press.

Levinson, D., Darrow, C., Klein, E., Levinson, M., & McKee, B. (1978). *The seasons of man's life.* New York: Knopf.

Lifton, R. (1986). *The Nazi doctors.* New York: Basic Books.

Marshall, V. W. (1979). No exit: A symbolic interactionist perspective on aging. *International Journal of Aging and Human Development, 9,* 345–358.

Mergler, N., & Goldstein, M. (1983). Why are there old people? Senescence as biological and cultural preparedness for the transmission of information. *Human Information, 26,* 72–90.

Mergler, N., & Schleifer, R. (1985). The plain sense of things: Violence and the discourse of the aged. *Semiotica, 54*(1/2), 177–199.

Meyerowitz, J. (1984). The adult child and the childlike adult. *Daedalus, 113*(3), 19–48.

Myerhoff, B. (1978). *Number our days.* New York: Dutton.

Myerhoff, B. (1982). Life history among the elderly: Performance visibility and re-membering. In J. Ruby (Ed.), *A crack in the mirror: Reflexive perspectives in anthropology.* Philadelphia: University of Pennsylvania Press.

Myerhoff, B., & Simic, A. (Eds.). (1978). *Life's career—aging: Cultural variations on growing old.* Beverly Hills, CA: Sage.

Neugarten, B. L. (1976). The future and the young old, *Gerontologist, 15,* 4–9.

Rose, N. (1990). *Governing the soul: The shaping of the private self.* London: Routledge.

Searle, J. (Ed.). (1979). *Expressions and meaning.* Cambridge, UK: Cambridge University Press.

Strathern, M. (1987). Out of context: The persuasive fictions of anthropology. *Current Anthropology, 28,* 251–281.

Trevarthen, C., & Logotheri, K. (1989). Child in society, and society in children: The nature of basic trust. In S. Howell & R. Willis (Eds.), *Societies at peace: Anthropological perspectives.* London: Routledge.

Turner, B. S. (1987). Aging, dying and death. In B. S. Turner (Ed.), *Medical power and social knowledge* (pp. 11–31). Newbury Park, CA: Sage.

Unruh, D. (1983). *Invisible life: The social worlds of the aged.* Beverly Hills, CA: Sage.

Winner, E. (1990). *The point of words: Children's understanding of metaphor and irony.* Cambridge, MA: Harvard University Press.

Woodward, K. (1980). *At last, the real distinguished thing: The late poetry of Eliot, Pound, Stevens and Williams.* Columbus: Ohio State University Press.

Woodward, K. (1991). *Aging and its discontents.* Bloomington: Indiana University Press.

Zola, I. K. (1982). *Missing pieces.* Philadelphia: Temple University Press.

CHAPTER 9

Epistemology, Expectation, and Aging

A Developmental Analysis of the Gerontological Curriculum

ROBERT KEGAN

TWO INTRODUCTORY VIGNETTES

While working on this chapter, I have also been shopping around for a Mazda Miata. I am about to be 50, and this handsomely designed but relatively inexpensive sports car, I had been thinking, might be just the special thing I would like to get myself for a present. Never having heard me express interest in owning such a car, my bemused wife sympathized with what she believed was my terror of growing old. She saw the gift I imagined for myself as a touching (or pathetic) effort to acquire externally the internal zip, flash, or grace I must feel was vanishing at 50. Psychologist though I might be, her depressing interpretation never occurred to me before she mentioned it. "Sometimes a cigar is just a cigar," I told her Freud once said. "But this isn't sometimes," she said. "You've never been about-to-be-50. And a sleek, fancy-looking cigar is not just a cigar."

She had me there. I had to admit a fancy sports car is not just another car. But actually, the Miata had quite a different meaning to me, one that had nothing to do with holding off a gloomy specter of waning power or attractiveness. (I don't claim any lifelong immunity to such a dread; it just didn't seem to be what this was about for me.) Forced to present my own "interpretation," I saw that driving this sports car was just a tiny further realization of a plan I had formulated and been carrying out since I was 40—to bring as much of the "vacation

ROBERT KEGAN • Graduate School of Education, Harvard University, Cambridge, Massachusetts, 02138 and Massachusetts School of Professional Psychology, Boston, Massachusetts 02132.

Handbook of Aging and Mental Health: An Integrative Approach, edited by Jacob Lomranz. Plenum Press, New York, 1998.

mentality" into my everyday life as possible, rather than waiting *until* (*until* the summer, *until* I retire, *until* I'm richer, *until* I'm more accomplished, *until* I deserve it). The "vacation mentality" (for me, this is a mix of breaking routine, taking pleasure, sensory adventuring, random contemplation, exuberance, appreciation, and, above all, having fun) is not the only delightful thread I have discovered in life but it is one I have noticed can be consigned to the fringes or the borders, or blocked off to its own domain (the *until*), when I have wanted to sew it thickly and regularly through the basic fabric of my life. The Miata looked to me like a little vacation mentality on wheels, and I happen to drive a car several times every day!

*   *   *   *   *

A friend who long ago turned 50 tells me, "You developmental psychologists have got it all wrong." "Many years ago," she says, "I'd been preparing for 'the empty nest.' I'd read the books. I knew when the last kid took off, and Burt and I were left there at the breakfast table staring silently at each other, I was going to have an 'empty nest depression' as advertised. It all made good sense to me, especially as a woman of my time, not having worked or developed a life outside the home, and having given up my drawing and painting to raise my kids and make a nice home for my husband and family, I figured that what you developmental psychologists had to say made a lot of sense."

"So let me give you a little tip," she continues. "I have discovered that the true meaning of liberation is when the last child goes off to college and the dog dies!" Far from anything like a depression, she was experiencing an extraordinarily vital new chapter in her late fifties, having opened an art studio, traveling all over the world (tax deductibly), purchasing paintings to sell in her store.

INDIVIDUAL AND CULTURAL CONSTRUCTIVISM

Of course, the idea that an era of the lifespan, like midlife, may be associated with crisis is not a fiction. Many people do develop a dread about the loss of youth and inevitability of old age, even fleeing into manic denial. Many do become depressed when the children leave home and the family feels empty. What the vignettes demonstrate first is that there is no one inevitable internal experience or personal meaning for the same set of circumstances. The identical situation of sending the last child off to college may trigger clinical depression or life-transforming liberation. This is an expression of the constructivist feature of human being. Organisms organize. Human organisms organize meaning. Reality doesn't happen up to us inherent in our experience. We construct the meaning or reality of our experience. What is true about the circumstances of midlife is surely true about the circumstances of old age as well. Even the most familiar litany of problematic challenges of later life does not contain within it a guaranteed meaning for the experiences of widowhood, retirement, sexual complications, physical decline and disease, dependency and hospitalization, dying. Why do some people construct more hopeful, life-expanding meanings for the same circumstances others construct in a life-contracting way?

The vignettes also demonstrate that however idiosyncratic our individual constructions of experience might be, the culture at large, or the culture's "discourse shapers" and knowledge communities, also participate in forming a public construction, even an expectation of how common circumstances will be commonly experienced. So my artist friend came to expect she should have an "empty nest depression." Just now, it seems to me, as an amateur observer of the gerontology field, we are awash in two competing collective narratives about how we might experience the circumstances of our old age.

By one account—a longer-lived and still prevailing account—the public story is essentially compensatory at best, or about adjustment to inevitable decline at worst. David Gutmann (1987) writes,

> The conventional psychology of aging is almost completely devoted to a study of its discontents: aging as depletion, aging as catastrophe, aging as mortality. At best the aged are deemed barely capable of staving off disaster but they are certainly not deemed capable of developing new capacities or of seeking out new challenges by their own choice (and even for the sheer hell of it). (p. 7)

The other, newer, countervailing account is also suggested in Gutmann's words. It implies that the later decades of life could be a context for the further flowering of our human capacities, a veritable "fountain of age," from which we are able to realize new depths of cognitive, emotional, interpersonal, and intrapersonal experiencing (Friedan, 1993).

Any widely held public story about how life will be or could be has the psychological effect of visiting upon the characters of the story a set of expectations for how the characters should be. Albeit in very different ways, one can find in each of these accounts of old age a kind of "disengagement theory" that carries an expectation at its core. The traditional, degenerative disengagement theory (Cumming & Henry, 1961) amounts to an expectation that we will retire, withdraw, step down, shrink the circle of our connections and influence when we are old. The countervailing, transformative "disengagement theory" amounts to an expectation that we will be able, in old age, to psychologically disengage from our own ego-driven, product-driven, ideologically bounded self-organizations in order to compose a more complex, more fluid, more reflective, more intimate self-organization. While these two sets of possibilities differ dramatically in their pessimism and optimism, they each make claims on the minds or psychologies of the elderly and therefore constitute "hidden curricula." What level of mental complexity is unwittingly expected in order for older adults to meet the expectations for greater dependency on the one hand, or the expectations for greater growth on the other? How well do the unrecognized epistemological demands inherent in these expectations match the self-complexity of older adults?

I've spent the last 20 years studying the mental structures by which people organize reality, and the evolution of these structures throughout the lifespan (Kegan, 1982, 1994). This work has included the development of a reliable interview-assessment procedure that identifies the level of complexity of an individual's prevailing "epistemological structure." The Subject–Object Interview (Lahey, Souvaine, Kegan, Goodman, & Felix, 1988) clarifies what aspects of meaning-organizing one has control over, can make use of, reflect upon (what is "object" in one's meaning-organizing), and what aspects control one, what aspects one is captive of, identified with (what one is "subject" to in one's meaning-organization). Longitudinal study shows that if people change the underlying structure of their meaning organizing, they do so in a developmental direction; that is, they differentiate from structures to which they were subject, thus making them object, and integrate these structures into a more complex organizational principle to which they are subject (Kegan, 1994). While much of this work throughout the world has focused on early and middle adulthood (the twenties through the fifties), virtually none of it, that I am aware of, has used my instrument specifically to study meaning making in old age. I am hopeful that a chapter such as this one might suggest a variety of researchable lines of inquiry into old age, from my model and method. Nonetheless, I am not going to let a little thing like the absence of data prevent me from making here what I will still claim is an empirically based argument that *neither of the popular "narratives of expectation" for old age square well with the epistemological realities of a large proportion of older adults.*

If for no other reason than to hold the reader's interest while a nongerontologist offers a model that may have some use to the gerontology field, I will take the ill-mannered position here that, without a smidgen of data from my perspective on old age, the evidence already exists that the traditional "degenerative" account of old age aims too low for a large percentage of older adults, and that the "fountain of age," "transformative" account aims too high for an even larger percentage. While both accounts are important, need to be kept in mind, and are fitting curricula for some, I will sketch the features of a third account that may actually be a more fitting curriculum for most. This third account is more optimistic than the first and more realistic than the second.

CONTEMPORARY ADULTHOOD: THE FIT BETWEEN MENTAL DEMANDS AND MENTAL CAPACITIES

Our research has identified three broad, qualitatively different, increasingly complex, epistemological systems to which the adults in our studies may have recourse (Kegan, 1994). It is usually possible to identify for any given subject a threshold of mental complexity beyond which one does not pass at that moment, and around which most of one's meaning–organizing takes place, a kind of "central tendency" in one's current reality–constituting. Although empirically we have been able to identify reliably five gradations of complexity between any two of these mental systems, thus permitting a quite discriminating account of the "central epistemological tendency" (Lahey et al., 1988), it will be sufficient for our present purposes just to distinguish between the three general systems themselves.

The first system I will call *the socialized mind.* This describes an order of consciousness that is able to think abstractly, identify a complex internal psychological life, orient to the welfare of a human relationship, construct values and ideals self-consciously known as such, and subordinate one's own interests on behalf of one's greater loyalty to maintaining bonds of association or group participation. These capacities are enabled by a gradual developmental transformation in which the general mental structure of "durable categories" (which cognitively creates a concrete world, e.g., or interpersonally allows one to recognize that others have a discrete point of view distinct from one's own) is no longer the organizational principle to which one is subject. As "durable categories" move from subject to object, a more complex general structure evolves which can coordinate or subordinate durable categories. Thus (e.g., cognitively), our thinking can now take the concrete as figure rather than ground, and we think more abstractly; or, interpersonally, we can now simultaneously hold our point of view with another's point of view and create a more reciprocal or mutual frame on human relationships. This new, more complex, "cross-categorical" structure permits the capacities of the socialized mind (see Figure 9–1). A variety of studies document the gradual evolution of this cross-categorical structure, usually in adolescence (Kegan, 1986; Villegas-Reimers, 1988; Walsh, 1989).

The structuring principles of the socialized mind make it a good fit with the

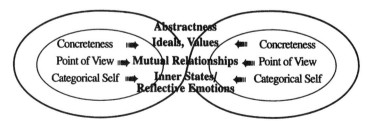

Figure 9–1. The transformation from durable categories to cross-categorical meaning making.

unrecognized epistemological demands inherent in our expectations of adolescents. We want adolescents to think more abstractly (hypothetically, propositionally, inferentially), take out membership in a community of interest larger than one, be interpersonally trustworthy, possess ideals, achieve a greater degree of emotional self-awareness. Although we do not realize it, all these capacities require the same central epistemological tendency—the "cross-categorical" structuring that brings into being the socialized mind. But how well does this epistemology do in meeting the mental demands inherent in our general expectations of adulthood?

This is the question I tackled in *In Over Our Heads: The Mental Demands of Modern Life* (Kegan, 1994), and the title alone suggests an answer. While beleaguered parents are relieved by the eventual and too gradual arrival of the socialized mind in their adolescent children, it is actually a poor match for the hidden curriculum of adult life. The psychological essence of socialization is that one becomes more a part of society because society has become more a part of oneself; that is, one internalizes, becomes identified with, is "made up by" the values, beliefs, definitions of the surround. The limit of the socialized mind is that it is choicelessly, unawarely "made up by" that to which it has become loyal or faithful. Subject to cross-categorical structures, it has no capacity to stand apart from the values, beliefs, expectations, or definitions of one's tribe, community, or culture and make independent judgments about them. Yet it turns out this is just what is required of us in contemporary adulthood.

In our role as parents, for example, we are expected to set limits upon our children, even to defy rather than identify with many of their wishes, an expectation the capacity for socialization alone will not be able to meet. We are expected to take charge of our families, establish rules and roles, create and manage boundaries between the generations, and monitor who and what from outside the family (including the television) is permitted to participate inside the family. All of these expectations require something quite different than being able to join with and internalize the surround; they require an ability to act upon the surround.

As partners in a long-term intimate relationship, we are expected to survive the inevitable end of the early, romantic phase of the relationship by developing a well-differentiated and clearly defined sense of self and a new conception of closeness built on the idea of two psychological wholes rather than two halves of one whole. At work, for example, we are increasingly expected to be more self-initiating, self-correcting, self-evaluating. As citizens of a diverse society, we are expected to contravene our tendencies toward ethnocentrism, to resist our tendencies to make "right" or "true" that which is merely familiar, to reflect on and evaluate the values and beliefs of our cultural inheritance rather than be captive of those values and beliefs. As psychotherapy clients, we are expected to "regard ourselves as the proper evaluators of our experience rather than regarding ourselves as existing in a world where the values are inherent in and attached to the objects of our experience" (Rogers, 1951), to learn the psychological myths or scripts that govern our behavior and reauthor them, rather than just use therapeutic insight for better understanding of why the script is as it is. As adult learners, we are expected to be self-directed, "examining ourselves, our culture and our milieu in order to understand how to separate what we feel from what we should feel, what we value from what we should value, and what we want from what we should want" (Grow, 1991).

All of these expectations call for an ability to transcend somewhat the captivity of socialization, to be ourselves actors upon the press of the surround. *The socialized mind* lacks an internal personal authority that acts on the values and expectations of the surround, independently decides about them, prioritizes them, measures them against one's own internally regulated ideology or value-generating system. Such a meaning–organizing system requires that cross-categorical structures themselves become objects of a qualitatively more complex "central epistemological tendency," which brings into being *the self-authoring mind* (see Figure 9–2).

The *self-authoring mind* is a much better fit with the general demands of adult life than the *socialized mind*, because the common thread running through these adult demands is for us to win some distance from an identification with the press of our cultural or psychological surrounds. We do this by creating an internal system, theory, or ideology that authorizes (or refuses to) the claims and expectations made upon us (rather than identifies with them). When we look, however, at the central organizing tendencies to which adults actually have

	SUBJECT	OBJECT	UNDERLYING STRUCTURE
The Socialized Mind	ABSTRACTIONS Ideality Inference, Generalization Hypothesis, Proposition Ideals, Values	Concrete	Cross-Categorical Trans-Categorical
	MUTUALITY/INTERPERSONALISM **Role Consciousness** **Mutual Reciprocity**	Point of View	
	INNER STATES *Subjectivity, Self-Consciousness*	Enduring Dispositions Needs, Preferences	
The Self-Authoring Mind	ABSTRACT SYSTEMS Ideology Formulation, Authorization Relations between Abstractions	Abstractions	System/Complex
	INSTITUTION **Relationship-Regulating Forms** **Multiple-Role Consciousness**	Mutuality Interpersonalism	
	SELF-AUTHORSHIP *Self-Regulation, Self-Formation* *Identity, Autonomy, Individuation*	Inner States Subjectivity Self-Consciousness	

LINES OF DEVELOPMENT	
K	COGNITIVE
E	**INTERPERSONAL**
Y	*INTRAPERSONAL*

Figure 9–2. The socialized mind and the self-authoring mind.

recourse, what we discover is that large percentages of adults (including large percentages of highly educated, middle-class adults) do not construct experience as complexly as *the self-authoring mind*. We find instead that among samples of adults (ages 20–50) who are socially favored (professional, highly educated, middle-class), about half do not construct experience as complexly as *the self-authoring mind*, and among samples reflecting a broader socio-economic range, about three-fourths do not (see Table 9–1).

The inability to construct experience as complexly as *the self-authoring mind* leaves one in an overmatched relationship to the demands of modernism. While *the socialized mind* is a good fit with fundamentalism or traditionalism (which requires the capacity to subordinate self-interest to the commonweal; to internalize, identify with, become faithful to the values of a homogeneous surround), modernism calls for the capacity to organize a personal psychological authority that can contend with, and act upon, ever-increasing heterogeneity. Yet as daunting as the demands of modernism may be, they do not constitute the only challenging curriculum contemporary adulthood faces. Ours is an age variously in the grip not only of traditionalism and modernism, but also of postmodernism as well (an influence we may one day understand well enough to characterize by what it is rather than only by what it is not).

Unlike modernism, the central mental demand of postmodernism is not a requirement to loosen our identification with the socializing influences that make us up, but to loosen our identification with the forms of authority we ourselves have made up. At the leading edge of many of our expert literatures (including, as we shall see, in gerontology) is a discourse that implicitly or explicitly calls upon us to develop a saving skepticism about what now appears as the pretension to wholeness or completeness in any single system or author-ity, be it psychological or sociopolitical, privately intrapersonal or publicly theoretical. Psychologically, this gathering discourse calls us to recognize the possibility of a bigger self that may compose a multiple of systems or ideologies rather than jealously holding onto one, identifying with it, and projecting the others and the opposites onto persons or institutions outside oneself.

This discourse is reflected in newer conceptions of leadership (Heifetz, 1995) or management (Argyris, 1993; Schon, 1987; Torbert, 1987) calling for an exercise of authority less on behalf of one's own vision and more on behalf of preserving a context in which many stakeholders can together bear the frustra-tion of fashioning a shared vision. It is reflected in new literature on dispute resolution commending the parties to consider that the conflict creates the disputants as much as the other way around, that the parties might seek not first to "solve their conflict" (thus preserving the illusion of the independence and wholeness of each side) but to let their conflict "solve them" (i.e., transform each side) (Chasin & Herzig, 1993). It is reflected in the social-constructivist discourse on the philosophy of curriculum, calling on us to consider that our disciplines as currently taught are essentially systems or procedures for authori-zing knowledge, inevitably partial and ideological, confusing internal consis-tency and the ability to account for all the data with objectivity or validity (Bruffee, 1993). Most recently, in the gerontological literature, it is reflected

Table 9–1. Distributions of Epistemological Systems among Adults

Epistemology	Composite (Studies 1–12) N = 282		"Full SES" composite (studies 1, 5, 11) N = 75		"Professional highly educated" composite (all but 1, 5, 11) N = 207		Bar-Yam study (13, a highly educated sample) N = 60	
5 (Self-transforming)	0	0%	0	0%	0	0%	0	0%
4–5	17	6%	2	3%	15	7%	6	10%
4 (Self-authoring)	97	34%	14	18%	83	40%	25	42%
3–4	91	32%	23	31%	68	33%	22	37%
3 (Socializing)	40	14%	9	12%	31	15%	7	11%
2–3	22	8%	17	23%	5	2.5%	0	0%
2	15	5%	10	13%	5	2.5%	0	0%

Study	Sample profile
1	12M, 12W; parents of 11- to 13-year-old sons; 1/2 clinic population; mean age = 39.45
2	20M, 20W; married couples, 28 to 55 years old; middle class
3	15M, 15W, 25 to 40 years old, highly educated
4	11M, 11W (each interviewed twice), 30 to 40 years old, professional, all with graduate degrees
5	24W, 19 to 30 years old, students at 2-year technical college
6	10M, 10W; married couples, 25 to 36 years old, highly educated, most have graduate degrees
7	20W, 28 to 50 years old, highly educated, 15 of 20 hold master's degrees
8	11W, 31 to 44 years old, middle class, majority hold college degrees or more
9	6W, 6M; owner/founders of small businesses; 31 to 66 years old, 11 of 12 college graduates
10	7M, 13W, parents of teens
11	27W, 40 to 49 years old, randomly selected from a single town, widespread educations
12	6W, 6M; 35 to 48 years old, six middle-class married couples; 10 of 12 college graduates; 5 of 12 advanced degrees
13	40 W, 20M; 25 to 55 years old; Americans in military service in Europe, their dependents, and civilians employed by military; all pursuing graduate degrees

in the countervailing, optimistic accounts of, or calls for, the development in old age of a less-bounded, more fluid self, friendlier to contradiction and paradox, oriented more to process than product, integrative rather than projective toward life's enduring polarities (bringing the masculine and the feminine together, e.g., the creator and the destroyer, the youthful and the aged) (Erikson, Erikson, & Kivnick, 1986; Friedan, 1993; Levinson, 1978).

Epistemologically, what is required to respond to these calls is a further voyage of subject to object. This time, the mental structure of complex system itself must gradually move from being the ruling, meaning-regulative principle to becoming an element in a more complex transsystemic or cross-systemic structure, a structure that can hold multiple systems simultaneously (see Figure 9–3).

		SUBJECT	OBJECT	UNDERLYING STRUCTURE

The Socialized Mind	T R A D I T I O N A L I S M	ABSTRACTIONS
		  Ideality
		  Inference, Generalization
		  Hypothesis, Proposition
		  Ideals, Values
		MUTUALITY/INTERPERSONALISM
		  Role Consciousness
		  Mutual Reciprocity
		INNER STATES
		  Subjectivity, Self-Consciousness
			Concrete
			
			Point of View
			
			Enduring Dispositions
			Needs, Preferences
				Cross-Categorical
				Trans-Categorical

The Self-Authoring Mind	M O D E R N I S M	ABSTRACT SYSTEMS
		  Ideology
		  Formulation, Authorization
		  Relations between Abstractions
		INSTITUTION
		  Relationship-Regulating Forms
		  Multiple-Role Consciousness
		SELF-AUTHORSHIP
		  Self-Regulation, Self-Formation
		  Identity, Autonomy, Individuation
			Abstractions
			
			Mutuality
			Interpersonalism
			
			Inner States
			Subjectivity
			Self-Consciousness
				System/Complex

The Self-Transforming Mind	P O S T - M O D E R N I S M	DIALECTICAL
		  Trans-Ideological/Post-Ideological
		  Testing Formulation, Paradox
		  Contradiction, Oppositeness
		INTER-INSTITUTIONAL
		  Relationship between Forms
		  Interpenetration of Self and Other
		SELF-TRANSFORMATION
		  Interpenetration of Selves
		  Inter-Individuation
			Abstract System
			Ideology
			
			Institution
			Relationship-
			Regulating Forms
			Self-Authorship
			Self-Regulation
			Self-Formation
				Trans-System
				Trans-Complex

LINES OF DEVELOPMENT	
K	COGNITIVE
E	**INTERPERSONAL**
Y	*INTRAPERSONAL*

Figure 9–3. The socialized mind, the self-authoring mind, and the self-transforming mind.

Such an evolution, should it occur, brings into being the third meaning-making system our research has been able to identify, what we call *the self-transforming mind* (since, unlike *the self-authoring mind*, it is not so much devoted to "self-formation"—the creation and buildup of the self as a single, ever-more-powerful "institution"—but to the self as a context for the transforming of one's psychological "institution").

The distinctions I draw here between the *socialized*, *self-authoring*, and *self-transforming* minds resonate with the work of several of the contributors to this volume. Gutmann's richly drawn distinction in this volume (e.g., between the "alloplastic extroverts," who look to and depend upon the psychological surround to compose themselves, and the "autoplastic introverts," who look to themselves as the source of their psychological design) may reflect, whatever their psychodynamic origins may be, the underlying epistemologies of the *socialized* and *self-authoring* minds, respectively. Although Gutmann could be understood to be making no normative claim here as to the developmental or maturational status of the two "types," I have it on good authority that this would be a misreading (I asked him!); he plainly intends to suggest that the "autoplasts" are developmentally further along than the "alloplasts."

Lomranz's heuristic concept in this volume of "aintegration," speaking to the dialectical capacities to embrace opposites, live with irresolvable contradiction, resist the temptation to truncate experience by making it all fit one coherent system, may reflect the metasystemic epistemology that underlies the *self-transforming* mind. By associating his conception with the work on "post-formal thinking," "dialectical operations," or Loevinger's "autonomous ego," he makes clear that he sees "aintegration" as a developmental "high art," a highly evolved way of organizing experience.

Hazan's call, in this volume, for a release from the mental captivity of the Aristotelian worldview also finds a response in my distinction between the *self-authoring* mind, a champion of modernism, and the *self-transforming* mind, a postmodern, post-Aristotelian meaning maker. As Hazan himself helpfully suggested (in our discussion of an earlier draft of this chapter), my work points to a disentangling of the conceptions of "identity" and "the self." The concept of "the self" (or "selfing") speaks to the lifelong, meaning–architecting process of human being; the concept of "identity" merely speaks to one of its products, however impressive that product may be, however much modernism may be in its thrall, however much we can misguidedly build a shrine to it as a realization of psychological development's fullest expression. The *self-transforming mind* suggests that the meaning–architecting activity of the self has further work to do even after it has constructed an "identity."

But how prevalent a phenomenon is the *self-transforming mind* as an empirical reality? From many studies of adults using the Subject–Object Interview (aged early twenties to late fifties), such as those in Table 9–1 and others, two findings are especially notable: First, *if people do make the move beyond the self-authoring mind toward the self-transforming mind, it is never before mid-life*. This finding should be of interest, especially, to those in what Friedan calls "the gerontological underground," who question the doctrine that later life

cannot be a time for further psychological growth, increasing complexification of
mind, or enhanced mental capacity. (As a matter of fact, a version of this
unhappy doctrine has long been visited upon eras of the lifespan considerably
younger than late life. Perhaps we are now able to entertain the possibility of
greater psychological growth in old age only because we have relatively recently
begun to defeat the notion that psychological development ends, for all practical
purposes, in adolescence!) Our studies confirm that some adults, and not before
midlife, do indeed develop a qualitatively more complex epistemological system that permits just the sort of psychological operations the optimistic account
of later life describes. These are qualitative complexifications of mind. They are
not compensatory strategies that enable one to get more out of the same mental
equipment; they are actual upgrading transformations of the equipment itself.

But the second finding (as Table 9–1 suggests) is that *the move beyond the
self-authoring mind toward the self-transforming mind appears to be relatively
rare among adults.* Only 5–10% of subjects constructed experience more complexly than *the self-authoring mind.* It is true, however, that these studies only
include those who have lived "the first 40 years" of adulthood. This percentage
could surely increase during the years after 60. For those who enter later life with
self-authoring minds, the optimistic call for us to drink from the fountain of age
is a usefully challenging but potentially achievable curriculum.

The self-transforming mind may be a rare phenomenon. But those who long
for more of its presence—for the recognition of our multiple selves, for the
capacity to see protracted conflict as a signal of our overidentification with a
single system, for the sense of our relationships and connections as prior to and
constitutive of the individual self, for an identification with the transformative
process of our being rather than the formative products of our becoming—might
well take heart in the phenomenon of our longer lives. The evolution of consciousness requires long preparation. A hundred years ago, the average American lived to an age we today call the middle of life, the middle forties. Today, the
average American lives more than 20 years longer, an entire generation longer for
each individual life. What might the individual generate given an additional
generation to live? Is it possible that more of us will construct *the self-
transforming mind* because we have found ways to increase the number of years
we live? And why exactly are we as a species increasing the number of years we
live? Is it possible we are living longer so that we might in fact evolve to a new
order of consciousness?

THE OLD-AGE CURRICULUM
AND THE MENTAL CAPACITY IT DEMANDS

It is not unuseful for our culture's visionaries to stand on the vanguard today
and trumpet the possibilities for a *self-transforming* old age tomorrow. Though
rarely attained, my research suggests these are not impossible goals (as the
remarkable exemplars such accounts typically parade before us demonstrate in a
less statistical, more three-dimensional fashion). And such accounts also serve

to dramatically challenge the more traditional portraits of debility, dependence, and passivity characterizing old age. Nonetheless, if we consider the tasks of aging in relation to the likely realities regarding the more common epistemological positions of aging adults, I think we will conclude that our primary gaze should be neither so low as the traditional, pessimistic portrait nor so lofty as the newer, optimistic one. *A more reasonable and more widely applicable gerontological position, it seems to me, would be to recognize that increasingly large percentages of the aging population will possess the capacities of* the self-authoring mind; *and a more reasonable and widely applicable aspiration would be to support the very large percentage of aging adults who do* not *yet organize their experience in a self-authoring fashion to do so.*

I say this because I think even a brief review of the broad tasks of aging (Newhouse, 1995) will suggest that it is *the self-authoring mind* that constitutes the implicit mental threshold for successfully handling this curriculum, a threshold many adults will not yet have reached in old age, and not having done so, will be "at risk" for poorer outcomes thereby. As elderly persons in post-industrial societies, we are frequently required, for example, to

1. Contend with widespread cultural disrespect and disregard for our ongoing value to society, and with social expectations of our stagnation and decline.
2. Give up a central identity formed around our work, career, or vocation, often at an arbitrary age and without our choice.
3. Surrender to others some considerable measure of authority, control, or influence over others and over ourselves and our own routines.
4. Change from a highly structured to a relatively unstructured existence.
5. Cope with the death of our spouse, friends, and other long-lived relationships.
6. Move from ready-made social relationships, personal identity, and purpose in life (e.g., through work) to having to create new friendships, identity, and purpose, often in unfamiliar locations.
7. Face "a marked decline in resistance to illness, a decline in recuperative powers, and increasing experience with bodily aches and pains" (Peck, 1956).
8. Not be an undue burden, financially or otherwise, on the caretaking resources of our family or society.
9. Face the inevitability that our living will come to an end.

Consider how differently those who face this curriculum with *the socialized mind* are likely to fare from those who face it with a *self-authoring mind*. It's true that *the socialized mind* might have an easier time relying and depending upon other persons and institutions to shape the routine and order of one's life, and might even be accepting of a powerfully communicated social expectation to disengage. But the same mental proclivity leaves one also internalizing, or breathing in, the toxins of disrespect and disregard in the cultural air toward the aged. This, by itself, is a pathogenic situation. Our first line of immunity in a psychologically toxic environment is our ability not to be defined by, or identified with, other people's negative or abusive characterizations and attributions of us. This ability requires *the self-authoring mind*. As wonderful as it might be for more elderly people to develop *the self-transforming mind* (and one can imagine how such a mentality might achieve the ego transcendence necessary to cope most successfully with the inevitable, permanent loss of the self), this most complex order of consciousness begins to look like more of a luxury in relation to the necessity of being able to distinguish oneself from the way one is being culturally defined, a self-authoring capacity.

This same necessity shows up in meeting the other demands as well. How well we can refashion our identities (e.g., in the face of retirement or widowhood) has to do with whether those identities were externally or internally conferred, an issue at the heart of the distinction between the *socialized* and the *self-authoring minds*. Consider, for example, these words from Lynn Caine's (1974) account of the personal journey of her widowhood. At the beginning of this painful but ultimately developmental journey, her loss was framed by *the socialized mind*, leaving her quite unable to master the curriculum she faced:

> Our society is set up so that most women lose their identities when their husbands die: Marriage is a symbiotic relationship for most of us. We draw our identities from our husbands. We add ourselves to our men, pour ourselves into them and their lives. We exist in their reflection. And then ...? If they die ...? It's wrenching enough to lose the man who is your lover, your companion, your best friend, the father of your children, *without losing yourself* as well. (p. 1, emphasis added)

The work of Gilligan (1982), Belenky, Clinchy, Goldberger, and Tarule (1986), and others, suggests that many women tend to orient to the world in a relational or connective fashion, "finding" the self in relation, while many men tend to orient in a more separated fashion, bringing a self known apart from relation to relation. If this is so, is the distinction between the *socialized* and the *self-authoring* minds merely a distinction between female and male styles, unwarrantedly favoring males with the preferencing designation of a more *mature* epistemology? Actually, the *styles* of our meaning making are orthogonally related to the *epistemologies* of our meaning making; it is quite possible, for example, to construct a *socialized* way of knowing in *either* a "connected" or "separate" voice. I discuss this more fully in *In Over Our Heads* (Kegan, 1994), but the point can be made by suggesting that, with very few substitutions, Caine's speech could as easily be rendered by a man with the same *socialized mind*:

> Our society is set up so that most men lose their identities when their job disappears. Work is a symbiotic relationship for most of us. We add ourselves to our jobs, pour ourselves into them. We exist in their reflection. And then ...? When we are forced to retire ...? It's wrenching enough to lose the source of your income, the routine and structure that has regulated your life, the social reference group you spend more time with than your own family, *without losing yourself as well*.

But Caine's journey into widowhood proved to be an evolutionary one. Her words at the end of her account suggest a change not just in how she felt but in who she was, a change in the organization of the self. Her newly emerging *self-authoring mind* permits her to master the curricular demand she before found beyond her reach:

I did not need a man for self-esteem any longer. And in a very strange way, this made me much less lonely. I no longer worried about whether or not a man—or a woman—liked me. My concern was with how I liked them, how they affected me, what kind of people they were. I no longer sought approval. I discovered that I was happy enough alone, *governing my own life now*. And I have modified that purposely: I am not "happy," but "happy enough." I am often lonely. I know what I'm missing, but I can cope with life. I find more pleasure in solitude. I am becoming a more serious woman. I want to write. I want to savor my children. I seek delights but my delights are different now. (Caine, 1974, p. 156; emphasis added)

Successful adjustment to the loss of spousal or vocational identity brings us back to our opening mystery as to why some people have an "empty nest" depression in midlife when the last child leaves home and some feel wonder-fully liberated. The issue here may have less to do with midlife and more to do with how the self is constituted in midlife. An "empty nest" depression in midlife may have a very similar architecture to the "empty bed" depression of a widow or widower in old age. The central question may be whether one is grieving only the loss of a precious other (what Freud would have called "mourning"), or whether one is grieving as well the loss of oneself (what Freud would have called "melancholia"). This question has everything to do with the difference between the epistemologies of the *socializing* and *self-authoring* minds.

Would the circumstance of constructing reality according to the epistemol-ogy of *the socialized mind* rather than *the self-authoring mind* compromise one's capacity to avoid being an undue burden on the emotional or financial resources of one's family or society? Very likely it would. It might not if one lived in the grip of a culture that provided a clear instructive address to just this issue (e.g., that the feeble elderly should separate themselves from the flock, drift off, and die of exposure or hunger, as I am told was the custom in some Native American tribes). In such a case, *the socialized mind* could meet the requirement not to be an undue burden, because by breathing the cultural air, one would unself-consciously take in the means to doing so. From a modernist perspective, we may imagine such a death, cut off from one's tribe and family, as lonely and shameful. From a traditionalist perspective, it is quite possible that such a person did not feel shamefully "sent away" at all, did not feel in the least alone, but psychologically surrounded by one's collective, faithful to it, well-integrated into it, carried off by it, borne away with it.

But the modernist world does not have a single address to this issue. At the same time we hear a call from various quarters not to be an undue burden, we see our society spending its treasure to support medical technologies and interven-tions that prolong life, even quite compromised life. We are told not to be an undue burden but we see our society prosecuting physicians who assist their patients in ending their lives.

And what of those who do still manage to live in a more traditionalist world, protected from modernism's confusing heterogeneity by the richly provided directives and traditions of their religious or ethnic collective? Their traditions are more likely to legitimate what we would regard as an "undue burden" than to mitigate against it. The elderly mother and her youngest daughter in the recent film, *Like Water for Chocolate*, are an extreme but still telling example. In her tradition, passed down for generations, the youngest daughter could not marry because it was her duty to care for her mother, a duty with which both mother and daughter were unself-consciously identified.

Countless less extreme but equally burdening arrangements exist between elderly parents and their children. What does it take psychologically (epistemologically) to avoid being an undue burden? Some may regard the very concept of "undue burden" as an outrageous indictment of the hyperindividualistic, anti-communal nature of modern life. But the hidden curriculum of modernism does institute the concept of individual rights and individual welfare; it does not completely subordinate the welfare of the individual to the welfare of the collective; it looks to balance the competing claims of individuals. And yet many elderly parents and their children are overmatched by this curriculum, collusively ensnared in overly burdening arrangements fueled by uncritically accepted expectations. What it takes epistemologically to avoid being an undue burden is an ability to construct the other (e.g., one's child) as a psychological whole, independent of oneself. It takes the capacity to separate from familial, ethnic, religious, or cultural expectations that would actually permit one to regard others uncritically as extensions of oneself. In other words, epistemologically, it requires *the self-authoring mind*.

TWO CONCLUDING IMPLICATIONS

A time-honored role for developmental psychology brought to the analysis of a school's curriculum is to inquire: What is it really you are asking of your students here? Are these expectations sensible, fair, or appropriate? What mental capacities in your students is your curriculum assuming, and are these assumptions warranted? If I were asked by the shapers of a "gerontological curriculum" what seemed to me the most appropriate fit between demand and capacity, I would say the following: While there is a value in evoking a picture of *self-transforming* developments in old age and thinking about how to support such development, a much greater constituency and a more compelling interest will be served by evoking a picture of *self-authoring* developments in old age, and thinking how to support these. The development of a capacity to separate the self from the socializing press of the surround, to create an internal personal authority, may be an absolutely crucial educational or mental health goal serving as a protective factor against decline and depression in old age.

Those with an interest in considering how educational and mental health settings for the aged can be fashioned to support gradual transformation from the *socializing* to the *self-authoring* mind will be helped by the work of constructive–developmental educators (e.g., Belenky et al., 1986; Daloz, 1987; Kegan, 1994; Taylor, 1991) and therapists (e.g., Carlsen, 1988; Kegan, 1994; Robbins, 1990; Rogers & Kegan, 1990) who have not necessarily addressed old age, but who have been working to support just this development among adults generally. Their work makes clear that the epistemological capacities I describe do not automatically unfold like some preprogrammed epigenetic code. Development proceeds (or fails to proceed) in contexts that are supportive (or thwarting) of the transformations of growth. Constructive–developmental educators and therapists look to the intentional fashioning of "holding environments" (Kegan, 1982, 1994), which make a setting rich in the elements that permit one to run the risks of leaving behind a familiar way of composing the self. While today's elderly population is only moderately using educational settings and underusing therapeutic and counseling settings, the baby boomers who will make up tomorrow's elderly population constitute a generation that is the greatest consumer of continuing education and psychotherapy in the history of the world. There is obviously not space to review this work in detail, but perhaps a single example will illustrate the care with which explicitly developmental educators or therapists try to attend to, and honor, the inevitable violations of faithfulness, loyalty, orthodoxy, or precious connection that persons experience when changing their (socializing) minds.

> I am sitting in my office with some loose time on my hands since one of my students can't make her appointment. Comes a knock on the door, and in walks Martha, a sixtyish, handsome woman, dressed for the late 19th century. Something about the expression on her face says that she would never do anything wrong. Although her reputation as a firm believer in Biblical Christianity precedes her, I have never met her, and I must say, I am curious.
>
> She tells me she is about to finish her Associate's Degree, and wants to go on for a degree in Education. She has to have the qualifications to help her get a job in the local Bible school. "There's a teacher there who plays favorites, and I don't think that's good," she told me. "I want to learn how not to play favorites."
>
> I explain to her that she won't have to be certified to teach in a private school, and go on to tell her what she will need to do. She seems satisfied. But then, as I think she is leaving, she reaches down into her purse and takes out a book. "There's one other thing I want to ask you about," she says, suddenly stern. The book in her hand is a standard health text. She opens it at a marker and slides the book across the desk toward me, her finger on a paragraph. "Just read that. Don't say anything. You don't have to say anything."
>
> It turns out to be some pretty explicit material about sexual behavior. I say nothing, and she then points to a picture on another page of two men holding hands. Beneath it is a discussion of homosexuality.
>
> She is shocked by it, she tells me. It is pure pornography. The whole book is a scandal. Useless. She tells me, scolding, that when she saw that she wanted to drop out of the course immediately. And then she begins to cry. Right there in my office! And I have never even met her before!
>
> I wait for the tears to slow down and then ask her if she has spoken to her teacher or to the community college staff about it. She replies that they just don't understand. It wouldn't do any good, she goes on. Then, at a forty-five degree angle, she asks, "Will your school be like this? Will I have to read this sort of trash in your program?"
>
> I assure her that she won't need to if she doesn't want, and that I can understand how deeply disturbing it is to her. I make a special effort to sympathize with her feelings about it and tell her again that she will not be forced to read what she feels is "trash."
>
> We talk on for some time about it and she vents about how disturbed she is. Finally, I say, "I do want to answer your question a little better about whether our school would be like this." And I say, "Our school will be the way you need it to be, Mrs. Findlay. But I have faith that as you get more schooling, you'll be less easily shocked by this sort of thing. I hope that you'll be more able to take it in stride. You don't have to believe it's

right, but I would hope that you can gain more distance from it so that it won't cause you so much turmoil."

She sits there and nods. She seems to be listening, though I feel a little as if I am giving her a lecture. As it happens, I spent part of the morning working with a student who was writing a paper comparing Frost's "The Hired Man" with the parable of "The Prodigal Son." So I am providentially able to quote chapter and verse from *The Bible.*

"Remember," I say to her, "that one of the remarkable things about Jesus is that he was able to go and speak to the publicans and the Pharisees right where they lived. He wasn't afraid to descend among them and witness to them; he went and spoke to the sinners and the wicked and the despised in the world. And he was able to love them, no matter how wicked."

She is definitely listening now. I feel a little hypocritical about this, but it's true. Jesus was amazing that way. I go on.

"Respectable people in the community were shocked by this," I tell her, "but not Jesus. He was able to see through their eyes. It wasn't a matter of whether he disapproved or not. He was just able to see as they saw and still love them. That's probably why he *did* love them. That was what was so amazing about him, Martha. He didn't have to agree with their homosexuality to find it in himself to love them."

She sits there for a moment. I can see she is still listening. All at once she straightens up, puts her Kleenex back in her handbag, and declares with surprising genuineness, "Well, yes. I guess I'm not perfect." We both laugh. We chat a little more after that, and I suggest that she go and talk with her Health teacher some more before she decides to drop out. Then, with a formal nod, morality back in place, she leaves the office. I'm left wondering what's happened. (Daloz, 1987, pp. 35–37, emphasis added)

The mentor neither disdains nor departs Martha's *socializing mind.* He does not require her to leave her loyalties at the gates of the university. He seeks rather to extend the gates to include her loyalties and in so doing allows Martha—not at her direction, but that of Jesus—to stay in school, to understand how school might be meaningful according to the terms with which she is still identified. Whether Martha will ever distinguish Jesus's authority from her own, only Martha can decide. In the meantime, should she find it agreeable, "higher education" of this sort can continue to offer her the opportunity to reflect on the terms of the authority to which she does feel bound.

The large numbers of aged adults who do not construct *the self-authoring mind* may suggest a clear educational or mental health goal for gerontology, since, I am arguing, this central epistemological tendency is the unrecognized threshold people need to meet to master the hidden curriculum of aging in contemporary society.

Alternatively, a second broad-gauged implication arises from considering the likelihood that an increasingly larger proportion of aging adults will construct reality in a *self-authoring* fashion. If this is so, it means there will be less and less acquiescence to cultural expectations for dependency and surrender of control in defining one's life among the elderly of tomorrow. It means there will be a much more publicly self-conscious exploration and invention of what life might be like in one's sixties, seventies, eighties, or nineties. In less than 10 years, the oldest members of the baby boom cohort will begin to turn 60. Significant proportions of this population will contend mightily against any social expectations that unwittingly, and dystonically, expect them to be in the grip of the *socialized mind.* While there are costs to facing a curriculum that is over one's head (predominantly borne by the beleaguered "student"), there are also costs to being saddled with one that is "under one's head." These costs will be borne by all involved. For many, "old age," over the next 30 years, is likely to become itself a culturewide context for ideological identification, personal empowerment, and the growth of the *self-authoring mind*, just as feminism, ethnic identification or sexual orientation served in the past and present. Where the "Grey Panthers" appear today as tiny and anomalous figures of elderly activity and self-assertion on the cultural ground, such public self-definition, more normalized, is likely to be a feature of the cultural ground itself.

Such developments could have highly liberating or highly disruptive results, and my guess is that we may see a good deal of both. I expect there will be a much more varied public "story" about what old age can be like, enabled by a capacity to separate from, and relate critically toward, established taboos and definitions. I think we will see a greater invention of living situations. And of dying situations. I think sexuality in later life will be a much more discussable, aboveground phenomenon. I think all social institutions—medical, religious, governmental, educational—will feel the pressure of *self-authoring* consumers who, rather than being shaped by the existing routines and self-definitions of such institutions, will feel entitled to make their own age-related demands, calling on such institutions to reshape themselves accordingly.

The story of higher education's relationship to the "older, returning adult student" is likely to be replayed in a variety of our institutions as a greater proportion of all our institution's constituencies is elderly: Originally, the adult student was on the margins of the campus and its consciousness, a guest of someone else's party. Increasingly, they are the reason the party is still going on. For the institutions, it is one thing to let new people into an ongoing party; the newcomers are the ones who must struggle to fit in. It is another thing to change the party; now, it is the institution that must struggle to fit.

The difficulties of greater self-authorship will not just be borne by threatened persons and institutions whose realities are being called into question. These are the difficulties that arise from the limits of *the socializing mind*; but there will also be difficulties arising from the limits of *the self-authoring mind*. The development of a greater "personal authority" in the psychology of the aged still leaves open the question of how this much more empowered constituency will resolve conflicts among its own members and with the generation of younger adults. The gradual emergence of greater self-authorship among the aging population may also be accompanied by new, protracted disputes, such as the specter of generational warfare over Social Security already on the horizon in the United States.

The twentieth century has come to be seen as a time in which we have become conscious of, and with great difficulty, gradually begun to redefine the meaning of, gender. It is possible that the twenty-first century may come to be seen as a time when we become more conscious of, and, with no less difficulty, gradually begin to redefine the meaning of elderly life. The new field of gerontology is itself an expression of this self-consciousness and the effort to author, rather than be authored by, the culture's definition of old age.

REFERENCES

Argyris, C. (1993). *On organizational learning*. Cambridge, UK: Blackwell Business.

Belenky, M. F., Clinchy, B. M., Goldberger, N. R., & Tarule, J. M. (1986). *Women's ways of knowing*. New York: Basic Books.

Bruffee, K. (1993). *Collaborative learning: Higher education, interdependence and the authority of knowledge*. Baltimore: Johns Hopkins University Press.

Caine, L. (1974). *Widow*. New York: William Morrow.

Carlsen, M. B. (1988). *Meaning-making: Therapeutic process in developmental psychotherapy*. New York: Norton.

Chasin, R., & Herzig, M. (1993). Creating systemic interventions for the sociopolitical arena. In B. Berger-Gould & D. H. DeMuth (Eds.), *The global family therapist* (pp. 149–191). Needham, MA: Allyn & Bacon.

Cumming, E., & Henry, W. (1961). *Growing old*. New York: Basic Books.

Daloz, L. (1987). "Martha meets her mentor," *Change Magazine*, July/August, pp. 35–37.

Erikson, E. H., Erikson, J. M., & Kivnick, H. Q. (1986). *Vital involvement in old age*. New York: Norton.

Friedan, B. (1993). *The fountain of age*. New York: Simon & Schuster.

Gilligan, C. (1982). *In a different voice*. Cambridge, MA: Harvard University Press.

Grow, G. (1991). Teaching learners to be self-directed. *Adult Education Quarterly, 41*, 125–149.

Gutmann, D. (1987). *Reclaimed powers*. New York: Basic Books.

Heifetz, R. A. (1995). *Leadership without easy answers*. Cambridge, MA: Harvard University Press.

Kegan, R. (1982). *The evolving self*. Cambridge, MA: Harvard University Press.

Kegan, R. (1986). The child behind the mask: Sociopathy as developmental delay. In W. II. Reid, J. W. Bonner III, D. Dorr, & J. I. Walker (Eds.), *Unmasking the psychopath* (pp. 45–77). New York: Norton.

Kegan, R. (1994). *In over our heads*. Cambridge, MA: Harvard University Press.

Lahey, L., Souvaine, E., Kegan, R., Goodman, R., & Felix, S. (1988). *A guide to the Subject–Object Interview: Its administration and analysis*. Cambridge, MA: Subject–Object Research Group.

Levinson, D. (1978). *The seasons of a man's life*. New York: Knopf.

Newhouse, M. (1995). *Successful aging and the development of the self*. Unpublished manuscript, Harvard Graduate School of Education, Cambridge, MA.

Peck, R. C. (1956). Psychological developments in the second half of life. In J. E. Anderson (Ed.), *Psychological aspects of aging* (88–93). Washington, DC: American Psychological Association.

Robbins, M. A. (1990). *Midlife women and death of mother*. New York: Peter Lang.

Rogers, C. (1951). *Client-centered therapy*. Boston: Houghton Mifflin.

Rogers, L., & Kegan, R. (1990). Mental growth and mental health as distinct concepts in the study of developmental psychopathology. In D. Keating & H. Rosen (Eds.), *Constructivist approaches to psychopathology* (pp. 103–147). Hillsdale, NJ: Erlbaum.

Schon, D. A. (1987). *Educating the reflective practitioner*. San Francisco: Jossey-Bass.

Taylor, K. (1991). *Transforming learning*. Unpublished doctoral disseration, Union Graduate School, San Diego, CA.

Torbert, W. (1987). *Managing the corporate dream*. Homewood, IL: Dow-Jones Irwin.

Villegas-Reimers, E. (1988). *Judgments of responsibility: Their relationship with self and moral reasoning in Venezuelan adolescents*. Unpublished doctoral dissertation, Harvard Graduate School of Education, Cambridge, MA.

Walsh, P. B. (1989). *Kegan's structural–developmental theory of sociopathy and some actualities of sociopathic cognition*. Unpublished doctoral dissertation, University of Pittsburgh, Pittsburgh, PA.

CHAPTER 10

An Image of Aging and the Concept of Aintegration

Coping and Mental Health Implications

Jacob Lomranz

INTRODUCTION

The field of social gerontology has grown enormously in the last decade. However, the abundance of theories, information, and publications leaves the reader somewhat bewildered. On the one hand, there are the many "medically influenced" publications that present "aging as a catastrophe, ... (the elderly) as damaged (and) incapable of new growth" (Gutmann, 1994, p. 9). On the other hand, social gerontology, with its branches of personality, cognitive, and social psychology, basically portrays a very positive picture of aging; it depicts the aged enjoying years of happiness and well-being as they move through outlined adult stages and tasks to be fulfilled. It is easy to arrange the publications in two piles labeled "optimistic" and "pessimistic." Given the ease of such an exercise, one wonders what gives rise to such divergent findings and theories? What are their overt and covert assumptions? Here, one is led to the underlying notions of human nature or the image of man.

In light of the given state of affairs, I dwell on two interrelated concepts: the image of man and the concept of aintegration (the prefix *a* denotes "not"). Both concepts should become part of the gerontological nomenclature, for "the particular kind of knowledge that arises out of the, gaps, inconsistencies and incongruities to the cultural (and psychological) perceptions of the old requires an appropriate language, one which addresses differences and contradictions

Jacob Lomranz • Department of Psychology and the Herczeg Institute on Aging, Tel Aviv University, 69978, Tel-Aviv, Israel.

Handbook of Aging and Mental Health: An Integrative Approach, edited by Jacob Lomranz. Plenum Press, New York, 1998.

rather than coherence and compatibility" (Hazan, 1994, p.6). I argue that many of the present psychosocial approaches and theories in gerontology are insufficient. Three main underlying reasons, embedded in their respective domains, are suggested for this. The first is the inappropriateness of scientific and cultural values related specifically to the image of human nature, which I suggest should be altered; the second is the insufficiency of dealing with the existential–cultural context as it pertains to the aged in society, which I propose to reconsider in a different light; third are the restricted and one-sided theoretical frameworks, which I juxtapose with the concept of aintegration. These issues are also relevant to the existence of human beings on all points of the lifespan.

I wish to emphasize that I do not intend to negate developmental, integrative principles, but rather to clarify and supplement them. I concur with the developmental orientation, depicted by Pepper (1942) as a "worldview" and conceive of lifespan development (Baltes & Baltes, 1993) in an "organismic–developmental" (Werner, 1948) and Lewinian perspective (Ziegler & Glick, 1986), as a series of qualitative reorganizations along specific principles. In that framework, I perceive human strength as a capacity to endure hardships and inconsistencies, enabling people to absorb events that do not make sense, to be bewildered cognitively and frustrated emotionally, and yet to maintain mental health. Perhaps a paradigmatic shift is necessary if we are to conceive of the human condition in its totality, including man's ability to age, suffer, enjoy, endure, and grow, all at the same time.

The area of mental health and aging (Gatz, Kasel-Godley, & Karel, 1996) has not yet reached its deserved position in either theory or application. This may be due to client, professional, as well as cultural factors (Gatz, Popkin, Pino, & VandenBos, 1985), but also because we have not created enough relevant concepts. It is with these needs in mind that the conceptualizations in this chapter have been conceived.

In the following pages, I summarize several major developmental lifespan conceptualizations and their implications. I then relate to existential incompatibilities, which these theories do not take into account. This will lead to underlying assumptions about human nature and the proposition for a composite image of man and the elderly. That image reflects a person's capacity for aintegration, a concept I define and explicate by focusing on its theoretical framework and root sources in psychology and human experience. Aintegration is then presented in a personality context, and its role in the experience of the aged will be demonstrated. Finally, implications for theory research, psychotherapy, and clinical methodology are suggested.

CONCEPTUALIZATIONS OF ADULTHOOD
AND AGING, AND THEIR IMPLICATIONS

I relate here only to the major lifespan conceptualizations that have had an important academic and professional impact, as reflected in all the basic textbooks on adulthood and aging. Similar principles underlie most of these conceptualizations: (1) They are based on life stages (e.g., Buhler, 1953; Erikson,

1959; Gould, 1978; Havinghurst, 1972; Levinson, 1978); (2) ages, with certain reservations, are designated for the stages (e.g., Buhler, 1953; Gould, 1978; Havinghurst, 1972; Levinson, 1978) reinforcing age-belongingness-to-stage positions; (3) conflicts, illusions (e.g., Gould) or tasks (e.g., Havinghurst) are postulated, often in polarized positions (e.g., Erikson), their resolution promising "successful aging" or integrity (e.g., Erikson, Havinghurst); (4) some of these tasks are psychodynamically based (e.g., Gould), others, socially (e.g., Havinghurst), still others combining the two (e.g., Erikson, Levinson); however the social orientation is heavily loaded in all; (5) the notions of "integration," "developmental tasks," "transitions," or "marker events" are utilized as concepts through which life changes, adjustment, and successful aging can be achieved; (6) it is often claimed that these must be encountered and resolved at specific times during the life cycle for normal development to occur.

I would like to devote particular attention to Erik Erikson (1959, 1963), since many of my critical remarks relate to his work. Among Erikson's many contributions is the view of epigenetically based ego development across eight stages, each constituting a psychosocial crisis to be resolved positively or negatively, with a resultant effect on a human tendency (e.g., love, caring, wisdom). The last stage, ego integrity versus despair, characterizes old age. According to Erikson, integrity will virtually evolve by itself as the successful resolution of all the previous crises. It requires an "acceptance of one's one and only life cycle and of the people who have become significant to it as something that had to be and that, by necessity, permitted of no substitutions" (Erikson, 1968, p. 139). Integrity also implies a sense of wholeness and completeness that can be gained by an introspective, self-examining process through which individuals are hopefully able to integrate a lifetime populated by successes and failures, affirm their past, and thus avoid despair, in which fear of death may be dominant. The person who accepts his or her past and has a sense of integrity accepts death as the inevitable end of having lived. Wisdom, related to the successful resolution of the final psychosocial conflict, is the virtue that comes at the climax of life, the culminating and integrative achievement of all previous stages and virtues. Erikson taught us that it is impossible to comprehend development without society and culture. His work is as rich in what pertains to culture as it is in ego psychology. Erikson's is a powerful vision, a synthesis of life as lived in human culture, as well as an "essentially hopeful, psychosocial ego psychology" (Kegan, 1982, p. vii).

What Do These Conceptualizations Signify?: Some Critical Remarks

Given the features of the various developmental lifespan theories, it is hard to see how they relate to the individual's uniqueness in society, and how they can contribute to clinical theory and interventions. The lifespan theories appear to be too simplistic, replete with overinclusions, oversocialized, almost like mechanistic articulations of concepts such as developmental tasks, age-designated life stages, and transitions. Therefore their generalizability and applicability to the elderly population at large is questionable. In terms of process, they anticipate disequilibrium, followed by conflict resolution and integration, leading positively toward successful aging. While they differ in their level of articulation and underlying assumptions, they have commonalities, which I examine with a critical eye.

1. It is assumed that one knows what aging is, so what remains is to identify its stages, tasks, and what makes it successful. Thus many theories seem to "put the cart before the horse," leading to inadequate rationality for studies, confusion in the formulation of questions, and bias research.

2. Although often termed *models and theories*, such conceptualizations do not meet the requirements of scientific theories. They are descriptive rather than prescriptive, do not differentiate between structure and process, and fail to explicate how development and change takes place.

3. They do not identify their underlying principles—whether, for instance, they are organismic, mechanistic, or psychoanalytic.

4. They are unable to explain, in a differentiated manner, individual change as a result of the person—environment interaction, nor do they define the active or passive role of the organism in structuring experience with regard to both the internal meaning—giving and the external manipulation of environmental circumstances.

5. They do not appropriately deal with characteristic core issues in developmental theory (Hayslip & Panek, 1989), such as the controversy regarding stages, the age—stage relationship, or how the elementist versus holistic approach applies to development.

6. They ignore the question of the relationship between qualitative versus quantitative change.

7. They do not elaborate their positions regarding the impact of nature versus nurture, determinism versus nondeterminism, or the place of biology.

8. They do not consider the relationship between various levels—physical, cognitive, and emotional—in the processes of development.

9. The impact of society is inadequately discussed. Indeed their normativity suggests a highly standardized society, whose standards reflect the priorities and values of the middle and upper classes. Moreover, they do not take into account the changing dynamics of societies and culture or the social reality encountered by the elderly.

10. The concept of development is used in diverse ways and given different meanings. Various frames of reference are employed: schematic—structural descriptions (e.g., Freudian or Piagetian), processes (e.g., response patterns, defenses, or coping styles), content of response (e.g., feeling fulfilled or integrity), and environmental or external demands (e.g., adjusting to retirement or loss of spouse).

It seems to me that a very important transposition occurs: When development in children is discussed, concepts are related to a structural and operational level; when it comes to aging, however, language is diverted from a structural to an experiential level. Furthermore, the limits of development are not defined. Is every motion equated with development? Should we equate "life" with "development," and if so, then what justifies duplication? Can a person be described as living fully, yet not necessarily developing? Finally, there is a value-laden double standard in the use of the term. Previously, *development* designated only the growth of children toward maturity. Now, it is used by many adult developmentalists to mean multidirectional, systematic, and expected change (Baltes, Reese, & Lipsitt, 1980). However, its use still is discriminative: When change denotes loss, one does not usually speak of development as in "She develops towards death." Rather, the term is associated with positive connotations. I believe this use of the term derives from an embedded Western value that attributes continuous growth to human beings, evoking an image of man racing toward limitlessness. Such an image, although relatively recent, now characterizes modern culture (Zoja, 1995).

All these shortcomings have serious implications. These developmental theories serve as messages and infer values and styles of living for the elderly. They present a one-sided, amiable picture of human nature, project unbased optimism, avoid sufficient exploration of life's difficulties, are oversocially grounded, diminish biological and psychological factors, and virtually "preach" adjustment before providing a comprehensive picture of developmental and coping processes.

Moreover, since the knowledge of what to expect of life is presumed, remedies for counteracting complexities are presented in almost a didactic and paternalistic manner like that typically found in books of popular psychology, mapping the road for the adult person to avoid depression, midlife or retirement crises, and achieve successful aging, as if there is only one way to age *successfully* (a term I propose we eliminate altogether).

In summary, these theories may harbor a negative potential for a wrong course in the science of adulthood and aging. These models propose, albeit indirectly, an epistemological stance that denies the importance of the complex experience of aging. While the various theories also relate to possible negative developments, for example, isolation, despair (Erikson), improper life structures (Levinson), and false assumptions (Gould), these are not sufficiently dealt with. In a sense, they are posited as the enemies to be avoided. The theoretical investment is in positive evolvement. One might use the metaphor of a marvelous sports team, powerful, convincing, attractive, and applauded. But against whom, we may ask, are they playing? How can the game be won if the opponent's power is unknown? I assume that the major theoretical foundation and support for these approaches stems, to a great extent, from Erik Erikson's legacy and forceful impact.

VICISSITUDES OF INTEGRITY
IN THE CONTEXT OF ADULT DEVELOPMENT

Integration, an inseparable part of developmental thought, generally denotes a process whereby a synthesis is created from differentiated, previously incompatible, parts or entities in the mind, resulting in the emergence of a new structure, all in the service of adaptive development and growth (e.g., Kegan,

1982; Piaget, 1980). Personality theorists have used the concept of integration in different ways. For some (e.g., Rogers), inconsistencies are a threat to the organization of the self, so in order to avoid personality breakdown a defensive process, such as integration, reorganizes personality structure. For some (e.g., Goldstein), integration relates to the total organism, while for others (e.g., Erikson, Loevinger) it appears to be a process. Unfortunately, *integration*, like *development*, is not always defined by those who employ the term. Despite Erikson's enormous contribution, a number of basic questions arise about his use of the concept. For Erikson (1963), integration, or integrity, in a person appears "only in him who in some way has ... adapted himself to the triumph and disappointments adherent to being, ... Only in him may gradually ripen the fruit of these seven stages. I know no better word for it than ego integrity" (1963, pp. 268–269). Disregarding, at this point, Erikson's stipulations for integrity, we still have to be clear as to its meaning. The problem may lie in the words *ego integrity*; while *ego* is a theoretical, structural construct, *integrity* is a human state (achieved perhaps by certain behaviors). The *Concise Oxford Dictionary* (1956) reflects diverse aspects when it defines *integrity* as "wholeness; soundness; uprightness, honesty, purity" but also defines *integration* as an act of "combining parts into a whole" (p. 620). Erikson, when claiming that elderly people should accept and integrate their past, focuses and describes their interpersonal and social level but does not elaborate this process in structural terms.

In point of fact, Erikson (1968) himself does not sufficiently elaborate the term *integrity*, stating "that for the state in which ... the fruit of the seven stages gradually ripens. I know no better word for it than integrity. *Lacking clear definition* (italics mine), I shall point to a few attributes of this stage of mind" (p. 139). Given its link to the trait of "wisdom," integrity has been accepted as a synonym for "successful aging," carrying immense implications as a value and evoking a certain image of the elderly person. However, integrity, as a condition for successful aging, is hard to accept. I would argue that a person may in fact attain Eriksonian integrity even in the absence of the conditions that Erikson formulates, that is, the acceptance of achievements as well as disappointments and that one's life was "something that had to be and that by necessity, permitted no substitution" (1963, p. 98). There is no necessary link between attaining "integrity" and wisdom and fearing death. People may feel that they have taken responsibility for their lives, yet still fear death, and vice versa. That elderly people should integrate their past and accept it (Erikson, 1963) has almost become a demand in light of the popularity of the "life review" recommended for all the elderly (Butler, 1963; Coleman, 1986). However, one wonders on what scientific basis such a claim is made, research being inconclusive (Lieberman & Tobin, 1983). Finally, in experimental terms, the attempts to measure Erikson's concepts have not been very successful (Walaskay, Whitbourne, & Nehrke, 1983). Peck (1968) claims that Erikson's last two stages are too global, and Clayton (1975) argues that rather than expect complete resolution of crises as the norm, it is more realistic to see individuals as "compromising" their way through the various crises. People do not always "accept" their past or "resolve" crises.

Erikson, it seems, provided us with only part of the aging puzzle, but unfortunately his impact may hinder us in our search for additional pieces. He was a great advocate of integrity, but his integrity lacks elaboration, is over-socialized, is only partly culturally updated, and is value biased. The association between aging and integration—integrity does not help us to comprehend what so many elderly persons actually experience as they age, and certainly should not be a condition of constructive life in old age. The life characteristics of the elderly person are such that acceptance and integration are often impossible.

AGING AMID EXISTENTIAL–SOCIAL INCOMPATIBILITIES

One wonders how the mentioned lifespan theories can convey the experience of human aging in society. How congruent is the aging process with modern society? Science, education, gender rights, and standards of living have all been revolutionized, but social structures still appear inflexible and are changing slowly, if at all. Let us consider certain implications of this state of affairs on sociocultural and personal levels.

Societal Blockades

At present, for many elderly, existence is accompanied by profound cultural disenfranchisement. More than 20 years ago, Irving Rosow (1974) claimed that the American culture does not provide the elderly with meaningful norms by which to live. Many retirees have stated that they experience "social death" (Guillemard, 1982, p. 230). Such problems, while varying in different social classes, are highly pronounced in most cultures, and it may be a grievous burden to age in a rapidly changing society.

Riley, Kahn, and Foner (1994) refer to these phenomena as a "structural lag," stating that

> there is a mismatch or imbalance between the transformation of the aging process from birth to death and the role opportunities or places in the social structure that could foster and reward people at the various stages of their lives. While the twentieth century has experienced a revolution in human development, there has been no comparable revolution in the role structures of society to keep pace with the ways people grow up and grow old. (p. 16)

Modern society provides the elderly with fewer "opportunity structures" (Merton, 1957) that are necessary to shape development so as to enhance the quality of human lives. The "goodness of fit" (Kahn, 1994) between individual needs, aspirations, and abilities on the one hand, and the expectations and opportunities provided by the social structure, on the other, is seriously distorted. The described predicament has far-reaching personal implications. Hazan (1994) emphasizes the tensions and paradoxes "emanating from irreconcilable tensions between images of the old, their own will and desires, and the facilities offered to them" (p. 2).

Personal and Interpersonal Blockades

The various roles of the elderly are all full of contradictions and paradoxes, as is reflected in some cogent domains.

Personal Realization. Many aged, knowing that chronological age is a poor indicator of will, desires, ability, vigor, mental competence (Suzman, Harris, Hadley, Kovar, & Weindruch, 1992), wisdom, and their compensating abilities (Baltes & Baltes, 1993), may experience how the realization of such productive potentials is being impeded, causing them to live with a cognitive and emotional schism and a sense of estrangement.

The Family. Once an integral part of a person's existence, the family is becoming less so for many of today's aged. A number of structural changes in modern family life (which may not hold for all ethnic groups) account for this (Hareven, 1994; Pearlin & Skaff, Chapter 14, this volume): unclear boundaries of the family structure; the privatization of the nuclear family, leading to a closing of households and increasing fragmentation; individualism—an emphasis on the individual rather than on the collective family needs and an exaggerated emphasis on love. In the past, family members were valued not merely for providing emotional satisfaction for each other but also for a wide array of services on the premise that a collective view of reciprocal familial obligations lay at the very base of survival. Ambiguity as to responsibility—the shift of responsibility for the care of older people from the family to the public sector—has generated confusion in aged persons and their kin as to the kind and limits of expected support.

Affect. Insofar as meaning is related to accomplishments and creativity, it provides a sense of worth and joy, feelings not sufficiently generated in the present conditions of aging. Attempts by the elderly to combat institutionally/socially imposed constraints are apt to fail, probably leading to further frustration, isolation, and depression. Many elderly are left with passive amusements and the consumption of material goods but without the driving force of meaning and accomplishment. Lazarus and Lazarus (1994) term as "existential emotions" those feelings that result from social–existential anxieties. These consist of anxiety–fright, guilt, and shame. Shame may also appear as a reaction to the failing body as well as to the exposure of the elderly person's condition. Blythe (1979) presents narratives in which the elderly convey resentment, due to the blocking of their desires, which they then learn to constrain. Others noted that many elderly experience a sense of resentment stemming from discrimination and inequitable distribution of social goods (Jonsen, 1992).

In conclusion, factors and processes of aging, like those mentioned earlier, constitute mental demands of modern life (Kegan, 1994) and have a major impact on the epistemological stance of many elderly. These factors may be the source of emotional and relational confusion, a sense of discord, estrangement, conflict, insecurity, bewilderment, and paradox. The existential predicament may serve not only as a potential source of stress, but it also weakens interdependence and sources of support. I do not wish to advocate a "deficit model" of aging, but only to stress that the elderly constantly feel that they are functioning below their potential. Given their existence, elderly persons, in metaphoric terms, may be required to accomplish a Herculean task but end up living like Sisyphus.

We thus come face-to-face with an unavoidable question: How can we possibly explain the optimistic lifespan theories if we take into account the totality of the aging ecology? It is misleading to construct global theories under the lamppost because there is light there, even if there are aged who fit the optimistic models of many theorists. Has optimism become a value embedded in science? What is in fact the image of human nature held by scientists in the field of adult development?

SCIENCE, HUMAN NATURE, AND THE IMAGE OF MAN

Theories and methods developed or adopted by scientists are contingent on their views of human nature and their image of man (Kenyon, 1988). The traits and orientation of scientists have a major impact on their products (Polanyi, 1958), and the work of Kuhn (1962) portrays science as scientists. The creation of a theory or body of research is often a melting pot of different, personal, scientific, ethical, and cultural needs (Lubow, 1977). A scientific community evolves its own norms, values, policies, and images of knowledge (Merton, 1957). These shared images may partly determine the nature of specific scientific products, and produce, perhaps as in our case, one-sided, at times contrasting, optimistic approaches to aging.

Values, Culture, and Images of Aging

Assumptions about human nature are essentially ontological suppositions that then serve as epistemological guidelines, eventually leading the theorist to focus on certain aspects of existence while perhaps ignoring others. The concept of human nature is expressed in the image of man. Images of man have been variously conceived and often reviewed (Lomranz, 1986). Moreover, there are relevant cultural differences within Western society, for example, pragmatism versus critical theory (Moody, 1988, 1992), as well as between East and West. Eastern philosophies, religions, and cultures, in contrast to Western culture, portray man as part of nature and life, which includes suffering and reincarnation. Eastern thought is much less dichotomous than the Western Aristotelian mode of thinking. That A could also be non-A would not constitute a dilemma for a Chinese philosopher. Another relevant cultural difference may be the American portrayal of human nature and image of man as opposed to the European, reflected in the histories of psychoanalysis and phenomenology/

existentialism. While ego psychology in the United States developed and focused on dimensions of adjustment, human capacities, growth, and psychosocial integration, the emphasis in Europe was more on object relations, the
intrapsychic, severe psychopathology, and the place of innate elements such as
the death instinct. In another example, we find the Europeans, under the same
banner of existentialism/phenomenology, dwelling on the essence of perception, the absurdity of life, and man's inherent continuous struggle with freedom, anxiety, loneliness, and death, while in America, these branches received
the added epithet of "humanism" and deal with peak experiences and self-
actualization, dismissing the question of the meaning of life (Moody, 1992). The
former reflect solemnness, fatalism, and pessimism; the latter reflect relief,
hope, and optimism. Do some of the theories in gerontology and lifespan development reflect American cultural values? And how does the aged person actually fit such images and values?

It should not come as a surprise that European images of man as well as those
of the human condition in general have been rejected in America (Cole, 1992;
Moody, 1992). The underlying assumptions and values in gerontology have for
the most part remained covert and insufficiently delineated. It seems that the
American way of life and the focus on self-actualization and youth have been
able to allocate only minimal space to the inherent hardships of life in general
and of aging in particular. This is even more pertinent now that we have
prolonged life but not always improved its quality.

In light of this, as we reconsider most of the lifespan theories, we must
conclude that they portray a rigid polarity of positive and negative stereotypes,
a moral code based on physical and materialistic control and success, on ratio-
nalism and Aristotelian logic, on pragmatism, activity, optimism, and on a
unidirectionality of integrated personal and social growth and an enlightened
society. At the same time, they reflect a denial of tragedy and death, a disregard of
multidirectionality, uncertainty, ambiguity, absurdity, social turmoil, misery,
mystery, or paradoxical situations. It is no wonder, therefore, that as theories
encounter life, the images of the elderly as portrayed in gerontology, by policymakers as well as in the public, appear disconsonant, conflicting, focused on
diverse levels (Labouvie-Vief, 1977; Marshall, 1980), riddled with extreme
stereotyping and reflecting positive and negative myths. Side by side with the
negative views are the innumerable books on the "golden years." We seem to
be in desperate need of a clear and balanced image of man in general and of the
elderly in particular.

A Composite Image of the Aging Person

If we consider the ideals of different cultures throughout history we realize
that taken together, they contain images of aging that reflect "the ineradicable
paradoxes of later life" (Cole, 1992, p. xxv). Aging has been perceived as a
source of both tranquillity and turbulence, as a state of wisdom and of cognitive
decline, as both rewarding and marked by suffering and pain, as both spiritual

growth and physical decline, as an object of honor and of insult, as a state of security and vulnerability, as both growth and decay. A composite image, like the one suggested below, does not tolerate a one-sided polarity or "either–or" approach but does allow for divergent simultaneous perspectives and alternatives. I would like to offer an image of human nature and the aged that may also be appropriate for gerontological research. The underlying assumption for this suggested image of humankind is that human beings are temporal, biological organisms, part of nature and of the processes of growth, development, loss, and decay, contextual in behavior, comprised of multidimensional systems, in a state of asynchronization, seeking balance, whose "being" involves a relational, social essence intricately interrelated to themselves and to their physical, human, and cultural surroundings. This "humanness" is self-propelled, and creates awareness, perception, consciousness, intentionality, realization, and creativity, but these may also be constricted by a sense of isolation, dualism, fatalism, and finitude. While continuously making meaning out of experience, conceiving their journey of life as their personal, perhaps mythical, narrative, they also are able to be content without interpretation or actualization, are able to cope and live with enigma, relativism, paradox, contradiction, meaninglessness, absurdity, and inconsistency.

This image, reflecting an orientation that needs to be further elaborated, has a broad sweep; it gathers and harvests the insights of many scientists, philosophers, psychologists, artists, and cultural sources. Such an image is multidimensional, complex, and postmodern, and thus shifts away from the absolute, universal, and unidimensional. It gives space to the human capacity to structure one's own life and encounter death (Kastenbaum, 1985). It allows one the latitude to concentrate on the different levels of progression or deficits in human life that occur at different times, and to consider compensations in specific contexts (Baltes & Baltes, 1993). It enables one to live with inconsistencies and with or without articulated meaning. Since it is composite, this image is able to contain the various complex, often paradoxical, processes occurring in old age. While this image of aging may seem far removed from that adopted by the abovementioned developmental theorists, it is supported by some important work on aging. These include, for instance, the lifespan developmental perspective emphasizing multivariate, multidirectional, multidetermined, and pluralistic components (Baltes & Baltes, 1993; Gatz, Chapter 4, this volume); comprehensive approaches adopted in longitudinal studies (e.g., Block, 1971); the dialectical approach (Reigel, 1973); work in the areas of personality, the self-concept, coping styles, adjustment, and change (Lieberman, 1975; Lieberman & Tobin, 1983; Peskin, 1987; Ruth & Coleman, 1996; Thomae, 1980); work, on ego mediators, cross-cultural gerontology (Gutmann, 1994), and on meaning-making processes (Kegan, 1982; Moody, 1992). As the thrust of my approach becomes clear, so does the obvious need to add a further, thus far, missing concept. Most of the gerontological literature, even that supporting the image of humankind I have outlined, does not fulfill all the conditions of that image. There is not enough emphasis on the limitations of thinking in polarities and absolutes, nor on the possibilities of cognition, perceptions, and feelings concerning ambiguity, inconsistency, absurdity, and paradox. In an attempt to meet the outlined basic condition of coping and human nature, I now introduce the concept of aintegration.

THE DEFINITION OF AINTEGRATION

Aintegration, a generic concept, is defined as a mental process and resultant state. As a functional coping capacity, it represents a level of mental organizational complexity in an individual's epistemological being. Adult developmentally seated, aintegration may or may not, depending on external or internal conditions and personal history, be activated and expressed in behavior. This ability to feel integrity without necessarily having integrated everything may be called upon at different times and in varying degrees, especially in situations of conflict, stress, and old age. Cognitively, aintegration, as conceived in the neo-Piagetian, postformal framework, is usually characterized by awareness but does not require "higher" mental functions or education. As affect, it presents an ability to withstand emotional strain as it reorganizes the impact of emotional pressure. As an attitude, it is part of a worldview, and as such it stands near postmodernism. Ingrained in a certain image of humankind, aintegration also carries a social evaluative component, and as such it connotes a person's stance in the face of the social predicament of aging and carries an existential worldview closer to European existential philosophy than to American individuality and pragmatism.

Aintegration should be conceived as a person's ability to feel well without necessarily having integrated all the various human biopsychosocial levels, or certain entities within each level (e.g., cognition, values, or affect), into an overriding whole. Aintegration entails a possible sense of inconsistencies, relativism, asynchronization, discontinuity, paradox, ambivalence, ambiguity, absurdity, and tolerance for contradictions. Inconsistency may cause anxiety and consequent efforts toward change and reintegration, but this is not necessarily always so. Aintegration enables one to cope not by manipulating incompatible entities of content and essence but by consciously living with such entities, while preserving well-being and experiencing "wholeness" or integrity. Contradictory states coexist. The person, especially the elderly, may experience an ability to consciously bear thoughts, emotions, events, and behaviors that seem inconsistent in personal, value, or cultural terms and yet be in a state of equilibrium, without feeling pressured, fragmented, or in need of a change in his or her state of mind; rather he or she functions appropriately and experiences self-content. Unwilling or unable to integrate inconsistencies, he or she may experience them dialectically or separately. Individuals may experience continuity regarding their identity (Gatz, Chapter 4, this volume) and Self, and yet experience aintegration.

Integration and aintegration should be conceived as independent orthogonal organizing principles and in contrast to the conventional view that regards integration as positive and nonintegration (aintegration) as negative.

THEORETICAL FRAMES OF REFERENCE
AND SOURCES OF AINTEGRATION

Current findings in quantum physics are inconsistent with traditional logic. The natural sciences have been plagued by implicit and explicit inconsistencies and contradictory theories, and that state has only recently been accepted. Can we accept such a state of affairs in human beings and in the social sciences as well? Perhaps not yet, since Western culture is built mainly on traditional logic in which the basic premise is the principle of the noncontradictory observation or postulates (i.e., A must always equal and be identical to A, and never to B). As a concept in discord with such traditional logic, aintegration requires elaboration. I attempt to elucidate the concept of aintegration by dwelling on its underlying theoretical sources as exemplified in four conceptual areas. These areas lend support to the concept of aintegration and show how the human mind is also familiar with the functional and attitudinal processes underlying aintegration.

Personality and Clinical Psychology

The branches of psychology dealing with human behavior have extensively been preoccupied by the question of what to do with "inappropriate," contrasting, and therefore disturbing stimuli. Major works have offered elaborate models for dealing with the problem, and are based mainly on the principles of integration and consistency, and on that basis, have elaborated processes leading to meaning making, cognitive dissonance, or congruency (e.g., works by Festinger, A. Freud, Hartman, Rogers). However, while these may explain many behaviors, explanations for other behaviors in the human repertoire as well as various substantive questions may be excluded. In point of fact, different psychological theories and research provide a sound foundation for aintegration by emphasizing duality, inconsistencies, paradox, and contradictions.

Clinical Theorizing. In clinical theory, the concept of paradox is attracting increasing attention (e.g., Modell, 1990). Freud's writings are suffused with the acknowledgment of paradox. For instance, transference love was real and unreal at the same time. Transference neurosis was understood as both a repetition of the past and also as a newly created illness. A basic paradox actually lies at the heart of the therapeutic process regarding the different levels of experienced emotionality that result from the juxtaposition and contrast of present objects (that which is happening now in the patient's life) and archaic objects (his or her parents, or significant others in the past). Therapists themselves also paradoxically represent both the potential danger of the past and the safety of the present. Winnicott (1971) makes a plea for accepting, tolerating, and respecting paradox. Part of the "impossible profession" is the therapist's need to cope with the paradox of attachment and nonattachment toward the patient. In addition, the therapist's function as a "participant/observer" is a dual, paradoxi-

cal task. Kumin (1978), like the neo-Piagetians, regards the acceptance of paradox as a higher developmental function. Baranger (1983) claims that it is essential during analytical work to conceive of every event as possibly having, simultaneously, alternative meanings. Modell (1990) claims that "most therapeutic
dilemmas are never really solved; they merely become less significant" (p. 130).
The question is how? Could it also result from an internal process enabling the
patient to achieve aintegration?

Self and Ego Psychology.   The paradoxical nature of the Self concept as
elaborated by James (1890) lies in the "I–me" and the "one in many Selves"
concepts. These represent an inconsistency between the assumption of the
unity of the Self and the different Selves we present in disparate situations. The
Self is both permanent and transient. People adhere to contrasting modes of
behavior. They, for instance, may hold to different private and public moralities
(Loevinger & Knoll, 1983). The Self is self-sustaining, yet contingent on social
roles. Various attempts have been made to solve these paradoxes: for example,
James sought an answer in the stream of consciousness; Goffman's (1959) presentations of the Self assume a variety of discontinuities connected by different role
Selves, as in the theater; Gergen and Gergen (1988) seek to overcome the paradox
by dwelling on a "self-narrative" and its story plot; Hermans and Hermans-
Jansen (1995) elaborate a "dialogical" Self; and Sarbin (1986) provides a basic
shift in the conceptualization of the Self with his distinction of narrative as a root
metaphor in human experience. The narrative view holds that it is the process of
developing one's changing life story that becomes the basis of all identity and
thus challenges any underlying concept of a unified or stable Self. Recent
clinical formulations of the Self weave a broad tapestry, claiming that "while
people certainly need a cohesive and integrated Self, they also need to accept,
tolerate and even enjoy confusion, contradiction, flux, lack of integration and
even chaos in their sense of who they are" (Aron, 1995, p. 203).

Tolerance of anxiety may often determine the ability to tolerate an inconsistency. Zetzel (1949) noted the positive value of being able to tolerate anxiety,
suggesting an "immune" effect in coping with stress and trauma. She employed
a similar approach in her study of the capacity to bear depression, arguing that
it is a prerequisite of maturation and an important ingredient in the ability to
withstand disappointment, loss, and frustration. Valliant (1993) categorizes defenses as mature and immature, and explicates how the mature defenses (anticipation, suppression, altruism, sublimation, and humor) contain the ability to
tolerate paradox, a capacity attributed to the autonomous ego.

Object Relations.   Behind Melanie Klein's work may stand a "European,"
existentially grounded perspective that views the struggles in life as complex,
continuous, and fierce. To illustrate some of her relevant concepts:

1. *Integration*: The mind is viewed as constantly operating in a splitting
and unintegrated manner: "More then any other analyst, Klein relinquished the
integrity of the mind" (Hinshelwood, 1994, p. 329). Integration becomes a continuous psychological task, but it does not mean making the different parts fit or

similar; "rather it means the more flexible choice of different aspects of the self" (Hinshelwood, p. 279). *Part objects*, elaborated by Bion (1962), sets forth the proposition that one may not always deal with the "whole" object or situation, and that such part-object relationships may be an initial state or approach, rather than the result of "splitting" or "repressing."

2. *Ambivalence:* The holding of conflicting feelings toward the same object (i.e., ambivalence) comes to the fore in the child's "depressive position" as he or she starts to differentiate between "good" and "bad" objects, an act causing anxiety and leading to ambivalence. Ambivalence has to be tolerated since it is a highly functional, lifelong process, necessary for developmental progress.

3. *Reparation:* For Klein, this is not a defense, but an "acceptance mechanism." Klein (1937) describes the healthy human capacity to carry heavy burdens, the capacity to tolerate painful feelings or loss and then find a way to make reparation. This is directly in line with the characteristics of aintegration. *Containing*, developed by Bion (1962), denotes a person's ability to be nuturant even if intensely negative feelings are projected onto him or her. The elderly, in particular, seem able to contain intense aggressive feelings directed at them from significant others or environments, usually without feeling revengeful or rebelling, thus showing a tremendous capacity to "contain." Taken together, the notions of reparation, containing, and holding reflect a quality of endurance among the aged that signifies strength and ability to tolerate incompatibility.

In recent object relation clinical theory, it is argued that the theory must be such that it is "able to sustain paradox, that it is, in Winnicott's (1971) terms, able to allow paradox to be tolerated, respected and left unresolved" (Aron, 1995, p. 198). Recently, relational theorists, in light of the postmodern critique, have been challenging traditional unitary notions, such as a core unified identity. Gender multiplicity and an emphasis on people as both unified, stable, and cohesive, and as fragmented and different from moment to moment are in keeping with the emphasis on deconstructing dichotomies, deconstruction of polarized concepts (e.g., male–female, identity–multiplicity, patient–therapist), and the acceptance of multiplicity. These perspectives are all being forwarded in recent clinical theory (Aron, 1995), in constructivist (Meichenbaum & Fitzpatrick, 1992) and narrative (Cohler, Chapter 11, this volume; Schafer, 1992) approaches.

Personality–Social Psychology.   Gatz (Chapter 4, this volume) notes wisdom as related to self-knowledge among the protective factors in coping with stress and illustrates this by quoting Betty Friedan's (1993) 80-year-old friend: "I am more and more myself. But I'm more comfortable with differences, not uptight about them…. Somehow … I am not anguished about my failures" (p. 572), clearly an example of adjustment that includes aintegration. MacDonald, Kuiper, and Olinger (1985) found that those who are mildly depressed are inconsistent when making self-descriptive judgments. As people get older, their ability to tolerate ambiguity increases. Investigations of self-esteem and the Self-concept have been reviewed (Baumeister, 1993), and when some of this data is considered from a clinical, mental health perspective (Tennen & Affleck,

1993), a number of interesting puzzles emerge. For instance, low self-esteem, even when extreme, does not necessarily lead to clinical depression. High-self-esteem individuals were found to be unresponsive to negative interpersonal feedback (Baumeister, 1993). People do display the ability to incorporate negative information but they do not always acknowledge all its implications (Lazarus & DeLongis, 1983), and may even hold on to positive self-illusions. Janoff-Bulman (1992) proposes that people can maintain illusory assumptions about themselves while at the same time accepting contrary information and evidence.

The style of novelists and artists has been defined (Cohen-Shalev, 1992) as "a tendency to strip down artifice.... The relative lack of distinction between fact and fantasy, autobiography and invention ... does not result in a harmonious resolution of these opposites, but rather in a coexistence that seems to transcend logical thought categories" (p. 297). Siebert (1983), in a study of traumatized war veterans, found that those who had handled that stress adequately, and even felt better prepared for future life through it, had psychological personality profiles that were biphasic and paradoxical in the sense that they did not "fit" or relate normatively. Many traits showed a combination of opposites, such as self-confidence and self-criticism, seriousness and playfulness, or introversion and extroversion. Siebert states that the paradoxical mix in these survivors enabled them to cope with and adapt to traumatic circumstances. As a result of aintegration, the elderly Self may be more fluid, open to contradictions and paradox (Kegan, Chapter 9, this volume).

Cognitive Psychology: Mature Thinking in a Postformalistic Framework

Cognitive psychology reveals findings indicating diverse modes of handling inconsistencies; for example, people with a "global-intuitive" cognitive style, as opposed to those with an "analytic" one, can tolerate inconsistencies and contradictions, and "intuitive," as opposed to "analytic" individuals, are unconventional and can live with doubt and uncertainty and even enjoy instabilities (Giora, 1991). I wish, however, to emphasize postformal thinking. Piaget revolutionized the study of thinking; Riegel (1973), after Perry (1970), provided breakthrough concepts in this area, positing dialectical operations as a higher, fifth-stage order, which is more pronounced in adults and the elderly, enabling them to synthesize life experiences and absorb contradictions. This may happen because many adults can understand the inherent changing and contradictory nature of reality and the subjectivity of knowledge, as well as the tensions that emanate from the different levels of organization and dimensions of reality (e.g., social vs. individual). A major thrust of Riegel's approach (1976) is an advocacy of dialectical psychology. His approach assumes four dimensions (inner-biological, individual-psychological, cultural-sociological, and outer-physical) that develop in the person but are often in different states of readiness as he or she interacts with the social world. Riegel's approach may also be related to many of the characteristics underlying the outlined image of human-kind and the concept of aintegration.

Dialectical Frameworks. Cognitive and developmental theoreticians have further articulated cognitive development in adulthood and devised models of adult cognition (e.g., Arlin, 1975; Kegan, 1982; Labouvie-Vief, 1977). Basseches (1980) developed and elaborated the characteristics of dialectical thinking and submitted them to empirical tests. Kramer (1983) conceived and investigated three adult, worldview-related thought processes: absolute, relativistic, and dialectical. Rybash, Hoyer, and Roodin (1986) formulated "contextualism," in which one "creates new principles based on the changing circumstances of life, rather than search for absolute universal principles that apply across all contexts and circumstances" (p. 39). There is no imperative connection between different contexts, or between past, present, and future in a contextualist or relativistic worldview (Pepper, 1942), a point also illustrated by posttraumatic persons.

A mechanistic worldview is basically integrative; it relies on formal opera-tional thinking (Reese & Overton, 1970) and on linear causality consistent with Aristotle's logic. The assumption of relativistic or dialectical thought or aintegra-tion would not square with such a scheme. Considering alternatives, a person may make a choice, but this does not automatically eliminate the alternatives he or she has considered (Chandler, 1975). As Kramer (1983) notes: "Relativistic and dialectic thought is believed to be more pragmatic in nature, as there is greater acceptance of life as it is, with all its contradictions" (p. 97). Dialectical thinking and relativism are generally agreed to be necessary for an adequate account of mature thinking, which can only be founded on postformal, and not just formal, operations. Furthermore, in the relativistic–contextualistic scheme, statements of conflicts (within systems) could be comprehended with no corre-sponding attempt at integration (Kramer & Woodruff, 1986).

It should be emphasized that the dialectical "fifth" or "final" stage (Riegel, 1973) of adult thinking does not eliminate or replace the previous stages of formal operations and linear causality. There are differences as well as sim-ilarities in the various theories of mature thinking outlined earlier. Nevertheless, these approaches increasingly focus on the stages of later adulthood (Basseches, 1980; Kramer & Bopp, 1989), revealing that (1) adult cognition reaches a further stage by the use of dialectics; (2) there is an acknowledgment of the relativistic, nonabsolute nature of knowledge; (3) there is an acceptance of contradictions in the thinking process; and (4) contradictions may or may not be integrated into novel constructions (Kramer, 1983). The emphasis on adult and mature thinking, as opposed to that of formal logical, operational thinking validated in childhood, may lead us to some basic assumptions: that integration based on formal opera-tions is developmentally prior to that of aintegration, and that only as people mature, confront life and accumulate experience do they also simultaneously develop the capacity for aintegration. Postformal thinking allows for contradic-tory positions and provides a reasonable basis upon which to further advance the concept of aintegration.

Traditionally, meaning making has correctly been related mainly to change in a positive sense, perhaps because it was related to children, young adults, and/or to end results of behavior that the "meaning-maker" frequently initiated. However, in relation to the aged, behavior is often imposed rather than initiated, and changes that occur are not always given meaning, especially when they are in the nature of loss. In this context, aintegration denotes the ability to absorb change without integrating, meaning making, or a feeling that one is becoming a part of a greater meaningful universal–social whole (Erikson, 1968).

Being in a World of Paradox and Double Binds.   The work of Bateson and his colleagues on paradoxes and the double bind have modified our thinking about certain aspects of human communications, interpersonal relations, and mental health. A paradox is defined as a "contradiction that follows correct deductions from consistent premises" (Watzlawick, Beavin, & Jackson, 1967, p. 188). This immediately signifies that we are not dealing here with "false" paradoxes based on concealed errors or deliberate fallacies. A paradox always presents a reality that includes a closed vicious circle and provides "double bind" statements that are often given on different levels of logic and dimensions of communication (verbal, nonverbal, emotional, etc.). A contradictory situation still contains an alternative. In the paradoxical situation, there is only the illusion that choice is possible. Usually, there can only be compliance.

Paradoxical situations and double binds arise for us all across the lifespan (they may be intensified in certain periods such as childhood and old age) and we are able to cope with them, perhaps better as we grow older (only in unusual cases will they lead to mental illness). In double-bind situations, no change can be generated if we remain within the system. Change can only come from stepping outside, disregarding a certain reality (often a difficult thing to do because of reality constraints, e.g., for a child or an aged person within the family circle). It requires the decision "not to play the game," to discount, to be indifferent and remove oneself from what is impinging on one, and yet keep one's peace of mind. The cognitive and emotional aspects of the double bind are only reinforced by the asynchronic nature of life as experienced by the elderly. The person's ability to deal with paradoxes and the double bind parallel some basic characteristics of aintegration.

Postmodernism, Existentialism, and Phenomenology

Postmodernism is a critical redirection of the traditional and the accepted on the basis of a revised understanding of human thought, art, science, and behavior. It actually addresses a condition of loss of faith in unified rational systems, in religion, and in science. Some common emphases and principles adopted by those who identify themselves as postmodernists are radical subjectivity, a focus on construction and deconstruction, an emphasis on text, on personal meaning and the narrative as an evolving process, on discontinuity, on working with fragmentary materials, on the différance, skepticism as to the possibility of an underlying consensus, a recognition of the inevitability of differences and incommensurabilities, the rejection of hegemony, disqualification of the pursuit of wholeness, skepticism about completeness, the rejection of "totality," the pursuit of liberation, and the changing character of the quotidian, the momentary nature of experience (Derrida, 1986; Lyotard, 1988). Many of the mentioned characteristics of postmodernism can be found in the defintion of aintegration and in the principles it elaborates.

Existentialism and *phenomenology*, conceived in their European forms as philosophical traditions, represent a set of attitudes and concepts concerning our comprehension of human beings: in temporality, as searching for meaning, free to choose, responsible for their mode of existence and not overly threatened by death. The existential characteristics of the human condition, however, include isolation, anxiety, loneliness, depression, freedom, meaninglessness and death, all of which are even more pronounced in adulthood and old age. Existentialism's range of definitions and diversity both in theory and clinical technique (May, Angel, & Ellenberger, 1958; Ryff, 1986) go beyond the scope of this chapter. However, certain basic relevant themes should be noted.

Ontology refers to the nature of Being (Heidegger, 1962). Yet "being" is inseparably bound up with contrasting elements. Kierkegaard (1957) and Sartre (1943) conceive contradictions and dialectics as being inherent to human existence, referring mainly to the person's sense of being as opposed to nonbeing, the contradiction between eternity and finality. Conditions such as isolation, loneliness, and despair are not necessarily considered pathological. Tillich (1952) wrote that as man is dehumanized, he reacts with the "courage of despair," thus attributing power to despondent and desolate situations. Sartre (1943) describes how despair may lead to the essence of man (i.e., his creative, responsible, self-accepting being). The problem of meaning-finding is defined as how to find meaning in a meaningless world. Camus and Sartre, following Schopenhauer, struggled with the nihilistic position, which led them to conclude that man himself must give meaning to his life. This is done mainly by rebelling against the "absurd" condition of life. Death, inseparable from human culture (Kastentaum & Kastenbaum, 1993), has been considered a major force in molding existence (Kierkegaard, 1957; Tillich, 1952). Heidegger (1962) believed that the realization of personal death moves a person to a higher mode of existence. In fact, the concept of life–death interdependence (Yalom, 1980) is fundamental, since one is meaningless without the other. These characteristics of existence may create anxiety, stress, or guilt, increasing the basic "ontological anxiety," a necessary condition inherent in existence (Heidegger, 1962), but to be separated from "neurotic anxiety" (Bugental, 1978). Existence therefore inevitably involves a sense of paradox and the absurd. Indeed, Nagel (1992) explains that "the absurd is a way of perceiving our true situation.... It results from the ability to understand our human limitations ... and we can approach our absurd lives with irony instead of heroism or despair" (p. 388). Nagel's approach is pertinent to the concept of aintegration, and I would argue that the elderly in particular are capable of experiencing the absurd without any accompanying despair.

Posttraumatic Survivors and the Holocaust

As indicated, various stressful life experiences may generate aintegration. The Holocaust survivors are one extreme example (Kahana & Kahana, Chapter 7, this volume). Many survivors, I maintain, had experienced aintegration during the Holocaust and continue to "practice" it in daily life, raising the question of how the trauma of the Holocaust, presenting extreme pain, dread, and horror, in memory and affect, persists in the mind of survivors after so many years of posttraumatic, yet adjusted, life. Most writers attempting to answer this question postulate that survivors hold, or held, "dual realities," different Selves or "multidimensional selves" (e.g., Lifton, 1983), which are explained on the basis of processes such as splitting, repression, fragmentation, dissociation, or other dissociative mechanisms (Herman, 1992; van der Kolk & Van der Hart, 1991). I contend that these types of explanations, based on the notion of the unconscious and "mind-splitting" operations, do not hold for all. Certainly, most survivors have not dissociated their horrible Holocaust memories during the past 50 years.

In our ongoing biographical studies on the long-term effects of the Holocaust among well-functioning Holocaust survivors (Lomranz, 1990, 1995), some striking findings have emerged regarding the inconsistencies and paradoxes that survivors reveal in relation to cogent domains of life and interpersonal behaviors. Among these findings are the following: (1) *Mourning*: Considered a prerequisite for overcoming loss, it is impossible for most survivors, yet this did not prevent them from adjusting well; (2) *Meaning*: While most survivors find meaning in endurance as well as in present life (e.g., Zionism, generativity), substantial numbers of respondents confronted this issue and unequivocally concluded that (quoted in narratives of survivors) "there is no meaning." A frequent statement is "to live after the Holocaust, it seems that either I am crazy or the world is." Hogman's (1985) survivor related to religion by stating, "I am comfortable with a lot of contradictions. I can't pray because I have a personal feud with God but I sent my children to Hebrew school" (p. 391). Integrating the Holocaust into the various dimensions of Self, values, and cultural beliefs remains problematic. Many feel their traumatic experience is incongruent with the prevailing cultural value system or ongoing modes of daily life (Janoff-Bulman, 1992). However, they live with this contradiction, are aware of it, and may nevertheless lead productive and well-functioning lives.

If the ability to reconnect verbally with the traumatic experience is considered crucial for recovery (van der Kolk & van der Hart, 1991), then what do the 50 years of continuous silence of adjusted survivors indicate? Many survivors insist that words cannot convey the horror and essence of their experience, and that the Holocaust is essentially incommunicable. Is continuity a condition for integrity? Most developmentalist and personality theorists would probably answer in the affirmative. However, it appears difficult for many survivors to assemble their life story into one continuous biographical line. They present their lives as having been disrupted and never reunited or reconnected. If the Holocaust is perceived as breaking the continuity of human experience, how can continuity still be the basis of one's self-image? Most of our subjects felt a strong sense of "integrity," but they resisted strongly, unyieldingly, when asked to affirm their past life in Eriksonian terms.

I hypothesize that the awareness of inconsistencies, dual realities, and paradox can still serve as an adjustive coping function for many people during and after stress. Survivors may function well in daily life while still remembering the unspeakable atrocities they have experienced, and cognitively keep their balance by realizing that this is an incomprehensible world. Under certain circumstances, people do not have to verbalize conflicts, can feel incoherent, do not have to repress or dissociate traumatic memories, and can experience existence as inconsistent and paradoxical. The long-term adjustment of Holocaust survivors confronts us with the realization that adjustment and well-being cannot always be comprehended in terms of their existing underlying theories. Aintegration may explain some of the paradoxical testimonies of survivors.

AINTEGRATION: OPERATIONAL PROFILE
AND PERSONALITY CONTEXT

The foregoing discussion offered theoretical frameworks that serve as essential sources of rationale and support for the concept of aintegration. Aintegration presents the mental complexity by which the epistemological demands in adults are coped with and met. Aintegration mediates between epistemology and ontology in the existence of the aged in society. As we have seen, aintegration is present in cognition, emotions, interpersonal relations, and behaviors. The well-functioning individual, conceived as both integrating and not integrating, provides a more comprehensive picture of the evolving Self. After having outlined conceptual sources, the next step should be experimental, that is, an attempt to verify the operational characteristics of aintegration such as (1) rejection of Aristotelian logic; (2) the ability to contain contradictions in one's Self schemata; (3) the capacity for postformal dialectic thought operations; (4) the ability to comprehend contradictions and relativism; (5) the emotional quality of sustaining ambivalence; (6) the ability to sustain ambiguity; (7) the ability to sustain complexity; (8) the ability to comprehend paradox; (9) the ability to step out of double-bind situations; (10) the use of internal, rather than external, sources for meaning making; and (11) the use of balanced worldviews and value positions.

The goal here would be to formulate a multidimensional personality profile reflecting the direction of these traits and behaviors. Such a profile would empirically emerge from identifying and relating these various traits that, as I hypothesize, have commonalities leading to a "profile of aintegration." The profile scores could differentiate between different people, at different points on the lifespan (e.g., perhaps aintegrative qualities may be constructive in old age, but harmful in young adulthood). A number of trait characteristics have already been operationalized [e.g., Basseches's (1980), dialectical schemata; Kramer & Woodruff's (1986) measures on contradictions and relativism]; some may be modified (e.g., tolerance for ambiguity) but many more still require operational formulations, hypothesis, and testing.

A Personality Context

While I referred to aintegration in descriptive and phenomenological terms, I suggest a multidimensional, developmental personality structure and configuration able to contain, and equipped to handle, the characteristics of aintegration. Conceptualizations regarding stress (Hobfoll & Wells, Chapter 5, this volume), developmental and dynamic ego psychology (Loevinger, 1976; Valliant, 1993), dynamic cognitive theory (Giora, 1991), developmental lifespan perspectives (Baltes & Baltes, 1993), existential psychology and the models of mind elaborated by Kegan (1994, Chapter 9, this volume) would all have relevancy for such a personality configuration. However, I conceive of Lewinian personality and field theory (Lewin, 1936) combined with Werner's (1948) developmental approach and the integration of these by Ziegler and Glick (1986) as the main basis for such a configuration. Lewin (1936) defines a person as a constellation of regions in a life space. His concepts of "life space," "permeability," "valences," "vectors," and "psychological ecology," as well as his emphasis on the degree of connectedness, firmness–weakness, fluidity–rigidity, interdependence, and differentiation of "regions" and "boundaries" all make it possible to explain the behavior of a person whose relation with the environment, as well as with him- or herself, is constantly changing and can endure inconsistencies, depending on the relationships between the regions in his or her psychological life space. For Lewin, as a Gestaltist, the importance lies in the way experience is organized rather than the content of specific experiences. Thus, even the most terrible, stressful memory can change from figure to ground, be invaded or be shut off completely, all depending on the state of the field, the qualities of the regions and boundaries and their position in the total life space. Werner (1948) presents an "organismic–developmental" model in which development is conceived as a series of qualitative reorganizations. Development here can be continuous or discontinuous, since meaning is always derived from the organization of the whole. The integrated model of Werner and Lewin presented by Ziegler and Glick (1986) may serve as the proper personality model explaining integrative as well as aintegrative processes. Thus, the study of personality in this perspective might become an avenue for a psychological coping and personality model in general, and specifically, when related to the phenomenon of incompatible existential spheres.

AINTEGRATION AND MENTAL HEALTH

This chapter argues for the acceptance of postmodern thinking in the discourse on mental health. Thus, particular focus should be on deconstruction theory, on the Self, not as a reified entity but as a narrative, on text, not as something to be interpreted but to be understood as an evolving process, and on the individual, to be considered within a context of personal and communal meaning (Lax, 1995). However, while postmodern thought builds its discourse almost exclusively on the interpersonal, social and communal (e.g., Gergen &

Gergen, 1988), I argue that it should be supplemented with the personal and the intrapsychic.

Generally, while aintegration, as part of a normal coping process, may be activated in response to many existential, perplexing, daily demands or stressful events, it would seem to be especially called upon in later life given the predicaments of aging as well the personality changes in old age that are posited by adult developmental theory (Ruth & Coleman, 1996). Vigorous elderly people are often prevented from being useful and finding meaning, but are conceived of as superfluous, discriminated against and constricted (Kahn, 1994). Although certain, sometimes successful efforts are being made to change this paradigm of "aging and society" (Riley et al., 1994), perhaps most elderly people living today are, to a greater or lesser degree, victims of such realities. The need for aintegration sometimes arises as many elderly persons who may feel vulnerable (Gatz, Chapter 4, and Solomon & Ginzburg, Chapter 6, this volume) confront the society's "lagging" realities and the unavoidable encounters with social roles, services, and institutions, which generally end unfavorably for them.

For many older people, aging is an enigma. Karp (1988) investigated what preretirement people think about aging and found that many termed it a "paradox." It was hard for them to convey the contradictions between how they felt about themselves, what was happening to their bodies, and how they appeared to others. The idea that they were as chronologically old as they actually were seemed foreign to them. The notion of "stranger" represented their feelings about aging. Aging was "psychologically near and distant at the same time" (p. 729). The inconsistencies, reflecting asynchronization, between body and mind, wish and its fulfillment, motivations and their realizations, produce disappointments and frustrations and often have a detrimental impact on the formation of the elderly Self. However, it should be emphasized that contrary to the past, the literature now suggests a controversy about the extent to which major depression differs across the lifespan and shows that cognitive and ideational symptoms such as guilt and self-reproach may be less common in late life (Gatz, Chapter 4, Katz, Chapter 21, and Niederehe, Chapter 18, this volume), perhaps indicating aintegrative processes.

Interpersonal existence in old age is often colored by constraints and the inability to react. For example, Jim delicately asks his son Bob if he is concerned about his inheritance, and Bob becomes so offended that Jim begins to doubt his suspicions, for which he has sufficient grounds. Or David tells his daughter that he knows she loves him, but since she does not visit him, perhaps there is a problem, to which she responds with a long speech to show him how wrong he is and goes on to complain that he constantly nags her. Thus, the elderly are often forbidden to acknowledge that a contradiction exists. Some maintain dignity by stepping out, as in the paradoxical situation, of circular fruitless argumentation, but many others may soon learn to become compliant (especially if power is on the other side, e.g., living in a home for the aged), abstaining overtly from independent thinking and from exercising freedom and control. The elderly are not openly rejected by their significant others or caretakers, but rather often encounter disconfirmations of their intentions, thereby stripping acts of their motives and consequences. The process underlying many such instances relegates the elderly to a world where they receive continuous disconfirmation of their ideas, wishes, thoughts, and opinions. In situations like these, if aintegration is not employed, the person may be led to doubts and lose all hope of ever having authentic communication with significant others; he or she may withdraw or experience helplessness and cultivate depression.

Psychological damage may arise when exposure to such inconsistencies and constrictions becomes repetitive and/or continuous, especially in children (Watzlavick et al., 1967). I do not believe that such exposure in the elderly necessarily renders them mentally ill, since, unlike children, many of them can, when needed, exercise aintegration. The following extracts from biographies and case histories may further demonstrate this.

Mr. C., aged 88, adjusted, married, and a grandfather, lives with the notion: "I have definitely not achieved in life what I really wanted to, but it's too late to change anything." He wanted to go to college but his father forced him into the family business, which was lost with the rise of the Nazis and so: "I had no career." He loved a woman to whom he never dared propose and has married and lived for 50 years with another woman, "also a good life, but...." The major event, 20 years ago, that "enriched" him in the sense that he became more "active—I started to read more, took courses and also became more politically involved," was the loss of his son in the Yom Kippur War. "I am not satisfied with my life, but what can I do," he says, with a thin smile." If I had a second chance I would do it all differently." This statement of a well-adjusted person should be related to the Eriksonian and life-review approaches.

Mrs. T., 78 years old, complains in therapy that her partner for the past 15 years does not understand her. She is alert and vibrant, and brings along pictures showing herself as a young woman with bare shoulders. "I am still there. I still feel that way, but I also feel old. I wish I could dance, but you see I can't even walk without the cane, and look how fat I have become. He can't have sex because of his heart condition and often I want it, and maybe more often I don't. Why is everything so split? It's irritating and confusing this way. You feel this and also its opposite.... If something is dead, okay, then you know, but this way you can't be sure.... You think I am old?" (She had an erotic transference to the 40-year-old therapist.) The notion of aintegration could be dwelled upon with her.

Nathan, 63, a successful salesman, is deeply involved in caring for his wife, a victim of Alzheimer's disease. He has been in various psychotherapies for the past 11 years. The presenting complaint concerned his caretaking duties and the resulting conflicts, but much of his therapy was usually focused on the guilt he felt about his son's death 25 years earlier. The son had been hospitalized for a long time in a terminal ward, in a coma, and it was unclear whether he would regain consciousness. Nathan, after lengthy deliberations, decided not to cancel a scheduled business trip abroad, and while he was gone, his son died. He felt guilty, continuously sullying his image as a father and his self-worth. At one point the therapist said, "You know, maybe this is just one of those things in life that nothing can be done about and you have to live with it." This made Nathan feel greatly relieved, and therapy continued constructively. Whatever one may choose to read into the therapist's intervention, it undoubtedly contained the message: "Well there is nothing you can do about it." Aintegration was a way of giving confirmation and form to a tormenting experience.

Hanna is a 70-year-old Holocaust survivor living on a *kibbutz*. She lost all her family, but survived work camps and Auschwitz. She recently wrote (Nisman, 1995), "With my memories I descend to a deep hole which I cannot understand, yet I belong to it (p. 20).... I can hardly believe that my past belongs to my life ... yet it's me living with all those terrible scenes together with a love for life.... The break in my life and then four decades of family building, then going back, the present and the past, and frustration and satisfaction.... These contradictions accompany me, and maybe everyone, along the course of my life. To know how to live with these contradictions, and within these inconsistencies—*is one's guarantee of a sense of wholeness in life* (italics mine).... I experience the inconsistencies within me: on the one hand, the ability to accept reality and the facts and on the other hand it is impossible.... One has to learn to live with contradictions and with the inconsistencies of life" (p. 61).

IMPLICATIONS FOR PSYCHOTHERAPY

In light of the characteristics of the aging process (e.g., internal and external changes, accumulated lifelong experiences, interiority and life review tendencies), the elderly person seems almost the perfect client for psychotherapy (Zarit & Knight, 1996). However, most therapists rarely engage in treating the elderly, and psychotherapy is far from being utilized as it should be for this population. This unfortunate situation and the reasons for it have been discussed elsewhere (e.g., Gatz et al., 1985). Here, I wish to emphasize that psychotherapy in a postmodern era has to include in its goals the study of how the capacity for accepting complexity and tolerating inconsistencies can evolve, be developed, and worked through. The following are two implications of psychotherapy relevant to the present discussion; one relates to a perspective, and the other to some basics in methodology.

Aintegration: A Perspective in the Psychotherapy with the Aged

Postmodern thinking minimizes the therapist's position as a knower and reinforces configurations in which both clients and therapists create a "therapeutic space" (Winnicott, 1971) and share responsibility for the therapeutic process. Different approaches to psychotherapy reflect different views about human nature, and the perspective from which behavior is viewed determines what problems are seen as meaningful and what kind of interpretations are made. However, therapists can only properly intervene if they are aware of their own knowledge and feelings about aging, and their image of the aged person. I presume that holding to the composite image of man suggested earlier, as well as to the perspective inherent in the concept of aintegration, may prevent therapists from slipping unchecked into a decremental outlook, allow them to have compassion for suffering, proper respect for helplessness, contradictions, and paradox, thereby increasing their chances of achieving an adequate relational interaction with an elderly client and better prepare them to facilitate self-creative aspects in their clients. They may be able to help their clients to foster change as well as to accept the inevitable, and may also reinforce elderly persons' paradoxical, humoristic, and playful aspects.

The basic body of advanced adult psychodynamic and cognitive clinical theory (e.g., Nemiroff & Colarusso, 1990; Woods, 1996; Zarit & Knight, 1996) should be supplemented by recent psychoanalytic approaches (Aron, 1995; Modell, 1990), further developmental concepts (Gutmann, 1994), phenomenology–existentialism and approaches to the deconstruction–construction of the narrative. Existentialism and phenomenology have an undifferentiated, unique, blend of theory and methodology, thus providing a high potential for the evolving issues of aging to appear directly. Yalom (1980) discusses the anxieties that accompany four basic conditions of existence–death, freedom, isolation, and meaninglessness–and elaborates their therapeutic potential. These existential conditions are even more accentuated in the second half of life. They represent basic life conditions of the elderly as well as cogent themes in clinical and social gerontology, and may provide direction to the geropsychotherapist. Thus, the existential orientation, dwelling on the "hardships" of life, may be particularly valuable to the therapist in helping the aged person to redefine his or her Self and life perspective.

Constructivism is a basic feature of psychotherapy. The geropsychotherapist may assist his historically rich client, as remembered events are given different meanings, to construct alternative life histories (Cohler, Chapter 11; Meador & Blazer, Chapter 22, this volume; Schafer, 1992) or multiple narratives (Hermans & Hermans-Jansen, 1995). In line with aintegration, therapists should be open to inconsistent, discontinuous life stories, and should be able to conceive of experiences for which the client, and the therapist, are unable to provide meaning. Meaning making, the life review, and autobiographical memory (Coleman, 1986; Haight & Webster, 1995; Ross, 1991) complement each other, are pertinent to psychotherapy, and can be further understood in narrative frameworks. In the past decade, social scientists have evinced a renewed interest in how Selves are discursively formulated within and through life stories, autobiographies, and other personal narratives (e.g., Gergen & Gergen, 1988; Neiser & Fivush, 1994; Schafer, 1992). Constructivism (Ryff, 1986), the biographical method (Alexander, 1990) and "narratology" (Sarbin, 1986) have all been the focus of theory, psychotherapy and research. Psychotherapy may thus be considered "rebiographing," or rewriting, the narrative (Irwin, 1996), as we basically live through stories and are lived by stories of our history and culture (Bruner, 1990; White & Epston, 1990).

Some Essentials of Psychotherapy and Aintegration

The following are some elementary methodologies that have a direct bearing on the composite image of man and aintegration:

Listening.   Gerotherapists may promote situations in which they find themselves listening to patients' "reports" rather than to direct stories told by elderly patients (Heaton, 1979). This may be due to the fact that the content brought by the elderly may be too distressing, boring, or create a sense of helplessness. Listening to "reports" with a "theoretical" ear, one too eager to construct formulations may not be conducive, while a conversation in light of the narrative with aintegration as a perspective may be.

Empathy.   The exercise of empathy may be hindered due to various factors, including the appearance of the elderly, physical disgust, countertransferential fears, and so on. In supervisory situations, younger therapists may attribute difficulties in therapy to age differences, and, in fact, elderly patients may relate to younger therapists with distrust. However, this may not be due to age differences as much as to a difference in worldview. A therapeutic relationship is impossible if a therapist is not open to and accepting of the hardships of later life and, albeit covertly, conveys to the patient the message "Keep smiling, be happy," as preached by popular culture and books on aging. In this way, the development of genuine empathy is impeded.

Language.   A therapeutic dialogue with the elderly requires an enriched language (Hazan, 1994, 1996) that contains aintegrative connotations. Language can be more direct and immediate with the elderly. The paradox deserves special attention. In daily life, paradox induces bewilderment but it also carries a forceful cognitive and emotional impact, providing, as in a creative process, a sense that we have learned something perhaps incomprehensible but also authentic. The use of paradox in therapy is familiar through the work of Milton Erikson (Weeks, 1991) as well as in the psychodynamic orientation (Modell, 1990). Valliant (1993) indicates how, through the patient's capacity for paradox and humor, therapists can utilize mature defenses and deal with conflicting material. Thus, what was recognized as a stalemate may become, through the use of paradoxical components, or the ability to step out of the paradoxical situation, an enlightening therapeutic experience. Metaphor, analogies, humor, contradictions, ambiguities, relativistic thinking, and stories, often considered the ingredients of creativity and art, may be of major value when aintegration is called for in psychotherapy.

The language needed to express the familiar and the understandable is more readily at our disposal than that required for the unknown, the awe-inspiring, the paradox, and the aintegrated. For Hazan (Chapter 8, this volume), the discourse on old age contains literal as well as metaphysical languages, both, being two sides of the same coin, derived from metonymical thinking. Derrida (1986) and Lyotard (1988) articulated the concept of the *différance*, the unacceptable language, which always includes tension between what is said and what is not said. This tension creates the potential for new understandings but also for internal pressures. People may find themselves in victimized situations as they experience feelings and thoughts for which they are unable to find recognition and direct expression, either because there is no appropriate vocabulary to express them, or because the vocabulary they use is not valid or is forbidden in their context. They may then be forced to express themselves in a distorted manner (e.g., paying visits to medical staff because of their need for attention). Such behaviors may occur in communities or institutions for the aged, where the possibilities for interaction and communication are often limited by cultural taboos, medical paradigms, or accepted images of elderly as defective, all ultimately preventing the elderly from expressing certain personal feelings or thoughts. This may be true also for younger, healthy, and educated gerontologists, who may not be able to listen or be sensitive to the "différance" in the elderly and their distorted or symbolic language. As therapists attempt to identify the meaning elderly patients convey to them, their sensitivity to these distinctions in language is crucial.

Self-Knowledge. Although a major goal in most psychotherapies, self-knowledge in the case of the aged client may be positioned otherwise. The elderly person may enter therapy to be helped in the difficulties of circumstantial living, and minimize the goal of finding out hidden truth about him- or herself. This reduced emphasis on self-knowledge may be irritating for some therapists. Aintegration would not attribute so much weight to "self-knowledge." Furthermore, in focusing on self-knowledge, the gerotherapist may err as to the termination of therapy. It is in fact striking how elderly patients may terminate therapy, when their therapists believe that this is premature. When, at the end of the second couple-therapy session, a 78-year-old husband responded to his wife's main complaint that he had stopped having sex with her by saying: "Oh, I thought you understood. After all, sex was not so great with us in the last 40 years so I assumed that now its time to stop, for you, too. Well, if you feel differently we'll see." The therapist prepared himself for the "real" work. The couple, however, decided not to continue and yet were observed in the home for the aged as more content and in greater harmony than during the entire previous year.

Affect and Drama in the Aged Self. If adequate, the elderly Self is different than that of the younger person, has given up the past perfectionistic, grandiose Self, and now tolerates imperfection and incompatibilities, recognizing that it is special, but not unique, and is able to accept the limitations, finitude, and complexities of life. Similar issues at different points on the lifespan may be experienced differently. At a younger age, when narcissistic involvement and threats to the Self are high, events are often experienced as extremely fateful, deterministic, and dramatic. In later life, reactions are often less dramatic. The worldview has perhaps been altered. In a three-generation family session in which the parents were extremely upset with their daughter's intention to marry a particular man, they turned to Grandma, confidently expecting her full support (Grandma was definitely not fond of her granddaughter's choice), but were astonished to hear her say, "Well, there are more important issues. At least both of them are healthy." Such positions often reflect the elderly's scale of values as well as the ability to live with inconsistencies. This may also signify a lifespan development in emotions and affect. "Dramas" in old age notwithstanding, in the main, the world is viewed in less dramatic colors, and perhaps contrasts, as in eyesight, have lost their edge. It would seem that in incidents such as that just cited, explanations implying that contradictions have been reorganized in a congruent "whole" are not satisfactory. Rather, as an aintegration, discrepancies remain; the person may have a sense of the tragic, but the emotional impact is different. This may also have implications on contexts in which gerotherapists can often "allow" themselves to put forward ideas, or nonlogical interpretations, with the anticipation that they will not be found "shocking." The experience and wisdom of many older people may "cushion" therapists by allowing them, for example, to make "mistakes" in interpretations, and so on.

Temporality.   Time is paradoxical and dualistic in nature, and it is important for therapists to be aware of this as well as of their own time perspective and attitude to time (Lomranz, Shmotkin, & Vardi, 1991). Therapists who recognize only linear time and do not comprehend its personal nature will be unable to feel empathy with the elderly patient who may experience the subjective, dualistic quality of time differently. The therapist's recognition of the patient's future time perspective is crucial. If the therapist holds to "objective" time notions only, has a "social clock" time orientation, is unable to comprehend relativistic and paradoxical aspects of time, it may hinder constructive psychotherapy with the elderly patient.

Relational Positions and Transference.   Therapist and client are engaged in deconstruction and co-construction of their interactions and understandings. The client's life is a text unfolding between them, and the therapist is always a coauthor/co-constructor of the story. It is usually not the lack of clinical experience but rather the often remarkable remoteness of the therapist from the world of the aged that accounts for most difficulties in working with the elderly, including a sense of threat. An experienced clinical group psychologist noted, "On the other ward I run a group of schizophrenics and I feel competent with them yet removed since I know I'll never be one of them. Here I am always aware that one day I'll be old like some of the group members and it makes it almost impossible for me to function as a therapist." We are reminded of the critical issue of the image of the elderly held by the therapist and his realization of the existential predicaments of aging.

With a more composite image in mind, it may be best to signify the relational positions between therapist and elderly patient with the term *comradeship* (David Gutmann, private communication), which denotes the relational quality of two persons struggling toward a common goal, emphasizes mutuality, and prevents the therapist from perceiving the elderly client as helpless. In contrast to the feeling of dependency that often characterizes the transference relationship, the stance of aintegration, as well as the acceptance of paradoxes, foster an atmosphere and relationship in which the two parties can experience more equality. This may require working against "transference love" and relinquishing the position of the "knower" and the paternalistic position in which so many therapists, working with the elderly, take refuge. Thus gerotherapists in particular, may have to relinquish features deeply ingrained in narcissism and usually supported by training and the professional clinical culture.

I have indicated the implications of several basic clinical themes stemming from the concept of aintegration and the composite image of the elderly, which are conducive to psychotherapy with the aged. Within the context of an appropriate approach, clinicians can experience gratification from their work with the elderly, as appreciation of wisdom, resiliency, and therapeutic success come to the fore.

CONCLUSION

As we age, the Self becomes more differentiated, and while it becomes clear that basic child-focused concepts (e.g., Oedipus, attachment, or holding environments) are actually lifespan concepts (Nemiroff & Colaruosso, 1990), additional concepts are needed to explain the novel abilities and mental capacities required by adult development and the challenges to adults in modern society. Aintegration, strongly related to both adult developmental theory and postmodernism, attempts to respond to such a need. I have attempted here to relate coping behavior, personality, mental health, and social criticism through the two major components of this chapter: the image of man and the concept of aintegration. While the present chapter serves as the basis of experiments on aintegration, the primary goal of this initial formulation is to suggest new avenues for our conception of human nature at large and specifically of the elderly. Further elaboration of the concept, experimentation, and application should find its place in the larger theoretical network of personality and clinical geropsychology.

REFERENCES

Alexander, I. (1990). *Personology: Method and content in personality assessment and psychobiography*. Durham, NC: Duke University Press.

Arlin, P. (1975). Cognitive development in adulthood: A fifth stage? *Developmental Psychology, 11*, 602–606.

Aron, L. (1995). The internalized primal scene. *Psychoanalytic Dialogues, 5*(2), 195–237.

Baltes, P., & Baltes, M. (Eds.). (1993). *Successful aging*. New York: Cambridge University Press.

Baltes, P., Reese, H., & Lipsitt, L. (1980). Life-span developmental psychology. *Annual Review of Psychology, 31*, 65–111.

Baranger, M. (1983). Process and non-process in analytic work. *International Journal of Psycho-Analysis, 64*, 1–15.

Basseches, M. (1980). Dialectical schemata: A framework for the empirical study of dialectical thinking. *Human Development, 23*, 400–421.

Baumeister, R. (1993). *Self-esteem: The puzzle of low self-regard*. New York: Plenum Press.

Bion, W. (1962). *Learning from experience*. London: Heinemann.

Block, J. (1971). *Lifes through time*. Berkeley, CA: Bancroft Books.

Blythe, R. (1979). *The view of winter*. London: Penguin.

Bruner, J. (1990). *Acts of meaning*. Cambridge, MA: Harvard University Press.

Bugental, J. (1978). *Psychotherapy and process*. Menlo Park, CA: Addison-Wesley.

Buhler, C. (1953). The curve of life as studied in biographies. *Journal of Applied Science*, *19*, 405–409.

Butler, R. (1963). The life review: An interpretation of reminiscence in the aged. *Psychiatry*, *26*, 65–76.

Chandler, M. (1975). Relativism and the problem of epistemological loneliness. *Human Development*, *18*, 171–180.

Clayton, V. (1975). Erikson's theory of human development as it applies to the aged: Wisdom as contraindicative cognition. *Human Development*, *18*, 119–128.

Cohen-Shalev, A. (1992). Self and style: The development of artistic expression from youth through midlife to old age in the works of Henrik Ibsen. *Journal of Aging Studies*, *6*(3), 289–301.

Cole, T. (1992). *The journey of life*. New York: Cambridge University Press.

Coleman, P. (1986). *Ageing and reminiscence processes*. New York: Wiley.

The Concise Oxford Dictionary. (1956). Oxford, UK: Clarendon Press.

Derrida, J. (1986). Différance. In M. Taylor (Ed.), *Disconstruction in context* (pp. 17–43). Chicago: University of Chicago Press.

Erikson, E. (1959). *Identity and the life cycle: Psychological issues*. New York: New York University Press.

Erikson, E. (1963). *Childhood and society*. New York: Norton.

Erikson, E. (1968). *Identity, youth and crisis*. New York: Norton.

Friedan, B. (1993). *The fountain of age*. New York: Simon & Schuster.

Gatz, M., Popkin, S., Pino, C., & Vanden Bos, G. (1985). Psychological interventions with older adults. In J. Birren & W. Schaie (Eds.), *Handbook of the psychology of aging* (2nd ed., pp. 755–785). San Diego: Academic Press.

Gatz, M., Kasl-Godley, J. E., & Karel, M. (1996). Aging and mental disorders. In J. Birren & W. Schaie (Eds.), *Handbook of the psychology of aging* (4th ed., pp. 365–382). San Diego: Academic Press.

Gergen, K., & Gergen, M. (1988). Narrative and self as relationship. *Advances in Experimental Social Psychology*, *21*, 17–56.

Giora, Z. (1991). *The unconscious and its narrative*. Budapest: T-Twins Publishing House.

Goffman, E. (1959). *The presentation of self in everyday life*. Garden City, NY: Doubleday.

Gould, R. (1978). *Transformations: Growth and change in adult life*. New York: Simon & Schuster.

Guillemard, A. (1982). Old age, retirement and social class structure: Analysis of the structural dynamics of the latter stage of life. In T. Hareven & K. Adams (Eds.), *Aging and life-course transitions: An interdisciplinary perspective* (pp. 221–243). London: Guilford.

Gutmann, D. (1994). *Reclaimed powers*. Evanston, IL: Northwestern University Press.

Haight, B., & Webster, J. (1995). *The art and science of reminiscing*. Washington, DC: Taylor & Francis.

Hareven, T. (1994). Family change and historical change: An uneasy relationship. In M. Riley, R. Kahn, & A. Foner (Eds.), *Age and structural lag* (pp. 130–150). New York: Wiley.

Havinghurst, R. (1972). *Developmental tasks and education*. New York: McKay.

Hayslip, B., & Panek, P. (1989). *Adult development and aging*. New York: Harper & Row.

Hazan, H. (1994). *Old age: Constructions and deconstructions*. Cambridge, UK: Cambridge University Press.

Hazan, H. (1996). *From first principles*. London: Bergin & Garvey.

Heaton, J. (1979). Theory in psychotherapy. In N. Bolton (Ed.), *Philosophical problems in psychotherapy* (pp. 177–196). London: Methuen.

Heidegger, M. (1962). *Being and time*. New York: Harper & Row.

Herman, J. (1992). *Trauma and recovery*. New York: Basic Books.

Hermans, H., & Hermans-Jansen, E. (1995). *Self-narratives: The construction of meaning in psychotherapy*. New York: Guilford.

Hinshelwood, R. (1994). *A dictionary of Kleinian thought*. London: Free Association Books.

Hogman, F. (1985). Role of memories in lives of World War II orphans. *Journal of American Academy Child Psychiatry*, *24*(4), 390–396.

Irwin, R. R. (1996). Narrative competence and constructive developmental theory: A proposal for rewriting the *Bildungsroman* in the postmodern world. *Journal of Adult Development*, *3*(2), 109–125.

James, W. (1980). *The principles of psychology*. New York: Modern Library.

Janoff-Bulman, R. (1992). *Shattered assumptions*. New York: Free Press.

Jonsen, A. (1992). Resentment and rights of the elderly. In N. Jecker (Eds.), *Aging and ethics* (pp. 341–352). Totowa, NJ: Humana Press.

Kahn, R. (1994). Opportunities, aspirations and goodness of fit. In M. Riley, R. Kahn, & A. Foner (Eds.), *Age and structural lag* (pp. 37–53). New York: Wiley.

Karp, D. (1988). A decade of reminders: Changing age consciousness between fifty and sixty years old. *Gerontologist, 28*(6), 727–738.

Kastenbaum, R. (1985). Dying and death: A life-span approach. In J. Birren & W. Schaie (Eds.), *Handbook of the psychology of aging* (pp. 619–643). New York: Van Nostrand.

Kastenbaum, R., & Kastenbaum, B. (Eds.). (1993). *Encyclopedia of death*. New York: Avon Books.

Kegan, R. (1982). *The evolving self*. Cambridge, MA: Harvard University Press.

Kegan, R. (1994). *In over our heads: The mental demands of modern life*. Cambridge, MA: Harvard University Press.

Kenyon, G. (1988). Basic assumptions in theories of human aging. In J. Birren & V. Bengston (Eds.), *Emergent theories of aging* (pp. 3–18). New York: Springer.

Kierkegaard, S. (1957). *The concept of dread*. Princeton, NJ: Princeton University Press.

Klein, M. (1937). *Love guilt, and reparation: The writings of Melanie Klein* (Vol. 1). London: Hogard.

Kramer, D. (1983). Post-formal operations? A need for further conceptualization. *Human Development, 26*, 91–105.

Kramer, D., & Bopp, M. (Eds.). (1989). *Transformations in clinical and developmental psychology*. New York: Springer-Verlag.

Kramer, D., & Woodruff, D. (1986). Relativistic and dialectic thought. *Human Development, 29*, 280–290.

Kuhn, T. (1962). *The structure of scientific revolutions*. Chicago: University of Chicago Press.

Kumin, I. (1978). Developmental aspects of opposites and paradox. *International Review of Psycho-Analysis, 5*, 477–483.

Labouvie-Vief, G. (1977). Adult cognitive development: In search of alternative interpretations. *Merrill–Palmer Quarterly, 23*(4), 227–263.

Lax, W. (1995). Postmodern thinking in a clinical practice. In S. McNamee & K. Gergen (Eds.), *Therapy as social construction* (pp. 69–85). London: Sage.

Lazarus, R., & DeLongis, A. (1983). Psychological stress and coping in aging. *American Psychologist, 38*, 245–254.

Lazarus, R. & Lazarus, B. (1994). *Passion and reason*. Oxford, UK: Oxford University Press.

Levinson, D. J. (1978). *The season of a man's life*. New York: Knopf.

Lewin, K. (1936). Dynamic theory of personality. New York: McGraw-Hill.

Lieberman, M. (1975). Adaptive processes in later life. In N. Datan & L. Ginsburg (Eds.), *Life-span developmental psychology: Normative life events* (pp. 135–159). New York: Academic Press.

Lieberman, M., & Tobin, S. (1983). *The experience of old age*. New York: Basic Books.

Lifton, R. (1983). *The broken connection*. New York: Basic Books.

Loevinger, J. (1976). *Ego development*. San Francisco: Jossey-Bass.

Loevinger, J., & Knoll, E. (1983). Personality: Stages, traits and the self. In M. Rosenzweig & L. Porter (Eds.), *Annual Review of Psychology* (Vol. 34, pp. 195–222). Palo Alto, CA: George Banta.

Lomranz, J. (1986). Personality theory: A position and derived teaching implications in clinical psychology. *Professional Psychology: Theory, Research and Practice, 17*(6), 551–559.

Lomranz, J. (1990). Long-term adaptation to traumatic stress in light of adult development in aging perspectives. In M. Stephens, M. Crowther, S. Hobfoll,l & D. Tennenbaum (Eds.), *Stress and coping in later-life families* (pp. 99–121). New York: Hemisphere.

Lomranz, J. (1995). Endurance and living: Long-term effects of the Holocaust. In S. Hobfoll & M. de Vries (Eds.), *Extreme stress and communities* (pp. 325–352). Boston: Kluver Academic Publisher.

Lomranz, J., Shmotkin, D., & Vardi, R. (1991). The equivocal meanings of time: Exploratory and structural analyses. *Current Psychology: Research and Reviews, 10*, 3–20.

Lubow, R. (1977). *The war animals*. New York: Doubleday.

Lyotard, J. (1988). *The postmodern condition: A report on knowledge*. Minneapolis: University of Minnesota Press.

MacDonald, M., Kuiper, N., & Olinger, L. (1985). Vulnerability to depression, mild depression and degree of schema consolidation. *Motivation and Emotion, 9,* 369–379.

Marshall, V. (1980). State of the art lecture: The sociology of aging. In J. Cradford (Ed.), *Canadian gerontological collection* (Vol. 3, pp. 76–144). Winnipeg: Canadian Association of Gerontology.

May, R., Angel, E., & Ellenberger, H. (1958). *Existence.* New York: Basic Books.

Meichenbaum, D., & Fitzpatrick, D. (1992). A constructivist narrative perspective on stress and loping: Stress inoculation applications. In L. Goldberger, & S. Breznits (Eds.), *Handbook of stress* (pp. 706–723). New York: Free Press.

Merton, G. (1957). *Social theory and social structure.* New York: Free Press.

Modell, A. (1990). *Other times, other realities.* Cambridge, MA: Harvard University Press.

Moody, H. R. (1988). Toward a critical gerontology: The contributions of the humanities to theories of aging. In J. Birren & V. Bengtson (Eds.), *Emergent theories of aging* (pp. 19–40). New York: Springer.

Moody, H. R. (1992). The meaning of life in old age. In N. Jecker (Eds.), *Aging and ethics* (pp. 51–92). Totowa, NJ: Humana Press.

Nagel, T. (1992). The absurd. In N. Jecker (Ed.), *Aging and ethics* (pp. 375–388). Totowa, NJ: Humana Press.

Neiser, U., & Fivush, R. (1994). *The remembering self.* New York: Cambridge University Press.

Nemiroff, R., & Colarusso, C. (Eds.). (1990). *New dimensions in adult development.* New York: Basic Books.

Nisman, H. (1995). *Soul and memory.* Kibbutz Ein Dor: Benei Shaul.

Pascual-Leone, J. (1983). Growing into human maturity: Toward a metasubjective theory of adult stages. In P. Baltes & O. Brim (Eds.), *Life-span development and behavior* (Vol. 5, pp. 117–156). New York: Academic Press.

Peck, R. (1968). Psychological developments in the second half of life. In B. L. Neugarten (Ed.), *Middle age and aging* (pp. 44–49). Chicago: University of Chicago Press.

Pepper, S. (1942). *World perspectives.* Berkeley: University of California Press.

Perry, W. (1970). *Forms of ethical and individual development in the college years.* New York: Holt, Rinehart & Winston.

Peskin, H. (1987). Uses of the past in the adult life-span. In G. Maddox & E. Busse (Eds.), *Aging the universal experience* (pp. 432–440). New York: Springer.

Piaget, J. (1980). *Experiments in contradiction.* Chicago: University of Chicago Press.

Polanyi, M. (1958). *Personal knowledge.* New York: Harper & Row.

Reese, H., & Overton, W. (1970). Models of development and theories of development. In Goulet & P. Baltes (Eds.), *Life-span developmental psychology* (pp. 397–416). New York: Academic Press.

Riegel, K. (1973). Dialectic operations: The final period of cognitive development. *Human Development, 16,* 346–370.

Riegel, K. (1976). The dialectics of human development. *American Psychologist, 31,* 689–700.

Riley, M., Kahn, R., & Foner, A. (Eds.), (1994). *Age and structural lag.* New York: Wiley.

Ross, B. (1991). *Remembering the personal past.* Oxford, UK: Oxford University Press.

Rosow, I. (1974). *Socialization to old age.* Berkeley: University of California Press.

Ruth, J.-R., & Coleman, P. (1996). Personality and aging: Coping and management of the self in later life. In J. Birren & W. Schaie (Eds.), *Handbook of the psychology of aging* (pp. 308–322). New York: Van Nostrand.

Rybash, J., Hoyer, W., &Roodin, P. (1986). Adult cognition and aging. New York: Pergamon Press.

Ryff, C. (1986). The subjective construction of self and society: An agenda for life-span research. In V. Marshall (Ed.), *Later life: The social psychology of aging* (pp. 33–74). Beverly Hills, CA: Sage.

Sarbin, T. (1986). *Narrative psychology: The storied nature of human conduct.* New York: Praeger.

Sartre, P. (1943). *Being and nothingness.* New York: Penguin.

Schafer, R. (1992). *Retelling a life.* New York: Basic Books.

Siebert, A. (1983, August). *The survivor personality.* Paper presented at the Western Psychological Association Convention, San Francisco, CA.

Suzman, R., Harris, T., Kovar, M., & Weindruch, R. (1992). The robust oldest old: Optimistic perspectives. In R. Suzman, D. Willis, & K. Manton (Eds.), *The oldest old* (pp. 341–358). New York: Oxford University Press.

Tennen, H., & Affleck, G. (1993). The puzzles of self-esteem: A clinical perspective. In R. Baumeister (Ed.), *Self-esteem: The puzzle of low self-regard* (pp. 241–261). New York: Plenum Press.

Thomae, H. (1980). Personality and adjustment to aging. In J. Birren & W. Schaie (Eds.), *Handbook of mental health and aging* (pp. 285–309). Englewood Cliffs, NJ: Prentice-Hall.

Tillich, P. (1952). *The courage to be*. New Haven, CT: Yale University Press.

Valliant, G. (1993). *The wisdom of the ego*. Cambridge, MA: Harvard University Press.

van der Kolk, B., & van der Hart, O. (1991). The intrusive past: Flexibility of memory and the engraving of trauma. *American Imago, 48*(4), 425–454.

Walaskay, M., Whitbourne, S., & Nehrke, M. (1983). Construction and validation of an ego integrity status interview. *International Journal of Aging and Human Development, 18*, 61–72.

Watzlawick, P., Beavin, J., & Jackson, D. (1967). *Pragmatics of human communication*. New York: Norton.

Weeks, G. (Ed.). (1991). *Promoting change through paradoxical therapy*. New York: Brunner/Mazel.

Werner, H. (1948). *Comparative psychology of mental development*. New York: Follett.

White, M., & Epston, D. (1990). *Narrative means to therapeutic ends*. New York: Norton.

Winnicott, D. (1971). *Playing and reality*. New York: Basic Books.

Woods, R. (1996). *Handbook of the clinical psychology of aging*. New York: Wiley.

Yalom, I. (1980). *Existential psychotherapy*. New York: Basic Books.

Zarit, S., & Knight, B. (1996). *A guide to psychotherapy and aging*. Washington, DC: American Psychological Association Press.

Zetzel, E. (1949). *The capacity for emotional growth*. New York: International Universities Press.

Ziegler, E., & Glick, M. (1986). *A developmental approach to adult psychopathology*. New York: Wiley.

Zoja, L. (1995). *Growth and guilt*. London: Routledge.

PART IV

Psychodynamics and Psychopathology in Later Life

The prevalence, diagnosis, and risk factors for psychopathology are major questions in the field of clinical gerontology (Gatz, Kasl-Godley, & Karel, 1996). Hans Loewald is quoted as stating that "those who know ghosts tell us that they long to be released from their ghost life and led to rest as ancestors. As ancestors they live forth in the present generation, while as ghosts they are compelled to haunt the present generation with their shadow life" (Mitchell & Black, 1995, p. 1). Part of elderly persons' mental health problem is how to release their ghosts while they are still alive, so that they may then rest as an ancestor. Some of the ways and processes that help them achieve that goal are presented in Part IV of this volume.

The work of Cohler (Chapter 11) incorporates psychoanalysis, the life course, aging, and the narrative. The author integrates aspects of adult developmental theory, characteristics of psychoanalysis adapted to the narrative process, sociohistorical and cultural components, literary criticism, the dialogue perspective, and reader response theory—all converging in the construction of the narrative and explaining change in the analysand. Adult development cannot be understood as linear and cumulative, as developmental stage theories have assumed (see Lomranz, Chapter 10); rather, it is constantly changing. The individual life story introduces continuity and order into a person's past and future life course (see Peskin, Chapter 13), affording him or her meaning and a sense of coherence (see Kegan, Chapter 9). Cohler clarifies how the narrative, as a rewritten life story integrating the various time dimensions, can be correctly grasped in a contemporary psychoanalytic framework. Psychoanalysis itself constitutes the situation, the manner, the means, and the process of telling and listening (often portrayed in psychoanalysis within the concepts of transference or enactment, empathy, and counterenactment) by which the person constructs his or her narrative. The cooperative effort of analyst and analysand enables the construction of a more coherent and "followable" life story (see Meador & Blazer, Chapter 22). Cohler actually elaborates the redefinition of psychoanalysis as a means of gathering evidence and building narratives rather than enacting an objective based on wishes and drives. It does not suffice to treat only the residual elements and to elaborate past nuclear conflicts. The elderly person's healing and change processes also dictate a focus on present life experiences and an analysis of the unique issues of aging. These, in addition to the relational quality between analyst and analysand, and the prolonged experience of time in therapy to construct a life story, are necessary in the analysis of elderly patients.

Gutmann (Chapter 12) conceives the function of the psyche as an immune system, its role being to preserve the consistency, continuity, and integrity of the Self, despite the flux of internal and external change. This psychoimmune system dynamically develops in a preserved, safe, environmental ecology and transitional space. Gutmann explains how adult development is achieved with the aid of a psychosocial "niche." However, the psychic immune system, like the bodily one, is prone to degenerate in later life. In light of that model, the author understands late-onset disorder not just as a result of the accumulation of losses and insults in later life, but as a result of specific, yet potentially reversible, attacks on the immune system that—perhaps from an earlier age—suffered from alternate poor rearing and developmental routes that turned the normal person into an at-risk survivor. Gutmann emphasizes a qualitative and subjective approach to stress and losses. Delineating transferential bonds, transitional space, alloplastic extroverts, and autoplastic introverts, the author eloquently discusses the psychodynamic developmental trajectories of the vulnerable, at-risk adult whose immune system served him or her well in earlier years but is unable to function adequately in later life as the supportive niche changes and defensive maneuvers can no longer operate. Gutmann's model of late-onset psychopathology enriches our lifespan understanding by integrating internal and external experiences along the life course in the histrionic, not the symptomatic, patient.

The basic question in every model of the mind and human behavior is what actually happens to our past life experiences. Is past experience just coded in the brain, erased, or does it continue to influence behavior? If so, then how? What is its impact, if any? Freud, in the last lines of his most ambitious but unfinished project, tackles the question "of the way in which the present is changed into the past" (Freud, 1949, p. 124). Peskin (Chapter 13), shifting the formulation of this question, demonstrates the influence of the present on the past and the uses of the past in adult development. He differentiates between the genetic viewpoint and adult psychodynamics, the latter possibly leading to new developments and definitions of the Self (see Kegan, Chapter 9). He expands on the different ways that the past figures in our lives and claims that during adult life transitions, changing organizations of the past may release new uses of long-standing but nonlinear, dormant capabilities. His model, which negates the linear causal chain of past-to-present axiom, is based on the primacy of current life purpose rather than on the primacy and immutability of the deterministic past. Such a model, based on a unique approach to the prediction of psychological health in longitudinal samples, provides new energies and potentials for novel endings to past problematic configurations and conflicts, and enables a more comprehensive definition of psychological health. Peskin's approach to adult-centered uses of the past credits the past with an elasticity reserved for narrative reconstruction and adult development, thus extending a modified psychoanalytic developmental psychology across the total lifespan, placing the concepts of relational autonomy and the narrative in an appropriate adult context (see Cohler, Chapter 11). Peskin's innovative model also has far-reaching implications for psychotherapy with adults and the aged. It departs from "historical truth" and genetic interpretations of childhood and moves to make it possible to realign primary relationships, rectify conflicts, provide "second chances" for conflict resolution, rediscover resources, and allow for novel late-life integration—all of which reflects how the second half of life organizes and harnesses new resources from the past for the present healthy emergence of selfhood (see Silver, Chapter 17).

REFERENCES

Freud, S. (1949). *An outline of psychoanalysis.* New York: Norton.

Gatz, M., Kasl-Godley, J., & Karel, M. (1996). Aging and mental disorders. In Birren & W. Schaie (Eds.), *Handbook of the psychology of aging* (pp. 365–383). New York: Van Nostrand.

Mitchell, S., & Black, M. (1995). *Freud and beyond.* New York: Basic Books.

CHAPTER 11

Psychoanalysis, the Life Story, and Aging

Creating New Meanings within Narratives of Lived Experience

BERTRAM J. COHLER

The notion that adult development is linear and cumulative—that is, that certain personalities are more "adult" than others—underlies stage theories of adult development. There is little empirical evidence for such orderly and progressive change, nor is there any agreement on the outcome.... From this perspective, lifespan development becomes individual life history, which in turn becomes a life story—an attempt by the individual to create a narrative given order and predictability only by the choices and decision making of that individual. The order in the course of lives lies, then, in the mind of the persons experiencing those lives, not in the observer. The goal of the study ..." (is) to explicate contexts and thereby to achieve now insights and new understandings" (Neugarten, 1984, p. 292). If adult personality demonstrates any order, then, it may not be the result a developmental trajectory but instead a reflection of the individual's attempts to maintain a sense of continuity. (Datan, Rodeheaver, & Hughes, 1987, pp. 162–163)

Datan et al. (1987), extending Neugarten's (1984) earlier observation regarding the significance of the manner in which persons recount the story of their lives, well portray both the manner in which contemporary psychoanalysis understands the course of life and emphasize the goal of psychoanalytic study of adult lives as a search for factors accounting for a presently constructed story of experience and the determinant of wish and action. The present chapter focuses on the significance of contemporary clinical theory within psychoanalysis, additionally informed by study within the human sciences, as a means for understanding the management of lived experience reflected in the successively

BERTRAM J. COHLER • Center for Aging, Health, and Society, University of Chicago, Chicago, Illinois 60637-1603.

Handbook of Aging and Mental Health: An Integrative Approach, edited by Jacob Lomranz. Plenum Press, New York, 1998.

rewritten life story from childhood to oldest adulthood. These life stories, told by the analysand to the analyst, provide the foundation for a shared effort at remaking accounts of lived experience in an effort to provide the analysand with increased sense of personal integrity and vitality.

Analyst and analysand maintain shared focus on the analysand's struggle to maintain a coherent or integrated life story, founded in the reenactment of that effort within the context of the analytic situation. Both the analysand's own presently experienced past, enacted anew within the unique context of the psychoanalytic situation, and the analyst's unique mode of listening and understanding this story contribute to the construction of a life story both more coherent and more "followable" (Ricoeur, 1977) than that told by the analysand at the outset of this unique collaboration. The analytic process is founded on empathy or use of vicarious introspection or empathy (Greenson, 1960; Kohut, 1959/1978; Schafer, 1959), fostered by the analyst's own personal analysis and continuing self-inquiry that makes possible continued resonance with the analysand's life story even as this story might evoke such anxiety or personal pain in the listener in a social situation that continued resonance with the story might be difficult.

The analytically informed listener employs a process of empathy or vicarious introspection (Kohut, 1959/1978; Schafer, 1959; Greenson, 1960) in an effort to understand the analysand's presently told account of lived experience. Indeed, what makes psychoanalysis a distinctive mode of inquiry within the human sciences, and what makes psychoanalysis so significant as a method of study relevant to ethnography, criticism, and the study of lives, as well as to clinical intervention, is precisely the analyst's ability to monitor his or her own self-state in order to continue "tasting" or experiencing the analysand's story even as this story evokes dysphoric affects (Devereux, 1967; Fliess, 1944, 1953; Moraitis, 1985).

Telling and listening to the life story in psychoanalysis, including the analyst's empathic resonance, take place within a particular culture and at a particular historical moment. Analysands growing to adulthood, becoming middle-aged, and growing older, lead their lives within a society that provides meanings used in fashioning a particular life story, but one which is markedly different both across generations or historical cohorts and also cultures (Kakar, 1990, 1995; Mannheim, 1923/1952; Hazan, Chapter 8, this volume). The process of retelling the life story, which is a result of a unique collaboration between a psychoanalytically informed listener and a teller, often experiencing psychological distress, must include this recognition of the continuing interplay of sociohistorical forces, changing relationship to means of production, and the particular changes in the life story, which are the result of the analysand's unique life circumstances as reflected in a particular story of the personal past.

THE CONSTRUCTION
OF THE PERSONAL PAST

Inspired by Riegel's (1979) reconceptualization of the process of development, which emphasizes the effort at continuing dialectical reintegration of lived experience, including both expectable transitions and eruptive, generally adverse, life-changes which may be beyond personal control (Bandura, 1982; Cohler, 1982; Gergen, 1977, 1994). From this perspective, a major task across the course of life involves "making sense" of life changes through continuing revision of the life story in ways that maintains sense of personal coherence over time (Bruner, 1987, 1990; Gergen, 1994). Failure to maintain this sense of continuity leads to feelings of fragmentation and disintegration of self such as is seen in psychotic states.

The life review, as portrayed by Butler (1963), is one example of this effort at the maintenance of personal meaning. Among older persons, there appears to be an effort at making sense of life as lived, creating an overall story of past experiences that makes "sense" in terms of presently valued goals and ideals. This effort at creating a consistent story of the life cycle must be understood in terms of both shared values and attitudes within particular cohorts and in terms of perceived place in the course of life (Cohler, 1982). As Lieberman and Falk (1971) have suggested, middle-aged persons use the life review in ways that are markedly different from the life review of late life: Reminiscence in midlife is used primarily in the service of mastery, with solutions for present problems sought by reviewing past solutions. Later in life, the life review appears much more important as a source of settling personal accounts, as a part of preparation for death (Grunes, 1980; Pollock, 1981).

Study of the means by which persons construct and maintain a coherent life story has become an issue of central importance for both the humanities and the social sciences, and an important point of connection between humanistic study and the disciplines of medicine (Antonovsky, 1987; Good, 1994; Hunter, 1991; Slaveny & McHugh, 1984). Study of the life story, making use of concepts of interpretation characteristic of criticism, within the humanities, together with methods and findings from social science study of lives over time, has led to renewed appreciation of the determining of meaning and coherence, the role of memory and present experience as the foundations of this narrative of the course of life, and the particular importance for the outcome of this process in the study of morale among older adults (Kegan, Chapter 9, this volume; Lomranz, Chapter 10, this volume).

Telling the Life Story

It is characteristic of the life course in contemporary society that persons strive to maintain a coherent account that fosters a sense of well-being. From earliest childhood through oldest age, persons successively rewrite this life story or personal narrative, striving to maintain meaning through construction of an understandable or "followable" narrative (Ricoeur, 1977). The fundamental issue in the study of lives concerns the manner in which persons attribute meanings to a presently experienced past and present, and anticipated future, resulting in a story of the life history that at any one point across the course of life preserves sense of continuity portrayed as the self (Kohut, 1981). Ricoeur (1977) has noted that

> narrative intelligibility implies something more than the subjective accountability of one's own life story. It comes to terms with the general condition of acceptability that we apply when we read any story, be it historical or fictional.... A story has to be "followable" and, in this sense, "self-explanatory."

This narrative or life story provides integration of presently experienced past and present, and anticipated future, including both expectable and eruptive life changes, into a consistent and integrated account of the course of life (Cohler, 1982). Freeman (1993) and Cohler and Freeman (1993) have suggested that lives may be considered as analogous to texts: Persons successively rewrite stories of their own development in order to take account of unpredictable, often adverse, experiences that require sense to be made of them in order to preserve sense of personal coherence over time. This perspective has been well demonstrated by Peskin (Chapter 13, this volume) and Peskin and Livson (1980, 1981), who similarly note the importance of the study of the life story as a narrative refashioned across the adult years, accompanying both expectable role changes across the course of life and also the very definition of time and finitude of life. Peskin's work and that of Lieberman and Falk (1971) shows that adults use the past in different ways and toward different ends across the middle years and into later life.

Telling the life story presumes that teller and listener are both embedded within a particular time that represents particular social and historical forces that determine the very manner in which the story is told. This focus on issues of telling and listening reflects a distinctive "interpretive turn" within psychoanalysis and the human sciences (Hiley, Bohman, & Shusterman, 1991; Rabinow & Sullivan, 1987; Rosaldo, 1993). What does endure over time is focus on the determinants of the enactment of a life story understood within presently active productive forces within the larger society. Theory may change, but the focus on questions about lives studied over time appears to endure.

Even as a reader of a subsequent transcript of that life story, including both the account of changing lives within a changing society and personal change across the psychoanalytic experience, the participating analyst has a quite different experience of the transcript than another reader; however, experience may itself change over time as a consequence of changing theoretical perspectives within both psychoanalysis and the human sciences (Kohut, 1979; Kracke, 1987). Readers always bring their own perspectives to the reading, just as to the telling of a story (Moraitis, 1985). That perspective within criticism known as reader response theory emphasizes the significance of the interplay between text and life history of the reader. Reader response theory, particularly as explicated by literary theorist Wolfgang Iser (1978), becomes central for this study of lives. Iser emphasizes the extent to which texts exist as a construction of the reader. The text may be thought of as a stimulus that leads to a particular response on the part of the reader seeking to make sense of that text. This dialogical focus (Bakhtin, 1981, 1986), takes into account explicitly the lived experience of the analysand and implicitly the lived experience of the analyst, as well as the place of both participants within culture and generation or history.

Implicit in Iser's portrayal of reader response theory is the use of the dialogic perspective emphasized in much contemporary study ranging from developmental psychology to criticism. Reflecting the second change across the past two decades in the study of social life, this emphasis upon the intrinsic intersubjective nature of social life, first explicated in the work of the Russian literary theorist, Bakhtin, and in the work of the Russian psychologists, Vygotsky (Vygotsky, 1924–1934/1987; Wilson & Weinstein, 1992, 1996) and Luria (1976), following in the tradition pioneered by Marx (1845), emphasizes the significance of human action as the foundation of meanings, among participants, either interviewer or interviewee, or writer and reader, in the construction of texts, including the life story as a particular kind of text.

Lives, cultures, and texts cannot be studied apart from both the relationship of teller and listener, and the social context and present sociohistorical circumstances of both teller or writer and listener or reader. This is well portrayed both in Kracke's (1987) account of changes in his understanding of fieldwork interviews in the context of changing theoretical perspectives within psychoanalysis, and Kohut's (1979) account of changes in his understanding of the case of "Mr. Z" from the perspective of two analyses similarly conducted at two points in time following contrasting theoretical perspectives. These changing theoretical perspectives, in turn, respond to changes within the larger society, including relationship of persons to means of production.

One example of such a change is well reflected in portrayals by Lasch (1978) and Gergen (1994) that ours is a time of particular pressure on concepts of self resulting from a world in which there is an overload of information, lack of clear values, and increased sense of personal and social dislocation, at least in part a consequence of downsizing of work, telecommuting, barriers interfering in person-to-person communication, and replacement of personal decision making by computers. This larger social change may be reflected in the emergence within psychoanalysis of an emphasis upon the self and the foundation and maintenance of the experience of personal coherence, as portrayed by Klein (1976), Kohut and his colleagues (Strozier, 1985), Stern (1995), and others.

The critic Hirsch (1976) has pleaded for recognition of "authoritorial intent" or recognition of the author's intended meaning for a text. Presumably, the author arranges events in a particular sequence, telling a particular story in a particular manner based on some intention. Hirsch is concerned that this intent fails to emerge when the task of constructing meaning is placed on the reader. However, as methods as disparate as clinical psychoanalysis, criticism, and ethnography have shown, there is a continuing dialogue between teller and listener, or between text and reader, with the very significance or meaning of an account shifting over time, in the context of additional elements of the story, new means for understanding stories, and such changes external to the text as shifts in theory used as an additional means for making sense of the story line, or additional life experiences (Iser, 1978; Kracke, 1987; Schafer, 1980, 1981). Hirsch's (1976) effort to appeal to authoritorial intent is understandable in terms of the anxiety generated by lack of certainty and fixed point of departure for interpretation (Devereux, 1967). It is important that we recognize this anxiety in order that we may be free to attend to the sequence of events comprising the text and focus on the task of interpretation in a manner akin to Freud's (1911/1958, 1914/1958) concept of "evenly suspended attention."

Psychoanalysis and the "Followable" Life Story

Riegel (1979) and Neugarten (1969) have both observed that understanding of change rather than continuity within lives over time is the most important issue in our study of the course of life. The important phenomenon to be understood is less stability or continuity reported within lives over time than change in experience of self and others with the passage of time. The very meanings that are made of the analytic experience itself change with the passage of time. As clinical reports of the follow-through of child analysis so clearly show, the very meaning of this clinical contact itself may change with the passage of time and with age (Cohen & Cohler, 1998). Furthermore, the very significance of the life story that is told across the years of clinical psychoanalytic collaboration shows a shift over time as a consequence of the manner in which analysand and analyst experience each other. The history of lived experience recounted in the first weeks of this analytic collaboration may bear little relationship with that recounted several years later at the conclusion of the formal psychoanalytic collaboration. What is of interest is precisely understanding those factors, reflected in the use made by particular persons of the larger symbolic world within which we all live, which might account for particular ways of experiencing change, rather than simply the fact of this change itself. Study of this change as lived experience provides important information more generally regarding the determinants of both personal and social change.

Particularly in Kris's (1956a, 1956b) later papers, and in the important posthumous essays of Novey (1968/1985), important questions were posed regarding the manner in which we understand the past. Most recently, detailed study of autobiographical memory (Singer & Salovey, 1993; Lindsay & Read, 1994) has supported Kris's initial concern regarding the manner in which we use the past. This study suggests that developmental perspectives may be more significant than those founded on mechanistic assumptions regarding the primacy of antecedent experiences and the ordered manner of the transformation of the past as continually active in the present. Furthermore, focus in the study of the use of the past must shift from concepts of an objective past as so often portrayed within psychoanalysis, even as later modified by Erikson (1951/1963, 1982/1985), to renewed focus on the manner in which the past is recounted, and the circumstances associated with telling the life story as a function both of the psychoanalytic setting and the relationship of teller and listener (Cohler & Cole, 1996; Schafer, 1992; Stone, 1961). Reconsideration of the manner in which the past is recalled within psychoanalysis raises serious question regarding the validity of assumptions that the past as recounted through dreams and recollection of memories may be regarded as anything more than reenactment within the analytic situation of the totality or actuality of the life history (Erikson, 1962/1964). From this perspective, it is important to reconsider assumptions such as that of Greenacre (1949) regarding the significance of reconstruction of the past in psychoanalysis, together with more recent discussion regarding the veridical nature of past memories (Lindsay & Read, 1994; Schimek, 1975; Singer & Salovey, 1993; Wolff, 1988).

The narrative of the course of life recounted at any one point in time across the course of psychoanalysis as more generally in telling the life story to an empathic listener, is comprised of meanings that are in turn determined by both shared life experiences and the organization of particular life circumstances, largely determined by events within family and community, all constructed in terms of presently salient realms of discourse or shared modalities of representing experience. Joint focus on the social context of the telling, and the listening, among these participants, together with concern with the meaning of just these social and historical consequences, provides information regarding not only personal change, but also social change.

The method of clinical psychoanalytic study is uniquely able to provide information regarding the dynamics of both personal and social change. It is in this sense that psychoanalysis is a method of significance not only for clinical intervention but also more generally for understanding lives in time and over time. The analysis of a man or woman who has experienced significant social change, such as taking place in contemporary Germany, provides an ideal manner for understanding the ways in which persons make sense of social change within their own lived experience. Experienced anew within the context of the transference emerging within the analytic relationship, the ways used by these men and women to cope with social change are represented within the analytic relationship as well. As a method of study, psychoanalysis may be able to provide important information regarding the interplay of the personal and social in the maintenance of a presently coherent narrative of lived experience (Nemiroff & Colarusso, 1985, 1990a).

Psychoanalysis may be best understood as a means of gathering evidence rather than a particular theory of wish and action; the process of psychoanalysis is one of recurring attention to the manner in which the life story is told (Schafer, 1958, 1980, 1981) within the context of the present relationship. This focus on relationship as the context within which a particular life story emerges reflects a so-called "constructionist" perspective, which focuses on experience within the life world (Schutz & Luckmann, 1973, 1989), as contrasted with an "essentialist" perspective. Rather, the clinical psychoanalytic approach is concerned with meanings that are presently fashioned regarding life experiences, recognizing that meanings shift overtime and with age. A similar point has been made by Lomranz (Chapter 10, this volume), focusing more generally upon the process of making (or refining) meaning across adult lived experience. Reports regarding expectable transference enactments across the course of life (Blos, 1980; King, 1980; Neubauer, 1980) provide important information regarding the manner in which persons maintain meanings of lived experience across the years from childhood to later life (Lomranz, Chapter 10, this volume). The psychoanalytic situation is able to offer a unique perspective regarding the dynamics of personal change, including use made of social and historical events as factors relevant to the creation of meanings over time regarding the significance of the presently remembered past, experienced present, and anticipated future across the course of life and into oldest age.

Psychoanalysis is but one occasion for the study of the personal past as experienced at any one point over the course of life (Nemiroff & Colarusso, 1990b). The process of recounting a life, whether in the form of personal documents, such as the diary, journal, or autobiography, or the telling to another, including both oral history or the psychoanalytic interview, becomes a means for constructing a narrative of the past or life story that provides for the reintegration of a presently recounted past (Berman, 1994; Kaminsky, 1992; Kotre, 1984). However, while writing and telling both assume an audience, the act of telling and that of writing may be somewhat different. The psychoanalytic process involves two participants involved in a relationship of some duration.

Psychoanalytic study of change over time emphasizes the manner in which the past is enacted anew in the present within the context of a particular relationship between analyst and analysand. Ironically, the findings from this psychoanalytic study have sometimes been founded more in Freud's prepsychoanalytic scientistic study (Sulloway, 1979) than in observation of the compulsion to repeat, as reflected in the transference or transference-like repetitions that are experienced anew between analyst and analysand. Gill (1976) and Klein (1976) both have noted that the fundamental contribution of psychoanalysis has been with meaning and intent rather than with phenomena beyond the experience-near observational perspective of the clinical interview. Gill and Klein both emphasize that to understand psychoanalysis as an epigenetic psychology is to misunderstand the importance of Freud's contributions, together with those of contemporary psychoanalysis across so-called theoretical "schools" emphasizing a two-person psychology (Gill, 1994). The particular collaboration between analyst and analysand, based on the analysand's present account of lived experience, provides the foundation for understanding psychological development over time.

NARRATIVES OF THE PERSONAL PAST:
TRANSFERENCE AS REENACTMENT

The dialogic perspective (Bakhtin, 1981, 1986), which includes the particular perspectives of reader and listener, or teller and reader, has important implications for psychoanalytic study of older adult lives as more generally in the study of lived experience across the course of life. The analyst, generally as listener, and the analysand, generally as teller, become participants in a process of shared listening and telling founded within the distinctive relationship made possible by the psychoanalytic situation, emphasizing nearly daily appointments at a regular time and place over the course of several years. Across the period of the analysis, focus is on understanding the analysand's distinctive mode of representing his or her life history in the presence of an active listener who, in turn, brings to this presentation or performance another distinctive life history, including his or her own personal analysis and heightened awareness of own contribution to the situation, which fosters that distinctive mode of listening termed by Kohut (1959/1978) "vicarious introspection" or empathy (Pigman, 1995; Schafer, 1959).

Analyst, Analysand, and the Construction of the Life Story

The clinical psychoanalytic situation is founded on the analyst's own personal analysis, together with continuing capacity for self-inquiry (Gardner, 1983), which makes possible empathic attunement with the analysand's life story. The analyst's own prior personal analysis fosters both increased capacity for self-understanding and the mode of reflective listening that is so central to the psychoanalytic process (Freud, 1911/1958, 1914/1958). Rather than responding with anxiety to the analysand's account of experience and the analysand's own enactment of this lived experience within the contest of the "new" relationship with the analyst who is friendly, but not otherwise involved in the analysand's life, the analyst assists the analysand to observe the impact of particular experiences upon wish and action in ways not previously recognized.

The distinctive aspect of psychoanalysis as a mode of listening to lived experience involves the analyst's capacity to "taste" (Fliess, 1944, 1953) or vicariously introspect (Kohut, 1959/1978) the analysand's accounts of earlier and present experience and to use this experience of the personal narrative or life story as a distinctive means of gathering information regarding the interplay of life experiences, social circumstances, and time or point in the course of life as factors shaping meaning and intent (Schafer, 1959). The concept of empathy is one of the least well-understood concepts within the human sciences. While the experience of "fellow-feeling" or empathy has informed inquiry in fields ranging from the humanities to psychiatry, as used within psychoanalysis, the term has much more specific application. Fliess (1944, 1953) and Jaffe (1986) have suggested that the activity of the analyst involves the experience of "tasting" these experiences of another and then the formation of an intervention based on this experience. This process, sometimes known as counteridentification (Fliess, 1944, 1953), or as concordant identification (Racker, 1968), represents an encounter with another's world of lived experience, has also been termed empathy, and has been more fully described by Schafer (1959), Greenson (1960), and Kohut (1959/1978, 1971). Kohut (1959/1978, 1971) notes that empathy is a method of study that may be used in a variety of contexts, from interrogation to psychotherapy, and represents a method of study distinctive to the human sciences.

As the fundamental method of clinical psychoanalysis, essential to the study of adult lives, the capacity to "taste" or experience and interpret tthe variety of enactments within the clinical situation facilies personality change through bringing previously unacceptable sentiments and intents into awareness as potentially subject to change. Freud's (1911/1958, 1914/1958) original concept of "evently hovering attention" implicitly assumed an experience-near collaborative process similar to that more thoroughly explored by Schafer (1959), Kohut (1959/1978, 1971), and Schwaber (1983) rather than the more experience-distant and scientistic role so often assumed as the ideal for psychoanalysis. Described by Kohut as "vicarious introspection," this cryptic description was later extended by Schwaber (1983) as "experience-near, immediate vicissitudes of the patient's state or affect, shifting defensive patterns and perceptual experience-seen as intrinsic to (rather than distorted by) emerging wishes, feelings, or defenses" (p. 523). Optimally, the analyst is attuned to the wishes, thoughts, and feelings of the analysand as a consequence of a process of listening to the analysand's narrative, experiencing the pain and joy of the analysand's life world, and fostering the analysand's enhanced self-awareness through integration, organization, and focus of this narrative, leading to an "interpretation" that further extends the analysand's range of self-observation and capacity for self-inquiry.

Transference and Countertransference, and the Nuclear Neurosis

Empathy, or concordant identifications with the analysand's narrative, founded on vicarious introspection (Fliess, 1994, 1953; Racker, 1968; Kohut, 1959) should be differentiated from complementary identification reciprocal to the analysand's account or countertransference. Countertransference is most often manifest as anxiety evoked within the analyst reciprocal to the analysand's narrative, determined by the aspects of the analyst's own unresolved nuclear neurosis (Reich, 1951/1973). Based on Freud's (1914/1958) concept of the transference, the psychoanalyst Annie Reich (1951/1973, 1966/1973) used the term *countertransference* to refer to intents and sentiments relevant to the analyst's own resolution of the nuclear neurosis stimulated by the experience of the analysand. As initially employed, the term *countertransference* did not refer to all manifestations of the therapist's personality as expressed within the therapeutic relationship, but only to those aspects of the experience of the analysand stimulated reciprocally to the analysand's own unresolved nuclear neurosis.

Founded in Freud's (1900/1958, 1910/1957a, 1910/1957b, 1914–1918/1955) concept of a "nuclear neurosis" or fundamental wish, deriving from the incest taboo present within the bourgeois Western family (Freud, in 1910/1957b referred to this nuclear conflict as the "Oedipal complex" in deference to Jung's views). Freud (1900/1958) maintained that the intensity of this wish leads to continuing search for satisfaction that is opposed by social reality in the form of demand for repression of this wish. Feelings of tenderness toward the mother, together with ambivalent feelings of love and resentment toward the father of early childhood, and socially defined prohibition against explicit recognition of this wish, which festers out of awareness, continue to seek satisfaction in a disguised manner through personally and culturally symbolically relevant means. Particularly as enacted within the context of the intense relationship of analysand and analyst, but within all of lived experience, the nuclear conflict of early childhood is presumed to lead to continuing effort to satisfy this wish across the course of life.

However, not just in childhood, but across the course of life, as seen in the enactment anew in later adult relationships of this wish stemming from early childhood, it once again seeks satisfaction. Partial satisfaction of the nuclear wish may be attained in a disguised form through a compromise formation that provides partial satisfaction yet meets the demands of social reality. Included among these compromise formations are dreams, slips of the tongue and other unintended actions, psychoneurotic symptoms (hysteria and the obsessional neurosis), creative activity or sublimation, and efforts at enactment through experience of self and other, which has been termed the *transference neurosis*. It was a part of Freud's singular understanding of the human condition that he recognized in the experience of all relationships similar disguised effort at the satisfaction of the nuclear wish as compromise formation.

Within the analytic situation, the fact that the analyst is not a person involved in the analysand's daily life provides a point of attachment for partial satisfaction of the nuclear wish in disguised form. The process of psychoanalytic treatment is designed to provide an interpretation of this nuclear wish experienced anew in the here and now of the psychoanalytic situation and, through recognition of the nuclear wish, to diminish the power of this wish in everyday life where repetition may lead to conflict, frustration, and disappointment in experience of oneself and with others. Ambivalence regarding the analysand's successful life attainments, feelings of competitive struggle engendered following the analysand's report of a love affair, and rivalry with other persons in the analysand's life for the analysand's affections would all be examples of countertransference evoked by particular analytic experiences (Kohut & Seitz, 1963/1978).

Beyond the Nuclear Neurosis: The Concept of Enactment

Across the last half century, with more detailed and systematic psychoanalytically informed study of the child's personality development across the first years of life, intensive developmental and clinical study has suggested that effort to satisfy anew wishes related to the nuclear wish was not the only mode of enactment evident within lived experience through oldest age. Efforts in adulthood to establish anew the security and dependence of the early caregiver–child tie have been recognized as additional modes of enactment of unresolved psychological issues from early childhood similar to those of the nuclear conflict (Mahler, Pine, & Bergman, 1975; Panel, 1973a, 1973b, 1973c; Winnicott, 1953, 1960). Kohut (1958/1978, 1977, 1984) has reformulated this continuing impact of childhood across the adult years in terms of a lifelong expectable effort to recreate the comfort and caring first associated in a nonspecific manner with the years of infancy and early childhood. Portraying a psychology of the self rather than that of psychological conflict, Kohut argues both for the experience of shame and disavowal, as well as guilt and repression, as an important sector of personality, and also for the study and interpretation of these "transference-like" enactments of idealization, mirroring, and experience of merger or twinship that are important in maintaining a sense of personal integrity and coherence when confronted across the adult years with both such expectable life changes as retirement and such unexpected adversity as personal illness or the illness, or loss, of beloved family members.

Extension of the concept of transference from its original understanding as the transference of the energy associated with the nuclear wish across the repression barrier through suitable disguise as a compromise formation to include issues associated with the experience of caregiving and attainment of sense of coherence suggests the need for some more general concept. Most recently, the concept of enactment has been proposed as a more inclusive concept in a number of clinical and theoretical reports by Jacobs (1986, 1991), McLaughlin (1991), Chused (1991), and a panel report of a meeting of the American Psychoanalytic Association (Johan, 1992). Based on Jacobs's (1986, 1991) discussion emphasizing the effort to satisfy unconscious (Oedipal) wishes out of awareness, the 1989 panel emphasized both the dramatic quality of enactments and the extent to which these dramatizations out of awareness determine the response of the other to the situation.

As portrayed by McLaughlin (1991) and Chused (1991), the experience of others out of awareness is characteristically expressed in action that has the additional significance of the impact of this action upon others. Underlying the formulation of this concept is recognition that we emplot all relationships with meanings based on the totality of experienced life circumstances and enact these meanings in fantasy, word, and deed. These meanings include the variety of ways in which persons experience others, not only in the realm of competition but also as a source of sustenance, comfort, and solace. Enactments are an essential aspect of all relationships across the course of life, in which the past is ever recreated within the present into oldest age (Nemiroff & Colarusso, 1990b). The extent to which these enactments facilitate or hinder therapeutic activity is largely a function of the analyst's capacity for continuing self-inquiry, which fosters increased awareness regarding these enactments.

Just as with the analysand's enactment in word and deed of experiences taking place across a lifetime, the analyst's response to the analysand's material reflects the analyst's own lived experience. Those aspects of the analyst's own experience not previously the subject of self-inquiry and understanding, presently out of awareness, may be reciprocally evoked by the collaboration between analyst and analysand. The analysand's bid for a mirroring or idealizing relationship may lead to the analyst's own feelings of lowered self-esteem and of being unworthy of such emulation. Kohut (1977) has cautioned against premature interpretation of these idealizing enactments, which could be experienced by the analysand as a break in empathy and lack of analytic understanding.

The analyst's own analysis provides a method for attaining enhanced awareness and understanding of enactments; personal therapeutic analysis is necessarily incomplete and enactments are inevitable, particularly as a consequence of work with the more troubled analysand. These more troubled older adult persons are particularly capable of evoking intense counterenactments and are frequently transferred to other therapists or modalities because of the anxiety that they evoke (Burke & Cohler, 1992). The patient preoccupied with issues of senescence and dying may evoke complementary concerns within the analyst also concerned with these issues (Nemiroff & Colarusso, 1985, 1990b; Racker, 1968): older analysands and their middle-aged and older analysts may be share concerns regarding the finitude of life and may both be dealing with issues of grief and loss. Nemiroff and Colarusso (1990b, p. 119) also report that issues of sexuality in the older patient may evoke complementary concerns on the part of the analyst who may be particularly troubled by the older analysand's expression of sexual wishes toward the analyst. An analogous process to the complementary response on the part of the analyst to the analysand's report of life experiences—so well portrayed by Devereux (1967)—may be observed more generally in the life-history interview, such as when the interviewer discussing incarceration in the camps and its aftermath with older survivors of *Shoah* experiences anxiety in response to the story that is narrated and seeks to avoid the discomfort induced by the participant's account of this experience.

Evocation of a variety of meanings of others for oneself is intrinsic within all relationships. Indeed, there is no "other" apart from one's own present experience of that other in terms of one's own lived experience. Use of one's own vicarious introspection (Kohut, 1959/1978) or empathy (Pigman, 1995; Schafer, 1959) provides a means for transforming meanings evoked by this "essential other" (Galatzer-Levy & Cohler, 1993) into enhanced understanding of oneself and maintenance of the capacity for bearing the lived experience of another. It is the anxiety that is evoked by the sense of experience of another that transforms evoked significance of another into those enactments that are detrimental to enhanced understanding in the consulting rooms, fieldwork, or in the confrontation with consulting room or field transformed into text. Clearly, continuing self-inquiry over time is essential in maintaining awareness of counterenactments and taking advantage of the experience of another as a means of fostering enhanced understanding.

Telling and Listening to the Life Story: Enactment and Empathy

Analysand and analyst jointly contribute to the presumably new life story that is constructed across the course of the analysis and permits the analysand an enhanced sense of personal congruity and vitality as contrasted with the analysand's life at the beginning of the analysis (Schafer, 1980, 1981) Analyst and analysand, as any teller and listener, live within the constraints of the larger social order. Consistent with Bakhtin's (1981, 1986) emphasis upon the dialogical perspective, shared understanding facilities emergence of a conversation between two participants. As Schafer (1980, 1981) has emphasized, the analysand's life history is a story co-constructed by analysand and analyst. The analyst's primary contribution is the capacity to bear anxiety as a consequence of his or her own personal analysis and continuing self-inquiry (Gardner, 1983), which fosters maintenance of empathy and a milieu in which the analysand is able to experience anew previously warded-off or disavowed aspects of experience and to construct a narrative of experience including these embarrassing or humiliating aspects of the life story (Basch, 1983; Freud, 1937/1964; Jaffe, 1986).

Furthermore, larger social and historical elements enter into this co-constructed life story, reflecting a dialogic process encompassing analyst, analysand, and the larger society: The nature of the life story presently constructed within analysis differs in a significant manner not only from that which would have been told at the beginning of the analysis but, across the course of the analysis, differs from a life story that might have been co-constructed by analyst and analysand at the inception of psychoanalysis in America early in the twentieth century, or that at the conclusion of World War II. This perspective is well demonstrated in Kohut's (1979) portrayal of the two analyses of "Mr. Z" over a period of two decades, which reflects changes taking place within psychoanalytic theory itself.

Finally, the psychoanalytic life story, as any life story, is a performance in which telling is a mode of acting (Kaminsky, 1992). Just as in the telling of life stories, more generally, gesture and speech, recognition of audience, and other aspects of performance are an intrinsic element of the life story that is both told and acted, with a teller and listener each bringing a history of meanings of experience emerging across a lifetime, and with varying capacity for self-inquiry, which is associated with variation in the capacity to listen to the study without experiencing such dysphoric sentiments that listening becomes particularly painful. The analyst's own personal analysis fosters listening at the outset that is both less burdened by personal pain and with enhanced capacity for self-inquiry and awareness of his or her own wishes and feelings greater than that of the analysand. As a result of collaborative inquiry, by the completion of the analysis, the analysand has acquired many of these same attributes and becomes both a different and more reflexive listener and teller.

PSYCHOANALYSIS, LIFE STORY, AND STUDY OF LATER LIFE

Freud was clearly troubled by issues of age and aging, and this concern led to pessimism regarding the success of psychoanalysis of older adults, whom he viewed (1905/1953b) as too complex in terms of the length of their life story, and as too rigid to profit from analysis. In the light of Freud's initial pessimism, it should be noted that a volume of case reports (Nemiroff & Colarusso, 1985, 1990a), together with Sandler's (1978) detailed report show that Freud's initial pessimism was not well founded. In Chapter II of *The Interpretation of Dreams* (1900/1958), demonstrating that his own dreams revealed the presence of a wish, Freud discusses his wish to be absolved for the responsibility of providing less than adequate medical care, and recounts the story of his work with an old lady, actually treated by another physician, but which Freud found personally disturbing. He notes that this troubling feeling reflects his distaste of aging, including his own aging. It is clear that this older woman, and his fear of working with older patients, reflects his own early life experience. The older women patient is a "stand-in" for two other women whom Freud views as "old," his nursemaids Monika Zajic and Resi Wittek, one or both of whom may have been involved in seduction of Freud during the time when he was between ages 2 and 4.

Recalling his early life in a letter to Fliess, Freud (Masson, 1985) portrays Monika as "ugly, elderly but clever," a Czech and a Catholic. Less is known about Resi Wittick, but it was Resi and not Monika who was a devout and practicing Catholic, and used to take the young Sigismund to Church, where he was terrified by the Mass. She must indeed have seemed elderly because his own mother, Amalie, was so young (age 20) when Freud was born (Krull, 1986). Freud had additional reasons to resent Resi Wittick, who was expected to provide the care for him that his own mother, grieving both her own mother's death and that of Freud's infant brother Julius, may have been unable to provide (Gay, 1988).

In the aftermath of these two closely spaced losses in this mother's life, Freud's mother may have withdrawn into her own grief, leaving the nursemaid as the particularly significant person in Freud's life. Anna Freud has reported that Monika was not in fact old, but only in her forties. However, for the young boy whose own mother was particularly young, a 40-year-old mother must have seemed "old" in the sense used by Freud in his letter. Resi, who is more likely than Monika the source of the reference to the ugly but clever woman referred to by Freud in his litter to Fliess, was somewhat older. Together, these two women are fused into a single image of the seducer for at least one, but perhaps both, as Freud reports in a letter to Fliess, were his "primary originator and instructuress in sexual matters (Freud, October 3; Masson, 1985).

Freud believed that he had experienced some seduction and accompanying erotic stimulation at the hands of his nursemaids, which may have provided the basis for his distaste of aging. As Kahana (1978) has noted, it is ironic that Freud so feared aging and loss of creativity, considering his long life and the remarkable creativity he showed in his own later life. However, not only was he hypochondriacal in his preoccupation with a presumed early death, but he disliked treating older patients. Krull (1986) reports that Freud's mother also disliked aging, and that she struggled until late in her life to look as youthful as possible. It may be suggested that at least a part of Freud's own distaste was related to the opposite feeling, engendered by the three women of his early childhood—his mother and the two nursemaids.

Freud clearly had strong sentiments regarding the older female patient whose treatment is recounted in Chapter II of *The Interpretation of Dreams*. This distaste was a major reason why Freud believed that psychoanalysis could be of little assistance for the older adult whose personality had crystallized to a point where change would prove difficult. It must be recalled, as Kahana (1978) has noted, that aging is much more characteristic of the population at the present time than in the late nineteenth century. Furthermore, at least at the outset, Freud understood the process of analysis as the recovery of memories rather than, as later (Freud, 1937/1964), the construction of a new life story. Indeed, for a long time, peer review manuals in psychoanalysis discouraged psychoanalytic intervention among middle-aged and older adults. This prejudice, founded on

Freud's initial pessimism, may be supported by the analyst's own fear of growing older, and of facing possible loss of energy, illness, or even confronting his or her own mortality. It is striking that not only have there been few reports regarding psychoanalysis among older adults, but also that these reports make little reference to the analyst's reciprocal experience in work with older adults.

It is only over the past two decades that psychoanalytic intervention has been extended to the second half of life, and much of that work has been founded on the reanalysis of persons who had been analyzed earlier in life, and who were presumably "prepped" by their earlier analysis to resume the free-associative work. Erikson's (1951/1963) effort to extend developmental perspectives in psychoanalysis across the course of life was an important impetus for reconsidering the significance both of the second half of life for the course of life as a whole, and for recognition of the important developmental changes taking place across middle and later life. At the same time, consistent with the observations of Lomranz (Chapter 10, this volume) Erikson's view of later adult life was somewhat biased by his immersion in bourgeois Western culture of a particular time and his own commitment to creativity as an essential goal of lived experience. Findings from developmental study such as that of Neugarten (1979) and her colleagues questioned assumptions that adults were less cognitively flexible than adults at younger ages. Finally, the reality of the aging of the population within Western industrial democracies highlighted the importance of better understanding psychological changes taking place even among the oldest old, over age 85, the most rapidly growing segment of the population.

Colarusso and Nemiroff (1979, 1981) have outlined issues important for psychoanalytic study among middle-aged and older adults. Of particular concern both in their own discussion, and in much study since, is the extent to which enactments of the life story observed within the psychoanalytic process are simply elaborations of the nuclear conflict of early childhood echoing across the course of life. Transference enactments stem from the manner and extent to which the nuclear conflict of early childhood was resolved. For example, Miller (1987) has reported on the analysis of a woman in her seventies. Transference enactments included continuing curiosity regarding the analyst's personal life, jealousy of the analyst's other commitments, and similar jealousy over the relationship with her women friends and their husbands and lovers. The analysis included reawakened longs for attention and sexual favors from her father and her male analyst, who she felt was withholding information from her. The last phase of her analysis focused on the need for continued vitality in order to be attractive to men, including her husband of 40 years. Concerns with wanting to be pregnant and living forever were prominent, together with dreams that she and her husband–analyst had a baby.

Without doubt, residual, transformed elements of this lifelong effort to resolve psychological conflict stemming from efforts to resolve the nuclear neurosis may be observed in the meanings that even older adults make of their relationship with their analyst. A 70-year-old man who feels competitive with his analyst for the attentions of the younger woman patient seen in the preceding hour, undue deference out of the concern that the analyst might be jealous of his attainments, or fear of the analyst's realization for expression of independent views are among the enactments from this early childhood experience common in the analytic situation. However, consistent with the "new look" on the course of development elaborated by Datan et al. (1987) within developmental study of adult lives, and by Nemiroff and Colarusso (1985, 1990b) with psychoanalysis, lives are transformed over time.

While residual elements of the nuclear conflict of early childhood may continue as salient within the story of even older adults, effort to reduce adult experience simply to early childhood experience fails to do justice to the complex nature of development across the adult years and into later life, fails to appreciate that the present story of lived experience includes not only the dialogic nature of the very telling of this story but also the extent to which meanings of lived experience are continually shaped by the interplay of personal life circumstances and the changing meanings attributed to lived experience as a consequence of social and historical change. At the same time, the analyst may be experienced in terms of such later adult issues as a grandchild (Rappaport, 1958), or the wise spiritual counselor, or Rabbi. The realities of physical changes related to aging—loss of vitality, illness, dissatisfaction with sexuality and, perhaps, memory problems—all become important in the analysis of older adults.

Extending King's (1980) discussion of enactments unique to the life story of the older analysand, and following Colarusso and Nemiroff's (1979, 1981) and Nemiroff and Colarusso's (1990b) discussion of five dimensions expectably salient across later life, enactments observed within lived experience of older adults, including the analytic relationship itself, include (1) fear of loss of personal and sexual potency and the impact of this sensed loss of potency on relationships; (2) displacement by preferred younger persons and threat of loss of self-esteem; (3) anxieties resulting from departure of children from home, together with a shift of concern from providing care to having care provided; (4) fear of becoming dependent on others and loss of physical mobility and independence; and (5) fear that death will cut short realization of important goals. Within the analytic situation, these five enactments become particularly salient as the analysand expresses fear that the analyst will prefer to work with younger analysands more personally attractive and interesting, both the wish and the fear of becoming dependent upon the analyst, and fear of loss, including worries regarding the analyst's own possible death, which would interrupt the analytic work before completion.

These enactments of lived experience relevant in understanding the psychoanalytic process among older adults and their analysts are clearly tied to adult concerns; while intertwined with concerns stemming from childhood, including the nuclear neurosis, and remade across a lifetime, experience of self and others across the years of middle and later life clearly introduces unique issues for analytic study and intervention. For example, Sandler (1978) describes the analysis of a man in his late fifties for whom sexual concerns appeared more loosely tied to fear of loss and death than to the nuclear neurosis, seen so often among younger adults. Clearly, enactments stemming from disappointments and losses of early childhood, including struggle for recognition from a mother grieving the loss of her own mother during the analysand's early childhood, all enter into the life story brought into the analysis. As Nemiroff and Colarusso (1990b) observe, "The developmental processes in adulthood are influence by the adult past as well as the childhood past (p. 101)."

The life story that is jointly constructed by analyst and analysand of the course of lived experience takes advantage of the analyst's concordant identifications (Racker, 1968) or ability to extend vicarious introspection or empathy as a means for observing the presence of these enactments. Founded on this ability to remain receptive to the analysand's enactments across a lifetime, and to bring them to the analysand's awareness, it is possible to explore the meanings of these enactments and to create a life story that is more coherent and shows greater vitality than that at the outset of the analytic experience. Clearly, the analyst's own ability to employ concordant identifications involves his or her own continuing self-inquiry, attentive to possible anxiety experienced reciprocally to the analysand's enactments.

The analysand's concern with issues of loss of independence, concerns about mortality and foreshortened lifetime, or family conflicts all pose particular demands upon the capacity to maintain vicarious introspection among analysts choosing to work with older adults and to the construction of this revised life story. Complementary identifications interfere in realizing this goal of assisting in the analysands' revised story of lived experience. These complementary identifications are employed by the analyst as a means of protecting him- or herself against anxiety consequent to the analysand's own personal struggles; focus on the analyst's enactments presented by older analysands largely in terms of repetitions of the nuclear conflict of early childhood may reflect such complementary identification. While such enactments may well be present, they are not present alone, and are expressed in ways consonant with the reality of the older adult's lived experience.

CONCLUSION

Contemporary focus on the self as the "vital pleasure" or center of activity designed to affirm a sense of personal integrity with experienced continuity in time and over time is only possible as a consequence of changing perspectives on personal development across the course of life (Klein, 1976). Pioneering psychoanalytic study has suggested the primacy of childhood as the determinant of later life experiences. As Datan et al. (1987) have so well argued, it is essential to expand horizons to a concern with the course of life as a whole. Furthermore, as Nemiroff and Colarusso (1990b) have suggested, childhood experiences may have a less privileged place in determining the course of adult lives than lived experiences across the adult years. The past continues to influence the present but not in a linear or cumulative manner. Rather, it is the past that is presently reworked or reconstructed, based on the totality of lived experiences, to that particular point that is significant as the personal past in influencing the present (Novey, 1968/1985; Schafer, 1992).

Historical and clinical study, together with review of findings from systematic community study of lives over periods of many decades, has called into question any perspective that assumes linear or even cumulative models for understanding personal changes over time. Rather, this study has called for renewed attention to the very manner in which the concept of life history or life story is constructed in contemporary society. Understanding regarding the course of life emerges out of a dialogue between presently existing productive processes and life circumstances of persons with particular pasts. Focus on the manner in which persons make sense of that past has replaced epigenetic perspectives, such as that initially portrayed by Abraham (1924) and extended by Erikson (1951/1963) as more appropriate in terms of both present conceptions of the course of life and of the means by which therapeutic change is realized within clinical psychoanalysis.

Furthermore, it is the process of constructing the life story that lends authenticity and integrity that has been portrayed as self. Self emerges within the matrix of presently recollected past and present experiences; to the extent that it is possible to fashion a story of the past that is both coherent and fosters the experience of personal vitality, persons are able to experience a vital self; interference in the construction of narrative of personal experience, founded either on a lifetime history of disappointment with those responsible for care or problems in the capacity to respond to this care, poses continuing problems in the maintenance of personal integrity. Adverse life changes may also be experienced as sufficiently catastrophic as to destroy sense of personal integrity or coherence. Revolution, widescale social conflict, and such terrible adversity as *Shoah* are among the large-scale catastrophes capable of such destruction of personal integrity. It is particularly instructive to study those persons able to remain resilient and to preserve sense of continuity even while experiencing these catastrophes.

Interventions within the psychotherapeutic setting are designed to restore sense of personal integrity and to foster enhanced sense of vitality and activity. Just as understanding of the course of development must be reconsidered in the light of contemporary social theory and practice, similar reconsideration must be given to the dynamics of the intervention process itself. The psychotherapeutic relationship itself must be understood as a collaboration between two participants focused together on the task of making sense of the analysand's presently recounted life story. This life story is both told and acted, and is experienced by each participant in terms of the totality of the life story of each participant.

Psychoanalysis differs from other psychotherapeutic modalities, particularly in terms of the manner in which the relationship itself between the two participants is reflexively used as a means of information. The analysand does not just narrate a story, but does so in a particular way, at a particular time, experiencing the analyst as a participant within this story in terms of particularly characteristic and significant employments. The analyst comes to understand the manner in which use is being made of the therapeutic process itself in terms of the manner in which the analyst "tastes" or is empathic with the analysand's communications. Reciprocal enactments on the part of each participant in the process become stories that themselves are told and performed by each participant. Indeed, as Schafer (1980, 1981) has suggested, the only aspect of the life that may be reconstructed is the history of the analysis itself!

If the process of psychoanalysis represents construction rather than the reconstruction of the life history as a *coconstructed story* of the life, it is important to understand what is "curative" or leads to therapeutic change as a result of telling the life story in dynamic psychotherapy and psychoanalysis. Without doubt, the co-construction of a life story that is both more coherent and also more vital and alive, and which leads to enhanced sense of vigor and confidence, plays an important role in the process of personal change. Again, this story is retold as a collaboration between analysand and analyst on the basis of the analyst's continuing empathic and careful listening to the analysand's story, including the story that is enacted within the therapeutic relationship.

Kohut (1984) has suggested that the very effort to understand and to be empathic with the experience of another has itself a restorative impact. Feeling understood and appreciated fosters enhanced courage to consider other, perhaps more shameful or painful aspects of the presently remembered past, and to make peace with that past as remembered and as told. It is in this sense that psychotherapy or psychoanalysis may be a "corrective experience," developing new confidence on the basis of the experience of being with another who is affirming and empathic over relatively long periods of time, and who is able to bear without returning to those painful memories and sentiments that are so difficult to bear by oneself.

This is a time of significant change in the understanding of the process of personal change both over time and in time, and also in the manner in which this process of change is portrayed. As the life story is first experienced over time and then recounted within the time of the psychoanalytic interview, or within other occasions where the life story might be told, present perspectives suggest that lives are governed by shared understandings founded on lived experience and represented in a story that follows culturally constructed conventions of beginning, middle, and end. Lives are like stories and are told within a variety of contexts. The telling is itself a performance of a particular sort, with living, telling, and reading stories joined together by common concern with the connection between a presently remembered past, experienced present, and anticipated future. What is so often termed *development*, across the course of life, into adulthood and oldest age, has been founded on assumptions regarding stages, processes of transformations, and cumulation that are difficult to support from within the present focus on lived experience.

In his review of Dr. Borg's life, recounted in Bergman's film *Wild Strawberries*, Erikson (1979) recounts the effort of an older scientist, on his way to receive university honors, to retell his life story as he passes familiar places on his journey. The film's title stems from the effort to make sense of the scientist's devotion to the lonely splendor of research rather than intimacy such as could have been realized with a young lady with whom he spent a day in his youth in the field of strawberries. The Bergman film well portrays the continuing effort into latest life to refashion the story of a lifetime; Butler (1963), Coleman (1986),

Neugarten (1979), and Cohler and Freeman (1993) have all suggested that the advent of midlife may add a note of urgency to this task. Making sense of the presently experienced past, of the recognition that more time has been lived than is left to be lived (Neugarten & Datan, 1974), and of remaking a life story that will provide a coherent account of lived experience appears to be a particularly significant issue across the second half of life, and especially into later life (Tobin, 1991).

Consistent with the position elaborated by Peskin (Chapter 13, this volume), psychoanalysis provides both a means for fostering a revision of the life story that leads to increased vitality and sense of coherence as contrasted with the life-story prior to beginning analysis, and a means for studying the manner in which the life story is successively reconstructed across the course of life. While issues regarding reminiscence, life review, and the life story appear to have particular salience across the second half of life, past reluctance to work analytically with older adults has limited psychoanalytic study of the life story in later life.

Parker (1972) has recounted her conversations with an older colleague making sense of her own lived experience within a difficult family situation, which shows the value of a psychoanalytic focus on the life story across the second half of life. Missing in Parker's account, but an important element of reports such as those of Sandler (1978) and Miller (1987), is the dual focus on the telling of the life story and the psychological use that is made of the listener or analyst, together with the focus on the analyst's reciprocal response to this story. Life stories reflect the joint effort of teller and listener to make meanings of lived experience and reflect the shared effort of each collaborator in the construction of this account, whether psychotherapeutic intervention or research account.

Study and intervention with adult lives might focus more directly on the experience-near dynamics of meaning reflected in presently told stories told about the course of life within the experience-near context of teller and listener, including analyst and analysand, rather than the more experience-distant effort to recast lives within epigenetic or cumulative representations of the purported course of life. The important focus of study should be the dynamics of the process of telling and listening, often portrayed in psychoanalysis within the concepts of transference or enactment and empathy and counterenactment. It is precisely this focus on the dynamics of the situation that is the hallmark of psychoanalytic inquiry and may become the foundation of a psychoanalytic study of lives across the course of adulthood and into oldest age.

REFERENCES

Abraham, K. (1924). A short study of the development of the libido, viewed in the light of mental disorders. In *Selected papers of Karl Abraham, M.D.* (pp. 418–501). London: Hogarth Press.
Antonovsky, A. (1987). *Unraveling the mystery of health.* San Francisco: Jossey-Bass.
Anzieu, D. (1986). *Freud's self-analysis* (P. Graham, Trans.). London: Hogarth Press.

Bakhtin, M. M. (1981). *The dialogic imagination* (C. Emerson & M. Holquist, Trans.). Austin: University of Texas Press.

Bakhtin, M. M. (1986). *Speech genres and other late essays* (V. W. McGee, Trans). Austin: University of Texas Press.

Bandura, A. (1982). The psychology of chance encounters and life paths. *American Psychologist, 37,* 747–755.

Basch, M. (1983). The perception of reality and the disavowal of meaning. *Annual for Psychoanalysis,* 11, 125–153.

Berman, H. (1994). *Interpreting the aging self: Personal journal of later life.* New York: Springer.

Blos, P. (1980). The life cycle as indicated by the nature of the transference in the psychoanalysis of adolescents. *International Journal of Psychoanalysis, 61*(2), 145–151.

Bruner, J. (1987). Life as narrative. *Social Research, 54,* 11–32.

Bruner, J. (1990). *Acts of meaning.* Cambridge, MA: Harvard University Press.

Burke, N., & Cohler, B. (1992). Countertransference and psychotherapy with the anorectic adolescent. In J. Brandell (Ed.), *Countertransference in child and adolescent psychotherapy* (pp. 163–189). New York: Aronson.

Butler, R. (1963). The life review: An interpretation of reminiscence in the aged. *Psychiatry, 26,* 63–76.

Chused, J. (1991). The evocative power of enactments. *Journal of the American Psychoanalytic Association, 39,* 615–639.

Cohen, J., & Cohler, B. (Eds.). (1998). *The psychoanalytic study of lives over time: Clinical and research perspectives on children returning to analysis in adulthood.* New Haven: Yale University Press (manuscript in preparation).

Cohler, B. (1982). Personal narrative and life course. In B. Baltes & O. Brim (Eds.), *Life-span development and behavior* (pp. 205–241). New York: Academic Press.

Cohler, B., & Cole, T. (1996). Studying older lives: Reciprocal acts of telling and listening. In J. M. Birren, G. M. Kenyon, J.-E. Ruth, J. J. F. Schroots, & T. Svensson (Eds.), *Biography and aging: Explorations in adult development* (pp. 61–76). New York: Springer.

Cohler, B., & Freeman, M. (1993). Psychoanalysis and the developmental narrative. In G. Pollock & S. Greenspan (Eds.), *The course of life: Vol. 5: Early adulthood* (Rev. ed., pp. 99–177). New York: International Universities Press.

Colarusso, C., & Nemiroff, R. (1979). Some observations and hypotheses about the psychoanalytic theory of adult development. *International Journal of Psychoanalysis, 60,* 59–71.

Colarusso, C., & Nemiroff, R. (1981). *Adult development.* New York: Plenum Press.

Coleman, P. (1986). *Aging and reminiscence processes: Social and clinical implications.* New York: Wiley.

Datan, N., Rodeheaver, D., & Hughes, F. (1987). Adult development and aging. *Annual Review of Psychology, 38,* 153–180.

Devereux, G. (1967). *From anxiety to method in the behavioral sciences.* The Hague: Mouton.

Erikson, E. (1963). *Childhood and society* (Rev. ed.). New York: Norton.

Erikson, E. (1964). Psychological reality and historical actuality. In E. Erikson (Ed.), *Insight and responsibility* (pp. 159–256). New York: Norton. (Original published, 1962).

Erikson, E. (1979). Reflections on Dr. Borg's life-cycle. In D. Van Tassel (Ed.), *Aging, death, and the completion of being* (pp. 29–67). Philadelphia: University of Pennsylvania Press.

Erikson, E. (1985). *The life-cycle completed: A review.* New York: Norton. (Original published, 1982)

Erikson, E. H., Erikson, J., & Kivnick, H. (1986). *Vital involvement in old age: The experience of old age in our time.* New York: Norton.

Fliess, R. (1944). The metapsychology of the analyst. *Psychoanalytic Quarterly, 11,* 211–227.

Fliess, R. (1953). Countertransference and counteridentification. *Journal of the American Psychoanalytic Association, 1,* 268–284.

Freeman, M. (1993). *Rewriting the self: History, memory, and narrative.* New York: Routledge.

Freud, S. (1958). *The interpretation of dreams. The standard edition of the complete psychological works of Sigmund Freud* (Vols. 4–5). London: Hogarth Press. (Original published 1900)

Freud, S. (1953a). Fragment of an analysis of a case of hysteria. In J. Strachey (Ed. and Trans.), *The standard edition of the complete psychological works of Sigmund Freud* (Vol. 7, pp. 7–124). London: Hogarth Press. (Original published 1905)

Freud, S. (1953b). On psychotherapy. In J. Strachey (Ed. and Trans.), *The standard edition of the complete psychological works of Sigmund Freud* (Vol. 7, pp. 255–268). London: Hogarth Press. (Original published 1905)

Freud, S. (1957a) Five lectures on psychoanalysis (The Clark Lectures). In J. Strachey (Ed. and Trans.), *The standard edition of the complete psychological works of Sigmund Freud* (Vol. 11, pp. 9–58). London: Hogarth Press. (Original published 1910)

Freud, S. (1957b). A special type of choice of object made by men (contributions to the psychology of love, 1). In J. Strachey (Ed. and Trans.), *The standard edition of the complete psychological works of Sigmund Freud* (Vol. 11, pp. 165–175). London: Hogarth Press. (Original published 1910)

Freud, S. (1958). Formulations on the two principles of mental functioning. In J. Strachey (Ed. and Trans.), *The standard edition of the complete psychological works of Sigmund Freud* (Vol. 12, pp. 215–226). London: Hogarth Press. (Original published 1911)

Freud, S. (1958). Remembering, repeating and working through: Further recommendations on the technique of psychoanalysis. In J. Strachey (Ed. and Trans.), *The standard edition of the complete psychological works of Sigmund Freud* (Vol. 12, pp. 146–156). London: Hogarth Press. (Original published 1914)

Freud, S. (1955). From the history of an infantile neurosis. In J. Strachey (Ed. and Trans.), *The standard edition of the complete psychological works of Sigmund Freud* (Vol. 17, pp. 7–122). London: Hogarth Press. (Original published 1914–1918)

Freud, S. (1964). Construction in analysis. In J. Strachey (Ed. and Trans.), *The standard edition of the complete psychological works of Sigmund Freud* (Vol. 23, pp. 257–269). London: Hogarth Press. (Original published 1937)

Galatzer-Levy, R., & Cohler, B. (1990). The selfobjects of the second half of life—an introduction. In A. Goldberg (Ed.), *The realities of the transference: Progress in self-psychology, 6*, 93–112.

Galatzer-Levy, R., & Cohler, B. (1993). *The essential other.* New York: Basic Books.

Gardner, R. (1983). *Self-inquiry.* Boston: Little, Brown and Atlantic Monthly Press.

Gay, P. (1988). *Freud: A life for our times.* New York: Norton.

Gergen, J. (1977). Stability, change, and chance in understanding human development. In N. Datan & H. Reese (Eds.), *Life-span developmental psychology: Dialectical perspectives on experimental research* (pp. 32–65). New York: Academic Press.

Gergen, K. (1994). *Realities and relationships: Soundings in social construction.* Cambridge, MA: Harvard University Press.

Gill, M. (1976). Metapsychology is not psychology. In M. Gill & P. Holzman (Eds.), *Psychology versus metapsychology* (pp. 77–105). New York: International Universities Press.

Gill, M. (1994). *Psychoanalysis in transition: A personal view.* Hillsdale, NJ: Analytic Press.

Good, B. (1994). *Medicine, rationality and experience: An anthropological perspective.* New York: Cambridge University Press.

Greenacre, P. A. (1949). A contribution to the study of screen memories. *The Psychoanalytic Study of the Child, 3/4*, 73–83.

Greenson, R. (1960). Empathy and its vicissitudes. *International Journal of Psychoanalysis, 41*, 418–424.

Grunes, J. (1980). Reminiscences, regression, and empathy: A psychotherapeutic approach to the impaired elderly. In S. Greenspan & G. Pollock (Eds.), *The course of life: Volume III. Adulthood and the aging process* (pp. 545–548). Washington, DC: U.S. Government Printing Office.

Hiley, D., Bohman, & Shusterman, R. (Eds.). (1991). *The interpretive turn: Philosophy, science, culture.* Ithaca, NY: Cornell University Press.

Hirsch, E. D. (1976). *The aims of interpretation.* Chicago: University of Chicago Press.

Hunter, K. M. (1991). *Doctors' stories: The narrative structure of medical knowledge.* Princeton, NJ: Princeton University Press.

Iser, W. (1978). *The act of reading: A theory of aesthetic response.* Baltimore, MD: Johns Hopkins University Press.

Jacobs, T. (1986). On countertransference enactments. *Journal of the American Psychoanalytic Association, 34*, 289–307.

Jacobs, T. (1991). *The use of the self: Countertransference and communication in the analytic situation.* Madison, CT: International Universities Press.

Jaffe, D. (1986). Empathy, counteridentification, countertransference: A review. *Psychoanalytic Quarterly, 55,* 215–243.

Johan, M. (1992). (Panel Reporter). Enactments in psychoanalysis. *Journal of the American Psychoanalytic Association, 40,* 827–841.

Kahana, R. (1978). Psychoanalysis in later life: Discussion. *Journal of Geriatric Psychiatry, 11,* 37–49.

Kahana, R. (1987). The Oedipus complex and rejuvenation fantasies in the analysis of a seventy-year-old woman: Discussion. *Journal of Geriatric Psychiatry, 20,* 53–60.

Kakar, S. (1990). Stories from Indian psychoanalysis: Context and text. In J. Stigler, R. Shweder, & G. Herdt (Eds.), *Cultural psychology: Essays on comparative human development* (pp. 427–445). New York: Cambridge University Press.

Kakar, S. (1995). Clinical work and cultural imagination. *Psychoanalytic Quarterly, 64,* 265–281.

Kaminsky, M. (1992). Introduction. In B. Myerhoff (Ed.), *Remembered lives: The work of ritual, storytelling and growing older* (pp. 1–99). Ann Arbor: University of Michigan Press.

Katz, J., & Associates. (1968). *No time for youth: Growth and constraint in college students.* San Francisco: Jossey-Bass.

Kaufman, S. (1986). *The ageless self: Sources of meaning in late life.* Madison: University of Wisconsin Press.

King, P. (1980). The life cycle as indicated by the nature of the transference in the psychoanalysis of the middle-aged and elderly. *International Journal of Psychoanalysis, 61,* 153–160.

Klein, G. (1976). *Psychoanalytic theory: An exploration of essentials.* New York: International Universities Press.

Kohut, H. (1978). Introspection, empathy and psychoanalysis: An examination of the relationship between mode of observation and theory. In P. Ornstein (Ed.), *The Search for the self: Selected writings of Heinz Kohut, 1950–1978* (Vol. I, pp. 205–232). New York: International Universities Press. (Original published 1959)

Kohut, H. (1971). *The analysis of the self: A systematic approach to the psychoanalytic treatment of narcissistic personality disorders.* New York: International Universities Press (Monograph 1 of the Psychoanalytic Study of the Child Series)

Kohut, H. (1977). *The restoration of the self.* New York: International Universities Press.

Kohut, H. (1985). Self psychology and the sciences of man. In C. Strozier (Ed.), *Self psychology and the humanities: Reflections on a new psychoanalytic approach by Heinz Kohut* (pp. 73–94). New York: Norton. (Original published 1978)

Kohut, H. (1979). The two analyses of Mr. Z, *International Journal of Psychoanalysis, 60,* 3–27.

Kohut, H. (1984). *How does psychoanalysis cure?* Chicago: University of Chicago Press.

Kohut, H., & Seitz, P. (1978). Concepts and theories of psychoanalysis. In P. Ornstein (Ed.), *The search for the self: Selected writings of Heinz Kohut, 1950–1978* (Vol. 1, pp. 337–374). New York: International Universities Press. (Original published 1963)

Kotre, J. (1984). *Outliving the self: Generativity and the interpretation of lives.* Baltimore, MD: Johns Hopkins University Press.

Kracke, W. (1987). Encounter with other cultures: Psychological and epistomological aspects. *Ethos, 15,* 58–82.

Kris, E. (1956a). The personal myth: A problem in psychoanalytic technique. *Journal of the American Psychoanalytic Association, 4,* 653–681.

Kris, E. (1956b). The recovery of child memories in psychoanalysis. *The Psychoanalytic Study of the Child, 11,* 54–88.

Krull, M. (1986). *Freud and his father* (2nd ed., A. J. Pomerans, Trans). New York: Norton.

Lasch, C. (1978). *The culture of narcissism: American life in an age of diminishing expectations.* New York: Norton.

Lieberman, M., & Falk, J. (1971). The remembered past as a source of data for research on the life cycle. *Human Development, 14,* 132–141.

Lindsay, D. S., & Read, J. D. (1994). Psychotherapy and memories of childhood sexual abuse: A cognitive perspective. *Applied Cognitive Psychology, 8,* 281–338.

Livson, N., & Peskin, H. (1980). Perspectives on adolescence from longitudinal research. In J. Adelson (Ed.), *Handbook of adolescent psychology* (pp. 47–98). New York: Wiley.

Luria, A. R. (1976). *Cognitive development: Its cultural and social foundation* (M. Lopez-Morillas & L. Solotaroff, Trans). Cambridge, MA: Harvard University Press.

Mannheim, K. (1952). The problem of generations. In K. Mannheim (Ed.), *Essays of the sociology of knowledge* (pp. 276–332). London: Routledge & Kegan Paul. (Original published 1923)

McLaughlin, J. (1991). Clinical and theoretical aspects of enactment. *Journal of the American Psychoanalytic Association, 39,* 595–614.

Mahler, M., Pine, F., & Bergman, A. (1975). *The psychological birth of the human infant.* New York: Basic Books.

Marx, K. (1845). The German ideology (pt. 1). In R. Tucker (Ed. & Trans), *The Marx–Engels reader* (2nd ed., pp. 146–200). New York: Norton.

Masson, J. (Ed.). (1985). *The complete letters of Sigmund Freud to Wilhelm Fliess, 1887–1904.* Cambridge, MA: Harvard University Press.

Miller, E. (1987). The Oedipus complex and rejuvenation fantasies in the analysis of a seventy-year-old woman. *Journal of Geriatric Psychiatry, 20,* 29–60.

Mink, L. O. (1965). The anatomy of historical understanding. *History and Theory, 5,* 24–47.

Moraitis, G. (1985). A psychoanalyst's journey into a historian's world: An experiment in collaboration. In S. Baron & C. Pletsch (Eds.), *Introspection in biography: The biographer's quest for self awareness* (pp. 69–106). Hillsdale, NJ: Analytic Press.

Nemiroff, R., & Colarusso, C. (1985). *The race against time: Psychotherapy and psychoanalysis in the second half of life.* New York: Plenum Press.

Hemiroff, R., & Colarusso, C. (Eds.). (1990a). *New dimensions in adult development.* New York: Basic Books.

Nemiroff, R., & Colarusso, C. (1990b). Frontiers of adult development in theory and practice. In R. Nemiroff & C. Colarusso (Eds.), *New dimensions in adult development* (pp. 97–124). New York: Basic Books.

Neubauer, P. B. (1980). The life cycle as indicated by the nature of the transference in the psychoanalysis of children. *International Journal of Psychoanalysis, 61,* 137–144.

Neugarten, B. (1969). Continuities and discontinuities of psychological issues into adult life. *Human Development, 12,* 121–130.

Neugarten, B. (1979). Time, age, and the life-cycle. *American Journal of Psychiatry, 136,* 887–894.

Neugarten, B. (1984). Interpretive social science and research on aging. In A. Rossi (Ed.), *Gender and the life course* (pp. 291–300). New York: Aldine.

Neugarten, B. L., & Datan, N. (1974). The middle years. In S. Arieti (Ed.), *American handbook of psychiatry: Vol. 1. The foundations of psychiatry* (pp. 592–608). New York: Basic Books.

Novey, S. (1985). *The second look: The reconstruction of personal history in psychiatry and psychoanalysis.* New York: International Universities Press. (Original published 1968)

Panel (M. C. Winesteine, Reporter). (1973a). The experience of separation–individuation in infancy and its reverberations through the course of life: I. Infancy and childhood. *Journal of the American Psychoanalytic Association, 21,* 135–154.

Panel (M. Marcus, Reporter). (1973b). The experience of separation–individuation in infancy and its reverberations through the course of life: II. Adolescence and maturity. *Journal of the American Psychoanalytic Association, 21,* 155–167.

Panel (I. Sternschein, Reporter). (1973c). The experience of separation–individuation in infancy and its reverberations through the course of life: III. Maturity, senescence, and sociological implications. *Journal of the American Psychoanalytic Association, 21,* 633–645.

Parker, B. (1972). *A mingled yarn chronicle of a troubled family.* New Haven, CT: Yale University Press.

Parsons, T. (1952). The superego and the theory of social systems. *Psychiatry, 15,* 15–26.

Peskin, H., & Livson, N. (1981). Uses of the past in adult psychological health. In D. Eichorn, J. Clausen, N. Haan, M. Honzik, & P. Mussen (Eds.), *Present and past in middle life* (pp. 154–183). New York: Academic Press.

Pigman, G. (1995). Freud and the history of empathy. *International Journal of Psychoanalysis, 76,* 237–256.

Pollock, G. (1981).. Reminiscence and insight. *Psychoanalytic Study of the Child, 17,* 278–287.

Racker, H. (1968). *Transference and countertransference.* Madison, CT: International Universities Press.

Rabinow, P., & Sullivan, W. (1987). The interpretive turn: A second look. In P. Rabinow & W. Sullivan (Eds.), *Interpretive social science: A second look* (pp. 1–30). Berkeley: University of California Press.

Rappaport, E. (1958). The grandparent syndrome. *Psychoanalytic Quarterly, 27,* 518.
Reich, A. (1973). On countertransference. In A. Reich (Ed.), *Annie Reich: Psychoanalytic contributions* (pp. 136–154). New York: International University Press. (Original published 1951)
Reich, A. (1973). Empathy and countertransference. In A. Reich (Ed.), *Annie Reich: Psychoanalytic contributions* (pp. 344–360). New York: International Universities Press. (Original published 1966)
Riegel, K. (1979). *Foundations of dialectical psychology.* New York: Academic Press.
Rosaldo, R. (1993). *Culture and truth: The remaking of social analysis* (2nd ed.). Boston: Beacon Press.
Sandler, A. M. (1978). Psychoanalysis in later life: Problems in the psychoanalysis of an aging narcissistic patient. *Journal of Geriatric Psychiatry, 11,* 5–36.
Schafer, R. (1958). How was this story told? *Journal of Projective Techniques, 22,* 181–210.
Schafer, R. (1959). Generative empathy in the treatment situation. *Psychoanalytic Quarterly, 28,* 342–373.
Schafer, R. (1980). Narration in the psychoanalytic dialogue. *Critical Inquiry, 7,* 29–53.
Schafer, R. (1981). *Narrative actions in psychoanalysis.* Worcester, MA: Clark University Press.
Schafer, R. (1992). *Retelling a life: Narration and dialogue in psychoanalysis.* New York: Basic Books.
Schimek, J. (1975). The interpretations of the past: Childhood trauma, psychical reality, and historical truth. *Journal of the American Psychoanalytic Association, 23,* 845–865.
Schwaber, E. (1983). A particular perspective on analytic listening. *Psychoanalytic Study of the Child, 38,* 519–546.
Singer, J., & Salovey, P. (1993). *The remembered self: Emotion in memory and personality.* New York: Free Press.
Slavney, P., & McHugh, P. (1984). Life stories and meaningful connections. *Perspectives in Medicine and Biology, 27,* 279–288.
Stern, D. (1995). *The motherhood constellation: A unified view of parent–infant psychotherapy.* New York: Basic Books.
Stone, L. (1961). *The psychoanalytic situation: An examination of its development and essential nature.* New York: International Universities Press.
Strozier, C. (Ed.). (1985). *Self psychology and the humanities: Reflections on a new psychoanalytic approach by Heinz Kohut.* New York: Norton.
Sulloway, F. (1979). *Freud, biologist of the mind: Beyond the psychoanalytic legend.* New York: Basic Books.
Tobin, S. (1991). *Personhood in advanced old age.* New York: Springer.
Vygotsky, L. (1987). *The Collected works of L. S. Vygotsky* (2 vols., R. W. Rieber & A. S. Carton, Eds.; N. Minick, Trans.). New York: Plenum Press. (Original published 1924–1934)
Wilson, A., & Weinstein, L. (1992). An investigation into some implications of a Vygotskian perspective on the origins of the mind: Psychoanalysis and Vygotskian psychology, Part I. *Journal of the American Psychoanalytic Association, 40,* 349–379.
Wilson, A., & Weinstein, L. (1996). Transference and the zone of proximal development. *Journal of the American Psychoanalytic Association, 44,* 167–200.
Winnicott, D. W. (1953). Transitional objects and transitional phenomena. In D. W. Winnicott (Ed.), *Collected papers: Through pediatrics to psychoanalysis* (pp. 229–242). New York: Basic Books.
Winnicott, D. (1960). The theory of the parent–infant relationship. *International Journal of Psychoanalysis, 41,* 585–595.
Wolff, P. (1988). The real and the reconstructed past. *Psychoanalysis and Contemporary Thought, 11,* 379–414.

CHAPTER 12

The Psychoimmune System in Later Life

The Problem of the Late-Onset Disorders

DAVID GUTMANN

INTRODUCTION

Since 1978 the faculty, staff, and students of the Older Adult Program at Northwestern Medical School have been studying the etiology, symptoms, and typical course of late-onset psychiatric disorders in middle-aged, young-old, and old-old men and women. For the author, these investigations have led to a still evolving but clinically useful conception: namely, that the various functions of the psyche constitute a de facto immune system, dedicated to preserving the consistency and continuity of the Self. When the immune system is in place, the individual experiences what Erikson (1952) has called a "self-sameness," and self-recognition in the face of flux and change; when the system fails, the result is self-fragmentation, as well as psychoses based on hectic attempts—"fevers of the soul"—to restore the lost continuity. In later life, immune systems—whether psychic or physical—tend to degrade. The late-onset disorders do not, as commonly assumed, result from the piling-up of nonspecific stressors and insults in later life; they result from specific, meaning-laden, and potentially *reversible* attacks on the psychic immune system itself.

DAVID GUTMANN • Department of Psychiatry and Behavioral Sciences, Northwestern University Medical School, Chicago, Illinois 60611.

Handbook of Aging and Mental Health: An Integrative Approach, edited by Jacob Lomranz. Plenum Press, New York, 1998.

QUANTITATIVE MODELS
OF LATE-ONSET DISORDER

The functional psychiatric disorders that have their first onset in later life pose challenging clinical and theoretical questions. For example, why do the afflicted elders, up to now reasonably stable, come unglued in this particular season of life? After all, our late-onset patients are for the most part survivors of much prior trouble: Following a difficult childhood, often involving the loss of one or both parents, they have persevered, they have lived long lives, sometimes marked by pain but also by reasonable degrees of love and work. These survivors have not succumbed to the thronging insults—economic depression, cultural revolutions, wars—of their earlier years. Why do they now decompensate, translating the "on-time," predictable troubles of the later years—illness, retirement, losses of kin and friends, and so on—into pathogens of clinical scale?

To such questions, the rather dismissive reply from conventional geropsychiatry comes phrased in the language of quantitative calculation: This argument holds that the increased rate of loss and insult in later life translates to greater psychological stress, and the added quanta of stress predict increased probability of mental breakdown. This is the "camel's back" calculus of psychopathology: The laden beast will endure until a critical mass of burden is reached; from then on, any additional straw will cause a decisive rupture of the bearing surface. This model does not specify the pathogenic properties of the destructive agents: Once the full load of bales is in place, any additional "straw," regardless of its special qualities, can bring about the sudden cracking of the dromedary's back. In this accountancy model of pathogenesis, quantity is all.

A QUALITATIVE APPROACH
TO PSYCHOLOGICAL STRESS

But the camel's back model does not conform with our clinical findings: When tracing out the causes of their disorders, middle-aged or older patients do tend to focus on the nature rather than the quantity of precipitating insults. Indeed, for specially predisposed individuals, a crippling arthritis or a slow-to-mend hip fracture can have a more catastrophic emotional impact than a potentially lethal cancer, or the deaths of kinsmen and friends. Thus, threats to motility can be more crippling, in the psychological as well as the physical sense, than a barrage of potential killer diseases—those, for example, that attack the heart rather than the joints. More to the point, we find that the great majority of elders—those who do not end up on our treatment services—tote their often considerable bales with resignation, even good humor, and without succumbing to late-onset disorders.

In short, it appears that "burden" is subjectively rather than objectively weighted: One man's meat is another man's poison. This being the case, no standard, "objective" catalogue of later life losses and insults—whether "on-time" or "off-time"—can steer our diagnostic studies toward correct, specific diagnoses or treatment plans. Meeting an older patient for the first time, we still have to ask the crucial "Why now?" question: "Why does this particular insult provoke in this person and at this time a pathogenic response?" Reaching for answers, we use the naturalistic, clinical interview to deconstruct the halo of idiosyncratic, often catastrophic, meanings surrounding an identified stressor—such as a painful arthritis—that might otherwise rank relatively low on any objective scale of "burden." Starting from the identified shock or insult, we typically open up the whole catalogue of traumatic memories and meanings that converge on this particular "straw" and are mobilized by it. From this starting point, we explore the patient's vital history: the private tally of trauma and mastery, of victories and defeats—how were victories gained or undone; how were defeats avoided, reversed, or invited?

In short, our clinical investigation of the immediate precipitant leads us into the crucial but usually overlooked historic self; we open up the charged personal narrative that is reactivated in the present by the current stress. Our clinical method often reveals the undercover agent that mediates between precipitants and symptoms, that forgotten historic person who can overburden seemingly minor stresses with idiosyncratic though catastrophic meanings. Pursuing this line, we usually find that the last straw breaks the camel's back not because of its added mass, but because, as construed by the historic person, the extra straw seems to weigh more than a whole bale.

THE PSYCHOIMMUNE SYSTEM

Repeating these exploratory and open-ended procedures patient by patient over the years, certain regularities begin to appear, and these point to larger principles driving adaptation and pathology in middle and later life. As a result, we have come to see the psyche as a kind of beleaguered organism, acting to preserve, despite the flux of internal and external change, regularities and consistencies that are vital to the self. More to the point, we find that it is clinically useful to look at the psyche as a kind of immune system, one that—like the body's immune system—is prone to degenerate in later life.

In the neonatal period, when the infant can no longer rely on the mother's antibodies, its own physical immune system is already in place to ensure the young organism's physical survival. But even in the extrauterine environment, the neonate's psychic immunity continues to be provided by the parents: In the face of a constantly changing extradomestic world, they keep the nursery as a neutral zone, characterized by relative calm and an absence of abrupt stimulation. Years will pass before the child develops the psychic capacities, built around the delaying functions of the ego, that reproduce, within its own self-boundaries, the sense of trustworthy continuity and predictability that the parents had once maintained for it in the home.

But while the physical and psychic immune systems emerge at different times, these two crucial structures appear to be in series with each other: Losses of physical health put heavy burdens on the psyche, and emotional disorders lay stresses on the body that the somatic immune system is not well equipped to handle.* Though they mobilize different agents and mechanisms, these two immune systems work toward equivalent ends: the preservation of a continuous, benign, and self-consistent internal environment in the face of unceasing and unpredictable change (see Staines, Brostoff, & James, 1993). Like many seeming banalities, "A sound mind in a sound body" might well turn out to be scientific truth.

Thus, the physical immune system acts through a variety of agents and functions to hold the internal bodily environment in a relatively pristine state: free of exogenous toxic agents—viruses, bacterial toxins, and so on—that could bring about infections or degenerative change in vital organs or systems. By the same token, in their immunizing role, the psychic functions also preserve the stability of a defined, boundaried environment, again in the face of continuously changing social and physical worlds. The integrity of the body is the responsibility of the somatic immune system; the integrity of the self is in the care of the psychoimmune system. The physical immune system monitors the boundaries of the body for potential invaders; in its turn, the psychoimmune system stands guard on the boundary between self and other, or between the familiar, daily self and its unconscious hinterland. This system acts through its various functions to moderate extreme mood swings; to separate fantasy, recognized as such, from the picture of external reality; to keep intruding thoughts out of consciousness, intruding stimuli out of perception, and intruding impulses out of behavior.

Thus, when the psychoimmune system and its boundaries are safely in place, when the "inside" will not be polluted by toxic influences from the "outside" (including the alien unconscious), then affection, attention, and action can safely shift to the exciting world beyond the self, and to the openings out there for productive, masterful action. As a consequence, the development and coordination of all the organs, senses, and effectors that serve external mastery and self-esteem can freely go forward. The appetites for exploration and change lead to new challenges, and these in turn can lead to the development of new stabilities in the form of matured executive capacities. These new forms of mastery, which lead to an expanded sense of self, are underwritten by—and augment—a relatively "immunized," trustworthy inner life.

In short, the experiences that give rise to inner stability also give rise to a realistic trust in the self, its persistence, its predictability, and its seasoned, tested resources. *Self-esteem* is another term for such trust: It is the assurance that the self is equal to whatever vicissitudes it will meet, or conjure up. According to the psychoanalyst Peter Giovacchini, (Personal communication) self-esteem is equivalent to the T-cell lymphocytes of the physical immune

---

*The somatic immune system's vulnerability to the burdened psyche is particularly evident at infancy and senescence, at the two ends of the life cycle. Thus, hospitalized babies routinely become depressed and can be carried off by diseases that most contented babies will shrug off. In later life, depression again degrades immune system microphagic cells (see Schindler, 1985; Schleifer, Keller, Siris, Davis, & Stein, 1985). By the same token, in later life, the counterdepressive stance appears to protect the immune system; thus, nursing home residents of a paranoid, extropunitive temperament are found to routinely outlive their intropunitive, depressive peers (see Hammond, 1991).

system. Thus, physically healthy individuals can go among strange peoples without suffering their diseases, while individuals holding equivalent psychoimmune protections can seek out, tolerate, and even relish the unfamiliar aspects of the world, without becoming estranged from themselves.

Transitional Objects in Transitional Space

The quality of self-esteem and the psychoimmune system associated with it develop along two lines: They are grounded in the tested assurance of mastery, and they rest also on internal "communities" of good presences, external in origin, that have become, through the alchemy of development, the essential architectures of self.

These vital "inner-world" resources ripen slowly. Using a cosmological metaphor, I digress briefly to trace their development. Starting out as infants, we are indeed like protoplanets; we exist at the center of a cosmos that is not composed of space, or of objects in space, but of an overriding, limitless mood: Freud's "oceanic sense." In cosmic evolution, the nuclei of future planets condense out of featureless nebular clouds, and in the evolution of self, the nuclei of other beings condense out of the primordial oceanic experience: These "presences" begin to define the social space that separates them. In this "transitional space," the domain and its component objects are blended, barely distinct from each other. This space comes to be peopled with what psychoanalysts (Winnicott, 1953; see also Giovacchini, 1993) term *transitional objects*—others who are only known insofar as they touch us, serve us, frustrate us, center on us. At that early stanza in development, the self–other distinctions (ego boundaries) are porous: The other is known as an extension of the self; the self is experienced as an extension of the other: "I am my Mommy's little boy." And in our transitional objects, we experience, in external guise, the emotions that these others arouse within us.

Self-Development and Transitional Space

Beginning to trust ourselves, and assuming that the trusted others will be on hand when needed, we can risk separating from them, and allow them to be distinct from us. Thus, as we continue to grow and individuate, we separate; forming personal boundaries, we firm up the distinctions between ourselves and those who sponsored the earliest stanzas of development. The transitional space recedes, away from our primary caretakers; they are left out there, beyond our self-boundaries, in their own space of "otherness." But the transitional space and its blended relationships are never finally abandoned: Receding, they carry with them the trustworthy qualities of parental figures, to be experienced as trusted qualities of the self. Thus, in psychologically mature individuals, the transitional space is retained within the self-boundaries: It becomes the arena of the inner life—of dreams and fantasies, and it is the interior ground on which the once external landscape of early, unboundaried relationships is reproduced.

In normal development, the ambivalence that pervades all intense relationships is muted by the generally benign parental role in child rearing and by the child's generally benign response to "good-enough" parents. These give the child its first experience of its own nurturing capacities. Ultimately then, the mothers and fathers who once combined love with discipline take up residence as constant presences. Given the merged, syncretic quality of transitional relationships, they will survive—as inner resources, idealized figments of the self— the demise of the real parents.

Ultimately, by making their strengths our own, we can separate from our parents, teachers, or mentors, and having loosened these ties, we can move ahead, trusting our own psychic stability, to shoot the rapids of the next developmental passage. Having established continuity internally, we can tolerate change, the contact with alien agents, as well as the toxic possibilities, within the self and outside of it, that new development and new ventures may bring into play.

Forming the Niche

Successful ego development not only restricts transitional space, but also uses it. Like most events in nature, developmental transitions do not, particularly at their outset, proceed smoothly. Driven by surgent, diffuse appetites, the person gropes toward those others who will mirror and sponsor the emerging potentials. Of necessity, and in order to make the first contact with those who reciprocate our own development, we extend transitional space beyond the ego boundaries. Within this transitional space, we create a rudimentary "community," composed of those persons who are given significance by the developmental advance, and who will sponsor its further progress. But as development proceeds, this blending of other with self is no longer automatic, the side effect of magical thinking and porous ego boundaries. With greater maturity, this union becomes reality-based, founded on learning from the other, on playing the "apprentice" role, so as to take in the competencies of instructors and mentors.

In this manner, a psychosocial "niche" forms around the growing individual, a structure created by the drives, appetites, and potentials that are active in the developmental process: It is composed of individuals who are "selected" by the emerging energies, and who will sponsor the transformation of these potentials into ego executive capacities. Like a ship taking form in a dry dock amid a forest of serving gantries, the young individual assumes mature physical and psychological "shape" amid its special thicket of concerned parents, siblings, teachers, and peers. Ships represent a special kind of immune system—against the rigors of the sea—and like the ship that has been built to swim by its own buoyancy, the individual will one day cut loose from its formative niche to survive—if need be—on its own and to become part of formative niches for oncoming generations. Put in another way, the successfully developing individual takes in good presences so as to eventually become a good, trustworthy presence for others.

IMMUNE SYSTEM BREAKDOWN: THE LATE-ONSET DISORDERS

But our at-risk survivors do not routinely put together these internal assemblages, these collectives of good presences. Early on, these future patients have been forcibly shunted to alternate developmental tracks, and while these afford some compensation for early childhood deficits, they could also lead to troubling outcomes in adulthood. From the beginning, as opposed to normotensive individuals, our late-onset patients are precocious survivors of early parent loss or abuse, family disruption, and major physical trauma. Whatever their nature, such formative tragedies could not leave their victims with an internal residue of good presences. The adequately reared child memorializes—in effect, *becomes*—the parental virtues that were exercised in its behalf, but to a much greater degree, the at-risk child is chronically in danger of becoming its own "bad" parent; that is, the failed parent becomes a portrait of the child's rage toward that same parent, and as the child lives out its version of the Stockholm syndrome and identifies with this caricatured aggressor, it becomes, in some hidden abscess of the self, a replica of the untrustworthy father and/or mother. That same survivor of poor rearing will always be plagued by the temptation to represent, actively, the same "badness" that had once been suffered passively. There is an unconscious push, which often brings on intense symptomatic reactions, to become, for example, the castrating or castrated father, the victimized or victimizing "witch mother."

But the strongest motive of at-risk survivors is to defend against and escape their own bad presences. Psychic immunity requires that these be repressed, kept out of consciousness and behavior; it also requires that the bases of self-esteem be located outside the self, rather than within its haunted, claustrophobic interior. The bad presence is too primitive and frightening to accommodate any benign possibilities; as a consequence, the unappeased hunger for nurture is split off, and seeks satisfaction through others, beyond the precincts of the self. Psychologically robust individuals retain their past internally, in the form of good objects, good presences; in turn, their outer-world niches complement their internal politics: they serve development and form bridges to the future. But the niches of our at-risk survivors are at odds with the inner world, and instead of serving new development, they are bridges back to a sentimentalized version of the past. The good early history is not stored internally; instead, the at-risk survivor attempts to reconstruct it in the outer world.

Transferential bonds are the links that bind the past to the future. Transferences are memorials to early primary relationships that have been lost in the objective sense but have never been relinquished and mourned in the subjective sense. *Via* the bonds of transference, the survivors try to reinstate the valued relationships that they have either lost or never known.

These lost relationships have never been subjected to what the psycho-analyst George Pollock (1961) has termed the "mourning–liberation process": They have not been acknowledged, grieved, and finally accepted, so as to make way for new encounters. In another sense, transferences represent an extension, beyond the psychological boundaries of the self, of subjective transitional space into objective social space—the "space of the other." Carrying transitional space beyond the physical boundaries of the self, the transferences replicate—as in early childhood—the linkage of self and other. *Via* the transferential linkages, transitional space is once again (as in the primitive ego) uncontained; breaching the self–other boundaries, the transferences attempt to restore the early fusion of the subjective and the objective, of fantasy and reality. Accordingly, when they discover others who conform to their transference-shaped expectations, the vulnerable survivors are comforted and stabilized: The transference fantasies have brought about and merged into a virtual reality, a *niche* wherein some lost condition of union has been restored. In this merger, the lost but unrelinquished relationships of the family of orientation are discovered (or rediscovered) in new social habitats, for example, the family of procreation.*

In summary, the survivor's niche does not serve to advance development. Instead, the survivor's niche serves a static condition: Its function is to maintain externally what has never been achieved internally—a panel of good, supportive, and unchanging presences. These allies compose the niche, and in so doing, immunize the self against the bad internal presence. But this protection is only temporary: The immune system of the at-risk survivor depends on transferences that can only be ratified by the changeful other. The niche that is meant to protect against catastrophic internal disruption is itself vulnerable to unpredictable, ungovernable change. The immune system of the at-risk person is a carrier of the very pathogen—catastrophic change—that it ostensibly guards against.

And when, for whatever reasons, the niche is degraded or lost, the at-risk elder loses his buffering distance from the bad object: the inescapable (because internal) malignant presence. Lacking the convoy of obliging others (including those who are willing to give an external face to the threatening internal presence), the at-risk person is finally left in claustrophobic confinement with his or her private devils: the castrating or castrated father; the guilt-slinging, abandoning or murderous witch-mother, and so forth. The special curse of later life is to be left alone, finally and inescapably, with the bad presence.

There are some clinically significant variations on this basic scenario. Thus, beginning in their earliest years, our late-onset patient group divides to follow at least two quite different developmental trajectories, each of which leads to niches and psychoimmune systems of special character and special vulnerabilities. Some at-risk survivors overcome their early, formative trauma *via* an

---

*A good metaphor for the habitat–niche relationship is provided by the African waterhole, in that it supplies water, the basic necessity of life to a whole range of herbivores, carnivores and omnivores, this resource constitutes a *habitat*. Within the habitat framework, each of the congregant species converts the general watering place into a species-specific design, a *niche*, for getting the life-giving water (while avoiding predators in the herbivore case, or while finding prey in the carnivore case). The life-sustaining water is a *given*, and each species spins its own necessary reality around it.

extroverted solution, based on fantasies of powerful providers and rescuers waiting for them in the outer world. By contrast, the introversive, autoplastic types
seek their redemption internally, in grandiose and narcissistic fantasies of their
own omnipotence. We first consider the alloplastic, extroverted individuals.

The Alloplastic Extroverts

Trustful children, convinced that caretakers and sponsors will always be
available to them, can separate and individuate. But the troubled early experience of at-risk extroverts does not lead to a condition of basic trust. Lacking
reliable others, they continue looking, even into later life, for the good mothers
and good fathers that they have never known, or that they had known too briefly.
Again, not having mourned and relinquished their lost caretakers, they have not
gone through basic maturational processes: taking in, letting go, and moving on.

These extroverts' yearnings, for the primary relationships that can finally
nourish and complete them, are expressed as persisting, compensatory fantasies
of love, nurture, and succor: in short, as transferences. The alloplastic extroverts will use these to create a projective ecology in which wives are experienced
as mothers, husbands as fathers—and in later life, under this sign, even grown
children can become the virtual "parents" of their own aging parents. *Via* their
ratified transferences, the family of procreation has been reconfigured to accommodate a lost and mythic family of orientation.

Paradoxically, these benign delusions are the keystones of psychic immunity. So long as the transference partners accept their assigned fantasies, so long
as they do not deviate from the unchanging expectations that have been mapped
on to them, then psychoimmunity—despite being externally located—is maintained, and the at-risk extroverts can endure the buffets of change and loss
without too much distress, and without recourse to psychosomatic illness. The
straws can pile up, but the camel's back does not break.

But in later life, the stubborn, persistent reliance on the transitional presence carries phase-specific risks. In early life, the transitional space is peopled
with nutritive personnel, usually parents in the grip of the Parental Emergency
(see Gutmann, 1994, Chapter 7), who are mobilized to meet the child's demands
for unstinting care. The child's imperial sensitivity, its awareness of being at
the center of its world, is confirmed by the immediacy and intensity of the
parent's regard and care. Unfortunately for them, senior persons, whether "normal" or "at risk," do not have this special charisma, the baby's capacity to charm
and mobilize a child-centered network in its favor. Instead, in the current
geriatric literature, those who minister to older people are generally referred to
as "burdened caretakers."

Thus, at-risk extroverts are doubly disadvantaged in later life: Their inner
life is apt to be persecutory rather than restorative, and their psychic provender
must come exclusively from real people, "out there." Inevitably—and particularly in later life—the niche of at-risk extroverts presents them with the same
crisis of trust that in early life had compromised their inner life. No matter how

loving or well-intentioned they may be, real people are prone to defect from their transference assignments. Reality finally overrides fantasy: Real people grow up, they find other loves or interests, they go away, they die. Finally, they reveal the tragic discrepancy between the imposed, virtual reality of the "carpentered" niche and the changeful, inconstant nature of real people, and real social worlds. In short, the patched-together niche is always in danger of regressing back to its original, amorphous "habitat" condition, to become, once more, "a world I never made."

The Autoplastic Introverts

By contrast to the extroverts, who continue to hunt through the world for some equivalent of the lost parent, the introversive types concede their trust mainly to themselves: to a narcissistic legend of their own omnipotentiality, or to an illusory and grandiose conception of their own complete self-sufficiency. Like the disappointed baby who, in Erikson's terms, "finds its thumb and damns the world," the introverts' essential, narcissistic legend is that they need nobody but themselves, that they have, in their own mind and in their own body, all the resources that they and their dependents might require. Their founding, grandiose myth of self is that they are their own parents, that they feed from the bottles that they alone have made and filled.

In their case, then, the introverts' transference is to *themselves*—to their own unrelinquished legend of all-inclusiveness and self-sufficiency. When they were very young, their primitive fantasies of omnipotence were sufficient to soothe and sustain them, but as they mature, the boundaries between fantasy and reality are tightened, and flagrant illusions, now recognized as such, are no longer believed. They no longer do the job of maintaining psychoimmunity. The legend, the founding myth of the self, is a fable that survivors tell themselves but that they can only believe if it is retold and confirmed by others. The myth of the self must be accredited in the world, by respected representatives from external reality.

Out of this population, introversive fantasists create their own version of the psychosocial niche: a theater, whose personnel comprise the audience to their psychodrama and the bit players willing to take special roles in it. Where the extroverts comb the world to locate appropriate vessels for their idealizing transferences, the introversive mythicists recruit those who will direct their idealizing transferences to themselves. Some of these groupies form the Greek chorus to the fantasist's special legend—they proclaim his virtues to the audience. Others of the fantasist's niche enact for their cameo parts in his contra-legend.

Thus, the mythicist lives on and by the legend of his complete fearlessness or self-sufficiency; it is these *others* of his niche who are needy—and, preferably, dependent on the mythicist. Where the mythicist is whole, these *others* are damaged, and they need him to be made whole; and where the mythicist is brave, these *others* are cowardly, needful of his courage and example. In short, the mythmaker uses selected others as self-extensions, to extract the dangerous, contralegendary aspects out of the self. In order to sustain the virtual reality of the founding legend, the mythicist exports these dangerous contents into the receptive members of the ambient niche, into the convoy that has been assembled to receive them. So long as the founding myth is maintained in its pristine form, albeit by an external bodyguard, then the psychoimmune system retains its integrity, and the introversive mythicist can endure, without significant pathology, the escalating insults of later life.

Losing the Niche: Alone with the Bad Presence

But the later years are not kind to either the physical or the psychic immune systems. In the autumn of life, the forces that attack niches are often stronger than those that bind them together. Older individuals lose access to the special social habitats—the family of procreation, the workplace, the playing field—out of which new psychosocial niches can be formed, or established ones regenerated. The nest empties, kinfolk and friends die, workers retire, and older individuals in any event get tired: They lack the energy to continually monitor, patch, and reassemble their straggling convoys.

When their niches degrade, at-risk elders are stressed in special ways: Mainly, they lose their *special* supply lines to their *necessary* emotional rations. For them, such deprivation counts for more than just one more straw added to the camel's back, more than the loss of accustomed comforts. The extroverts, for example, lose the confirmation, in their families of procreation, of the unsurrendered but never satisfied dreams that were spawned in their families of orientation. Thus, when their postparental wives come out of the closet, concentrate on their own development, and refuse to mother their aging husbands, these men suffer more than inconvenience and missed meals. In their case, their worst fears have caught up with them: They are finally confronted by the separation from the maternal presence that they had always avoided, and by the shamed awareness of themselves as helpless, needy babies. The result can be a significant, sometimes suicidal, depression, or more commonly, a chronic psychosomatic disorder. The hospital inpatient unit, with its corps of concerned, TLC-giving nurses is richly furnished with potential "mothers." The hospital can become the last habitat for maternal transferences; as such, it can be readily formed into the last niche of the aging "mother's son."

When, in their turn, the introversive mythicists lose their particular niche—their bodyguard of admirers, dependents, and selected enemies—they lose a vital illusion: that their founding legend of the self is accredited by significant others. The believers, the upholders of the survivor's virtual reality, pass and fade, but the personal legend, though left unsupported, is rarely abandoned. Instead, the mythicist finally sees the dream for what it is and always has been: a fantasy, and a persecutory one at that. As one older patient put it, "I'm not the man I used to be—and I never was." The fantasy persists, but now only to remind the mythicist that it was never anything but a lie.

Deprived of their credible legend, the introversive mythicists are at risk for becoming either depressed or psychotic. Absent their myth, there is nothing—now including themselves—that they can trust. Moreover, the legend that has lost the tonus of reality is replaced by its opposite: the Bad Presence that has been waiting in the psychic wings. Finally, they are in danger of discovering, in themselves, the terrible presences that they had always exported to others: the *helpless baby*, the *needy one*, the *castrated one*, the *coward*. Under great pressure to restore the virtual reality of their myth (and to counter the depression that follows its loss), the introversive mythicists will often distort their awareness and spin a delusional caricature of their actual circumstances: There is nothing wrong with them; they are still perfect; others have plotted their downfall, and when their evil designs are thwarted, that perfection will again shine forth. *Via* the paraphrenic delusion, irreversible losses are transformed into reversible ones: "If the mayor would make my neighbors stop poisoning me, I would be okay again." Through such flagrant distortions, the credibility of the personal myth is preserved, but at the price of reality and sanity.

CLINICAL ILLUSTRATIONS

Ernest Hemingway

This great but vulnerable writer provides a classic example of a later-life suicide whose habitat was in good shape—he was rich, famous, and free of lethal disease—but whose niche had failed to preserve the integrity of his special legend.

Hemingway had been raised by a self-dramatizing mother who was both jealous and admiring of the special powers of men. She went out of her way to diminish Hemingway's father (like his famous son, he, too, was a suicide), and she alternated between treating her little son as a hero, and as the virtual twin sister of her oldest daughter.* Reacting strongly against this virtual castration, young Ernest was heard to announce, in his third year, the legend that from then on was his life's *motif*: "Ain't afraid of nothin'." True to this legend, he threw himself into danger: in wars, in the hunt, and even in the bullring. Within these habitats, he created niches: He found those who would teach him how to be brave, those who would acknowledge his courage, and those who, because of their own fearfulness, would depend on him to be fearless. In more peaceful settings, and particularly in his later years, he sought out younger women as lovers and admirers: To him, they were always "daughter"; to them, he was always "Papa." Clearly, the domains of danger provided occasions for living out his myth, for demonstrating "Ain't afraid of nothin'." Meanwhile, the satellite

*Thus, the Hemingway family albums show little Ernest, aged 2, togged out in the frilliest of baby drag outfits. Written in his mother's hand, the subscript title reads "Summer Girl."

system of young "daughters" provided Hemingway with occasions for living out his antimyth: Through young, nubile women, he could remove from himself (while at the same time contacting) the "daughter" that his mother had imprinted, early on, in his psyche. Thus, Hemingway was plunged into a late-onset psychotic depression by the loss of two essential niches: His presumably invulnerable, hypermasculine boxer's body had been weakened to the point of impotence by heavy drinking and by wounds, and he could no longer find adoring, sexually compliant "daughters" to hold his feminine aspect for him, outside of himself. Finally, he was left alone with the bad presence, the *internal* daughter. Thus, Hemingway's final works—*Across the River and into the Trees* is a notable example—feature the theme of intense sexual love between a battered but admirable older soldier and an adoring young woman: Typically, she loves him for his scars, and she demands that he call her "daughter."*

But Hemingway's attempts to restate his myths and reify his niche through literary creativity could not save him for long. When his body and his social worlds no longer bolstered the legend, his final recourse was to alter reality through paranoia: He accused his wife of reducing him to pauperhood, and he was completely convinced that the IRS was about to jail him for income-tax fraud. Money equals phallic power, and in his delusions Hemingway had projected his inner sense of masculine depletion into the external agents that were out to rob him of this fiscal/phallic essence. But the paranoia did not finally succeed in staving off depression, and Hemingway, the hunter, found his last prey: At the age of 61 he blew his own head off with a sporting gun.

The Taxi Driver

This pathogenic pattern is not restricted to celebrities. At Northwestern's Older Adult Unit, we recently treated a suicide attempter whose early history was similar to that of Hemingway. He, too, had been raised by a mother of aristocratic pretensions, who felt that she had married beneath herself, and who elevated her only son above his father in her esteem. But sons require fathers to aid them in separating from the mother, and Oedipal victors like our patient may have freed themselves from their weak fathers at the cost of binding themselves forever to their strong mothers. They can never escape the shameful feeling that they are in reality no more than a figment of their mothers.

Like Ernest Hemingway, our patient fought against the bad maternal presence by creating a heroic, *macho* myth, by serving that myth, and by recruiting

---

*Hemingway's most poignant book on this theme was published posthumously as *The Garden of Eden*, written following his divorce by "First Daughter"—the writer Martha Gellhorn. The book begins by describing an idyllic honeymoon on the Edenic Cote d'Azur, but quickly degenerates into nightmare as the young bride becomes obsessed by her wish to have sex as a man (with her husband as the "woman"), and by her wish to turn him—via matching haircuts, hair dyes, and shared suntan sessions—into her identical twin. Once the external "daughter" has been lost, Hemingway's internal "daughter"—his mother's "Summer Girl," his sister's twin—pushes for expression and liberation.

others to form a protective niche around it. Thus, he was an athletic star in high school, and as an infantry officer in Korea, he won the coveted Silver Star. Returning to civilian life, he joined an advertising firm and rose rapidly to executive status. But—again, like Hemingway—this driven man needed challenge and danger more than he needed status. In order to serve his own "Ain't afraid of nothin'" myth, he dropped out of his highly paid CEO position and went back into "combat." He took a job as a Chicago cab driver, specializing in the inner-city runs that white drivers ordinarily shun. Arming himself, he even welcomed and successfully fought off the occasional mugging attempt. Back at the "front," once again "on point," the patient was, for a while, stabilized.

However, his wife was not. In her middle years, imbued with the self-assertion of the postparental woman (see Gutmann, 1994, Chapters 5 & 6), she became impatient with her husband's lack of ambition and conventional success, and went for it on her own: She opened a trendy boutique that took off and did well. The phallic essence—money—had passed to the wife; she was no longer the holding ground for the patient's feminine side, and the patient was left alone with his demons—himself as "mama's boy," himself as a figment of the powerful mother. In this regard, his Rorschach was one of the strangest that I have ever seen: For him, each stimulus card called up the same idiosyncratic imagery: sagging bags full of foul, stinking liquids that had been stamped on and burst. Clearly, the patient felt possessed by something soft and corrupt; in his case, he tried to kill the invading "feminine" presence with a lethal slug of lye.

CONCLUSION: TREAT SYSTEMS, NOT SYMPTOMS

In summary, as they lose their necessary confirmations, whether found in themselves or in others, the long maintained psychic immune systems of the at-risk individuals—the extroverts as well as the introversive mythicists—are compromised. Self-psychology doctrine holds that loss of the personal narrative leaves the person devastated, without internal structure. But we have found that the real pathogen is not postnarrative emptiness, but the emerging antinarrative, the bad presence that has been concealed behind the accredited legend of the self. Left alone with the bad presence, these patients then become catastrophically vulnerable to further change and loss.

Thus, it is only at this relatively late point in pathogenesis, when the psychic immune system can no longer manage the inner demons, that the conventional camel's back model becomes relevant. It is only then, when the real damage has already been done, that the at-risk individual is ripe to be undone by the last straw, by the psychological equivalent of opportunistic infections.

Conventional geropsychiatrists and geropsychologists have missed the point; they still confound effects with causes, the incidental fevers with the full disease process. If they troubled to study the predisposed, historic patient, they might discern the qualitative roots of disorder and recognize that the late-onset psychopathology begins—as in AIDS—not with exposure to the latest insult (the psychological equivalent of the opportunistic infection) but with the degradation of the psychoimmune system itself. On the physical side, internists begin to control AIDS not by treating Kaposi's sarcoma—at that advanced stage, no cure is as yet possible—but by concentrating on the opening stanza of the illness: the viral attack on the immune system per se.

Applying this logic to psychogeriatrics, we hold that it is not enough to treat the incidental symptoms of late-onset depression, anxiety, or paranoia; we should study—so that we can eventually reconstitute—the protective structures and functions of the late-onset patient's psychoimmune system. To this end, we have to place the historic rather than the symptomatic patient at the forefront of our research and treatment. How one might do this is a matter for another paper.

REFERENCES

Erikson, E. (1952). *Childhood and society*. New York: Norton.

Giovacchini, P. (1993). *Borderline patients: The psychosomatic focus and the therapeutic process.* Northvale, NJ: Aronson.

Gutmann, D. (1994). *Reclaimed powers: Men and women in later life*. Evanston, IL: Northwestern University Press.

Hammond, J. (1991). *A case study of the relocated: A detailed examination of residents and their family caretakers during a radical change*. Unpublished doctoral dissertation, Northwestern University, Evanston, IL.

Pollock, G. (1961). Mourning and adaptation. *International Journal of Psychoanalysis, 42*, 341–361.

Schindler, B. (1985). Stress, affective disorders, and immune function. *Medical Clinics of North America, 69*(3), 170–197.

Schleifer, S., Keller, S., Siris, S., Davis, K., & Stein, M. (1985). Depression and immunity. *Archives of General Psychiatry, 42*, 243–252.

Staines, N., Brostoff, J., & James, K. (1993). *Introducing immunology*. London: Mosby.

Winnicott, D. (1953). Transitional objects and transitional phenomena. In D. Winnicott, *Playing and reality* (pp. 1–26). London: Tavistock.

CHAPTER 13

Uses of the Past in Adult Psychological Health

Objective, Historical, and Narrative Realities

HARVEY PESKIN

THE GENETIC VIEWPOINT AND ADULT DEVELOPMENT: FRIENDS OR STRANGERS?

If being adult is being fully grown up, then *adult development* is something of an oxymoron. But not if we take it as we take adult entertainment: intended only for adults; not suitable for children. We begin with this bit of conceptual hyperbole to highlight the sense that development in adulthood marches to a different drama than in childhood. Nevertheless, just as there is obviously no well-developed child apart from a well-developing one, there is no well-developed adult. Such, essentially, was Jung's (1933) complaint to Freud: not against the validity of libido theory itself, but with Freud's failure to recognize that the second half of life ("the psychology of the afternoon," Jung called it) had passed beyond the aims of psychosexuality to follow now utterly new directions and seize new terms of being, rather than to stay put, protecting the winnings of the first half ("the psychology of the morning") from dwindling any further.

The second half of life—whether catalyzed by the giving and fostering of life by procreation and parenting (Benedek, 1959), or by the ebbing of parenthood when such life matures (Gutmann, 1987), or by the compelling awareness of physical decline, death, and loss (Butler, 1963; Jaques, 1965; Kernberg, 1980; Pollock, 1961), or by a kind of Jungian biological clock—proceeds through existential realms that rely, it would seem, on the first half only to finish or interrupt its various youthful missions so that it, the second half, can get on with the journey toward new definitions of the self.

Adult development, then, is not a holdover of belated youth, but a good-enough term, suitable to and instigated by any or all of the aforementioned catalysts, that indicates (borrowing from Kegan, Chapter 9, this volume) the self-authoring and self-transforming potential of the adult to move beyond the socialized-mindedness of youth and adolescence; at least, to stand apart from conventional wisdom; at best, to recognize the paradoxes and contradictions of socialization, using them to animate new and reanimate past experience.

The discontinuity or even estrangement between early and late life in some of these by now familiar scenarios of adult development inevitably raises the issue of whether the reputed formative years of youth and adolescence are formative of only a short-lived space in the lifespan. If so, then where are the formative influences of later adult development to be found? Surely, the determinants of who one is becoming in late life would seem much closer at hand, more palpable, and hence more open to change than searching for them in the dim past. It is probably not fortuitous that interest in the historical truths and genetic interpretations of childhood has declined in analytic treatment as analytic respect for the developing adult has increased. In this light, there is some irony that elders' ready interest in reminiscence and life history has been devalued as symptomatic of living in the past, hence escapist and unreliable, rather than as integral to the unfolding of character in late life (Butler, 1963; Erikson, 1950).

Freud showed no particular regard for the older adult's accessibility to the past. On the contrary, Freud (1905) discouraged analytic treatment for the middle-aged (beyond 50) on the very grounds of their declining "elasticity" to sort through "the mass of material" for the relevant experiences in the early past. Such a position, of course, is merely self-fulfilling, since it also discourages serious empirical test of its truth. For researchers, such as Neurgarten (1968), who have made middle and late adulthood a subject of serious study, the conscious awareness of past experience in shaping behavior becomes increasingly dominant over adulthood. From our adult-development perspective, Freud seems to have been overprotecting his claim to a generic psychosexual theory by thus distancing himself from clinical testimony that could point to the contrary (e.g., Jung's path) or to the necessity for theory revision for the later lifespan. (Jung's thinking, of course, was no less self-fulfilling in withdrawing interest from the younger patient. A self-psychology for the first half of life was a Jungian nonsequitur that awaited theorists from the current, less ageist period, e.g., Winnicott, Kohut.) The high price of barring such evidence is evident in the sparseness of a developmental psychoanalysis for the whole lifespan and skepticism that psychoanalysis can regain its own elasticity to develop cogent concepts for it. But there is otherwise today a sea-change of attitude, for psychoanalysis has moved from insouciance to vigorous catch-up in more openly and evenhandedly confronting a question that its own neglect had once foreclosed: Is there a need and place for a psychoanalytic developmental psychology of the lifespan?

   The conceptual antagonism between youth and adulthood is doubtless one of the countless residues of culture's infiltration of theory. But nothing in adult development requires divesting the influence of the past on later personality. The threat to classical theory rather lies in doubting its vested interest in unalterable past/present relationships that do not comport with the changing nature of adulthood. Around life transitions from adolescence to aging, changing organizations of the past may release and potentiate new uses of long-standing but dormant capabilities. Such a conceptual trend represents a departure from the classical psychoanalytic view of the primacy and immutability of antecedent experiences in determining adult psychological health. Next to the classical model exist, then, new genetic models based rather on the primacy of current life purpose.

   F. Scott Fitzgerald could have been capturing the mood of orthodox psychoanalysis toward adult development when he taunted that there are no second acts in American lives. Yet if the essence of drama is that the second act rewrites the first with the energy of a new creation, then so might the second half of life rework the first half. If narrative is the current metaphor for psychic reality, then drama is the analog for lifespan development. Each act or half of life uses and is used, replenishes and is replenished by the other act or half. This contemporary position constructs a stage for second acts and second chances on which the cast of characters from life's first half is assembled for creating new energies and new endings. This chapter adduces uncustomary empirical evidence for this new model from the objective past of longitudinal study—specifically, for the selective potency of the actual past as a function of adult age and family stage. Such evidence credits the actual past with an elasticity usually reserved for narrative reconstruction.

   This chapter seeks to revive for adult development the flagging relevance of the genetic viewpoint by drawing on the methods and findings of lifespan research from longitudinal samples. Specifically, this review of my own and my colleagues' work deals with the prediction of psychological health in the longitudinal sample of the intergenerational studies (IGS) observed from adolescence to age 60 (Eichorn, Clausen, Haan, Honzik, & Mussen, 1981). This work traverses three versions of the genetic viewpoint, each more attuned to developmental process than the one before: (1) the linear order of behavioral consistency and continuity for which longitudinal study is best known and which reflects the quasineurobiological sequence of cause and effect in classical psychoanalytic theory; (2) the less frequented and more complex order of nonlinearity and transformation that indicates specific stage action and interaction; and (3) the reordering of the causal direction itself, shifting to the influence of the present on the past, and, necessarily, to the person as the center of action. This last version—to which we give the chapter's title—is also the latest and largest paradigmatic shift, having laid in wait for us to collect midlife and late-life follow-up data before it could reveal itself. These versions of the model and phases of the research are roughly attuned to the evolution of psychoanalytic theory from a child-centered to an adult-centered ethos.

SUITABILITY OF LONGITUDINAL STUDY
FOR TESTING GENETIC VIEWPOINTS

Given that reliable clinical and behavioral observation is its strong suit, longitudinal study has been curiously underutilized or unrecognized for investigating the efficacy of genetic models in psychoanalysis. Strong suited it may be, but it is short on psychoanalytic suitors and rather an unwanted stepchild to more ideographic methods of psychic reality of the past (such as memories, narrative, constructions, and reconstructions) that require no underpinning in objective reality. Cohler's reviews (1980, Chapter 11, this volume; Cohler & Galatzer-Levy, 1990) of longitudinal studies are rather a recent exception, with the essential conclusion that a consistent and continuous course of development is not prefigured by earlier developmental events. But scouting for such linear consistency is only one version of the genetic approach in psychoanalysis. Unfortunately, the unique power of longitudinal study to be a testing ground for behavioral consistency had come to stand for its entire power, both by longitudinal researchers themselves and by the ambience of American ego psychology, occupied with the stability of conflict-free spheres of personality. In effect, behaviors failing to show high stability over time were likely to be regarded as merely inconsistent and unpredictable (euphemistically called "change," as in the oft-read phrase, "consistency and change"), the outcome of observer error resulting from the welter of the uncontrollable events of living. In short, inconsistency was uninteresting, and certainly inexplicable.

But as longitudinal research has grown up and faithfully ages with its study sample, the reach of early development into the adult lifespan becomes progressively measurable and increasingly sophisticated. The complexity of statistical inference afforded by over-time data collection provides findings more subtle than linear and cumulative outcomes of past experience for which, in any case, evidence is unimpressive. The lack of findings for linear associations is hardly, then, a final answer to the question of the influence of the objective (i.e., consensually observed) past on the present. Our research has usefully pursued relationships that are no less orderly for being nonlinear. Accordingly, such findings have demonstrated the efficacy of longitudinal study for nonlinear genetic models in psychoanalysis that deal with comprehensible transformations of personality. (In addition to the studies on psychological health, we refer here to our research on behavioral change in adolescence for subsamples posited to be more or less ready psychosexually for the onset of puberty [Peskin, 1973].)

Moreover, with multiple adult follow-ups, complex associations are compounded, for when prediction is no longer confined to a single outcome age, there is an abundant yield of changing predictors that no single outcome age can represent well. Such associations cannot, then, be so inertly attributed to the influence of the past on the present, since both past and present are themselves in motion, requiring us to seek new conceptual ground. By this time, one realizes how much longitudinal study has left the straight and narrow of its traditional bent for linear research and has come of age.

This précis seems now rather self-evident looking back on our empirical studies over three follow-up points from early to late adulthood. But our work hardly seemed so as we felt our way hesitantly from follow-up to follow-up, perhaps analogous to Freud's (1920) own observation that on looking back, one's development feels coherent and continuous, but proceeding forward—as in longitudinal prediction—the chain of causation is hardly self-evident, indeed, even (Freud said) impossible to predict. Our research has often been just such an experience of groping, without the guide of clear-cut hypotheses hardwired from theory to data. Yet the research urged itself on by a growing sense that the recovery of the past in psychoanalytic treatment had a statistical counterpart in the rich empirical data of the IGS. As one entered into this surprisingly subjective research process, the investigator's self-invented orchestration of where and how to organize the statistical data also has felt curiously like the pursuit of narrative truth between analyst and analysand that Cohler (Chapter 11, this volume) and others (Schafer, 1983; Spence, 1982) have described.

Classical Linear Model of Causation

We give the following exemplar from a larger statistical "case history" from the IGS archives. The researcher who conceives of the genetic model as upholding the primacy of antecedent experience could choose to organize his work, as we did at first (Livson & Peskin, 1967), by comparing the predictive power of earlier and later age periods. We proceeded this way by correlating behavior ratings at each of four separate time periods (ages 5–7, 8–10, 11–13, 14–16) with a global index of psychological health at age 30 that measured how closely an individual approximated an ideal portrayal of a psychologically healthy person. The index was simply the correlation between each participant's adult personality profile on the 100-item California Q-sort and an "ideal" Q-sort of psychological health composited from the independent and highly consensual ratings of four clinical psychologists. In addition to excluding explicit psychopathology, the ideal healthy Q-sort highlights capacity for work, satisfying relationships, sense of moral purpose, and realistic perception of self and society. Findings were indeed sparse for the linear genetic model. Only preadolescent behavior (ages 11–13) in both sexes predicted adult psychological health. Thus, results showed neither the primacy of earlier behavior nor of behavior from the closest-to-adulthood period (ages 14–16), while predictive gaps ("sleeper effects") appeared in the series of correlations, reflecting the uncertainty of continuous development (Cohler, Chapter 11, this volume; Kagan & Moss, 1962).

Transformative Model of Causation

On next choosing to fit a genetic model of nonlinear order that did not require primacy of early experience, we proceeded in a second study (Peskin,

1972) to multiply predict adult psychological health from behavior across the early periods rather than within each separate period. Here, we were not, as before, interested in comparing the predictive power of separate age periods, but in the ways in which age periods carry forward or otherwise transform the effects of prior periods. Results revealed a new abundance of predictions, linear and nonlinear. Perhaps the most startling was the revelation that a so-called "sleeper effect" could be a real effect gone unnoticed, being masked statistically by its opposite effect in the previous time period. Where a stable behavior at two periods actually predicts to adulthood in opposite directions, the prediction of the later period will appear reduced or washed away, since simple correlations from the later time necessarily sum and confound effects of the earlier period. If, however, the significant earlier prediction has been removed, then the later one will be free to emerge with reversed sign. This removal can be easily accomplished with multivariate correlational techniques, such as partial correlation. (Several of Kagan & Moss's original sleeper effects, based on zero-order correlations, revealed just such a powerful effect after their findings were recalculated by partial correlation; cf. Livson & Peskin, 1980.) Such statistical interventions may be likened to recovering the past in the psychoanalytic treatment of adults where the welter of lived experience initially obscures the onset of developmental lines.

We present a vignette of such peeling a sleeper effect into its separate age effects. What first appeared in the IGS sample as the failure of an adolescent behavior (ages 14–16) to predict adult outcome from zero-order correlations was transformed into a significant multiple prediction with opposite signs of the beta weights at each age period. Thus, in our first study, psychological health for females at age 30 was associated with *independent* behavior at ages 11–13 but not at ages 14–16. In our second 1972 study, in which multiple correlations were calculated across periods, *dependent* behavior at ages 14–16 now predicted high psychological health at age 30, certainly a remarkable shift of function for a relatively stable trait. The research had then uncovered an interesting reversal of dependence–independence between adjacent age periods that increased the prediction of adult psychological health over either stage alone. Such transformations readily constitute evidence for an interstage, developmental order, but not for unpredictability. As we will discuss, they also may be more abundant in late adulthood.

Uses-of-the-Past Model

As we said, the third version of the genetic model (i.e., the influence of the present on the past) could make itself known only with the arrival of new adult follow-ups. From one adult age to the next, the often considerable change in the amount and substance of predictions of psychological health called into doubt the linear causal chain of past to present. Since such change indicated that a single, unalterable adulthood was no longer tenable, it has been reasonable to support the model's third version: Healthy adult functioning determines the relevant resources from the past, with such resources being altered as the tasks of healthy functioning themselves alter. We summarize now how such coordination of adult psychological health and adolescent resources is organized at each follow-up age or stage (e.g., parenthood vs. postparenthood).

The index of adult psychological health was predicted, via multiple correlation, by each Q-sort item rated separately in early (junior high school) and late (senior high) at each of the three adult ages. This analysis was undertaken for two cohorts at each follow-up age: for the Berkeley Guidance Study (GS) at ages 30, 40, and 52; for the Oakland Growth Study (OGS), at ages 37, 47, and 60. Q-sorts were made by clinicians from intensive interviews of the participants at each follow-up.

A continuous view emphasizing the primacy of earlier experience would be indicated by a larger yield of past–present correlations the nearer they were in time, with a declining influence of the past as the time between them widened. This pattern was not found (Peskin & Livson, 1981). In three of the four subsamples analyzed (males and females of the GS and OGS cohorts), the number of Q-sort items in adolescence that significantly predicted adult psychological health climbed from earlier to later adulthood (Figure 13–1). Past–present asso-

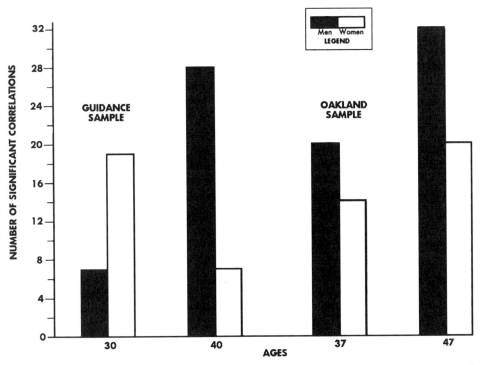

Figure 13–1. Number of significant correlations between adolescent Q-sort items ($P = 100$) and Q-sort measure of adult psychological health.

ciations, then, did not diminish, but increased with age. Such evidence for the
new accretion of psychological resources at later points in the lifespan disputes
the contention (Costa & McCrae, 1994) that development is essentially finished
by age 30. The uses-of-the-past research design provides an approach to the completion of personality growth that does not rely, as do Costa and McCrae, on the
customary method of behavioral stability. Thus, although the index of psychological health is indeed significantly stable between the IGS sample follow-ups,
its adolescent behavioral correlates are nonredundant, even—as reported below—
reversing the direction of prediction from one follow-up to the next. Certainly,
this changing composition of psychological health makes a strong case for the
open-endedness of personality growth into late adulthood (Peskin, 1987).

Nor does the statistical pattern of Figure 13–1 support either Freudian or
Jungian-styled renditions of the past, since both models agree (from quite different premises) that growing older is associated with the decline of past–present
continuity. Rather than decline, the past becomes available for psychological
transformation the more it becomes *past*. This truism may contain a useful truth
if it is understood as a developmental line of *having a past*: the recognition and
acceptance of the past as a part of oneself, whereby the past is invested with a
sense of ownership, and with it, the properties of ownership to organize—to
master, guide, and otherwise make use of—our experience. This view comports
broadly with post-Freudian constructions of life history, where the passively
received and uncohesive past (via the plethora of childhood identifications)
becomes increasingly organized and animated by the self-regulation of personal
identity and internalization (Erikson, 1950; Loewald, 1980a). In this sense,
passing time might render the past not dimmer but more luminous (more
structured in the traditional terms of ego psychology, or more in reach of one's
subjectivity in the terms of social constructivism). The concept of life review
(Butler, 1963), not as living in the past but as purposeful confrontation of one's
mortality, can readily be seen as the culmination of this developmental line.
Furthermore, the feasibility of dynamic psychotherapy in late age is more readily
apparent since, by this line of having a past, life history becomes less resisted,
more available, and "experience-near" to the older patient than the younger.
Freud's own practice with helping the younger patient recover crucial gaps in
life history may well have caused him to dismiss such availability of the past to
the older patient as a too large and distant "mass of material" rather than to
formulate it as inchoate signals of the patient's striving to reorganize (rather
than primarily to recover) life history usefully.

Adolescence itself is a period where the issue of self-ownership, if you
will, is prominent. One might conjecture that for the young adulthood of the GS
males at age 30, still in the individuating throes of young adulthood (Levinson,
Darrow, Klein, Levinson, & McKee, 1978), adolescence is a past not yet passed (or
a past-not-yet-past) and thus not yet sufficiently self-possessed to confirm the
developmental distance one has come and the strides one has made. Moreover, it
may be too early for them—all new parents or recently married by age 30—to be
drawn to attributes of adolescent mastery until later goals, especially the reality
of settling down vocationally (beyond marriage and parenting) come into

sharper focus. The discontinuity of past–present relations for these young men at this point may then suggest that males' adolescent preparation for young adulthood is ambiguous and provisional.

But 10 years later at 40—the on-time age for the established and instrumental man—the men come closer to their own adolescence, finding there abundant wellsprings of healthful adult self-esteem, authority, and mastery (Figure 13–2).

ADOLESCENT BEHAVIORS

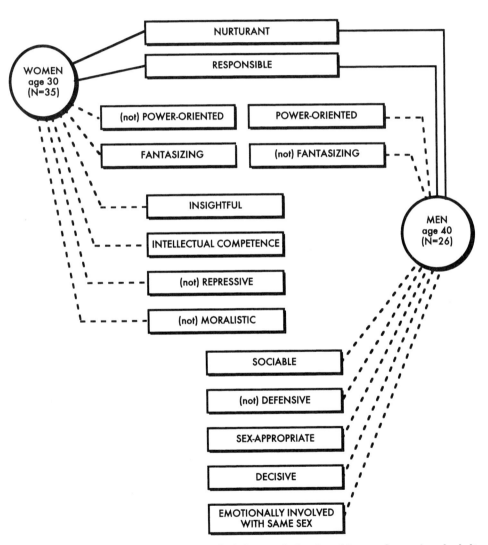

Figure 13–2. Significant correlations of adolescent behaviors (*Q*-sort clusters) and adult psychological health: women at age 30, men at age 40.

(Note that all Figures are based on the significant findings of 19 Q-sort item dimensions.)*

Psychological health of GS women follows an opposite path, clearly drawing more from the adolescent past at age 30 than 40 (Figure 13–3). Women at age 30 are almost all mothers of preschool-age children, and, indeed, the adolescent resources for adult psychological health seem of a kind that nourishes the maternal function: emotional openness, competence, nurturance, and even-handedness. This use of the past for parenting recurs at age 40 only for those women who give birth again in the intervening 10 years. Those who have not given birth again during this time period show no correlations of psychological health with adolescent behaviors. Thus, for those mothering young children at both 30 and 40, past–present continuity is strong, in keeping with the socialization for parenting that occurs during female adolescence. Meanwhile, for women at 40 who have had no more children in the intervening 10 years, the lack of any significant past–present correlations suggests that adolescence no longer provides resources for these women who are past the intensive years of parenting young children. For them, adolescent support, guidelines, or energies for the parental imperative (Gutmann, 1987) leave off much before the imperative is over, suggesting both role ambiguity in later parenting and new attunements to changing goals or directions even while the parental function itself remains intact. Since in this research we are always dealing with adult psychological health, discontinuity between past and present (as in this women's subgroup) should disabuse us of the notion that continuity alone is normative and healthful.

The age 30–40 gender reversal in using the past (males from less to more; females from more to less) is yet more sharply drawn when the genders are compared on past–present correlations for adults parenting younger and older offspring. As Figure 13–3 shows, the mother of the young child (at ages 30 and 40) is well prepared by her adolescence to function healthfully, whereas the mother of the older child is not so provided. For men, the contrary holds (Table 13–1). At age 40, it is clearly the healthy father with an older last-born child (10 years and over) who draws from his adolescence those traits congruent with the established, decisive, and instrumental man. Such past resources for the quintessential active mastery of the parental imperative seem to "lock in" only as the older child's own maturing instrumentality becomes congruent with the father's. Lesser congruence with the younger child may delay the father's use of such adolescent capabilities (Table 13–1). For the older child, one might also discern a

---

*The large yield of Q-sort findings was managed more conveniently by cluster analysis. A common solution for the early and late adolescent Q-sorts yielded 11 oblique clusters accounting for all the reliable covariance among the items and defining important dimensions of personality. These clusters have also been successfully tested for fit within each of the "component groups" (two sexes × two cohorts × two adult age periods). In addition to the clusters, eight single items quality as separate "dimensions" in that they (1) neither define a cluster nor have their variance "explained" by any combination of the 11 clusters and (2) show sufficiently high interjudge reliability. Hence, the 19 (11 plus 8) Q-dimensions from which the results of Figures 13–2, 13–3, 13–4, and 13–5 are drawn.

For Figures 13–2, 13–3, 13–4, and 13–5, the separate effects for early and late adolescence are given in Peskin and Livson (1981).

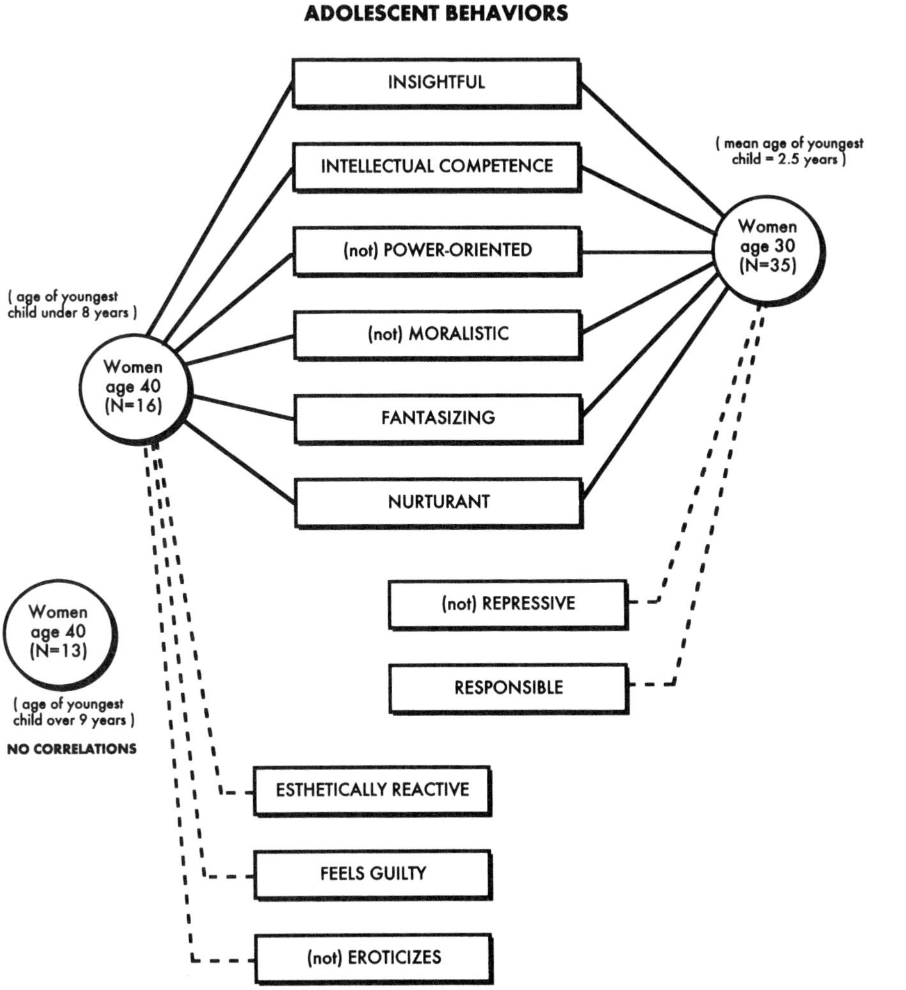

ADOLESCENT BEHAVIORS

Figure 13–3. Significant correlations of adolescent behavior and adult psychological health: women at age 30 and 40 with younger and older last-borns.

kind of rotation of parental labor, whereby the healthy father draws amply on past resources for active parenting as the healthy mother's need for such support from her past recedes.

We turn now to the older cohort of the OGS. Between ages 37 and 47, healthy men draw from adolescence affectively softer, generative, inward-seeking, and cognitive resources (Figure 13–4). Here is clear support for the development of the self in life's second half that substantiates a conceptual model positing the relevance of early life history for the healthful attainment of late-life goals. Our findings converge with those of Gutmann (1987; Florsheim & Gutmann, 1992) working with intrapsychic assessment methods (e.g., projective tests and mem-

Table 13–1. Relationship of Adolescent *Q*-Sorts to Psychological Health by Age of Last-Born

Guidance Study Men age 40			Oakland Growth Study Men age 47		
Q-sort dimensions			*Q*-sort dimensions		
	N	R		N	R
Younger (≤ 9 years)	12		Younger (≤ 13 years)	17	
Responsible		.70**	Responsible		.86****
(Not) somatizing		.59*	Nurturant		.71***
Moralistic		.57*	Esthetically reactive		.65***
Nurturant		.56*	Intellectually competent		.62***
Intellectually competent		.52*	Self-insightful		.57**
			(Not) power-oriented		.57**
Older (≥ 10 years)	14		Older (≥ 14 years)	17	
(Not) defensive		.74***	(Not) somatizing		.51**
Decisive		.65**			
Sex-appropriate		.64**			
Power-oriented		.59**			
Sociable		.58**			
Does not feel guilty		.53*			

*$p < .10$
**$p < .05$
***$p < .01$
****$p < .001$

ory), and thus make a yet stronger case for later-life psychodynamics. Like such intrapsychic measurements, behavioral evidence, if gathered longitudinally, also escapes the snares of superficial compliance and social correctness. In this regard, the contribution of our findings is to represent midlife interiority as actualizing later-life psychological health rather than as a normative lifespan change. Normative change is an indistinct, catch-all category that can subsume, mimic, or confound quite similar behaviors that are quite disparate in origin, aim, or meaning. For example, manifest passivity in males after the parental imperative can be read in such markedly different ways as healthful interiority and androgyny or aging disengagement. Distinguishing between these meanings can obviously be helped by ascertaining the psychological health of the manifestly passive adult. By comparing, as we do, healthy and unhealthy psychological adaptation within a same-age cohort, we seek to filter out such extraneous meanings as socialization to aging or aging itself, leaving intact Jung's and Gutmann's attribution of new vitality, rather than compliance or decline, to the postparental self.

Too few of the OGS males had arrived at postparenthood by age 47 to separate the effects of age from this last family stage. However, past–present correlations for fathers of older and younger last-born children (Table 13–1) suggest that early family stage is strongly associated with male interiority at midlife. Almost all of the significant findings of male interiority (Figure 13–4, left

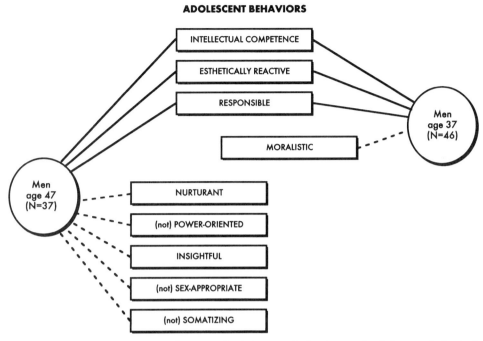

Figure 13–4. Significant correlations of adolescent behavior and adult psychological health: men at ages 37 and 47.

side, and Table 13–1) are attributable to fathers of younger children (age 13 and below). Fathers of older children show no apparent use of the past, which does not, of course, dispute the decline of active fathering in late or postparenthood. Rather, these findings indicate that interiority may be a vital aspect of active parenting in midlife, particularly evoked by younger children. Just as active parenting for younger fathers (age 40) may be drawn to (and by) the instrumental needs of older, more mature children, the active parenting of older fathers may be drawn to (and by) the nurturant needs of their smaller offspring. Such a relational—including parental—aspect of interiority (Lieberman & Peskin, 1992) has been rather overlooked in the literature, an offshoot perhaps of the failure to treat active parenting itself as a developmental line with age-specific expressions along the adult lifespan. Given that we are dealing here with parents who are psychologically healthy, relational interiority may represent a dimension that integrates rather than separates the first and second half of life. (In Jung's version [1933] of the second half of life, a relational interiority is indeed an oxymoron.) An overview of our findings leads then to this conjecture: that what makes up active parenting is constructed by the reciprocity of parental age and children's stage, so that each—age and stage—will seek out and be found by the other.

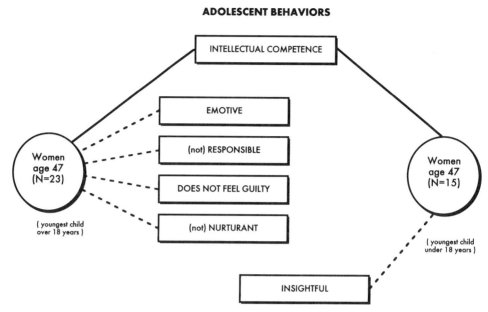

Figure 13–5. Significant correlations of adolescent behavior and adult psychological health: women at age 47 with youngest child older and younger than age 18.

The uses of the adolescent past in postparenthood could be investigated for the OGS women at age 47. When this cohort is partitioned by family stage (Figure 13–5), the postparenting women draw more from adolescence than those still in the late-parenting era, perhaps again an indication of women's role ambiguity when the parental function declines. Next, as Gutmann's model would predict, women whose last-born is over 18 years old seem now to have greater access to resources pertaining to personal autonomy that betoken the turn to the postparental and extrafamilial: In adolescence, they had been intellectually competent, emotive, not responsible, did not feel guilty, and were not nurturant.

Does counting the past statistically, in the way we have done, bear on recounting the past narrationally? Narration has at once a shared and a unique base that gives the listener a sense of understanding and the teller a sense of being understood. Significant statistical trends necessarily lose the unique differences within a cohort while capturing what its members share at a particular point in time. We propose, however, that our findings, by being based on multivariate methods, strike a balance between the opacity of sample averages and the nuances of life history. They "tell" the narrative of the cohort—of shared age, gender and family stage—in which the individual life history is currently embedded. Such shared age–stage narratives, in terms of how the adolescent past is used and transformed for present adaptation, seem distinctive for mothers of young children irrespective of mother's age; for mothers in postparenthood; for fathers, at age 40, of older children; for fathers, at age 47, of younger children.

Uses of the Past in Adult Psychological Health 311

Conversely, the past seems relatively opaque and unavailable for young men of age 30; for mothers of older children; for fathers, at age 40, of younger children; for fathers, age 47, of older children.

Uses of the Past at and after the Midlife Transition

For the third and most current IGS follow-up, we summarize analyses that underscore the past as a reserve for replenishing the older adult's thrust to experience current and future life fully. Our focus, of course, stays on past–present discontinuities, which Emde (1985) rightly considers our most important and provocative findings, because such results establish the adult-centered, uses-of-the-past orientation with more certainty. Discontinuity itself is a catch-all for findings that meet more or less rigorous tests of confidence. For example, the break in a continuous series of correlations by itself can be as much measurement error as evidence for discontinuity. But the reversal of findings from a positive to negative sign is more persuasive, especially if the variable in question is reliable and stable. It is in such reversals in the third follow-up that we are especially interested.

1. Since the second follow-up, behaviors that had previously predicted psychological health in one direction have switched significantly to the other direction. Healthy GS men at 40, it will be recalled, had drawn upon past resources of instrumental dispositions, much in keeping with becoming established in the world. Now at age 52, healthy GS men change this use of adolescence dramatically on three dimensions: They reject the appearance of masculinity in adolescence, favoring inner psychological states invested in fantasy and unconventional thinking. This use of adolescent inwardness at midlife is much like the OGS men's use of adolescence at age 47 (Figure 13–4) and again in line with midlife interiority posited by Jung, Gutmann, and Levinson. (Since most of the GS sample at age 52 are in postparenthood, a comparative analysis of early–late parenting with the OGS males could not be undertaken.)

2. The number of adolescent Q-sort predictors of psychological health at these later ages, removed from adolescence by yet 12 more years, remain at a level high enough to merit extending the uses of the adolescent past further into middle age. That is to say, there is no drop-off of statistical relationships with distance from adolescence, indicating that recency does not account for the findings. At age 52, the psychological health of GS males and females approximates the number of predictive items as the OGS male and female samples had shown at age 47. For the OGS males and females at age 60, the level of prediction approaches the number of predictive items yielded at age 37. It is worth noting that this count is based on the same computational procedure discussed earlier in regard to correcting for sleeper effects. Here, the statistical prediction of psychological health was honed to this third age (52 or 60) of follow-up by holding constant, i.e., removing the possible confounding effects of psychological health scores from the preceding two adult follow-ups.

3. With additional follow-ups, the predictors of later psychological health

could be broadened to include early adult behavior along with adolescent behavior. Since the uses-of-the-past model gives priority to relevance rather than to timing alone, the model is strengthened if the remote adolescent antecedents neither reduce nor are reduced (or washed away) by early adult antecedents. The actual timing of experience should not then be decisive to the ease of its recovery. Moreover, including recent predictors might add way stations to help identify the transformative processes that bring the past into harmony with current purpose.

We proceeded to calculate multiple correlations of psychological health at age 52 for GS and at age 60 for OGS using now three predictors: early adolescence, late adolescence, and the first adult follow-up (30 for GS; 37 for OGS). (Again, the confounding influence of the preceding adult age was removed by partialing.) The early adult predictor did not reduce or replace the contribution of the adolescent predictors but tended overall to increase prediction by its inclusion. What Cohler (Chapter 11, this volume) and Nemiroff and Colarusso (1990) assert from clinical observation clearly pertains to our own findings: that the importance of youth neither diminishes nor is diminished by the importance of adulthood.

4. The inclusion of early adult predictors also helped to delineate a more complex causal chain over the first half of life. The most compelling example of such complexity was the large yield of predictive reversals between and among the three predictors of psychological health at age 60. For men, these reversals enlisted all three predictors. For example, a highly significant prediction of health at age 60 followed from this sequence of antecedents: dependability in early adolescence, undependability in late adolescence, and dependability again at age 37. Other examples include undefensive in early adolescence, defensive in late adolescence, and undefensive again at age 37; productive in early adolescence, unproductive in late adolescence, productive again at age 37. For women, reversals involved two predictors of psychological health at age 60, for example, submissive in late adolescence and unsubmissive at age 37; lacking autonomy in late adolescence and autonomous at age 37; reluctant to act in late adolescence, not reluctant to act at age 37. Note in these findings that late adolescence contributes to the prediction of psychological health by the expression of seeming problematic behaviors, for example, undependable, defensive, and unproductive for males; submissive, inautonomous, and reluctant to act for females. Here, one may sense the experimental enactments of a negative identity—Erikson's (1950) moratorium—during late adolescence that are relinquished in early adulthood.

Opposite Uses of the Past in Later Adulthood

Reversal effects offer no simple interpretation as might be possible for single predictors. The abundance of reversals at age 60 draws our attention to the relation of such transformations to aging. We wonder, for example, whether the past at this time does not so much yield up fresh resources for late-age mental health as it allows equal access to once discordant (e.g., submissive–autonomous) facets of personality and the opportunity for new transformative experience. More than any of our findings, the drawing on the opposites of a behavior strongly suggests a "bundle of transformations" rather than an "inventory of elements" (Piaget, 1970). Taking from opposite poles of a behavior may reveal the more complex and necessarily less orderly origins of psychological health in late middle age. Lomranz's (Chapter 10, this volume) concept of "aintegration" nicely captures the beneficial welter of this bundling. The reversals of our later-age samples suggest that *having a past* now consists not only of a capacity to expand and use one's inventory of past elements but also to recruit and reconfigure elements that have been kept apart. The older adult may call upon such more complex use of the past in order to revise long-held internalizations (Loewald, 1980a) for the present and for the impending future of late age.

RELATIONAL AUTONOMY IN LATER ADULTHOOD

Autonomy and relatedness, surely developmental antonyms in adolescence and early adulthood, may be the most far-reaching of late-life "aintegrations." Autonomy in the first half of life, especially in the independence seeking of youth and young adulthood, is normatively situated in the psychic distancing and separation from family, whereas striving for autonomy in late adulthood is essentially relational, situated in object choices within the social network of generational and intergenerational role responsibilities, entitlements, and attachments. Especially in the elderly, such autonomy may also include choosing for oneself on whom to depend. In the later years, separating in order to establish selfhood may itself take on a relational quality in realigning primary relationships rather than in detaching from them. The older adult seeks, then, to sustain or recoup autonomy within the very family arena where his or her autonomy has also been thwarted. For psychoanalysis, this capacity of *related autonomy* (Lieberman & Peskin, 1992) acknowledges a new integration, arising late in the lifespan, that rectifies the uncompromising elements of the original Oedipal dynamics in a manner that was unavailable to the younger adult still locked in conflict with them. This capacity may offer the older adult opportunity for rediscovery of resources in the past that had been lost in the competitive family tumult of the first half of life. With such a capacity, it is the older adult, contra Freud, who can confront Oedipal issues with new cogency to transcend the conflict between Oedipal ambition and attachment. A psychoanalytic psychology of late life would posit this emergence of Oedipal resolution that allows the individual wider boundaries of self-exploration.

Clinical observations of this late-life capacity are not commonplace. Indeed, beyond the concept of androgyny, this capacity in late life for new integrations of conflictual elements is relatively unacknowledged. Rather, the domains of relatedness and personal autonomy in late life tend to remain at odds as before. The Jungian-based ethos in adult development tends to situate the full expression of the self outside the relational sphere of mutual responsibilities and human interdependency. Indeed, most theorists (Erikson, of course, is a notable exception) view the relational sphere in late life as diminishing, whether from a Jungian base of increased introversion, interiority, or disengagement, or from a Freudian base of strengthened (or threatened) narcissism. That the parental imperative severs relatedness and selfhood into the first half/second half of life has become a forceful tenet of adult development. But as we have indicated, our findings (Table 13–1) suggest that this split may be too absolute: For the older (age 47) fathers of younger children, resources of selfhood may actually enhance and be enhanced by the parenting function. It may well be that older parents are capable of integrations less available to younger parents (like the GS men at age 40).

In the psychoanalysis of older patients, the emergence of this capacity may be more apparent. Several clinical vignettes suggest the concept:

• A patient's long-standing disdain for her late mother was considerably moderated after the patient's menopause had begun. From then on, the patient could allow that her mother may have envied her, hence admired her, for achievements in youth and adolescence. Here, competitiveness and attachment, kept apart in the early adulthood of Oedipal-related envy and guilt, came together in a way that culminated in a dream of the patient longing to tell the dead mother about entering menopause (Bemesderfer, 1996; Peskin, 1995).

Menopause too has become a stage for the second acts and second chances of late life to shed species responsibilities, so that the women can come to be, as Ursula LeGuin (1990) put it, "pregnant with herself." How different from the Freudian-based view of menopause as irrefutable loss of femininity, itself founded on an infantile sense of inferiority. For the latter view, then, menopause is an atrophy of development; for the former, it is a trophy. But in either case, late life finds no new way back to the past. For the former, the early past contains the familiar Jungian irrelevance; for the latter, it continues the familiar Freudian inexorability. The capacity for late-life integrations of past and present proposes a third position that sets aside the polarized competition between exclusive child- and adult-oriented positions. In our rendition of Bemesderfer's (1996) case, such integration allowed the patient to recover seeming opposite resources from the past long lost in the lifeless relationship to the mother.

• Loeward himself (1980b), in introducing his well-known paper on the waning of the Oedipus complex, honors his mentors by sharing credit with them for his original contributions to psychoanalytic theory. The younger patient, whose case the article goes on to cite, presents a sharp contrast to Loewald's own integration of exceeding yet staying attached to his teachers. The patient remains in the grip of the young adult's Oedipal conflict, wishing yet fearing father's defeat in the same intellectual field as the patient. Between Loewald and his patient is the contrast of lifespan narratives on the use of the past in Oedipal resolution. For the younger patient, relatedness to father threatens his autonomous standing as an independent scholar; for the older analyst, a step forward in autonomy brings him yet closer to his mentors. While the young adult supplants the father, the older adult succeeds him.

- Kernberg's (1980) discussion of normal narcissism in middle age addresses the capacity of the healthy adult to draw on the childhood past for overcoming envy when others have more than oneself. Middle-age envy for lost youthfulness is mitigated by one's capacity in childhood and elsewhere to have enjoyed the older person's good fortune, and now, in older age, to return to oneself this enjoyment of youth's good fortune.

OBJECTIVE, HISTORICAL, AND NARRATIVE VOICES IN LIFESPAN DEVELOPMENT

The scientific weakness of the classical linear model should encourage not only ahistorical alternatives, but also stronger interest in the innumerable ways that the actual past figures in our lives. Obviously, the three ways—the linear, transformational and uses-of-the-past models—presented in this chapter are not exhaustive, but rather exemplars in a wide span of more nuanced possibilities. The past as being reworkable threads through all three voices of the objective, historical, and narrative. The greatest allowance for recasting the past is reserved, of course, for narrative, since the suspension of disbelief is its essential nature. The reworkable past is an idea that does not come so ready-made for the objective voice of longitudinal study or the historical voice of psychoanalytic theory. At their inception, neither voice had made conceptual provision for the past as a changing reserve for present and future life. In psychoanalysis, we see the idea cogently fought for and hard won in both Erikson's (1950) concept of identity and in Loewald's (1980a) view of internalization and therapeutic change, where adult development goes hand in hand with recasting the actual past under the impctus of personal relationships. Similarly, it has been the aim of our research to free objective longitudinal study from its conventional service to the fixed linear model only. As our statistical juxtaposing of genetic models in this chapter has demonstrated, longitudinal study proves to be surprisingly versatile and hardly restricted to uncovering an unalterable past—given appropriate multivariate method and a rich enough assessment of multiple adult ages.

Freud's disclaimer (1920) of any higher knowledge of historical reality beyond what memory could recover is a sobering reminder that longitudinal prediction has had no privileged status in the validation of psychoanalytic theory. Far from it, given Freud's astonishing certainty that confirmation must come from historical reconstructions. One can imagine Freud saying about predictive research what he once said on the occasion of being sent an empirical doctoral dissertation proving the existence of repression: "*Ganz amerikanish.*"

Yet, also *ganz narrisch* (entirely nonsensical) are those theories and therapies of narrative that would cavalierly "retrofit" past to present, slighting the critical, even if elusive differences between telling and fictionalizing a life story. Between one's past as actually lived experience and one's past as an invention of one's projections lies the existential stuff of literature and psychoanalysis. Indeed, it often seems to be the chief occupation of literature—from Doonesbury to Othello—to plot what lures us to forget the distinction between the actual and the invented past. (From comedy, we take Gary Trudeau's wonderful strip in which Mike Doonesbury is chastising Zonker for embellishing the past beyond anything that really happened in their youth. Zonker, sedatively and blithely self-exempted from the real world, replies, "We're not getting any younger Mike. You gotta grab the past while you can.")

The embellishment of the unalterable facts of life doubtless drives the mechanisms of both neurosis and creative psychological health. In our research, adolescent data longitudinally collected, however, make the case not for the retrofitted embellishment of the past, but rather for the use of past experience as existing in a realm outside of one's personal control. It is indeed the power of longitudinal study that its data do exist outside of such control. It is not like a half-finished painting that, still wet, can always be touched up (to borrow Hofstadter's [1996] felicitous image for George Sand's forgeries of her old letters), but an unretouchable one ("as in old letters ... already lived ... and understood" [Rilke, 1996]) whose intrinsic worth can be more fully known, accepted, and used for the very reason that it is allowed to survive outside of one's self-fulfilling omnipotence. (More than once have our objective data been mistaken for adults' recollections of their adolescence.) Owning one's past in the sense of possessiveness is, therefore, supplanted by owning up to one's past, in the sense of granting it a fuller—more objective, complex, and autonomous—voice. The life review of late adulthood, as rendered by Butler (1963), is of such an accountable rather than convenient past, but no less deeply owned. Our results pertaining to the statistical reversals of past usage in later adulthood likewise point to the maturing of a more complex holding of the past. Indeed, we wonder whether the three voices of the past converge in late adulthood as never before. Our formulations here treat the past much as Winnicott (1969) treated object development: from an initial state of omnipotent control of the mother ("object relating") to the capacity to use ("object usage") the mother once she comes to survive and exist for the child outside of its control. Like the mother, the past comes to be owned no longer only as a mirror; rather, its unalterable autonomy prompts the child to reach for more complex relations with it.

While openly skeptical of what we now call narrative truth, Freud (1920, 1937a) recognized that it might come closer to the psychic reality of historical truth than to objective truth, for actual longitudinal knowledge simply could not foretell toward which direction the patient's life would turn. Near the end of his life, Freud (1937a) implied another consequence of this linkage between the historical and narrative voice: that the historical might be alterable after all, with fresh recoveries of the past in the wake of new and unforeseen "active conflicts" of adult life. This may have been Freud's friendliest, if short-lived, brush with adult development, with the past as multifaceted, nonlinear, and likely capable of being remembered veridically. As Strachey indicates in his editorial notes, Freud did not return to this idea that would surely have placed the classical dominance of the (psychosexual) past in jeopardy. We would like to think that our findings pointing to the uses of the actual past for adult purpose expand on Freud's abandoned idea by suggesting that the second half of life organizes and shepherds new resources from the past for the healthy emergence of selfhood, much as infantile sexuality is organized for the psychosexual purposes of the first half. Perhaps if we knew what resources Freud at age 81 called on from his past to originate and then to abandon this nascent idea, we might have a better sense of the active conflicts in his own late life over the future of psychoanalysis after him and without him.

REFERENCES

Bemesderfer, S. (1996). A revised psychoanalytic view of menopause. *Journal of the American Psychoanalytic Association*, *44*, 351–369. (Suppl. [Female Psychology]).

Benedek, T. (1959). Parenthood as a developmental phase. *Journal of the American Psychoanalytic Association*, *7*, 389–417.

Butler, R. (1963). The life review: An interpretation of reminiscence in the aged. *Psychiatry*, *26*, 65–76.

Cohler, B. (1980). Developmental perspectives on the psychology of the self in early childhood. In A. Goldberg (Ed.), *Advances in self psychology* (pp. 69–115). New York: International Universities Press.

Cohler, B., & Galatzer-Levy, R. (1990). Self, meaning, and morale across the second half of life. In R. Nemiroff & C. Colarusso (Eds.), *New dimensions in adult development* (pp. 214– 260). New York: Basic Books.

Costa, P., & McCrae, R. (1994). Stability and change in personality from adolescence through adulthood. In C. Halverson, G. Kohnstamm, & R. Martin (Eds.), *The developing structure of temperament and personality from infancy to adulthood* (pp. 139–150). Hillsdale, NJ: Erlbaum.

Eichorn, D., Clausen, J., Haan, N., Honzik, M., & Mussen, P. (Eds.). (1981). *Present and past in middle life*. New York: Academic Press.

Emde, R. (1985). From adolescence to midlife: Remodeling the structure of adult development. *Journal of the American Psychoanalytic Association*, *33*, 59–105.

Erikson, E. (1950). *Childhood and society*. New York: Norton.

Florsheim, P., & Gutmann, D. (1992). Mourning the loss of "self as father": A longitudinal study of fatherhood among the Druze. *Psychiatry*, *55*, 160–176.

Freud, S. (1905). On psychotherapy. In J. Strachey (Ed. & Trans.), *The standard edition of the complete psychological works of Sigmund Freud* (Vol. 7, pp. 255–268). London: Hogarth Press.

Freud, S. (1920). The psychogenesis of a case of homosexuality in a woman. In J. Strachey (Ed. & Trans.), *The standard edition of the complete psychological works of Sigmund Freud* (Vol. 18, pp. 145–172). London: Hogarth Press.

Freud, S. (1937a). Constructions in analysis. In J. Strachey (Ed. & Trans.), *The standard edition of the complete psychological works of Sigmund Freud* (Vol. 23, pp. 255–270). London: Hogarth Press.

Freud, S. (1937b). Analysis terminable and interminable. In J. Strachey (Ed. & Trans.), *The standard edition of the complete psychological works of Sigmund Freud* (Vol. 23, pp. 209–254). London: Hogarth Press.

Gutmann, D. (1987). *Reclaimed powers*. New York: Basic Books.

Hofstadter, D. (1996). *The love affair as a work of art*. New York: Farrar, Straus & Giroux.

Jaques, E. (1965). Death and the mid-life crisis. *International Journal of Psychoanalysis*, *46*, 502–514.

Jung, C. (1933). The stages of life. In C. Jung (Ed.), *Modern man in search of a soul*. New York: Harcourt, Brace & World.

Kagan, J., & Moss, H. (1962). *Birth to maturity*. New York: Wiley.

Kernberg, O. (1980). Normal narcissism in middle age. In O. Kernberg (Ed.), *Internal world and external reality* (pp. 121–134). New York: Aronson.

LeGuin, U. (1990). The space crone. In R. Formanek (Ed.), *The meanings of menopause* (pp. i–xxv). Hillsdale, NJ: Analytic Press.

Levinson, D., Darrow, G., Klein, E., Levinson, M., & McKee, B. (1978). *The season of a man's life*. New York: Knopf.

Lieberman, M., & Peskin, N. (1992). Adult life crises. In J. Birren, R. Sloan, & G. Cohen (Eds.), *Handbook of mental health and aging* (pp. 119–143). New York: Academic Press.

Livson, N., & Peskin, H. (1967). The prediction of adult psychological health in a longitudinal study. *Journal of Abnormal Psychology, 72*, 509–518.

Livson, N., & Peskin, H. (1980). Perspectives on adolescence from longitudinal research. In J. Adelson (Ed.), *Handbook of adolescent psychology* (pp. 47–98). New York: Wiley.

Loewald, H. (1980a). On internalization. In H. Loewald (Ed.), *Papers on psychoanalysis* (pp. 69–86). New Haven, CT: Yale University Press.

Loewald, H. (1980b). The waning of the Oedipus complex. In H. Loewald (Ed.), *Papers on psycho-analysis* (pp. 384–404). New Haven, CT: Yale University Press.

Nemiroff, R., & Colarusso, C. (1990). Frontiers of adult development in theory and practice (pp. 97–124). In R. Nemiroff & C. Colarusso (Eds.), *New dimensions in adult development*. New York: Basic Books.

Neugarten, P. (1968). Adult personality: Towards a psychology of the life cycle. In P. Neugarten (Ed.), *Middle age and aging* (pp. 137–147). Chicago: University of Chicago Press.

Peskin, H. (1967). Pubertal onset and ego functioning. *Journal of Abnormal Psychology, 72*, 1–15.

Peskin, H. (1972). Multiple prediction of adult psychological health from preadolescent and adolescent behavior. *Journal of Consulting and Clinical Psychology, 38*, 155–160.

Peskin, H. (1973). Influence of the developmental schedule of puberty on learning and ego functioning. *Journal of Youth and Adolescence, 2*, 273–290.

Peskin, H. (1987). Uses of the past in the adult lifespan. In G. Maddox & E. Busse (Eds.), *Aging: The universal human experience* (pp. 432–440). New York: Springer.

Peskin, H. (1995). Discussion of "A revised psychoanalytic view of menopause" by S. Bemesderfer. San Francisco Psychoanalytic Institute. Unpublished.

Peskin, H., & Livson, N. (1981). Uses of the past in adult psychological health. In D. Eichorn, J. Clausen, N. Haan, M. Honzik, & P. Mussen (Eds.), *Present and past in middle life* (pp. 153–181). New York: Academic Press.

Piaget, J. (1970). Structural analysis in the social sciences. In C. Maschler (Ed. & Trans.), *Structuralism* (pp. 97–119). New York: Basic Books.

Pollock, G. (1961). Mourning and adaptation. *International Journal of Psychoanalysis, 42*, 341–361.

Rilke, R. (1996). *Rilke's book of hours*. New York: Riverhead.

Schafer, R. (1983). *The analytic attitude*. New York: Basic Books.

Spence, D. (1982). *Narrative truth and historical truth*. New York: Norton.

Winnicott, D. (1969). The use of an object. *International Journal of Psychoanalysis, 50*, 711–716.

PART V

The Family in Later Life

Family relations are a vital aspect of life in old age and largely determine the mental health and quality of life of the elderly. The late-life family is almost unknown territory that only recently is receiving the attention it merits in gerontological research. There is an urgent need to develop research and conceptual guidelines. The discrepant findings and unresolved questions in this field may be attributable to theoretical and methodological shortcomings. Never before have families been as heavily populated with older persons, and familial relationships—including multigenerational ones—last longer than in any previous period in history (Aizenberg & Treas, 1985). However, the various rapid, multidimensional, cultural changes, including those in norms and societal roles, have as great an impact. These may all be potential sources of stress and mental illness. The chapters in Part V address these aspects and cogent research needs in the field as well as their mental health implications.

Pearlin and Skaff (Chapter 14) map out and interrelate cogent stressors to which the late-life family is potentially exposed and the modes with which these may be theoretically dealt. They discuss the structural interconnectedness of conceptual constructs from a number of perspectives: the stress process, role theory and sociocultural organizations, and life-course theory. The authors attempt to develop perspectives for the study of family stress in late life and thus analyze the context of the stress process in the triple framework of interactions within the family, interactions outside the family boundaries, and with the family as a mobilizer of support, resources, and coping. Pearlin and Skaff explicate how structural forms, role composition, social and economic circumstances, and biological imperatives of aging all interplay and influence late-life family trajectories. They specify the interpersonal dynamics of family role sets and trace their interrelated effects with the contextual circumstances of such dynamics. They elaborate the notions of "stress proliferation," and "moderating resources," the dialectics of conflict and caring, and the differentiation in the concept of support. Pearlin and Skaff explicate the various aspects of the marital role set, the parent–child role set, the transfer of external stressors to the family interior, and the family as a possible source of support and buffer to mental illness. The authors propose conceptual guidelines that can be followed in delineating inside and outside origins of stress (see Silver, Chapter 17). Their novel approach is a dual one: They attempt to comprehend how the characteristics of the stress process can provide an understanding of the elderly in the family and how the family dynamics can generate stress, as well as integrating these two aspects. This approach leads them to present a number of cogent family, late-life issues that have not yet been properly investigated.

Interpersonal relationships are foundations to mental health. Relationships in old age (Hansson & Carpenter, 1994) in general and in the family in particular are crucial. Unfortunately, we lack evidence that relates attachment theory to the mental health of elderly family members. Cicirelli (Chapter 15), responding to this scientific void, investigates the effects of adult attachment on mental health in the aging family. Attachment theory (Bowlby, 1969) captures both the personal and the interpersonal elements of human behavior and, as Cicirelli notes in his thorough review, can enhance the explanation of adult behavior. Beginning from the cornerstones of mental health and the characteristics of the aging family, through the evolution of attachment as a life-span concept, Cicirelli leads the reader to his seven formulated propositions, which, theoretically and methodologically, imply a link between aging family attachments and mental health. The experience of the aging family calls for continuous adaptation to change and adds specific implications to the dynamics of attachment, which will include unique characteristics such as developmental tasks, lifelong attachment histories, and multigenerational contexts (see Lieberman, Chapter 16). The propositions Circirelli formulates expand the relevancy of attachment theory based on his analysis of the characteristics of adult attachment. That analysis includes the concepts of secondary attachments, multiple attachments, hierarchical attachments, and reciprocal attachment (see Peskin's concept of "relational autonomy" in Chapter 13) in the family system, shifts and mix of attachment styles—all of which capture and convey the ongoing processes, intricacies, dynamics, and complexity of attachment as it develops and changes as people grow old. When thus characterized, attachment in later life certainly has implications for the quality of living and mental health of the elderly in his family. Research as well as psychotherapeutic implications are an integral part of Cicirelli's chapter.

Lieberman (Chapter 16) claims that macrotheories and sociological approaches dominate family studies, and that these, while valuable, are not helpful in selecting specific variables and in hypothesis testing on the level of midrange family approaches. His work attempts to do just this; he has developed a framework for studying the role of the multigenerational family in coping with the chronic illness of one of its members. Lieberman focuses on a general model and its measurement strategies. A review of the field discloses that there are scant empirical data available on (1) the specific family characteristics that affect the management of elderly ill, (2) how the demand characteristics of different chronic diseases affect families differently, (3) how family ethnicity/culture affects these processes, and (4) what standard should be utilized to assess effective family management of disease. The author reports on his research project that endeavored to shed light on these questions. Family functioning and how it affects the course of the illness of the elderly within the family is investigated in relation to four areas: (1) *Worldview*, shared values of the family;

(2) family *structure and organization*; (3) the family's methods of *regulating emotions*; and (4) the family's strategies of *problem solving and decision making*. The specific variables in each of these areas are related to the course of illness, functional decisions, service use, well-being, strain, health, family system, and characteristics and functioning of the total multigenerational family. Lieberman emphasizes the differences between families and the consequences of these differences for Alzheimer patients. While the major focus of most research until now has been on aspects of the primary caregiver, Lieberman also investigates the total multigenerational impact in a novel conceptual and methodological manner. His findings suggest that the multigenerational family's management of the elderly ill has a powerful and consistent impact over time. This work contributes to the development of family-based therapeutic interventions by suggesting new techniques and models of intervention. Finally, Lieberman provides a unique contribution to applications of family concepts to intergenerational families with ill members.

The fact that most research on the aging family has been culturally bound has limited the generalizability of theoretical statements and research findings, and has restricted the formulation of conceptual questions in this important area. The cross-cultural work of Silver (Chapter 17) reduces these limitations as it sheds light on the cogent issues of attitudes toward family responsibility, aging, and well-being in later life on the basis of a broad, life-span (ranging from ages 18 to 92) study of aging in Japan and the United States.

Silver's work explores how the Self of the elderly is culturally organized through prescriptive norms, categorizations, ideologies, and historical circumstances, how structural positions shape the Self, and how the links between theoretical and methodological assumptions affect the meaning and scope of research findings. The meaning of important concepts and processes (such as norms of familial and economic responsibility toward aging parents, familial identity, familial and social obligations, lifelong friendships, autonomy, individuality, attachment, sacrifice, satisfaction with society, personal and social well-being, the image of aging, and desirable ways of living in old age) can all be differentiated and illuminated through cross-cultural perspectives. This work—drawing upon a variety of sociological, cultural, and psychological conceptualizations, and reflecting methodological caution and sophistication as well as contextualization, value, and language analysis—is able to analyze the tension between emotional caring and social isolation, thus providing a better understanding of well-being and images, sometimes contradictory, of aging. Silver demonstrates that beneath the image of older people conforming to normative expectations, there is a layer of needs and feelings that go counter to existing social norms (see Hazan, Kegan and Lomranz, Chapters 8–10, respectively). The author presents theoretical formulations involving a micro–macro synthesis as interrelations of the family context with other social institutions, norms, and values. Silver suggests that the older person's marginalization leads to social and emotional withdrawal from younger generations, yet the high levels of satisfaction point to an emergent transcultural sense of Self among older people in modern society. Silver's work challenges the definition of aging as a linear process of deterioration, loss, and depression, as well as the idealization of aging, and facilitates alternative aging models.

REFERENCES

Aizenberg, R., & Treas, J. (1985). The family in late life: Psychosocial and demographic considerations. In J. Birren & W. Schaie (Eds.), *Handbook of the psychology of aging* (pp. 169–189). New York: Van Nostrand Reinhold.
Bowlby, J. (1969). *Attachment and loss: Vol. 1. Attachment.* New York: Basic Books.
Hansson, R., & Carpenter, B. (1994). *Relationships in old age.* New York: Guilford.

CHAPTER 14

Perspectives on the Family and Stress in Late Life

LEONARD I. PEARLIN AND MARILYN M. SKAFF

INTRODUCTION

This chapter is organized around what we regard as the three principal functions of the family within the context of the stress process. First, the family is an arena in which stressors are generated by the problematic interactions of its members. Second, in their multiple social roles outside the family boundaries, family members may encounter problems that impact adversely on relationships and activities within the family. Third, the family is a social group able to mobilize resources in support of its members as they contend with life problems, regardless of the source of the problems (Pearlin & Turner, 1987).

The family, of course, is not a static entity. Its composition, its inner life, and the social and economic circumstances surrounding it are in a constant state of change and development as its members move across the life course. Among these changes are the stressors it confronts and the resources it is able to muster. Necessarily, then, a comprehensive examination of the functions of the aging family in the stress process needs to be located within a life-course framework (Elder, George, & Shanahan, 1996).

Because relatively few studies are directly aimed at illuminating the stressful circumstances surrounding the family life of older people, our discussions are not as fully based on empirically established knowledge as we would like. There is a fairly substantial body of research that, while not directly concerned with the issues considered in this chapter, has implications for them. Where appropriate, we draw freely from this research. On balance, however, this chapter is less a review of the somewhat limited knowledge of exposure to difficult

LEONARD I. PEARLIN AND MARILYN M. SKAFF • Department of Sociology, University of Maryland, College Park, Maryland 20742-1315.

Handbook of Aging and Mental Health: An Integrative Approach, edited by Jacob Lomranz. Plenum Press, New York, 1998.

life conditions of older family members than an effort to develop perspectives for the study of family stress in the later stages of the life course.

Any exploration of social stress and its processes, we submit, must eventually turn its attentions to the family. More than any other social institution, the family stands at the critical junctures of the stress process. It is the site of intense experiences and of highly emotionally charged attachments of considerable duration; it is the institution that binds people to both preceding and succeeding generations (Bengtson, Rosenthal, & Burton, 1990), and it provides much of the meaning and many of the markers of life-course change (George, 1996). Moreover, as we discuss in greater detail throughout this chapter, the family can be the setting out of which severe stressors surface, the arena in which many of the stressors arising outside its borders are acted upon and negotiated, and, finally, the place where people may find the strength and the means to confront their problems without damage to their own well-being and to move forward with their lives. Although family conflict is surprisingly rare or ephemeral in light of the rich opportunities for its occurrence, when it does surface, its effects can be highly distressing. Because family relationships typically occupy an emotionally central place in people's lives, their conflictual disruption can be powerfully stressful.

Despite the broad interest in the family by social scientists, including both stress and life-course researchers, there is a good deal of ambiguity as to what the family is and how it is best studied (e.g., Fisher, 1982). A detailed discussion of these issues would carry us astray. However, it should be noted that a number of family forms that are now quite prominent were in earlier years far less common. Familiar examples include the increasing number of families comprised of children and a single parent, or of blended or merged families, those where parties to a second marriage bring their respective children into the same household (Johnson & Barer, 1987). These kinds of changes can create confusion not only for researchers whose conceptions of the family have not kept pace with their structural variety, but also for all of the present and former relatives who need to restructure their identifications and behaviors. As we discuss later, reconstituted families can create role ambiguity for the grandparental generation where there may be few standards that would guide this restructuring.

In addition to the variety of their forms, their composition, and their role differentiations, the study of families is complicated by differences in their social and cultural backgrounds and their economic resources. These kinds of differences are particularly evident when we observe the hardships and challenges people face as they enact their family roles (Turner, Wheaton, & Lloyd, 1995). Thus, advanced age and the stressors it entails are very different for people whose economic welfare is assured than for those who must engage in economic brinkmanship. We know, too, that social class has a pervasive effect on the relationships and interactions among family members. For example, fathers in middle-class occupations are likely to value independence and foster self-direction in their children, while working-class men place greater emphasis on obedience and are more likely to employ physical discipline (Kohn, 1969). All in all, then, the social, cultural, and economic characteristics of family members need to be taken into account in detecting the stressors to which people are exposed and in observing the quality of their transactions.

What we wish to emphasize in this discussion is that the structural forms and role composition of families and the social and economic circumstances in which they are embedded can influence the life-course trajectories of families and their members. These kinds of influences, along with the biological imperatives of aging, make the family, the interactions among its members, and the challenges that confront them highly dynamic and differentiated. It is understandable that the study of the family and its relationships can entail a number of complexities, some of which may not be consistently recognized. In large measure, we believe, these complexities reflect the richness of family life and the subtle and manifold ways in which its interconnections with the larger society influence the well-being of family members.

A BRIEF REVIEW OF THE STRESS PROCESS

Throughout this chapter we make frequent reference to the stress process. We have written extensively on the conceptual framework underlying this process, and here, we only address its major features (e.g., Pearlin, 1989; Pearlin, Lieberman, Menaghan, & Mullan, 1981). First, as the term *process* implies, the stress process framework treats stress not simply as a response to a noxious stimulus, but as involving a number of closely interrelated circumstances such that a change in one results in a change in others.

A driving element of the process entails *stressors*, which refer to conditions that put to test the adaptive capacities of individuals. Stressors may be in the form of life events, changes that have clear temporal origins, or they may reside in the enduring and threatening conditions of daily life. With regard to eventful stressors, some are closely tied to the life cycle and its transitions, such as marriage, the birth of children, the advent of grandparenthood, retirement, widowhood, and the deaths of age peers. These events are highly predictable and, typically, represent situations for which we are socialized (George, 1993; Pearlin, 1982). For this reason, perhaps, their consequences are usually not deleterious (Pearlin & Lieberman, 1979), although they may certainly impose the need for restructuring activities and relationships. In general, events that are unexpected are more stressful than those that are scheduled (Thoits, 1983). Examples of events for which there is little or no socialized expectation include the death of a child, involuntary job loss, one's own divorce or that of one's child, or the "premature" death of a spouse. The repercussions of such "unscheduled" events can be quite severe and exert adverse effects on well-being (Pearlin & Lieberman, 1979).

The more enduring stressors can grow out of a variety of life domains, including problematic aspects of daily roles, such as job, friendships, marriage, or parenthood (Pearlin, 1983; Wheaton, 1995). There is some indication that the more importance individuals attach to the role or status in which the stressors arise, the greater will be its stressful impact (Krause, 1994). It is well documented, too, that emergent roles, such as those involving long-term care-giving, can be a source of enduring stress (Aneshensel, Pearlin, Mullan, Zarit, & Whitlatch, 1995; George & Gwyther, 1986; Pearlin, Mullan, Semple, & Skaff, 1990; Zarit, Orr, & Zarit, 1985). And, we suspect, chronic stressors may also be linked to disparities between the goals to which people are driven and their movement toward the achievement of the goals. It will be noted that these examples pertain to stressors that arise out of social and economic life and do not include idiosyncratic and randomly occurring stressors, like the hapless person struck by lightning. Such stressors may indeed be important to individuals, but they are of limited interest to scholars primarily concerned with stressors that surface within the context of major institutional roles.

Two aspects of eventful and chronic stressors are of special relevance to aging and the life course. One is that stressors, whether eventful or chronic, tend to generate other stressors. Divorce, for example, may lead to a serious reduction in economic resources (Pearlin & Johnson, 1977), involuntary job loss may result in marital conflict (Pearlin et al., 1981), or the engulfing demands of a caregiving role may result in problems at work (Pearlin, Aneshensel, & LeBlanc, 1997). In each instance, and there are many more examples that can be offered, there is a contagion of stress, where an initial stressor gives rise to additional stressors. Once established, these secondary stressors, as we refer to them, can be at least as potent as the initial or primary stressors. We use the term *stress proliferation* to describe the process whereby constellations of secondary stressors may be generated by those that are primary.

The array of stressors that occurs and proliferates at one point of the life course may be quite different from those that appear at later points. To a substantial extent, therefore, we cannot derive an accurate picture of the demands and stressors of later life by projecting forward those that were observed to be present at an earlier point (Pearlin & Skaff, 1996). One of the challenges of stress research is linking changes in the stressors to which people are exposed to the changing conditions of life as people age (Pearlin & Skaff, 1996). As indicated earlier, this task is further complicated by the fact that life-course changes are not only the consequence of increased age but also of the interplay of age with social and economic statuses of individuals. Concretely, we can assert that the configurations of stressors across the life course will vary for men and women, for professional workers and manual workers, for the rich and poor, and so on. There are multiple pathways to late life, and the stressors people encounter depend substantially on the paths they are traversing (Dannefer, 1987).

Another major component of the stress process concerns *outcomes*. Outcomes refer to the effects of stressors, especially effects that indicate some adverse consequence of exposure to the stressors. The outcomes typically considered are those reflecting on individuals' mental or physical health, although gerontologists also examine such outcomes as life satisfaction, quality of life, or "successful aging" (Baltes & Baltes, 1990). The status characteristics of people may influence the ways in which they exhibit outcomes, just as they influence the stressors to which they are exposed. To illustrate, there is evidence that depression is a more common outcome among women than men, while among men, stress is expressed more frequently in alcohol abuse and aggressive behavior (Aneshensel, Rutter, & Lachenbruch, 1991).

The final component of the stress process to be discussed in this brief overview concerns *moderating resources*. It is typically the case that people exposed to the same stressors are not affected by them to the same extent: Some may appear to escape being harmed, and others to be seriously damaged. This may be because people exposed to the same primary stressors are embedded in different secondary stressors. But it may also be a result of possessing different resources that function to minimize the negative impact of the stressors (Pearlin, 1991). Coping repertoires, protective self-concepts, and—of critical relevance to older people—social support are among the resources that are considered to be able to moderate the otherwise harmful effects of stressors. Again, the status characteristics of people may be associated with their access to effective resources.

The stress process, then, provides a useful conceptual framework for observing the critical conditions and experiences of family members across the life course and for interpreting variations in the impact of these conditions and experiences on their well-being. In this chapter, we make frequent reference to elements of this process as we focus on individuals within the contexts of their family life.

THE FAMILY AS A SOURCE OF STRESS

It is useful to think of the family as comprised of multiple role sets (Merton, 1957). The notion of role set calls attention to the fact that there cannot be a role without there also being a complementary role. Thus, one is not a mother without a child, a husband without a wife, a son without a parent, a niece without an aunt or uncle, and so on. A plethora of unspoken rules and normative expectations serve to guide the interactions between the participants of the role set. Within the family, normative expectations help to structure and stabilize interpersonal relationships over time, in this way providing some of the underpinnings of continuity.

We again emphasize that the normative rules and expectations that structure relationships within family role sets are by no means uniform for all strata and collectivities of society. On the contrary, expectations commonly vary under a number of circumstances, including the gender and ages of the interacting parties. The rules also vary with the situational context in which the interactions are occurring. For example, a grandparent might be amused at the mischief of the grandchild in the privacy of the home but demand a different deportment when in more public settings.

Finally, and very pertinent to this chapter, rules and expectations are not frozen in time but are constantly subject to redefinition. In part, redefinition is driven by the sheer aging of actors making up the family role sets and the corresponding alterations in their needs, capabilities, and autonomy. Changes in expectations also result from role or status transitions among one or more parties to the role set. Thus, a marked shift in expectations governing the relationship of parents and a child can be observed on the occasion of the marriage of the child or the passage of the child into the labor force. Still other changes in expectations come about more subtly as a consequence of broad socioeconomic and cultural changes. The continued financial responsibility of older parents for their adult children, for example, may vary with the expansion or contraction of opportunity structures in the society.

The treatment of the role sets as a unit of analysis, and an awareness of the normative expectations undergirding them, is a useful vantage point for understanding the family as a source of stress. Briefly, where expectations break down or are not shared in a complementary way, stressors in the form of conflict between members of the role set may emerge. It can be reasoned that family harmony depends, at least to a substantial extent, on the ability of family members both to recognize and legitimate each other's reciprocal expectations and to be motivated to act in accordance with such expectations. Given the number of role sets typically found in families, and given their complexities and subtleties, it is understandable that the family has a formidable potential for stressful conflict. What is surprising is that there is not more severe and lasting conflict than appears to be the case. We assume that in the course of family life, deviations from an ideal of harmony occur with some frequency, but whatever conflicts might result from such deviations are usually healed over quite quickly and without lasting damage to the relationships.

The Marital Role Set

Nevertheless, when conflict does surface and becomes chronic, it stands as a potent stressor to those exposed to it (Pearlin & Schooler, 1978). The family role set that has commanded most attention in this regard is that of wives and husbands. Findings from studies of marital satisfaction and its antecedents have generally found that interference with the closeness and solidarity of marriages is likely to be stressful to couples, including those in late life (Tower & Kasl, 1996). However, there is a tendency for stressors of all types to decline with age (e.g., Turner et al., 1995), including stressors in the marital relationship (e.g., Aldwin, Sutton, Chiara, & Spiro, 1996). Indeed, it is not only a reduction in conflict that can be observed in older couples but also an increase in positive interactions (Treas & Bengtson, 1987). There are several speculative explanations for the relative harmony seen among late-life couples, each helping to illuminate possible lifespan associations with marital stress.

First, of course, it can be recognized that any comparison of the prevalence of marital stress among younger and older couples reflects the attrition of failed marriages; that is, the older group has already been purged at earlier stages of many stressful unions through separation and divorce. A second, though not contradictory, explanation is that the conditions of life actually tend to become easier as people enter into the older age ranks, thus easing the pressures on the marital role set. Young couples face a great deal of entry work that is typically challenging. They are engaged in the rather lengthy process of mutual discovery, a process that occasionally yields unpleasant surprises, and they are establishing themselves in the labor force and securing an economic foothold.

They are also having and raising children, something that demands the restructuring of the marital role set and the changing of prior expectations. Because the mother–child and father–child role sets are structurally integrated by the marital dyad, the transactions that take place in marriage affect those in the parental roles and vice vera. Thus, marital conflict can arise when child care for one or both parents is problematic, when the parents employ different disciplinary measures for different perceived transgressions, or when they espouse different goals or values for the child (Pearlin & McCall, 1990). Along with the arguments that young couples have over the use of their financial resources, differences in their definitions of socialization responsibilities and practices are common sources of stressors within the marital role set.

We suggest, then, that older couples experience less conflict than the younger because many of the potentially stressful and divisive tasks that they faced earlier are no longer salient (Aldwin et al., 1996; Pearlin, 1980). In addition, people whose marriages survive to mid- and late life may have become more adept at dealing with marital problems. Thus, some people may learn to reduce conflict by aligning their behaviors so as to make them more congenial to their partners' expectations. Others, perhaps more often, seek accommodation not by changing behavior but by changing expectations, so that they are in closer accordance with the realities of their partners' behavior. This kind of accommodation may be particularly common among older cohorts subscribing to role definitions emphasizing conflict avoidance over self-assertion.

In attempting to provide some explanation for the observed decline in marital stress across the life course, we do not mean to create the impression that advancing age inevitably brings with it marital bliss. Some conflicts that arise early in marriage occasionally persist into middle and late life, where they may be no less stressful than they previously were. Even deeply troubled marriages may continue because of moral commitments to the insolubility of marriage or because of the social compression exerted on the marital relationship. In the latter instance, the marriage persists out of consideration of the trauma that dissolution would have on children, grandchildren, parents, or friends. As such marriages continue into late life, we suppose that the parties to them become increasingly resigned and inured to the disappointments and hardships the marriage embodies. In such instances, overt conflict might be minimized as people become reconciled to maintaining the relationship.

In addition to conflicts that are carried along as baggage as the marital partners traverse the life course, there are other marital strains that tend to be particularly associated with later life. It is notable in this regard that normative life-cycle transitions, such as the emptying of the nest as children depart from the household, are usually not found to be sources of marital strain (e.g., Barber, 1980). Retirement from occupational life, too, is not by itself particularly stressful (Midanik, Soghikian, Ransom, & Tekawa, 1995). However, it has been suggested (Szinovacz, 1984) that in dual-earning families, retirement decisions are interactional, and where there is a failure to coordinate the timing of retirements, tension between the marital pair might result. Similarly, retirement might bring with it the expectation of change in the division of household labor, and conflict can arise should the expectation not be fulfilled (Schafer & Keith, 1981). In general, nevertheless, scheduled eventful changes do not have stressful effects (Pearlin & Radabaugh, 1985).

There are circumstances other than scheduled life-cycle changes that surface in late-life marriages, some of which can severely impact on the marital role set. We refer specifically to the emergence of long-term caregiving that is necessitated by the illness or impairment of one of the marital partners. This is a contingency that can impose on the marital role set the profound restructuring of expectations and behavior (Pearlin & Aneshensel, 1994).

In a real sense, of course, caregiving is an inherent feature of the exchanges that normally go on in marriage. But in instances of severe and permanent impairment, as in the case of Alzheimer's disease, there is a suspension of the reciprocities that previously were expected (Antonucci & Jackson, 1990; George, 1986). As the impairment progresses and the very self of the impaired marital partner is transformed, and as the expanding demands of caregiving come to engulf the spousal caregiver, it is possible to chart a steady elevation of strains on the caregiver (Skaff & Pearlin, 1992). Although there are other exigencies that might create strains in late-life marriage, such as diminished sexual appetites or aptitudes, there is probably no situation that so totally restructures the marital relationships as when one partner comes to have asymmetrical responsibility for the life of the other.

The Parent–Child Role Set

Like stressors that are rooted in marital relationships, those involving the interactions between parents and children probably decrease as people advance over the life course. Indeed, parent–child conflict and that found in marriage are often closely connected. As suggested earlier, the integration of these two role sets is such that the transactions that take place in one of them often affect those that take place in the other. It is probably unlikely that parents have conflict-free relationships with each other while they are at war with their children, and it is equally unlikely that parents who are mired in a lasting conflict with each other enjoy harmonious relationships with their children. The close connections between the parent–child and wife–husband role sets are reflected in the fact that adult children tend to have more distant relationships with parents having a history of marital conflict (Webster & Herzog, 1995).

It is useful, or course, to examine parent–child role sets independently of their interface with other family relationships. Across the entire life course, there are changes in what Bengtson and Achtenbaum (1993) refer to as "the changing contract across generations" in the title of their book. During the years that parents are actively involved in the care and socialization of their children, they are likely to be concerned about such issues as the children's school performance, conformity to and participation in household routines, recognition and acceptance of parental authority, and the regulation of friend-ships and social life. As the child ages and the bonds of dependency weaken, there is a restructuring of the parent–child role set and the expectations that underlie its interactions.

At the time children move out of the parental household and assume greater responsibility for own lives, the salience of problems that might have peppered their earlier relationships with their parents largely recede and are replaced by other concerns. This restructuring is particularly apparent when adult children form their own families and are engaged in the kind of entry work with which their parents were involved a generation earlier. During these times, parents are able to form a clearer picture of the directions of their children's life-course trajectories. The judgments they make of these trajectories depend on the kinds of expectations and hopes they entertained for their children. For example, parents may be anxious as to whether children took a suitable spouse, whether they chose the "right" occupation, if they are likely to achieve the financial success or to attain other statuses that the parents had envisioned, whether they are observing the moral or religious precepts to which they had been socialized, if their lifestyles involve elements of which there is disapproval, such as exces-sive drinking, and so on. There may be some separation of parents from the lives of adult children, but most parents remain indefinitely responsive to and emo-tionally involved in their children's lives. They continue for the entirety of their lives to feel the pangs of their children's pains as well as the satisfactions of their children's uplifts.

Of a different order is the impact on the parents of adverse events that might befall their adult children. As Aldwin (1990) points out, the negative events that strike those close to us can also affect our own well-being. This is probably nowhere more true than in relationships between parents and children. Among the events that can adversely affect parents are children's divorce or separation, injuries and health problems, or—most serious of all—the death of a young relative. The transmission of pain and stress from younger to older family gene-rations does not stem only from adverse events, it should be noted. Thus, many parents of advanced age find themselves destined as lifelong caregivers to adult children impaired by various mental and physical health problems (Greenberg, Seltzer, & Greenley, 1993; Tobin, 1996). It is clear that the well-being of one family generation is not insulated from the travails of the other.

Similar areas of discomfort potentially arise where there are grandchildren. Here, too, the grandparents might be host to numerous concerns, some, perhaps, identical to those that they had in the course of the development of their own children. For example, older people who have lost a grandchild face a triple blow: They grieve for the grandchild, for their child who has lost a child, and for themselves and their lost future with the grandchild (Ponzetti & Johnson, 1991). Divorce, too, can create some unwanted disruption of grandparent–grandchild relationships. Occasionally, divorce either breaks or attentuates the relationship, particularly where the grandchild is young and requires the par-ent's mediation. Adult grandchildren, by contrast, usually maintain relation-ships with their grandparents on their own (Cooney & Smith, 1996; Johnson & Barer, 1987). We can speculate that there may be some ambiguity of the grandparental role when grandchildren acquire stepsiblings following divorce and remarriage. In such merged families, one or more children in the household are unrelated to the grandparent. Although this is certainly not a rare situation, it would seem that the norms governing grandparents' relationships with the children of their sons and daughters are clearer than those that guide their interactions with children in the household unrelated by blood. This lack of clarity, in turn, could conceivably contribute to the creation of cross-cutting resentments and conflicts. Given the increase in the prevalence of such households, these are hardly esoteric issues.

Differences between parents and their adult children are usually not expressed in overt conflict; if older parents are, in fact, critical of their children, they are typically silent critics. The restructuring of the role set that has taken place by the time families reach this life stage imposes limits on the conditions and extent to which parents can intercede in the lives of the children. Unlike during their children's preadult years, parents lack the legitimacy required to intervene in the lives of their adult and independent children. Whatever pain and grievance parents might have, intervention could very well evoke a challenge to their right to judge or, in the extreme, create a risk of estrangement. Consequently, the stressed parents of adult children are usually condemned to silent suffering, able only to seek, but not necessarily find, comfort in their spouse.

At a still more advanced arc of the life course, other points of friction between parents and children occasionally surface. We particularly call attention to instances in which children assume responsibility for the needs of their parents that, because of encroaching physical or mental limitations, parents are no longer fully able to satisfy by themselves. The friction occurs in cases where the child assumes greater responsibility than is necessary—or than the parent thinks is necessary. This can pose a threat to the remnants of independence that the parent wishes to protect and nurture, the result being that the well-meaning children might unwittingly find themselves at loggerheads with their parents.

The foregoing discussions of family relationships seek to trace out the conceptual guidelines that can be followed in searching for intrafamilial sources of stressors and to provide illustrations of such stressors. The principal notion around which these guidelines are developed is that of role set and, in this regard, we have limited our focus to the husband–wife and parent–child role sets. Although the family domain and the interactions that go on within it are by themselves potentially fertile grounds for the generation of stressors, they are not the only grounds. Some of the stressors to which family members are exposed have their origins in conditions residing in nonfamilial roles and statuses. It is this matter that we now consider.

The Transfer of External Stressors to the Family Interior

It is likely that family stressors most commonly arise out of problematic relationships of family members sharing the same role set. Yet, some of these stressors may be rooted in conditions lying outside the family. Such stressors may then penetrate family role sets in ways that are disruptive of them. The structural underpinning for the transfer of extraneous stressors to the family domain lies in people's multiple roles. Just as individuals are actors in multiple role sets within the family, they are the incumbents of different roles outside the family. They are workers, friends, volunteers in community associations, and members of religious congregations. The conditions that prevail in these various roles are integrated in the experiences of the single incumbent of the roles. Thus, although the enactments of one's multiple roles are often separated in time and space, the actor may carry the experiences of one role into the expectations of another (Wheaton, 1990).

From a stress process perspective, the structural interconnectedness of different roles means that the hardships that arise in one role may proliferate to hardships in other roles. For example, responsibilities for caregiving to an impaired relative or close friend can result in stressful problems on one's job (Aneshensel et al., 1995; Pearlin et al., 1997). As noted earlier, we refer to this process as stress proliferation. Most research that has examined the proliferation of external stressors into the family is limited in two related ways: (1) It is largely confined to the effect of occupational experiences on marital and parental relationships; and (2) because it deals with people still in the labor force, it is primarily concerned with families that are in the earlier stages of the life course (e.g., Menaghan, 1994).

The inattention to proliferated stress into older families cannot be taken to mean that such families are free of stressors whose origins are external to the immediate family arena. Economic hardships, ambient neighborhood threats, and anxious encounters with the medical care system are concerns that may surround older families with greater intensity or frequency (Pearlin & Skaff, 1995). We may also speculate as to whether "the cost of caring" is greater in older families. There is some evidence that people, particularly women, can be stressed by their sheer emotional involvement in the problems and frailties of friends and other age peers (Kessler & McLeod, 1984). To the extent that there may be an increase with age in the frequency with which such involvements occur, it would represent a stressor associated with late life. What is currently unknown is whether this kind of externally generated stressor impacts on family role sets as well as on individuals.

Similarly, little is known of the impact on late-life family relations of the death of friends and relatives, although it is something that on the face of it merits attention. For example, social relationships that previously might have involved interaction among couples now includes one couple and one single, a rather radical change in the structural composition of the relationship. Casual observation, moreover, indicates that the surviving couple may be called upon for responsibilities that had been those of the deceased person, such as chauffeuring, household repairs, and shopping. Again, we must leave to conjecture how the restructuring of social relationships occasioned by death or impairment affects the marital and other family relationships.

It is clear from the previous discussions that there are gaps in the research into external stressors that might adversely affect the family relationships of older people. Nevertheless, there is no reason to suppose that such relationships are somehow immune from proliferated stressors. In families actively engaged in occupational life, and whose children are in school and involved in their own peer relationships, conditions and experiences outside the family domain can set off a chain of stressors within it. While this kind of process can be assumed to ease off in late life, it should not be assumed that it disappears. Future research would be better guided by the understanding that in older families, too, the stressors that we observe in family role sets can have their origins outside as well as inside the family.

The Family as a Source of Support

Fifty years ago, the prevailing sociological theories foresaw a decline of family solidarity (Parsons & Bales, 1955). It was reasoned that in industrialized societies, the family was no longer a unit bound by its economic activities; instead, its sole function was reproduction and socialization. According to this reasoning, social mobility, geographic dispersion, and occupational specialization would contribute to the weakening of ties between adult children, now engaged in their own reproductive and socialization activities, and their aging parents. Subsequent research has consistently belied these predictions; all indications are that family attachments are stronger and more durable that those of any other social institution (e.g., Litwak, 1960). Moreover, family solidarity encompasses its older as well as its younger members (Lebowitz, 1978; Troll & Bengtson, 1992).

Some of the stressors, both those arising directly from family interactions and those spilling over from conditions outside the family, may enhance the solidarity of a role set. Other stressors, as we have been emphasizing, function to separate and divide the incumbents of the role set. One of the remarkable aspects of family life is that even those locked in continuing conflict may be deeply committed to the well-being of their adversary. Where the family is concerned, conflict and caring often have an independent presence. We have evidence that this is the case with marital partners (Pearlin & McCall, 1990), and we suspect that it may be even more the case where children and aged parents are concerned.

Given the strength of its bonds, it is understandable that the family is a major source of emotional and instrumental support for people. Indeed, access to such support by older people is thought to be an essential ingredient for their successful aging (Mancini & Simon, 1984). Obviously, then, the absence of support can be a problem for those in late life, a problem that may be particularly severe for the oldest-old. The convoy of close associates, as it has been described (Kahn & Antonucci, 1980), is sinking. Many of the circle of family and friends who traversed the life course together have died, in some cases to the point where nothing remains of the circle. Even many of one's younger relatives and friends may no longer be alive. Thus, the demography of death can assault the sources of support of older people.

Moreover, surviving children and grandchildren may not be suitable substitutes for the deceased who formerly provided support. The reason is suggested by research showing that the most effective emotional support is given by those who are experientially similar to the recipients of support. People who have been through the same ordeals as the recipient of support are the best donors of effective support (Suitor & Pillemer, 1993). No matter how eager younger family members may be to give emotional support, the age gap between them and their very old relatives is also a critical experiential gap. We should note that the shortcomings of *emotional* support provided by experientially disparate relatives do not necessarily extend to deficiencies in the instrumental assistance they give to older relatives. This, of course, is abundantly clear in the many cases where adult children are caregivers to their impaired parents.

Despite the constrictions of networks from which older people draw support, especially the parts of their networks comprised of age peers, probably most older people have access to some sources of emotional support. In marriages that survive into late life, one's spouse is likely to remain as a major supportive figure, although husbands may benefit more than their wives from spousal support (Antonucci, 1994). Moreover, there is no reason to suppose that people stop augmenting their networks as they approach old age. It is more likely that as some sources of support are lost, others are newly added.

Of course, there is a difference between the availability of supports and the quality of the supports that are available. Thus, although there has been some interest in failed support (Rook, 1984), little is known of the conditions and interactions that make supports supportive. It is, however, possible to make some observations from inquiries into younger populations (Pearlin & McCall, 1990). For example, in attempting to assist their aged relatives, well-meaning family members may rely too heavily on directive advice or on emphasizing the shortcoming or inabilities of the elder, thus inadvertently diminishing that person's self-esteem. Probably the most common cause of failed support directed to elders is the usurpation of the recipient's sense of control or mastery over important elements of his or her own life. It is well established that when people are stripped of mastery, they become highly vulnerable to the stressful conditions of their lives (Pearlin et al., 1981; Rodin, 1986).

There is an interesting twist to old people as the beneficiaries of support. It may be that the effects of *giving* support by old people compensate for whatever decrease there is in their *receipt* of effective support. In a study of a national sample of households in which an aged parent was residing in the home of an adult child, Speare and Avery (1993) found that the parent was more often a source of support to the younger generations than the other way around. What is potentially noteworthy here is that the giving of support may be as beneficial as the receiving of support, because the donor of support is able to nurture a sense of what Rosenberg and McCullough (1981) refer to as *mattering*. We believe that mattering, the flip side of social support, is an unstudied issue of considerable importance. It is reasonable to assume that old people who are able to continue to matter to the well-being of loved ones are less damaged by not being the recipients of support. At any rate, it is well to recognize that even as support "convoys" of older people begin to disappear, they may continue to be donors of support to the younger echelons of the family. The sense of mattering that might stem from their support giving may help to alleviate the sense of loss that would otherwise burden them.

DISCUSSION

We have sought in this chapter to provide some sense of the rich variety of stressors to which the family is potentially exposed and how the supportive resources of the family can serve to blunt the impact of these stressors. It is a complex undertaking, partly because it depends on an amalgamation of constructs from several perspectives: the stress process, role theory and social organization, and life-course theory. The large life-course literature is somewhat weighted toward the lives of younger families and is thus limited in its ability to illuminate the stress process in late-life families. However, the complexities in the subject matter and the gaps in the research literature notwithstanding, there is a substantial base of knowledge and theory to guide the consideration of the multiple functions of the family in the stress process: as a direct source of stressors, as the arena in which stressors arising outside the family become family stressors, and the family as a source of support in easing the deleterious outcomes of stressors.

In identifying stressors whose origins are within the family, we emphasized some of the problematic interactions that can be found in the everyday lives of very ordinary family relationships. The role set, which refers to multiple actors in complementary roles, is a useful intermediate construct for the specification of stressors stemming from family relationships. Conceptually, the notion of role set lies between the individual as the unit of analysis, which is not always appropriate for the study of families, and the entire web of family relationships, a system that can mire us in its complexity. We assume that there is a structure to role-set transactions; that is, the actions and reactions of incumbents assume a more or less stable form resting on mutually legitimized expectations. When these expectations are violated or no longer accorded legitimacy, conflict may ensue.

Our identification of stressors anchored in family role sets is admittedly limited. First, it is limited by an emphasis on husband–wife and child–parent role sets, excluding, for example, relationships with siblings, cousins, aunts and uncles, and so on. The explorations of stressors anchored in the role set are further limited by looking primarily at potential interpersonal conflicts resulting from disparities between the expectations of one or more parties to the role set and their behavior. Because of these limitations, the stressors that were discussed cannot be thought, nor were they intended, to represent an exhaustive inventory of stressors generated within the family domain. Instead, they should be regarded as but a sample of the universe of late-life family stressors.

No matter how intense family attachments are or how important they are to people, the family and its relationships do not exist in a contextual vacuum. Consequently, we cannot fully understand the family life of either aged or young people by fixing our attention solely on its interpersonal transactions. Family members have status placements and roles in systems and institutions that interface with and affect inner-family relationships. The economic and social statuses of family members, including their ages, have a bearing on the form, quality, and stressfulness of the interactions that take place in the confines of the family. Therefore, although in some respects each family is different from all other families, in other respects, each may be similar to families having similar status placements. Moreover, family members have roles in other major institutions: They are job occupants, members of religious groups, participants in voluntary associations, and residents of neighborhoods. The difficult life conditions that people may be exposed to within the context of their statuses and roles help to form a range of understandings and dispositions that, in large measure, underlie the stressors that may arise in family relations. A frustrating occupational life, for example, or the involuntary loss of a job—two extrafamilial conditions that have been most closely studied for their effects on family relations—may proliferate into intrafamilial conflicts or other stressors.

Finally, it needs to be underscored that the family is in a constant state of flux; whatever its continuities, it is an institution in which relationships at one moment in time may be quite different than those at another. Shifts in surrounding social, economic, and historic conditions, as well as the inexorable alterations that occur with aging and movement along the life course, make the family a most dynamic setting of social life. This means that we cannot project from what we know of young families to predict with acceptable accuracy the stressors and strengths of older families. The prevalence of stressors is likely to be lower at the latter stages of life, as we discussed, and the nature of the stressors is also likely to be different for contrasting age cohorts. Moreover, because of cohort differences, we cannot assume that the families of the old in the 1990s will inform us about families of the same age in the 2020s. These kinds of changes add to the complexity of identifying stressors that are associated with the family life of old people.

However, although the prevalence and nature of stressors may change with the life course and differ among historic cohorts, it is our assumption that the *processes* involved in the generation and moderation of family stressors will remain the same. In future decades, as now, these stressors and many of the conditions that buffer their effects can be specified by examining the interpersonal dynamics of family role sets and tracing the effects of contextual circumstances on these dynamics. The contemporary refinement of our theories and our conceptual frameworks, and the development of long-term longitudinal research into *aging* rather than into the aged, will enable us to appreciate better the dynamic interrelationships between the life course and the stress process.

ACKNOWLEDGMENT: This work was supported by the first author's MERIT award, MH42122.

REFERENCES

Aldwin, C. M. (1990). The elders life stress inventory: Egocentric and non-egocentric stress. In M. A. Stevens, S. E. Hobfall, J. N. Crawther, & D. L. Tennenbaum (Eds.), *Stress and coping in later-life families* (pp. 49–69). New York: Hemisphere.

Aldwin, C. M., Sutton, K. J., Chiara, Q., & Spiro, A. (1996). Age differences in stress, coping and appraisal: Findings from the normative aging study. *Journal of Gerontology, 51*, P179–P188.

Aneshensel, C. S., Pearlin, L. I., Mullan, J. T., Zarit, S., & Whitlatch, C. (1995). *Profiles in caregiving: The unexpected career.* New York: Academic Press.

Aneshensel, C. S., Rutter, C. M., & Lachenbruch, P. A. (1991). Social structure, stress, and mental health: Competing conceptual and analytic models. *American Sociological Review, 56*, 166–178.

Antonucci, T. C. (1994). A life-span view of women's social relations. In B. J. Turner & L. S. Troll (Eds.), *Women growing older* (pp. 239–269). Thousand Oaks, CA: Sage.

Antonucci, T. C., & Jackson, J. S. (1990). The role of reciprocity in social support. In B. R. Sarason & G. R. Pierce (Eds.), *Social support: An interfactional view* (pp. 173–198). New York: Wiley.

Baltes, P. B., & Baltes, M. M. (1990). Psychological perspectives on successful aging: The model of selective optimization with compensation. In P. B. Baltes & M. M. Baltes (Eds.), *Successful aging: Perspectives for the social sciences* (pp. 1–34). Cambridge, NJ: Cambridge University Press.

Barber, C. E. (1980). Gender differences in expressing the transition to the empty nest: Reports of middle aged and older women and men. *Family Perspectives, 14*, 87–95.

Bengtson, V. L., & Achtenbaum, W. A. (1993). *The changing contract across generations.* New York: Aldine de Gruyter.

Bengtson, V. L., Rosenthal, C., & Burton, L. (1990). Families and aging: Diversity and heterogeneity. In R. H. Binstock & L. K. George (Eds.), *Handbook of aging and the social sciences* (3rd ed., pp. 263–287). San Diego: Academic Press.

Cooney, T. M., & Smith, L. C. (1996). Young adults' relations with grandparents following recent parental divorce. *Journal of Gerontology, 51*, S91–S95.

Dannefer, D. (1987). Aging as intracohort differentiation: Accentuation, the Matthew Effect, and the life course. *Sociological Forum, 2*, 211–236.

Elder, G. H., George, L. K., & Shanahan, M. G. (1996). Psychosocial stress over the life course. In H. Kaplan (Ed.), *Perspectives on psychosocial stress* (pp. 245–290). San Diego: Academic Press.

Fisher, L. (1982). Transactional theories but individual assessment: A frequent discrepancy in family research. *Family Process, 21*, 313–320.

George, L. K. (1986). Caregiver burden: Conflict between norms of reciprocity and solidarity. In K. G. Pillemer & R. S. Wolf (Eds.), *Elder abuse: Conflict in the family* (pp. 67–92). Dover, MA: Auburn House.

George, L. K. (1993). Sociological perspectives on life transitions. *Annual Review of Sociology, 19*, 353–373.

George, L. K. (1996). Missing links: The case for a social psychology of the life course. *Gerontologist, 36*, 248–255.

George, L. K., & Gwyther, L. P. (1986). Caregiver well-being: A multidimensional examination of family caregivers of demented adults. *Gerontologist, 26*, 253–259.

Greenberg, J. S., Seltzer, M., & Greenley, J. R. (1993). Aging parents of adults with disabilities. *Gerontologist, 33*, 542–550.

Johnson, C., & Barer, B. M. (1987). Marital instability and the changing networks of grandparents. *Gerontologist, 27*, 330–335.

Kahn, R. L., & Antonucci, T. C. (1980). Convoys over the life course: Attachment, roles, and social support. In P. B. Baltes & O. G. Brim (Eds.), *Life-span development and behavior* (Vol. 3, pp. 253–286). New York: Academic Press.

Kessler, R. C., & McLeod, J. D. (1984). Sex differences in vulnerability to undesirable life events. *American Sociological Review, 49*, 620–631.

Kohn, M. L. (1969). *Class and conformity: A study in values.* Homewood, IL: Dorsey Press.

Krause, N. (1994). Stressors in salient social roles and well-being in later life. *Journal of Gerontology, 49*, P137–P148.

Lebowitz, B. D. (1978). Old age and family functioning. *Journal of Gerontological Social Work, 1,* 111–118.

Litwak, E. (1960). Geographic mobility and extended family cohesion. *American Sociological Review, 25,* 385–394.

Mancini, J. A., & Simon, J. (1984). Expectations of support from family and friends. *Journal of Applied Gerontology, 3,* 150–160.

Menaghan, E. G. (1994). The daily grind: Work stressors, family patterns, and intergenerational outcomes. In W. R. Avison & S. H. Gotlib (Eds.), *Stress and mental health: Contemporary issues and prospects for the future* (pp. 115–147). New York: Plenum Press.

Merton, R. K. (1957). The role set: Problems in sociological theory. *British Journal of Sociology, 8,* 106–120.

Midanik, L. T., Soghikian, K., Ransom, L. J., & Tekawa, I. S. (1995). The effect of retirement on mental health and health behaviors. *Journal of Gerontology, 50,* S59–S62.

Parsons, T., & Bales, R. J. (1955). *Family, socialization and interaction process.* Glencoe, IL: Free Press.

Pearlin, L. I. (1980). The life cycle and life strains. In H. M. Blalock, Jr. (Ed.), *Sociological theory and research: A critical approach* (pp. 349–360). New York: Free Press.

Pearlin, L. I. (1982). The social contexts of stress. In L. Goldberger & S. Breznitz (Eds.), *Handbook of stress* (pp. 367–379). New York: Free Press.

Pearlin, L. I. (1983). Role strains and personal stress. In H. B. Kaplan (Ed.), *Psychosocial stress: Trends in theory and research* (pp. 3–32). New York: Academic Press.

Pearlin, L. I. (1989). The sociological study of stress. *Journal of Health and Social Behavior, 30,* 241–256.

Pearlin, L. I. (1991). The study of coping: Problems and directions. In J. Eckenrode (Ed.), *The social context of coping* (pp. 261–276). New York: Plenum Press.

Pearlin, L. I., & Aneshensel, C. S. (1994). Caregiving: The unexpected career. *Social Justice Research, 7,* 373–390.

Pearlin, L. I., Aneshensel, C. S., & LeBlanc, A. J. (1997). The forms and mechanisms of stress proliferation: The case of AIDs caregivers. *Journal of Health and Social Behavior, 38,* 223–236.

Pearlin, L. I., & Johnson, J. S. (1977). Marital status, life-strains and depression. *American Sociological Review, 42,* 704–714.

Pearlin, L. I., & Kohn, M. L. (1966). Social class, occupation, and parental values: A cross-national study. *American Sociological Review, 31,* 466–479.

Pearlin, L. I., & Lieberman, M. A. (1979). Social sources of emotional distress. In R. Simmons (Ed.), *Research in community and mental health* (pp. 217–248). Greenwich, CT: JAI Press.

Pearlin, L. I., Lieberman, M. A., Menaghan, E., & Mullan, J. T. (1981). The stress process. *Journal of Health and Social Behavior, 22,* 337–356.

Pearlin, L. I., & McCall, M. E. (1990). Occupational stress and marital support: A description of microprocesses. In J. Eckenrode & S. Gore (Eds.), *Stress between work and family* (pp. 39–60). New York: Plenum Press.

Pearlin, L. I., Mullan, J. T., Semple, S. J., & Skaff, M. M. (1990). Caregiving and the stress process: An overview of concepts and their measures. *Gerontologist, 30,* 583–594.

Pearlin, L. I., & Radabaugh, C. (1985). Age and stress: Perspectives and problems. In B. H. Hess & E. W. Markson (Eds.), *Growing old in America* (3rd ed., pp. 293–308). New Brunswick, NJ: Transaction Books.

Pearlin, L. I., & Schooler, C. (1978). The structure of coping. *Journal of Health and Social Behavior, 19,* 2–21.

Pearlin, L. I., & Skaff, M. M. (1995). Stressors and adaptation in late life. In M. Gatz (Ed.), *Emerging issues in mental health and aging* (pp. 97–123). Washington, DC: American Psychiatric Press.

Pearlin, L. I., & Skaff, M. M. (1996). Stress and the life course: A paradigmatic alliance. *Gerontologist, 36,* 239–247.

Pearlin, L. I., & Turner, H. A. (1987). The family as a context of the stress process. In S. V. Kasl & C. Cooper (Eds.), *Stress and health: Issues in research methodology* (pp. 143–165).

Ponzetti, J. J., & Johnson, M. A. (1991). The forgotten grievers: Grandparents' reactions to the death of grandchildren. *Death Studies, 15,* 157–167.

Rodin, J. (1986). Aging and health: Effects of the sense of control. *Science, 233*, 1271–1276.

Rook, K. S. (1984). The negative side of social interaction: Impact on psychological well-being. *Journal of Personality and Social Psychology, 46*, 1097–1108.

Rosenberg, M., & McCullough, B. C. (1981). Mattering: Inferred significance and mental health among adolescents. In R. G. Simmons (Ed.), *Research in community and mental health* (Vol. 2, pp. 163–182). Greenwich, CT: JAI Press.

Schafer, R. B., & Keith, P. M. (1981). Equity in marital roles across the life cycle. *Journal of Marriage and the Family, 43*, 359–367.

Skaff, M. M., & Pearlin, L. I. (1992). Caregiving: Role engulfment and the loss of self. *Gerontologist, 32*, 656–664.

Speare, A., & Avery, R. (1993). Who helps whom in older parent–child families. *Journal of Gerontology, 48*, S64–S73.

Suitor, J. J., & Pillemer, K. (1993). Support and interpersonal stress in the social networks of married daughters caring for parents with dementia. *Journal of Gerontology, 48*, S1–S8.

Szinovacz, M. (1984). Changing family roles and interactions. *Marriage and Family Reviews, 7*, 163–201.

Thoits, P. G. (1983). Dimensions of life events that influence psychological distress: An evaluation and synthesis of the literature. In H. B. Kaplan (Ed.), *Psychosocial stress: Trends in theory and research* (pp. 33–104). New York: Academic Press.

Tobin, S. S. (1996). A non-normative old age contrast: Elderly parents caring for children with mental retardation. In V. L. Bengtson (Ed.), *Adulthood and aging: Research on continuities and discontinuities* (pp. 124–142). New York: Springer.

Tower, R. B., & Kasl, S. V. (1996). Gender, marital closeness, and depressive symptoms in elderly couples. *Journal of Gerontology, 51*, P115 –P129.

Treas, J., & Bengtson, V. L. (1987). The family in later years. In M. B. Sussman & S. K. Steinmetz (Eds.), *Handbook of marriage and the family* (pp. 625–648). New York: Plenum Press.

Troll, L. E., & Bengtson, V. L. (1992). The oldest old in families: An intergenerational perspective. *Generations, 16*, 39–44.

Turner, R. J., Wheaton, B., & Lloyd, D. A. (1995). The epidemiology of social stress. *American Sociological Review, 60*, 104–125.

Webster, P. S., & Herzog, A. R. (1995). Effects of parental divorce and memories of family problems on relationships between adult children and their parents. *Journal of Gerontology, 50*, S24–S34.

Wheaton, B. (1990). Where work and family meet: Stress across social roles. In J. Eckenrode & S. Gore (Eds.), *Stress between work and family* (pp. 153–174). New York: Plenum Press.

Wheaton, B. (1995). Sampling the stress universe. In W. R. Avison & I. H. Gotlieb (Eds.), *Stress and mental health: Contemporary issues and prospects for the future* (pp. 77–114). New York: Plenum Press.

Zarit, S. H., Orr, N. K., & Zarit, J. M. (1985). *The hidden victims of Alzheimer's disease: Families under stress.* New York: New York University Press.

CHAPTER 15

A Frame of Reference for Guiding Research Regarding the Relationship between Adult Attachment and Mental Health in Aging Families

Victor G. Cicirelli

PRELIMINARY CONSIDERATIONS

Objectives

The overall objective of this chapter is to provide a frame of reference for carrying out research using concepts from attachment theory to help understand the connection between interpersonal relationships and mental health in aging families. By frame of reference, I mean a collection of ideas that can be used to guide further thinking in a particular domain. My intent is to formulate propositions based on existing attachment theory and research that will suggest directions for future research regarding attachment between aging family members and its contribution to their mental health.

As a result, the chapter first focuses on attachment rather than on either aging families or mental health per se. Second, the focus is on the elderly family member (i.e., the focus is on the influence of the aging family on the mental

VICTOR G. CICIRELLI • Department of Psychological Sciences, Purdue University, West Lafayette, Indiana 47907.

Handbook of Aging and Mental Health: An Integrative Approach, edited by Jacob Lomranz. Plenum Press, New York, 1998.

health of an elderly family member rather than on the mental health of the aging family as a whole).

Evidence already exists that families do influence the mental health of the elderly. For example, the existence of a confidante (whether the confidante is a family member or a friend), or the presence of family members in an elder's social convoy can provide support and facilitate the mental health of elderly family members (Antonucci, 1994; Keith, Hill, Goudy, & Powers, 1984). On the other hand, some aging families may ignore, isolate, alienate, or abuse elderly family members (Gelles & Cornell, 1990), increasing their vulnerability to mental disturbance. What is needed is research based on more general theoretical notions that will account for both phenomena. I feel that attachment concepts or theory offer this possibility.

Mental Health

Both mental health and mental illness are somewhat nebulous terms for which there is no standard definition. An individual's mental state may be regarded as a point on a continuum between good mental health on the one hand and mental disturbances on the other; they are often indexed by life satisfaction and psychological symptomatology, respectively. Considered from a medical model, mental health is often viewed as the absence of mental disease or symptomatology, whereas mental illness is viewed as a level of mental disease or symptomatology severe enough to warrant treatment. From a functional adequacy model, mental health is regarded as the ability to successfully carry out everyday tasks and cope with problems in life, regardless of symptoms; mental illness is seen as an inability to function adequately. Finally, mental health is seen by some from a growth model, implying continuing development toward higher levels of adaptation and self-actualization and deepening integration of the personality (Butler, Lewis, & Sunderland, 1991).

Overall, mental illness is less prevalent among the elderly than among younger persons, although rates of cognitive impairment (various forms of dementia and delirium) are higher. Most frequent mental illness conditions among the elderly, in addition to cognitive impairment and confusion, include anxiety disorders, depression, paranoia, and suicidal tendencies (Rabins, 1992; Wykle & Musil, 1993).

The Aging Family

As lifespan continues to increase in the future, families will become more important to older people who outlive those contemporaneous family members and friends ordinarily expected to provide social support. Elders may have little choice but to depend more on the remaining younger members of the aging family if they are to avoid isolation and facilitate their mental health for the help they need over the longer time period in which they will live.

Studying the influence of the aging family depends on first defining what constitutes the family. The criteria for what constitutes a family are important, as they determine the kinds and number of people who may have close and influential relationships to aging family members and a commitment to help them.

The traditional nuclear family of a married couple and their biological children is easy to define on the basis of biological and legal criteria. When one considers extended families consisting of ascending, collateral, and descending kin, additional criteria are needed to determine who should be included or excluded (e.g., those in a direct vertical line of descent, those living in the same household or in close proximity). It becomes still more difficult to define a family when the criteria have broadened to deal with such social and cultural changes as surrogate motherhood, serial marriages, and quasifamilies of people living together in the same household. For simplicity of discourse in this chapter, the discussion will refer to a more or less traditional extended family.

The family also has to be considered from the perspective of a particular individual and along a continuum of time. The family of a child consists solely of collateral and ascending kin of siblings, parents, aunts and uncles, and grandparents, as well as various cousins. As time passes, the family of a young adult is likely to have added a spouse, children, nieces and nephews, but may have lost one or more grandparents. In contrast, the family of an old person is unlikely to contain any ascending kin (parents, grandparents, aunts and uncles) and may have already lost the spouse, some siblings, and cousins.

However, the aging family has certain characteristics that are unique and may lead to influences on family members that differ from those found in younger families. It consists of many individuals with a long relationship history with one another, individuals in the same role for extended periods of time (e.g., a woman may occupy the role of mother for 70 years or more), as well as individuals added to the family through births and marriages. Whereas the young adult faces the developmental tasks of finding a mate, beginning a new nuclear family, and establishing a career, the older adult faces dealing with events and developmental tasks more unique to this period of life, such as retirement, widowhood, and chronic disease. The changes over time in family membership, roles, and developmental tasks have implications for the amount of social support that the aging family is able to provide to an elderly family member (Brubaker, 1990).

In regard to the objectives of this chapter, it is possible to conceptualize all types of families as a set of personal relationships between individuals. The influence of the aging family on an older person's mental health will depend to a greater or lesser degree upon the quality of these family relationships. The question then becomes, "Can attachment concepts or theory give us a perspective that can lead to better understanding of these relationships?"

Restated, the purpose of this chapter is to further extend the aforementioned thinking and explore the possible contribution of attachment to understanding the connection between close relationships and mental health in the aging family.

ATTACHMENT RELATIONSHIPS

Before continuing further, I review basic concepts of attachment theory in infancy and adulthood for the reader who may not be familiar with this field of study. (Because there is a large literature in this area, only a few relevant studies are cited where appropriate rather than attempting a literature review.)

Infant Attachment

Development of Attachment.   Briefly, attachment theory, as developed by Bowlby (1969, 1979) and Ainsworth (1982), holds that attachment in infancy and childhood is an affectional bond that involves a desire to be physically close to a specific person (the mother or primary caregiver), leading to a system of attachment behaviors that maintain a set goal of proximity, which in turn is associated with feelings of emotional security and comfort; there is distress if the infant is separated from the attachment figure and joy upon subsequent reunion.

From the perspective of evolution, infant attachment occurs as a means of protecting the infant's survival, and consequently the species. Attachment as a motive is a hereditary predisposition to seek and maintain proximity or closeness to the mother; when separated from the mother, the infant shows distress to elicit caregiving behavior or physically moves toward the mother by using limited motor behavior to attain proximity. Simultaneously, there is a hereditary predisposition on the part of the mother to provide care, and as infant and mother reciprocally interact, the infant eventually establishes an attachment to the mother (or other primary caregiver), and the latter also bonds with the infant.

Attachment Concepts.   The *attachment figure* is the individual to whom the infant has become attached, and who provides a secure base from which the infant can move to explore the environment, and a safe haven within which he or she can experience security and comfort. Infant–mother attachment is called primary attachment and serves as a prototype for other concurrent or future secondary attachments.

The *attachment behavioral system* is the set of behaviors that serves the function of establishing and maintaining proximity to an attachment figure to experience emotional security and comfort. It also regulates behavior to restore proximity and reunion after separation from the attachment figure. The infant is born with genetically determined behaviors that serve as signals to elicit the mother's attention (e.g., crying when hungry or wet). New behaviors emerge as the child develops and eventually become coordinated into a homeostatic system that serves the purpose of seeking and maintaining proximity to the mother. Any separation perceived as being a greater distance than what is acceptable to the infant will activate the behavioral system to restore the appropriate distance (e.g., calling for the mother or crawling toward her). Also, if the infant perceives a threat from the environment, or feels under too great a stress, the attachment behavioral system will be activated. The set goal regarding an acceptable distance from the attachment figure can vary, depending upon the availability of the attachment figure and the degree of perceived threat in the environment.

As the infant and mother interact over time, the infant develops an *internal working model*, which is a subjective representation or mental representation of the self, the mother (attachment figure), and the relationship between them (Bretherton, 1992). The working model includes information about the extent to which the mother is sensitive, responsive, and consistent in relation to the infant's needs, and guides the child's behavior with the mother and others.

Attachment Styles. Attachment style refers to the child's typical overt pattern of attachment behaviors and reflects individual differences in the manner of attachment. Each infant develops a characteristic pattern or type of attachment behaviors depending on the content of the internal working model as well on temperament and ongoing experiences. Ainsworth (1982) identified three infant attachment styles: secure, insecure–anxious/ambivalent, and insecure–avoidant. Although additional attachment styles have been identified (e.g., Main, Kaplan, & Cassidy, 1985), only the original three styles are discussed here.

When the mother is consistently available, warm, sensitive, and responsive to the infant's needs, the infant tends to develop a secure attachment style. In secure attachment, the infant approaches the mother with positive feelings, protests and feels distress upon separation, but feels relieved and happy to see the mother upon reunion.

When the mother is inconsistent in her care, alternately loving and rejecting, the infant tends to develop an insecure–anxious/ambivalent attachment style. The infant experiences heightened feelings of anxiety regarding the mother, with anxiety increasing upon separation; he or she continues to be upset upon reunion. The infant displays fear, crying, and clinging behavior, is overpreoccupied with finding security with the mother, but is ambivalent in his or her feelings and may be hostile during reunion with the mother.

If the mother is aloof, withholding feelings and rejecting the infant, the infant tends to develop an insecure–avoidant attachment style. The infant may suppress feelings upon separation, and show a reduced attempt to make contact with the mother upon reunion. There is a tendency to deny the need for the mother and attempt to become more self-reliant.

Multiple Attachments. In addition to the attachment to the mother, attachment relationships can develop to the father, siblings, grandparents, and others important in the child's life. However, attachment to the mother is regarded as unique and primary in importance (Bretherton, 1992; Collins & Read, 1994). By contrast, attachments to other family members may fulfill only some of the functions of an attachment relationship. The internal working model also contains information about the child's relationship with these secondary attachment figures.

Adult Attachment

Most psychologists agree that attachment does not end in childhood, but continues in some form throughout life (Feeney & Noller, 1996; Sperling & Berman, 1994). The study of attachment in adulthood has proceeded in various directions, reflecting researchers' areas of interest. Developmental psychologists have been concerned with such topics as the intergenerational transmission of attachment styles (Main et al., 1985), the continuity and stability of attachment relationships throughout life, and the relation of adult attachment to the care of aging parents (Antonucci, 1994; Cicirelli, 1993). Social psychologists have been interested in the development of new attachments in late adolescence and adulthood, primarily in romantic relationships and relationships with a mate (Hazan & Shaver, 1987). Clinical psychologists have focused on the association of disturbed attachment patterns and mental health problems (Parker, 1994; West & Keller, 1994).

However seemingly disparate the various research interests, most agree on certain core principles. First, types of attachment behavior patterns found in adult relationships are basically similar to the attachment styles found in the infant's relationship with the mother. In this sense, infant attachment styles are prototypes for later relationships. Second, given the existence of an internal working model, it is assumed that relationships in childhood are abstracted to a generalized working model of relationships, stored in memory, retrieved, and applied to other relationships in adulthood. Third, the form of attachment behaviors is changed in adulthood with less emphasis on direct proximity or contact (except to the mate) and more emphasis on symbolic attachment, and occasional visits or calls; stressful situations and those involving threat will activate the need to gain security by contact with attachment figures.

Characteristics of Adult Attachment. Adult attachments are secondary attachments; that is, they are perhaps less stable and may involve changing and substituting attachment figures, as in serial romantic relationships. Beyond this, certain attributes of both childhood and adulthood attachment are discussed in sources scattered throughout the attachment literature. As they seem more relevant in adulthood, I review them here.

Multiple attachments seem to be more extensive and important in adulthood, involving the attachment to a mate, attachments to parents, siblings, and other family members, as well as attachments to a few close friends. In late adolescence and young adulthood, the relationships to a love interest resembles an attachment process (e.g., Hazan & Shaver, 1987). When this attachment deepens into a permanent commitment to one another, involving mutual love, sexual attraction, and caregiving, the attachment to a mate is often the most important one in adult life (Hazan & Zeitman, 1994).

Hierarchical attachments occur in adulthood, because family attachments may be ascribed with long attachment histories compared to voluntary attachments, and the individual may be involved in attachment relationships that have different degrees of importance. The working models for these relationships can be viewed as forming a hierarchy (or order of preference) of attachment relationships (Collins & Read, 1994).

Reciprocal attachments also occur in adulthood. In childhood, the child has a bond to the mother, and vice versa, but this bond is asymmetrical in nature; the mother is in a caregiver role and is viewed as stronger, wiser, and more capable. Later in life, especially in adulthood, many attachments are reciprocal and symmetrical; that is, both members of an adult family dyad have an attachment to each other and view the other as capable and caring. However, not all attachments are reciprocal, as one dyad member may have a strong attachment to a second dyad member who feels only an affectional relationship (not an attachment) toward the first. Reciprocal attachment relationships may involve individuals who have the same or different attachment styles (e.g., secure–secure, secure–anxious/ambivalent); the attachment style of each is influenced by the partner's attachment style (Feeney & Noller, 1996).

In short, adult attachments can be characterized as multiple, hierarchical, and reciprocal relationships.

Adult Attachment Styles. There is some continuity of infant attachment styles into adulthood. In adult relationships, one can find patterns of attachment behavior representing certain attachment styles that are similar in many ways to the patterns of behavior observed in infant–mother attachment relationships. However, different investigators using a variety of assessment methods have identified different sets of styles, for example, the secure, preoccupied, and dismissing styles identified by Main et al. (1985), or the fourfold styles of Bartholomew and Horowitz (1991). Others (e.g., Collins & Read, 1990) have identified basic dimensions underlying attachment styles.

As in childhood, the generalized working model is an abstraction from the mental representations (attachment styles) stored in memory for each of the individual's attachments. Although the generalized working model in adulthood is heavily dependent on the prototype working model of attachment to the mother in childhood, it is also influenced by the separate working models of other attachments, which may differ in attachment style. The generalized model is applied to guide behavior when forming new relationships, whereas specific working models are applied in existing relationships.

Stability and Change in Attachment Styles. Once the prototypic attachment style is developed in childhood, it has considerable stability over time as various attachment behaviors and behaviors in new relationships tend to occur somewhat automatically. In their review of studies of stability of attachment styles over periods from 1 week to 4 years, Feeney and Noller (1996) found overall stability rates ranging from 67% to 80%, with stabilities highest (80–88%) for secure attachments and lowest (11–58%) for anxious–ambivalent attachments. Although some instability may be due to unreliability of measurement, it appears that one's attachment style can be changed as a result of new relationship experiences or losses, new interpretations of past attachment-related events, and so on (e.g., a secure person involved in a negative relationship may become insecure).

Attachments as a Profile. Attachment styles has traditionally been viewed as a relatively stable trait, with the prototype style applied to each new attachment relationship. Others (e.g., Hazan & Shaver, 1987) have viewed attachment style as a relationship, which varies with the attachment figure. However, given the existence of multiple attachments and evidence of differing attachment styles in relation to different attachment figures, one might reconcile the trait and relationship conceptions by viewing the individual as having a *profile* of attachment styles (i.e., a set of attachment styles), with one style the dominant style (e.g., a given individual may have a high degree of a secure style, a moderate degree of an insecure–ambivalent style, and a low degree of an avoidant style). The dominant style would be activated in certain relationships, with other attachment styles activated as appropriate in other relationships. In short, there would now be a profile of potential attachment styles, reflected in an individual's multiple and different attachments styles in relation to different individuals. A "generalized attachment working model" would thus contain some kind of resultant of the multiple styles. The notion of profile allows one to reconcile the idea of having a generalized attachment style, and simultaneously having specific (and possibly different) attachment styles with specific attachment figures. Such a theoretical conception also could help to account for the seeming instability of attachment styles.

Reciprocal Attachments in the Family System. According to Hazan and Shaver (1987), attachment styles in reciprocal attachments can be additive or interactive. Within the family, an individual's views of the self and a particular attachment figure are made more positive or negative by the views of the self in relation to other family members (Senchak & Leonard, 1992; Simpson, 1990). (For example, a father's insecure attachment to his wife may become less insecure if he has a secure attachment to a sister and daughter. This reduction in insecurity may be influenced not only by secure attachments to other attachment figures, but also the degree of importance regarding these other attachments, the gender of the attachment figures, and other aspects of the family context. It may also be influenced by the attachment styles of family members to each other; for example, the father's relationship to his wife may be different if the wife and sister are avoidant than if they are securely attached to one another.) Furthermore, the attachment of an individual to a given family member will also be influenced not only by the combination of that individual's attachment styles, but also by the number of attachment relationships within the family boundary compared to the number of nonattachment relationships. In short, the degree and style of attachment of one family member to another depends upon the family context (i.e., the network of attachments linking various family members). From a systems perspective, various family dyadic attachments exist and each dyad may influence the other. Thus, within the family dynamic system, attachments are interactive and contextual.

Extending Attachment Concepts to the Aging Family

The concepts of adult attachment outlined earlier apply to the aging family as well. However, unique aspects of the aging family may further influence attachment relationships. In aging families, the long relationship between family members implies a long attachment history. Such longevity could lead to a more stable attachment style (whether it is a secure or insecure one), and it may be more difficult to modify such an attachment relationship. On the other hand, the long history of the relationship could allow time for reinterpretations of the attachment relationship, leading to shifts in attachment styles.

Aging families are also multigenerational, which can involve a greater diversity and complexity of attachment relationships, including those to other generations and affinal kin. The situation is still more complex if there is divorce and remarriage, with reconstituted or blended families. In such a situation, one would expect a larger hierarchy of attachments, with the relative importance of these attachments to the individual extending over a wider range. Furthermore, reciprocal attachments may involve more varied combinations of attachment styles since a greater diversity of people would be involved.

Aging families face different developmental tasks (e.g., retirement, widowhood, illness) and demands for everyday living than younger families; resulting stresses and strains between family members may lead to a shift in the degree and style of attachment between some family members. The symmetrical nature of reciprocal attachment relationships may shift in response to the functional deficits of old age; the attachment figure (perhaps an adult child) will be seen as stronger and more capable, with the elder seen as weaker and needing care.

Finally, aging family members face the loss of major attachment figures through death, reducing the number of multiple attachments but increasing stress and adjustment problems. The attachment hierarchy of the elderly person is likely to be quite different than it was in middle adulthood; parents, siblings, and the spouse may all be dead. The mix of the attachment styles applying to the remaining relationships in the hierarchy may be quite different than before. Thus, a person with a predominantly secure attachment style in middle adulthood may shift toward a predominantly insecure–ambivalent style in old age if he or she has insecure–ambivalent attachment styles with the remaining living members of the hierarchy.

RELATION OF ATTACHMENT TO MENTAL HEALTH AND MENTAL ILLNESS

Infancy and Childhood

Existing evidence indicates that a child's attachment style to the primary caregiver is related to behaviors indicative of mental health or mental illness.

In childhood, secure attachment to the mother has been related to such positive qualities as a long attention span (Main, 1983), sociability with unfamiliar adults (Main & Weston, 1981), open and effective communication with parents (Main, Tomasini, & Tolan, 1979), and low levels of distraction and need for discipline (Bus & Van IJzendoorn, 1988).

On the other hand, insecure attachment (either anxious–ambivalent or avoidant) to the mother has been related to distractibility (Bus & Van IJzendoorn, 1988; Erikson, Sroufe, & Egeland, 1985), and hostility and aggression (Erickson et al., 1985; Lyons-Ruth, Alpern, & Repacholi, 1993; Main et al., 1985). In adolescence, insecure attachment has been related to lack of competence in interpersonal relationships, dysphoria, and depressive symptomatology (Batgos & Leadbeater, 1994). It should be pointed out, however, that the foregoing relationships are moderate at best, and that many intervening factors can influence the development of mental illness. The best conclusion seems to be that a poor early attachment relationship with the mother may make a child more vulnerable to mental health problems later on.

Adulthood

In adulthood, as well as in childhood, evidence exists linking attachment styles to mental health or mental illness. Research findings indicate that whereas secure attachment is related to subjective well-being, insecure attachment (anxious/ambivalent, avoidant) is related to various aspects of mental disturbance. Among these are depression and depressive symptomatology (Carnelley, Pietromonaco, & Jaffe, 1994; Parker, 1994; Roberts, Gotlib, & Kassel, 1996), personality disorders (West & Keller, 1994), posttraumatic psychological distress (Mikulincer, Florian, & Weller, 1993), and suicidal behavior (Adam, 1994). Sperling and Lyons (1994) outlined a model for psychotherapeutic interventions in which they attempted to correct dysfunctional mental representations of attachment and alter the defenses maintaining these representations.

Basic Propositions: Aging Family Attachments and Mental Health

Thus far, there is no evidence relating attachment concepts or theory to the mental health of elderly family members within the context of aging families. However, it seems logical to extend the knowledge about the relation of attachment to mental health in younger adults to include aging families. In doing so, I want to make more explicit a frame of reference that will suggest problems and approaches for research in the future.

Proposition 1. An individual perceives a set of individuals as family within a boundary determined by that individual's conception of family. Within this boundary, family relationships are ascribed; attachments may develop from the extensiveness and nature of interactions between individuals. Thus, in studying attachment and mental health between aging family members, it is important to determine just who is included in the family.

Proposition 2. As the individual interacts with these family members over time, a hierarchy of attachments develops, which can be either stable or changing. It would be important to interview subjects to determine the relative importance of each of their attachments to different attachment figures, and to determine changes over time. This sort of information may have implications for mental health.

Proposition 3.   Over time (beginning early in life), certain family members become very important attachment figures. To the extent that secure attachment exists and has a cumulative effect, the elderly family member should build up a reservoir of felt security and consequently be better adjusted. The researcher would want to determine whether greater felt security in an individual results from having multiple secure attachment relationships, and whether such felt security declines following the death of significant attachment figures.

Proposition 4.   Although attachments have a reasonable degree of stability, they are subject to change over time, especially in response to critical life events. Certainly, the researcher should attempt to determine stability of attachment in relation to the unique critical life events of the aging family.

Proposition 5.   Reciprocal attachments in an aging family dyad should be explored for their effect on each dyad member. It is especially important to determine differences in effects when dyad members' attachment styles are the same or different.

Proposition 6.   Within the aging family as a whole, the researcher should explore the influence on each family member due to multiple reciprocal family attachments. The researcher could also conceptualize the aging family as a dynamic system in which the components are family dyadic attachments (each dyad being assessed in terms of degree of attachment, effects of combinations of attachment styles), and the reciprocal interactions of all the dyads on one another over time. Chaos theory would possibly apply to such a nonlinear dynamic system, in which the dyadic relationships change in an unpredictable manner.

Proposition 7.   The mental health or mental illness of an elderly family member would be a function of the number of attachments to other family members, the different degrees and styles of each attachment relationship, and the additive or cumulative effect of the combinations of attachment styles in each of the dyads. One should no longer think in terms of the effect of a single attachment relationship with one attachment figure on an older person's mental health, but rather the effects on that person's mental health of multiple attachment relationships among dyads made up of aging family members.

CONCLUSIONS

This chapter has provided a frame of reference in terms of a set of ideas or propositions based on family attachment relationships that would suggest future directions of research in dealing with mental health in aging families. We already know that close relationships between family members lead to more positive mental health rather than mental disturbances. What is needed is a good theory to help explain how interpersonal relationships affect the mental health of older people within the context of ongoing aging families. Attachment concepts seem to hold promise not only as an explanatory framework, but also eventually as a useful theory when empirical work has actually been done in this domain.

REFERENCES

Adam, K. S. (1994). Suicidal behavior and attachment: A developmental model. In M. B. Sperling & W. H. Berman (Eds.), *Attachment in adults: Clinical and developmental perspectives* (pp. 275–298). New York: Guilford.

Ainsworth, M. D. S. (1982). Attachment: Retrospect and prospect. In C. M. Parkes & J. Stevenson-Hinde (Eds.), *The place of attachment in human behavior* (pp. 3–30). New York: Basic Books.

Antonucci, T. (1994). Attachment in adulthood and aging. In M. B. Sperling & W. H. Berman (Eds.), *Attachment in adults: Clinical and developmental perspectives* (pp. 256–272). New York: Guilford.

Bartholomew, K., & Horowitz, L. M. (1991). Attachment styles among young adults: A test of a four-category model. *Journal of Personality and Social Psychology, 61,* 226–244.

Batgos, J., & Leadbeater, B. J. (1994). Parental attachment, peer relations, and dysphoria in adolescence. In M. B. Sperling & W. H. Berman (Eds.), *Attachment in adults: Clinical and developmental perspectives* (pp. 155–178). New York: Guilford.

Bowlby, J. (1969). *Attachment and loss: Vol. 1, Attachment.* New York: Basic Books.

Bowlby, J. (1979). *The making and breaking of affectional bonds.* London: Tavistock.

Bretherton, I. (1992). Attachment and bonding. In V. B. Van Hasselt & M. Hersen (Eds.), *Handbook of social development: A lifespan perspective* (pp. 133–155). New York: Plenum Press.

Brubaker, T. H. (1990). An overview of family relationships in later life. In T. H. Brubaker (Ed.), *Family relationships in later life* (2nd ed., pp.13–26). Newbury Park, CA: Sage.

Bus, A. C., & Van IJzendoorn, M. H. (1988). Mother–child interactions, attachment, and emergent literacy: A cross-sectional study. *Child Development, 59,* 1262–1272.

Butler, R. N., Lewis, M., & Sunderland, T. (1991). *Aging and mental health: Positive psychosocial and biomedical approaches.* New York: Merrill.

Carnelley, K. W., Pietromonaco, P. R., & Jaffe, K. (1994). Depression, working models of others, and relationship functioning. *Journal of Personality and Social Psychology, 66,* 127–140.

Cicirelli, V. G. (1993). Attachment and obligation as daughters' motives for caregiving behavior and subsequent effects on subjective burden. *Psychology and Aging, 8,* 144–155.

Collins, N. L., & Read, S. J. (1990). Adult attachment, working models, and relationship quality in dating couples. *Journal of Personality and Social Psychology, 58,* 644–663.

Collins, N. L., & Read, S. J. (1994). Cognitive representations of attachment: The structure and function of working models. In K. Bartholomew & D. Perlman (Eds.), *Advances in personal relationships* (Vol. 5, pp. 53–90). London: Jessica Kingsley.

Erickson, M. F., Sroufe, L. A., & Egeland, B. (1985). The relationship between quality of attachment and behavior problems in preschool in a high-risk sample. *Monographs of the Society for Research in Child Development, 50*(1-2, Serial No. 209), pp. 147–166.

Feeney, J., & Noller, P. (1996). *Adult attachment.* Thousand Oaks, CA: Sage.

Gelles, R. U., & Cornell, C. G. (1990). *Intimate violence in families* (2nd ed.). Newbury Park, CA: Sage.

Hazan, C., & Shaver, P. R. (1987). Romantic love conceptualized as an attachment process. *Journal of Personality and Social Psychology, 52,* 511–524.

Hazan, C., & Zeitman, D. (1994). Sex and the psychological tether. In K. Bartholomew & D. Perlman (Eds.), *Advances in personal relationships* (Vol. 5, pp. 151–177). London: Jessica Kingsley.

Keith, P. M.. Hill, K., Goudy, W. J., & Powers, E. A. (1984). Confidants and well-being: A note on male friendship in old age. *Gerontologist, 24,* 318–320.

Lyons-Ruth, K., Alpern, L., & Repacholi, B. (1993). Disorganized infant attachment classification and maternal psychosocial problems as predictors of hostile–aggressive behavior in the preschool classroom. *Child Development, 64*, 572–585.

Main, M. (1983). Exploration, play, and cognitive functioning related to infant–mother attachment. *Infant Behavior and Development, 6*, 167–174.

Main, M., Kaplan, N., & Cassidy, J. (1985). Security in infancy, childhood, and adulthood: A move to the level of representation. *Monographs of the Society for Research in Child Development, 50* (1–2, Serial No. 209), 66–104.

Main, M., Tomasini, K., & Tolan, W. (1979). Differences among mothers of infants judged to differ in security. *Developmental Psychology, 15*, 472–473.

Main, M., & Weston, D. R. (1981). The quality of the toddler's relationship to mother and to father: Related to conflict behavior and the readiness to establish new relationships. *Child Development, 52*, 932–940.

Mikulincer, M., Florian, V., & Weller, A. (1993). Attachment styles, coping strategies, and posttraumatic psychological distress: The impact of the Gulf War in Israel. *Journal of Personality and Social Disorders, 64*, 817–826.

Parker, G. (1994). Parental bonding and depressive disorders. In M. B. Sperling & W. H. Berman (Eds.), *Attachment in adults: Clinical and developmental perspectives* (pp. 299–312). New York; Guilford.

Rabins, P. (1992). Prevention of mental disorder in the elderly: Current perspectives and future prospects. *Journal of the American Geriatrics Society, 40*, 727–722.

Roberts, J. E., Gotlib, I. H., & Kassel, J. D. (1996). Adult attachment security and symptoms of depression: The mediating roles of dysfunctional attitudes and low self-esteem. *Journal of Personality and Social Psychology, 70*, 310–320.

Senchak, M., & Leonard, K. E. (1992). Attachment styles and marital adjustment among newlywed couples. *Journal of Social and Personal Relationships, 9*, 51–64.

Simpson, J. A. (1990). Influence of attachment styles on romantic relationships. *Journal of Personality and Social Psychology, 59*, 971–980.

Sperling, M. B., & Berman, W. H. (Eds.). (1994). *Attachment in adults: Clinical and developmental perspectives.* New York: Guilford.

Sperling, M. B., & Lyons, L. S. (1994). Representations of attachment and psychotherapeutic change. In M. B. Sperling & W. H. Berman (Eds.), *Attachment in adults: Clinical and developmental perspectives* (pp. 331–347). New York: Guilford.

West, M., & Keller, A. (1994). Psychotherapy strategies for insecure attachment in personality disorders. In M. B. Sperling & W. H. Berman (Eds.), *Attachment in adults: Clinical and developmental perspectives* (pp. 313–330). New York: Guilford.

Wykle, M. L., & Musil, C. (1993). Mental health of older people: Social and cultural factors. In M. A. Smyer (Ed.), *Mental health and aging* (pp. 3–17). New York: Springer.

CHAPTER 16

Multigenerational Families and Mental Illness in Late Life

Morton A. Lieberman

The popular indoor sport by academics of browsing Medline would yield little in searching for studies of aging, mental illness, and the family. The absence of a robust yield does not signify that this is an unimportant topic; rather it bespeaks a serious oversight.

Formal family research began in the 1950s. The emphasis was on the "traditional" family, with theory and empirical research based on an image of the isolated nuclear family living in the suburbs. Almost exclusively, family research focused on nuclear families that contained a mother and father and several dependent children. Multigenerational families, in which the first generation is elderly, has been a relatively ignored area of research. This has slowly changed in the last two decades. However, a perusal of the first *Handbook of Aging and the Family*, published in 1995, reflects the limitations of both theoretical thought and empirical research.

Family studies targeting the elderly are almost exclusively about the sociology of the family: roles, exchange, and propinquity. It is the study of changing cultural views of what constitutes the family, or it is the study of the history of the family and the changes over lengthy periods of time. Macrotheories predominate. Family systems theory, symbolic interactionism, and developmental theory are the most frequently used global perspectives for observing family life. Family development theory views the family through a role structure lens; it sees the individual family members as sharing a complex and mutually constructed history that impinges on current interactions and interpretations. Its

Morton A. Lieberman • Aging and Mental Health Program, Center for Social and Behavioral Sciences, University of California at San Francisco, San Francisco, California 94143.

Handbook of Aging and Mental Health: An Integrative Approach, edited by Jacob Lomranz. Plenum Press, New York, 1998.

emphasis is on the family as it moves through time, beset with a number of events that can trigger changes: development of the individual, changed roles of one or more individuals, changed participation in an external system or relationship, new expectations placed on the family from the community, or changed definitions of the situation. A second general approach, family stress theory, was developed to account for how families respond to stressful events. It is, of course, associated with Hill (1949), whose initial statement of the model included some event generally adverse and unexpected that interacts with the family's ability to cope with that event, including available resources and sources of social support, and the family's particular understanding that life changes, including both objectively and subjectively defined elements, resulting in the creation of what at least some family members view as a crisis, role strain, role overload, or conflict.

Unfortunately, although these perspectives provide a lens for viewing family operation, they do not aid in selecting specific variables for study of family characteristics that could provide hypotheses for testing the influence of family on concerns of the investigator interested in mental health outcomes. Midrange family theory fills the gap left by the abstractness of global theory. Appreciating the immense complexity of family life, midrange approaches describe how families work by focusing on well-defined domains of family life, for example, the Olson, Russel and Sprenkle (1989) circumplex model and Reiss's (1981) family belief model. Walsh (1982) has noted the important absence of family models that integrate "midrange" approaches, because (1) each theorist focuses on favored family characteristics, (2) each interprets the literature of the others selectively, and (3) the models, although internally coherent, do not provide the operational mechanisms that facilitate integration.

My colleague, Larry Fisher and I, set out about 5 years ago to develop a framework for studying and understanding the role of the multigenerational family in addressing chronic illness. The impetus to immerse myself, in what for me was a new field of inquiry, was the result of a few simple studies I conducted on Alzheimer patients. In one, we found (Lieberman & Kraemer, 1992) that the severity of the illness and its presumed impact on the family caregivers did not predict subsequent institutionalization. Rather, some characteristics of the caregiving relationship did. In a subsequent study of 3,000 patients, I found that despite enormous efforts on the part of 9 Alzheimer Centers in California to link families to services, only about one in five recommended services were ever used by the family within a year after the recommendation. In both studies, income, education, and gender of the patient did not affect these findings.

What impacted on service use and decisions to institutionalize a patient? We began to explore the effects of the family on such decisions. To date, we have focused on families in which one member of the first generation has Alzheimer's disease (AD). Although more strictly a neurological disorder, the psychiatric symptoms that are associated with patients who are so diagnosed is common (e.g., 20% were delusional, 40% manifested hallucinations). The fact that it is a chronic, progressive illness requiring a variety of adjustments by all family members makes this, in our perspective, an ideal candidate for study. We have plans to expand our work , examining the other scourge of old age, depression, and eventually comparing these two illnesses to crippling arthritis, a high-demand illness that does not involve the profound changes in the persona of the patient.

Our studies were set in a context of previous studies and constructs. Based on a wide variety of surveys, it is well documented that intergenerational family relationships are a central bond for the psychological and physical well-being of the parental generation. Approximately 80% of all elderly have living children, and 78–90% of all older people with living children see their children once a week or more often (Shanas, 1979). There is much evidence that a mutual helping relationship between parent and child continues throughout life (Bengtson, 1989).

A number of researchers of the traditional family have reported findings that suggest characteristics of the family as a unit are predictive of its ability to respond to a major health crisis over time: for example, diabetes (Hauser, Jacobson, Wertlieb, Brink, & Wentworth, 1985), cancer (Soccorsi, Lombardi, & Paglia, 1987), and cardiovascular disease (Medalie & Goldbourt, 1976). For example, family beliefs, structures, and styles have been associated with compliance with medical regimens (Rissman & Rissman, 1987), frequency of hospitalizations (Doane & Diamond, 1975), use of health care facilities (Schor, Starfield, Stidley, & Hanks, 1987), and postillness recovery (Medalie & Goldbourt, 1976). In general, the following family variables have received the most attention and have demonstrated the most consistent links with poor health: low family cohesion, high family conflict, too rigid or too permeable family boundaries, low levels of family organization, distant or hostile family affiliative tone, criticalness, lack of clear communication, and poor spousal support (Fisher, Ransom, Terry, Lipkin, & Weiss, 1992).

An overview of the family and health literature (e.g., Campbell, 1986; Gillis, 1989; Ransom, 1981) suggests that

1. Certain characteristics of the family show strong and consistent associations with various health outcomes.
2. The most powerful findings are associations between the aforementioned family characteristics and response to the diagnosis, the management, course, severity of disease, and the rate of relapse. Little evidence exists associating family variables with the etiology of disease.
3. Specific family characteristics are seldom associated with specific disorders.
4. The main characteristics of the disease, whether it is acute or chronic, and the stage of the family life cycle in which the disease occurs, interact with family functioning to affect patient and family member health and well-being. There is some evidence to suggest that family characteristics are associated with a willingness to make use of supports offered by extended family and health care resources.

The knowledge base was developed on the traditional family, parents, and dependent children, and not on the modified extended multigenerational family. If we look to studies of such families struggling with a chronic illness of an elderly family member, little exists to guide our explorations. Despite the rapid proliferation of empirical studies examining the relationship of family members to AD patients, the vast majority of such studies have not addressed the family as an integrated system responding to and being affected by the presence of the illness. Cohler, Grover, Borden, and Lazarus (1988) suggested that the best documented empirical evidence is of the relationships between patient characteristics and caregiver burden.

In recent years, there has been an increased focus on considering family variables as important in understanding family management of the disease (or lack thereof) and decisions to institutionalize. Some studies report that emotional support from siblings (Horowitz, 1985) and other relatives (Zarit, Reever, & Back-Peterson, 1980) mediate the caregiver's strain. Other studies document the problem of conflict and disturbed relationships between caregivers and their siblings. Brody (1989) reported that 45–60% of primary caregivers complained that their siblings failed to help as much as they should. Matthews and Rosner (1988) found that sibling conflict is sometimes exacerbated to the point that responsibilities can no longer be shared. Overall, the central focus of "family" research in caregiving for frail elderly centers on family conflict (Abel, 1989; Archbald, 1982; Frankfather, Smith, & Caro, 1981; Haussman, 1979; Smith, Smith, & Toseland, 1991). Stuifburgen (1990) reported that those families she characterized as involving "structured conflict" perceived a greater impact of illness than those she characterized as "cohesive." Pearlin and Hall (1990), viewed family conflict as a secondary stressor and reported a relatively small effect size. In a recent study, Strawbridge and Wallhagen (1991) reported that 40 of 100 adult children caregivers experienced serious conflict with other family members. They found that family conflict correlated with higher perceived caregiver burden and poorer reported health. Despite the rapid proliferation of empirical research on psychosocial aspects of chronic illness in the elderly, however, only a small number of studies have addressed the family as an integrated system, responding to and being affected by the presence of chronic disease.

The following characteristics and problems articulate the current state of knowledge about the family and chronic disease in the elderly: (1) Much family research uses data based on the perceptions of one family member rather than family-centered data; (2) most studies assume that the primary burden and the effects of caring for the patient fall on the defined primary caregiver exclusively; (3) most caregiver studies do not study differences in family relationships. Generalizations about the caregiving burden across members of the same family are difficult to make. The studies that do take into account differences in relationship suggest that the processes and procedures used, as well as the impact on the caregiver, are different for spouses compared to offspring.

We began with the realization that there were relatively little empirical data available on (1) the specific family characteristics that affect management of ill elderly, (2) how the demand characteristics of different chronic diseases affect families differently, (3) how family ethnicity/culture affects these processes, and (4) what standards should be utilized to assess effective family management of the disease.

Proposed is a general prospective on the family in which there are four issues regarding their functioning and particularly how such functioning affects the course of the illness of the elderly within the family: (1) *worldview*, a shared view in values common to a family, (2) the family *structure* and *organization*, (3) the family's methods of *regulating the emotions* of its members, and (4) *problem-solving* and decision-making characteristics of the family.

Our studies of families have, as yet, not addressed many important questions. We have not examined how the modified extended families of three generations, or more, not necessarily in the same household, differ from families in which there are younger children still living in a household. This chapter focuses on the general model and its measurement strategies in examining multigenerational families. A series of studies on the way the family is structured, the way it goes about making decisions, the way it regulates emotions, and its shared view of the world affects the course of the illness, decisions about dealing with the chronic illness, well-being, health, and role functioning of all members of the family across generations are summarized. The central concern is with individual differences among families and the consequences of these differences for these various outcomes.

This chapter also examines a number of methodological issues, something that cannot be easily escaped once a decision is made to study multigenerational families. Our studies began with direct observation of family interaction as members struggled with the care recommendations made by our Alzheimer center. A pilot based on 15 families suggested that, despite our view that this is an ideal method logistically, it was impossible to generate a large enough sample. We turned to intensive interviews and questionnaires to generate data. The immediate problem confronting an investigator who undertakes this strategy is how to take these individual responses of various family members and generate "family scores," the unit of analysis. Furthermore, it soon became clear that there were systematic differences among family members in their view of the family. Systematically, the first-generation non-ill spouse in the family setting, the grandmother or grandfather, had the most optimistic view of the family; the adult children had a somewhat middling position, and, invariably, the in-laws, the spouses of the adult children, had a less benign view of how the family operated. It is tempting to see their view as most accurate, since they are acting much like informants who are somewhat outside the system. There is no ultimate test of accuracy; rather, we take an empirical view and ask the question whose description of the family better serves the prediction of our hypotheses.

THE STUDIES

Our research over the past 5 years, with over 350 families of AD patients, has shown that characteristics of the family interact with the demands for care posed by AD to affect (1) the physical health and well-being of all family members, not just the primary caregiver; (2) the marriages of adult offspring; (3) the use of community-based services; (4) the follow-through on recommendations made by health care professionals; and (5) the decision to institutionalize.

We followed families in two studies for 3 years. In each study, one member of the first generation was diagnosed as being demented and at the time of our study was living independently with his or her spouse and/or adult children.

THE SAMPLES

Study sample 1 (consecutive patients and their families meeting sample criteria) was drawn from the four San Francisco Bay Area university-based Alzheimer Clinics developed and supported by the State of California, Department of Health. Study 2 sample patients were drawn from all nine California Alzheimer centers.

Each clinic sees an average of 130 new patients and their families per year for diagnostic and management/care planning; most families are followed for reevaluation every 12 months. The clinics are multidisciplinary: Their diagnostic procedures include a neuropsychological, family, medical, psychiatric, and social evaluation, as well as advanced diagnostic imaging procedures. Also, the patient's behavior and environment are assessed by a home visit by a clinic staff member. Each patient's evaluations are reviewed in a clinical case conference to arrive at a consensus diagnosis and care plan. Three to 4 weeks after the staff conference, family members attend a feedback meeting in which diagnostic information and recommendations for management and care are discussed.

Inclusion criteria for the studies included the following: (1) The patient met the NCCHD diagnostic criteria for probable or possible Alzheimer's or vascular dementia; (2) in study 1, the patient was living with a spouse in a community setting; in study 2, patients living alone or with children or relatives were included. In addition, for Study 1, we restricted the sampling frame based on the following criteria: The patient's spouse was capable of providing some modicum of care, defined as Activities of Daily Living/Instrumental Activities of Daily Living (ADL/IADL) tasks; at least one adult offspring provided "help" as judged by the clinic based on the family interview; at least one offspring was married; and at least one offspring had a child living in the second-generation household. The Study 2 sampling frame was not restricted by the previous criteria. In both studies, no restrictions were placed on social class or number and severity of patient problems.

In Study 1, only non-Hispanic whites were included, and all members of the family were invited to participate. Study 1 included 97 families, composed of 67 men and 30 women diagnosed as having probable or possible Alzheimer's or vascular dementia, their 97 spouses, 201 offspring, and 97 inlaws. In Study 2, minority families were recruited as well, as only select families members were

Table 16–1. Sample Characteristics of Study 1

	Patient	Spouse	Offspring	In-law
Age mean	69.8 (7.6)	68.5 (7.7)	40.2 (7.7)	42.3 (7.2)
% women	32%	68%	63%	41%
% college	30%	44%	53%	61%
Marriage length	—	42.6 yrs.	13.7 yrs.	—
Number of children	—	3.5 (1.4)	1.6 (1.3)	—
Care-hours mean	—	*	6.2 (10.9)	3.9 (8.6)
Care-strain mean	—	21.5 (5.5)	21.0 (5.1)	18.3 (4.1)
Functional mean	—	29.6 (7.3)	30.4 (7.1)	30.5 (7.0)
Problem behavior mean	—	17.1 (10.0)	17.9 (10.8)	18.3 (12.0)
Troubled mean	—	15.6 (9.9)	13.0 (10.3)	10.8 (10.6)

*Primary caregiver/spouse was not asked the number of hours spent in caring for ill spouse.

invited to participate. Study 2 included 247 families: 96 spouses, 203 offspring, and 146 inlaws (married to another offspring, not the offspring respondent). Characteristics of the samples are shown in Tables 16–1 and 16–2.

Comparability of Our Samples to Populations of Alzheimer and Vascular Dementia Patients

The study sample was compared to the 5,000 cases evaluated by the state-funded Alzheimer Clinics. Approximately 86% of all clinic patients were diagnosed as having possible or probable Alzheimer's or vascular dementia; 49.1% resided with a spouse in the community, and 87.2% received some ADL/IADL care from their spouses. Three broad classes of community-based patient living arrangements represented more than half of all patients: patients who lived with their spouse, with spouse and children, and with children only. Controlling for age and gender, a Multivariate Analysis of Covariance (MANCOVA) compared the effects of living arrangements on selected patient characteristics. The patients from the three types of living arrangements did not differ on the defining characteristics of dementia, level of mental status, or degree of functional deficit. Thus, the data from this study can be generalized to patients who live in community settings with their families or, if they live alone, have family members involved in their care.

We also compared the California AD population to the data from the 1982 National Long-Term Care Survey (Stone, Cafferata, & Sangl, 1987). The 1982 survey examined elderly care recipients who required ADL/IADL care, and was not restricted to a specific disease. Mean scores for the California Alzheimer's clinic population and the National Survey Population, respectively, were 74.5 versus 77.7 for age, 63% versus 60% females, 55.2% versus 51.3% married,

Table 16–2. Study 2 Population Characteristic of Cases Used for Sampling Cases Seen at the Nine DHS Centers, 1993–1995

Characteristic	Population $N = 2,606$	Sample $N = 252$
% men	35.1	37.8
% women	64.9	62.2
Mean years schooling	11.79 (4.22)	11.84 (4.16)
% married	43.7	58.7
% divorced, separated	13.1	24
% widowed	39.1	34.2
% single	3.5	0
% living alone	22.2	16
% living with spouse only	34.8	48.9
% living with spouse plus others	7.1	8
% living with relatives	23.3	20.4
% living with nonrelatives	3.1	3.6
% institutional settings	9.8	3.1
Asian	4.9	4.9
Filipino	1.0	0
Hispanic	11.8	11.6
Afriacan American	8.7	3.6
Non-Hispanic whites	72.3	79.6
Other	1.4	0
% SSI*	17.4	16
Primary caregiver—% spouse	38.1	51.7
% son	9.5	12.4
% son-in-law	.3	0
% daughter	23	21.1
% daughter-in-law	1.8	3.3
% other relatives	6.2	1.4
% friends	2.5	0
% neighbor	.5	0
% no one	11.5	7.2
Secondary caregivers—% family	54.3	55
Secondary caregivers—% nonfamily	7.1	13.8
Mini mental status examine	18.06 (7.37)	16.18 (7.39)
Blessed Roth dementia rating scale	4.81 (3.52)	4.64 (5.75)
Mean number psychiatric symptoms	6.61 (5.15)	5.97 (4.79)
Delusions, hallucination present	33%	37.3%
Mean number of neurological signs	1.79 (2.37)	1.50 (2.04)
Mean number of other illnesses	2.18 (1.80)	2.11 (2.08)
Primary syndrome—dementia %	83.2	100
% possible—probable Alzheimer's	61.4	80.7
% possible—probable vascular	6.8	12.4
% mixed etiology	13	7
% etiology undetermined	8.6	0
% depression	2.3	0

*(68.8% of the respondents did not report income).

33.2% versus 41.3% widowed, 11.2% versus 3.6% divorced/separated, and 3.9% versus 33.1% never married. Living arrangements for the two populations were 45.3% versus 39.5% with spouse, 8.3% versus 35.7% with spouse plus children, and 24% versus 10.7% living alone. The California Alzheimer's group contained fewer never-married respondents and more respondents living alone, compared to the national study.

ANALYTICAL STRATEGIES

Our overall analytical strategy was to evaluate first the effects of more traditional predictors, entering family characteristics as the last step in regression equations. Examined were

Patient Characteristics

These include income, age, education, and gender.

Severity of Disease

Seven measures, drawn from the evaluations undertaken by the Alzheimer's Clinic, were used to assess this construct. Included were (1) Level of Cognitive Disturbance (Mini-Mental State Exam [MMSE]; Folstein, Folstein, & McHough, 1975); (2) Level of Functioning (Blessed–Roth Dementia Rating Scale [BRDRS]; Blessed, Tomlinson, & Roth, 1968); (3) Number of Psychiatric Symptoms (psychiatrist's rating of the number and intensity of nine psychiatric symptoms, e.g., delusions, severe depression); (4) Number of Neurological Signs and Symptoms (neurologist's rating of the presence of nine indicators, e.g., agnosia, gait disorders); (5) Other Health Problems (physician's rating of the number of major illnesses based on a history and physical examination); (6) Problem Behaviors (clinical nurse's rating after a home visit of 10 current difficulties faced by the family in caretaking, e.g., self-care, memory/cognitive, harmful to others); and (7) Length of Time since Onset of Dementia Symptoms (clinician's rating based on interview with family members).

These seven indicators were submitted to a principal components analysis (PCA) with oblique rotation. Two well-constructed components emerged that accounted for 55% of score variance. Factor 1 reflected behavioral aspects of the illness and contained high loadings on Psychiatric Symptoms (.81), Problem Behaviors (.77), BRDRS (.60) and Other Illnesses (.56). Factor 2 reflected cognitive aspects and included high loadings on the MMSE (.78), Neurological Symptoms (.66), and Length of Dementia Symptoms (.65). As expected, the two components were moderately correlated ($r = .24$). Both were used in the analyses described below.

Illness Demands

These include demands posed by patients on family members. These scales include:

Perceptions troublesomeness (frequency of 17 patient problem behaviors, alpha = .85).

Being suspicious or accusative
Being constantly restless
Not recognizing familiar people

Functional ability (16 items, alpha = .94).

Can he or she get to places beyond walking distance?
Can he or she manage own money?
Can he or she take own medications?

Family Characteristics

Fisher, Ransom, Terry, Lipkin, and Weiss (1992b) developed a family assessment framework after an extensive review of the literature that identified those family characteristics that were consistently related to health outcomes. The framework comprises four "domains" of family life. Worldview (beliefs, values, sentiments), Structure/Organization (closeness, orderliness), Emotion Management (tone, style of affect regulation), and Problem Solving (skill, style, effectiveness). We have adapted selected variables from each family domain based on their work. Each selected variable has shown significant relationships with a variety of outcomes, and each has undergone extensive psychometric study with AD and non-AD families.

Two methods of measurement, questionnaire and telephone interview, were used to assess the domains of family life, and two levels of measurements were utilized: family characteristics based upon each respondent, and family level ratings of all family members.

Family Structure/Organization (person-level). This was assessed by questionnaires including the following:

Organized Cohesiveness (13 questionable items; alpha = .841). Combination of degrees of family togetherness and level of organization and structure. At one end are chaotic families, whose members do not spend much time together; at the other end are families who plan activities and have set roles, and so on, and whose members spend time with each other.

Family members spend much of their free time together.
In our family we are alike in how we think and feel.

Boundary Ambiguity (Boss, Wayne, Horbal, & Mortimer, 1990; five questionnaire items; alpha = 770).

> I am not sure where our ill family member fits in the family.
> It feels like the family has already lost our ill family member.

The two interview indices are

Number of Family Routines and Rituals: exact rater agreement = 65%
Presence of Family Isolates and Deviates: the degree to which the family identifies isolates and deviates among its members; exact rater agreement = 75%.

Family Worldview

Child–Adult Separation (Q-4 items; alpha = .688).   Refers to clear generational boundaries appropriate to developmental level. Parents are not too overly involved with children. Children are not too overly involved with adult issues. There is a sense of separateness in the family between children and parents.

> Our family believes that adults must have a life separate from the children.
> Our family believes that it is very important for adults to spend time away from the kids.

Life Engagement (Ransom, Fisher, & Terry, 1992; Q-10 items, alpha = .803).   Family support for moderate risk taking, preference for variety over sameness, and tolerance of difference versus consensus. Refers to a tendency to engage the world, try new things, and enjoy differences among people.

> Our family prefers friends who are always doing new things.
> It is okay in our family for everyone to have a different point of view.

Family Coherence (Ranson, Fisher, & Terry, 1992; Q-13 items; alpha = .877).   Refers to viewing life as comprehensible, meaningful, and manageable. A view in the family that one's destiny can be controlled to some extent, and that members can cope effectively with what life has to offer.

> Getting what our family wants requires pleasing those people above us.
> Our family believes that most things usually work out well.

Religion Scale (Q-4 items; alpha = .876).

> How important was religion in your day-to-day living over the past year?
> To what degree do you feel that religion has been an influence in your life?

Family Emotion Management.
Five questionnaire scales and eight interview indices present the emotional measures based on the measures that demonstrated independence from the other emotional management questionnaires and interviews. We have elected to explore this family domain in somewhat greater detail than the others because of the variety of underlying emotional themes that often are operative in these families.

Criticalness (Shields, 1992; Q-7 items; alpha = .822).

Use of criticalness and judgmental behavior.
My family approves of most everything I do.
My family is always trying to get me to change.

Emotional Distancing (Q-4 items; alpha = .811).   This occurs when family members tend to pull way from each other during times of stress. It could occur with one or two members or with everyone. The tendency is, however, to move away during disagreements rather than working things out.

> When there is a disagreement between two of our family members, they tend to pull away from each other instead of working it out.
> One or more of our family members seem to work or stay busy most of the time, with little time left to spend with the family.

Family Problem Solving.   This area was assessed by two questionnaire scales and six telephone interview indices. Each respondent was asked to describe a situation in which the family had to make a decision regarding the ill family member. A series of interview probes were then asked about the processes and feelings of each family member in the process, their satisfaction with the decision, the family, and external resources they used in arriving at the decision. Raters then used this information to construct a series of ratings. The telephone interview indices include

> *Intrafamilial Instrumental Support* (100%)
> *Disruptiveness of Family Problems* (80%)
> *Style of Decision Making* (100%)
> Ability to Manage Now (80%)
> Ability to Use New Information (80%)

The scales and indices reflect the family's ability to solve problems, its style of decision making, its ability to process new information, and the disruptiveness of unresolved problems (Reiss, 1989). In addition, the questionnaires assessed two problem-solving scales:

> *Express Opinion* (tolerance of family members expressing their opinion, 5 items, alpha = .840; Bloom, 1985)
> *Family Problem Solving* (effectiveness of family problem solving, 5 items, alpha = .740; Epstein, Baldwin, & Bishop, 1983).

Family-Level Family Characteristics.   We have also developed a series of Global Family Ratings, based on the questionnaire scales and telephone interview indices of all family members. This rating format was developed to reflect the family as a unit and to reduce the contamination that can occur when self-report scores from the same respondent are used as both the independent and dependent variables in the same analysis. The method is particularly useful with families who are dispersed or not easily gathered together. We have developed 17 Global Family Ratings that have particular relevance for families with a member with AD. One rater interviewed all members of the same family using the person-level scales and has available the scored questionnaire scales of each respondent. When all the data for a given family were collected, the rater reviewed the material, constructed an internal representation of the family unit based on his or her experience with the family and family theory, and rated the family on the family-level indices.

We list 17 Global Family Ratings and the integrator reliabilities. The Global Family Ratings for *Structure/Organization* are (numbers in parentheses below refer to the correlations between two raters based on 32 families used in a study of family characteristics and health care utilization in a primary care setting): Organized Cohesiveness (.80), Orderliness (78%), *Sex-Role Traditionalism* (.74), *Splits, Isolates, Deviates* (.84), and Family Cutoff (.67). Global Ratings for family *Worldview* are *Family Coherence* (.72), *Life Engagement* (.68), and *Religiousness* (.78). For family *Emotion Management*, the Global Ratings are *Current Family Stress* (.82), *Avoidance of Affect* (.67), *Emotional Tone* (.72), *Emotionally Aversive* (hostility, guilt, criticalness; .70), and *Positive Conflict Resolution* (reflecting use of compromise, discussion, etc., and excluding use of guilt induction, intimidation, etc.; .78). For *Family Problem Solving*, the Global Ratings are *Problem-Solving Effectiveness* (.74), *Problem-Solving Activity* (general level of activity devoted to the task; .66), *Style of Decision Making* (democratic, autocratic; .78), and *Instrumental Help* (.80).

Outcome Measures

Marital Strain: The Marital Strain Scale was originally developed by Pearlin and Lieberman (1978) on a large, random, normative sample (14 items, 4-point agree–disagree scale; alpha = .923). Illustrative items are "My spouse is affectionate to me, is a good sexual partner, brings out the best in me, spends money wisely, is someone I can really talk with about things that are important to me." Based on a large, random sample, interviewed 5 years apart, the validity of the marital scale was demonstrated by Menaghan and Lieberman (1986), who reported that high marital strain at Time 1 predicted subsequent divorce and separation. Furthermore, elevated marital strain was associated with elevations in depression and poorer health.

Parental Strain: This measure is based on two dimensions—worries and problems (Mullan, 1981); separate items were used depending on the age of the children (12 items for each, average alpha = .86).

Caregiver Strain: The Care–Burdens scale, developed by Niederehe and Fruge (1984), was used to assess offspring's subjective reactions to the demands of the illness. This 11-item scale (alpha = .82) asked, using a 4-point response alternative (*Almost always, Much of the time, Once in a while, Never,* or *Almost never*) such questions as the following: Do you feel embarrassed over your family member's behavior? Are you afraid of what the future holds for your family member? Do you feel you have lost control of your life since your family member's illness?

Health and Well-Being.

Somatic Symptoms is a list of 13 common problems developed by Ware et
al. (1984).
Anxiety/Depression was developed originally by Derogatis (1974) and modified by Pearlin and Lieberman (1981). It contains 22 items (alpha = .82).
Well-Being is a 9-item scale developed by Bradburn (1969; alpha = .94).

Service Use. We indexed the use of both formal and informal services over the last 3 months and family follow-up of clinic recommendations for services. Utilization of all services by the patient and family for the previous 12 months was recorded by the Clinics at Baseline. At the follow-up evaluations, every 6 months, respondents were asked which services were used. In both cases, a standard list of 20 services was employed. We then calculated the number of services recommended by the Clinic at Time 1 that were utilized by the family by Time 2. For example, if the clinic recommended that the caregiver attend a support group, follow-through on that service was scored positively if, indeed, the caregiver attended at least one session of a support group during the Time 1– Time 2 interval. This procedure was repeated for all types of services. Thus, service use was calculated for the 6 months prior to the evaluation, and follow-through on clinic recommendations was recorded for the year following the evaluation.

Because of the low frequency of service use in some categories of service, and the low intercorrelation among the types of services used, we constructed three indices to reflect groups of services based on their target and function. Patients–families who used one or more services within a particular group of services received a 1 and those that did not use any service within that group received a 0. The three indices are

Patient Services: those directed at modification or management of the patient's dementia-related problems (e.g., use of psychotropic medication, be-havioral programs for toileting, restructuring of safety features in the home).

Caregiver Task Services: those directed at the caregiver to relieve some of their caretaking burdens by temporarily reducing demanding and time-consuming care (e.g., use of a homemaker, transportation, respite, etc.).

Caregiver Psychological Services: those directed at caregivers' feelings of stress, providing a vehicle for modifying how they experienced the problem psychologically (e.g., support groups, counseling, and psychotherapy).

Institutionalization: defined as a permanent change in living arrange-ments from previous community living.

Informal Help by Family Members: Respondent were interviewed about the things they do to help the ill family member and the primary caregiver. Specifically, we focused on eight areas of task help: shopping, financial errands, transportation, personal care, food preparation, clothing care, home maintenance tasks. They were asked, if, during the past 6 months, they had provided that specific help, and if yes, how frequently. Frequency was coded as daily, 2–6 times per week, once per week, 1–3 times per month, and occasionally.

RESULTS

Effects on Health and Well-Being

We found, using cross-sectional data, that managing an elder with AD was associated with health and well-being of spouses, offspring, and offspring spouses (in-laws) (Lieberman & Fisher, 1993). Using 12 indicators of family functioning, grouped into three behavioral domains of family life, Worldview, Structure/Organization, Emotion Management, we found that adult offspring and in-laws displayed variations in anxiety/depression, somatic symptoms, and well-being as a function of qualities of the family system (Fisher & Lieberman, 1994). For example, adult offspring from AD families rated high on Parent–Offspring Separation, frequency of Family Rituals, and Tolerance of Family Conflict reported better health and well-being scores than offspring from families rated low on these family descriptors, even after controlling for severity of patient deficit and respondent gender (see Figures 16–1 and 16–2 for family characteristics and health outcome measures).

A second study (Fisher & Lieberman, 1994) examined the consistency and change in family and health relationships over time. We asked how characteristics of the family unit at Time 1 either exacerbate or buffer the stress of patient care from affecting the health and well-being of adult offspring of AD patients by Time 2. We found that (1) the number of hours per week that adult offspring devote to patient care is significantly associated with offspring health and well-being both at Time 1 and Time 2, whereas the severity of patient disorder is unrelated to offspring health and well-being at either point in time; (2) most characteristics of the family from each of the three family domains assessed at Time 1 show consistent relationships with health and well-being both at Time 1 and Time 2, even after controlling for the effects of care hours, gender, education, and severity of patient disorder; (3) aspects of Family Emotion Management (Family Avoidance of Conflict, Family Guilt Induction) assessed at Time 1 are linked with significant reductions in offspring health and well-being over time; and (4) Family Avoidance of Conflict is associated with adult offspring vulnerability to the effects of increasing patient-care distress over time. These characteristics of the family reflect its beliefs about affecting and managing life's problems (protective function), its tendency to fuse intergenerational boundaries (nonprotective function), its degree of family closeness and interlocking organization among family members (protective function), and the amount of

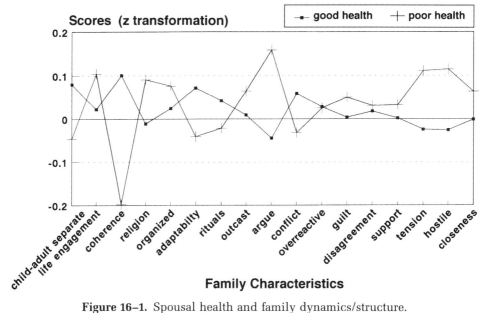

Figure 16–1. Spousal health and family dynamics/structure.

underlying tension and hostility among family members (nonprotective function). These findings suggest the powerful and consistent role over time played by the multigenerational family in response to managing an elder with AD. It also emphasizes the important effects of caregiving on family members other than the primary caregiver.

Marital Relations

In another study (Lieberman & Fisher, unpublished) using the same family descriptors, we found that qualities of the family system either exacerbated or contained the stresses of caregiving from cascading through the family system to affect non-disease-related family roles, in this case adult offspring-in-law marital role functioning. For example, in-laws reported high Marital Strain in their marriages to adult offspring of AD patients when the adult offspring came from families rated high on Emotional Distance, low on Parent–Offspring Separation, or had a member who was rated as over or underreacting to the disease. The study found that chronic illness in a family member, such as dementia in the parental generation, is significantly associated with non-disease-related family-role functioning in the second generation. The severity of the patient's illness and the degree of perceived burden experienced by offspring in caring for the ill parent are independently related to marital relationship strain.

Three aspects of these findings are noteworthy. First, in no case is a domain of family variables directly associated with marital strain; the effect occurs

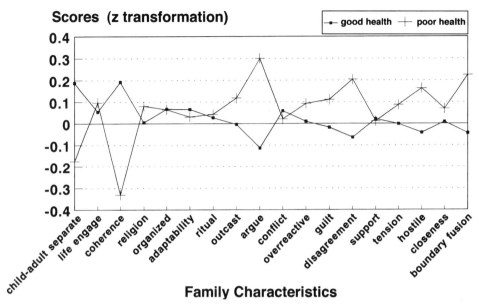

Figure 16–2. Children and family characteristics: Effects on health.

only in conjunction with level of offspring–caregiver strain. This suggests that caregiver strain is related to other family member role performance. In this case, the association operates through the experience of the family member who is at the interface between the two family systems: the family of origin (with the ill family member), and the family of choice. The "effect" of family characteristics, therefore, may not be seen directly, but only under conditions of low caregiver strain. Similar findings have been reported by Reiss and Oliveri (1980). Of particular interest is the finding that the family variables are not associated with the caregiver strain–marital strain relationship when caregiver strain is high, but only when it is low. This suggests that the negative effects of high caregiver strain on other family-role behaviors cannot be reduced by protective aspects of the family environment.

Second, only two of the three family domains interact with caregiver strain significantly in their association with marital strain: Family Worldview and Family Emotion Management display significant associations with in-law marital strain, whereas Family Structure/Organization does not. This reminds us that family characteristics are not a "homogeneous vector" (Coyne, 1987), an undifferentiated, unitary construct that operates in an all-or-none fashion. Rather, we see that "the family" is a complex of interrelated and often systematized processes, some of which are related to adaptation to some diseases, and some of which are not. The present findings concur with their earlier results, indicating the relative importance of how families construct their shared views of the world (Family Worldview) and how they regulate the emotional life of the family (Family Emotion Management).

Third, if we speculate a causative link among the variables, all but one of the significant Caregiver Strain by Family Characteristics interactions suggest that the family variables may serve a protective function; that is, the family variable may buffer the negative effects of caregiver strain from affecting the second generation's marriage. Families that have clear and firm intergenerational boundaries (Child–Adult Separation), that do not experience emotional distance among family members, and that do not have a family member who is judged to be either over- or underreacting emotionally to the disease are better able to limit the effects of the disease and its management from impinging upon the role functioning of family members. The interaction with Family Coherence suggests a similar protective function. The interaction with Family Life Engagement, however, indicates the opposite finding: Life Engagement is associated with an exacerbation of the relationship between Caregiver Strain and Marital Strain in the offspring–in-law marriage.

This suggests to us that family variables need to be viewed within the context of the demand characteristics of the disease (Rolland, 1987). Family Life Engagement reflects family support for variety over routine and repetition, encouragement of differences among family members verses sameness and agreement, and acceptance of moderate levels of risk taking, all of which would appear to be positively related to family adaptation. Our data suggest, however, that this apparently positive family characteristic is associated with negative consequences for the family. Upon reflection, however, it is reasonable to assume that a family that scored high on Life Engagement would have difficulty tolerating the often confining, long-term management routines required for the care of a family member with a debilitating chronic illness, especially when the family has little control over the course of the disease and the increased demands for care over time. The requirements for care run counter to the family's ethic of variety and action. Therefore, it is important to consider the patterns of family belief and function in conjunction with the particular demands placed upon the family by an acute or chronic disease when exploring the ability of the family and its members to manage over time. Different families have different sets of skills; these variations enable some families to function well in some settings but not necessarily in others.

Parenting

Our interest was in the impact of the illness of the grandparent, the family's reaction to managing the illness, and how this impacted on the third generation. Unfortunately, we could not gain access to these children, and we only have some information on how the second generation, the parents, functioned in their role as parents. Using a similar analytic strategy, first statistically removing the effects of demographic characteristics and illness severity, we did find a significant effect on the parenting role of the structure and dynamics of the family (defined of course not as the nuclear second generation but of the modified extended family) on parenting. Families that were low on coherence, did not practice large number of family rituals, and were low on support impacted on how well the parents performed in their role vis-à-vis their minor children.

Thus, how the multigeneration family with an elder with AD operates as a unit (i.e., its beliefs, structures, and qualities of emotion management) was associated with both offspring health and well-being and how offspring and in-laws functioned in non-disease-related family roles. These studies identify the multigenerational family system as a crucial social unit in caregiving and suggest that the health-related effects of AD go far beyond the primary caregiver to include adult offspring, in-laws, and others.

These family variables are similar to those identified in studies of other chronic diseases. For example, Antonovsky and Sourani (1988) showed that their measure of Family Coherence was related to the ability of injured or chronically ill males and their wives to adapt to the stress of disease in the family; Blechman and Delemater (1993) showed that family closeness and clear intrafamilial organizational structures were associated with good blood-glucose control in child and adolescent diabetics; and Doane and Diamond (1994) sum-marized the affective style literature, which indicates that family patterns of criticalness, guilt induction, and intrusiveness are major predictors of the course and rate of relapse of major psychiatric disorders. Thus, the family qualities that display consistent relationships with health and well-being over time in families caring for an elder with AD are similar to those found in studies of other chronic disease. This suggests that important qualities of the family that are related to health and well-being may not be disease specific. Instead, a basic set of family qualities are probably important for responding effectively to most demands for care, tempered by the family's life stage, other stresses, and perhaps some of the unique characteristics of each disease (Rolland, 1994).

Management of the Illness

We examined two indirect measures for evaluating the impact of the family on the way the family managed the disease. In all the clinics we studied, considerable effort was invested in helping families create and put into opera-tion a care plan. Family conferences were a help, with as many family members as could be induced to participate. A detailed set of recommendations were made, and specific sources of services were identified. As mentioned previously, only about one in five of these recommendations were followed through, within a year of the conference. Characteristics of the patient, the illness, and so forth had little predictive power in distinguishing characteristics that made for follow-through. Thus, we asked what role the structure and dynamics of the family played in this.

In a comparison of families following through on clinic recommendations versus not following through, our findings were as follows:

Families that did not follow through on recommendations were characterized by more closeness among family members, less detachment, fewer disagreements among family members in how to manage the illness, and showed changes over time, indicating that people grew close to one another. They also shared activities and enjoyed being with one another in these activities, and showed considerably less tension (80% of the families were scored as nontense compared to only 18% of those who followed through on recommendations). They were rated as much more expressive of affection and love within the family situation.

In contrast, those who follow through on recommendations were less close, much more detached, experienced high levels of disagreement in how to manage the illness, and appeared to be less able to enjoy activities with one another. One variable that does not fit the pattern of emotional regulation is that those who did not follow through on recommendations did use guilt more frequently to control the behavior of other family members compared to those who did follow up on recommendations.

The role of the family appears to be clearly implicated in whether the family will or will not follow through on recommendations made from the clinic. Although at first glance the direction of the findings seem counterintuitive, namely, families that did not follow through on the recommendations were families that on many of the parameters we measured appeared to be functioning much better in problem solving, in the emotional life of the family, in the levels of closeness and sharing, and so on, compared to the families that followed through. However, reflection on the nature of external services and family "health" would suggest that the results are consistent with general family theory, to wit, better functioning families do have the resources within themselves to deliver services and to take the complex situation of the care of a chronic illness such as dementia that makes complex demands. A well-functioning family is more likely to turn to its own resources than external ones.

Could it be that the clinic, in making and helping families carry out recommendations, perceived differences in the family and pursued with more vigor their recommendations with families they perceive as not functioning as well or being overwhelmed, and that the reason for the relationship between family characteristics and the carrying out of clinic recommendations may be mediated by this characteristic differential of the way the clinic treated the family and their recommendations? Unfortunately, we have no direct evidence to examine this alternative. However, we do have a variety of scores that may reflect family-member distress around the caregiving role—their perceptions of how disturbed the patient was, how troublesome his or her behavior was, the amount of strain they experienced in a caregiving role, as well as variety of measures indexing each individual's well-being, ranging from measures of mental health (anxiety and depression), physical health, positive and negative affects, and role strain in the major role areas beyond the caregiving one. An analysis of these characteristics comparing family members where recommendations were not carried out as opposed to those where they were carried out, and analyzing the information by individual scores, namely, the spouse's, the offspring's, and the in-laws's, we find no compelling evidence that the family members who follow through on recommendations were systematically different than those who did not on the basis of such scores.

The Amount of Help Provided by Second-Generation Family Members

The amount of task help (shopping, errands, financial management, laundry, personal care, cooking, and home maintenance) were examined. Every 6 months, the second-generation family members were interviewed and asked to describe the things they did for their parent–parent-in-law during the past few weeks. We found that the amount of help provided did effect the primary caregiver—the more help, the lower their depression and anxiety.

What factors affect the amount of help provided?

Step 1 entered the distance the children lived from the parent, their gender and education level; Step 2 was a series of dimensions assessing the functional competence and types of problems manifested by the ill family member. Step 3 entered the amount of professional services currently used by the patient and the primary caregiver. In Step 4, the family dimensions were entered, in effect controlling for the previous three steps.

We found that

1. The second generation's gender and education impacted on the amount of help children provided. Women and those with higher education provided more help.
2. Hyperactive patients and those experiencing difficulty in common household tasks were provided more help, and as anticipated, the more competent the patient, the less help was forthcoming.
3. The more professional services were used, the more the informal help was provided.
4. Families that were high on child–adult separation did not have clear-cut Generational Boundaries and were not Coherent provided less help.

Institutionalization

Similar analyses were carried out to understand the effects of the family on decisions to institutionalize. After controlling for demographic characteristics, the severity of the illness, the use of community services, and the stresses and strains on the primary caregiver, family characteristics proved to have a significant impact on the decision. Families whose worldview endorsed a highly religious explanation of the world and illness, who were structured and organized but low on adaptability, who avoided conflict, and who had family members who were label in their reactions to the illness, were more likely to institutionalize the patient within a year.

THE PRACTICAL SIDE
OF STUDYING FAMILIES:
DEVELOPING NEW MODELS OF INTERVENTIONS

Most intervention studies have been directed at alleviating one or more of the problems experienced by the primary caregiver in caring for a frail elderly person (Schultz, Visintainer, & Williamson, 1990). The results of these interventions, however, have been mixed. In overview, a recent review of intervention studies that used control groups found that interventions directed at caregivers of frail elderly showed either nonsignificant findings or modest effect sizes when results were significant (Zarit, 1990). Thus, there are no consistent data to suggest that interventions to reduce the burdens of care targeted exclusively at the primary caregiver have been successful. Based on our studies and the findings of current intervention strategies, we believe an approach for multigenerational families struggling with an elderly family member suffering from a chronic illness may well be a method of choice.

Following World War II, the earlier view of family therapy disorders of individuals across the lifespan were as a function of disturbances in early parent–child relationships, and treatment was primarily directed at the patient with the presenting problem evolved to form the foundation for the development of "family therapy," which consists of both a way of thinking about the social context of clinical problems (e.g., Bateson, Jackson, Haley, & Weakland, 1956; Lidz, Fleck, & Cornelison, 1965) and a method of treatment. The underlying premise is that a pathological process inherent in the family system underlies the display of symptoms in one or more family members. Consequently, treatment methods target the family unit. For example, methods focus on changing family structure, boundaries, alliances, beliefs, communication, and so on. Although originally developed for the treatment of schizophrenia, the family therapy movement was quickly generalized to the treatment of other mental and behavioral disorders of children, adolescents, and adults.

In recent years, family-based techniques have been applied to the treatment of problems arising from the presence of chronic disease in the family. Applied primarily to chronic illnesses in children and adolescents (Drotar, 1992), the premise is that management problems are a function of poor family functioning and ability, and changing the family will modify the stresses and strains inherent in managing a disabling and chronic disease. By and large, methods of family intervention that emerge from this orientation are of four types: (1) those that focus on the individual, usually the patient, as a vehicle for changing behavior in the family setting; (2) those that provide "support" to family members in the form of social contact; (3) those that educate family members about the disease; and (4) those that deliver clinical care to the family as a unit in either a single- or multifamily group setting (e.g., case management and therapy; see Akamatsu, Stephens, Hobfoll, & Crowthers, 1992, for a review).

Although clinicians have recognized the importance of the family in managing chronic disease, family therapy techniques have been infrequently applied to this context historically for two important reasons: (1) Family models assume that pathological family processes "cause" management difficulties, and they do not emphasize that the disease affects family life profoundly and influences basic aspects of family operation and relationship; (2) because of this orientation, family models do not facilitate collaboration between the family and the health care provider. In the family therapy approach, the provider is viewed as the family's therapist, whose goal is to change the system. Consequently, the application of family concepts to chronic disease has been relatively slow to develop (Jacobs, 1992).

An alternative to the traditional family therapy model began with a series of studies initiated by George Brown and his colleagues in the United Kingdom. Brown was interested in the determinants of its course (i.e., what happens to the illness once it is established). In a series of studies, he and other researchers showed that the affective climate of the patient's household predicted rate of relapse. Similar research has been undertaken with families of chronically depressed and obese patients, with similar results. Also, Coyne & Smith (1992) have shown a parallel family pattern in spouses of post-myocardial infarct patients. The findings demonstrate that specific aspects of family climate and relationships affect the management of a chronic disease, without the necessity of positing that the management problems are the result of long-standing, dysfunctional family processes.

This research led Anderson, Griffin, Rossi, Pagonis, Holder, and Treiber (1986a) to extend earlier work on a family-based program of intervention for managing chronically ill patients. Called the psychoeducational model, its central notion is that the family and other natural social groups can be trained to create an interactional environment that compensates for the problems that arise in managing functional disability in one member of the group. In many ways, this model is not family therapy at all, but rather a flexible, family-focused strategy for treating the effects of a disabling and chronic illness in the family. The model consists of three parts. First, it emphasizes the centrality of creating a functional collaborative treatment system in which family members engage as partners with health care providers. Second, in a series of family meetings, either in a single family or multifamily group format extending over time, information about the disease, its cause, course, and effects on the patient and other family members is presented and discussed in detail until a common frame of reference is established among and between family members and health care providers. Third, four areas of family life are assessed clinically and, through collaborative group discussion, changes are suggested and implemented. In the specific program suggested by Anderson and colleagues, the areas include personal and generational boundaries, clarity and consistency of family communication, family structure and organization, and family problem solving and coping. Discussions focus on current management problems, specific goals and plans are made, and evaluation is addressed directly (see MacFarlane, 1991, for a summary). Since many management problems are related to high family stress, inconsistent and unclear family messages to patients and family overinvolvement, disagreement, and conflict, modifications developed in the model for use with schizophrenic and depressed patients can be easily applied to families struggling to manage chronic disease in the elderly. The effectiveness of the approach in reducing rates of relapse and other management-related problems among family members has been well documented (Falloon et al., 1982; Leff, Kuipers, Berkowitz, & Sturdgen, 1982).

However, we know of no empirically evaluated, systematic, psychoeducational program for families of ill elderly.

Toward the Future

1. General theoretical models only point the way; they are currently too broad to answer the specific questions of who, how, and what effects.

2. The impact of the multigenerational family on the management of the chronic illness, and the impact of the illness on the physical and mental health, and role performance of all family members across generations is real.

3. Needed are midlevel theories that must have their specifics firmly embedded in empirical research. Our findings clearly reflect specifics; to try and conceptualize "good" and "bad" families is an exercise in futility. The effects of family functioning on all family members and the ability of the family to mitigate distress is not the same issue as the ability of the family to proceed sensibly in managing the welfare of the patient. Traits stereotypically associated with positive family characteristics, such as life engagement, may be characteristic of well-functioning families in their ordinary life course, but, as found in the particular crises confronting them in caring for a chronic illness in the first generation, such characteristics are not helpful.

4. Based on our findings, it is not too large a step to suggest that our field needs to develop family-based therapeutic interventions. Although the models are there for the traditional nuclear family, the need is to push ahead with them in working with multigenerational families.

5. Finally, in the education of clinicians, the lack of input of family models and techniques is glaring and needs correction.

REFERENCES

Abel, E. (1989). *Love is not enough: Family care of the frail elderly.* Washington, DC: American Public Health Association.

Akamatsu, T. J., Stephens, A. P., Hobfoll, S. E., & Crowther, J. H. (1992). Family health psychology. Washington, DC: Hemisphere.

Anderson, C. M., Griffin, S., Rossi, A., Pagonis, I., Holder, D. P., & Treiber, R. (1986a). A comparative study of the impact of education versus process groups for families of patients with affective disorders. *Family Process, 25,* 185–206.

Anderson, C. M., Hogarty, G. E., & Reiss, D. J. (1986b). Schizophrenia and the family. New York: Guilford.

Anderson, C. M., Reiss, D. J., & Hogarty, G. E. (1986). *Schizophrenia and the family.* New York: Guilford.

Antonovsky, A., & Sourani, T. (1988). Family sense of coherence and family adaptation. *Journal of Marriage and the Family, 50,* 79–82.

Archbald, P. G. (1982). The impact of parent-caring on women. *Family Relations, 32*, 39–45.

Bateson, G., Jackson, D. D., Haley, J., & Weakland, J. (1956). Toward a theory of schizophrenia. *Behavioral Science, 1*, 251–264.

Bengtson, V. L. (1989). The problem of generations: Age group contacts, continuities, and social change. In V. L. Bengtson & K. W. Schaie (Eds.), *The course of later life: Research and reflections* (pp. 25–54). New York: Springer.

Bloom, B. L. (1985). A factor analysis of self-report measures of family functioning. *Family Process, 24*, 225–239.

Blechman, E. A., & Delameter, A. M. (1993). Family communication and Type I diabetes: A window on the social environment of chronically ill children. In R. E. Cole & D. Reiss (Eds.), *How do families cope with chronic illness?* (pp. 1–24). Hillsdale, NJ: Erlbaum.

Blessed, G., Tomlinson, B. E., & Roth, M. (1968). The association between quantitative measures of dementia and of senile change in the cerebral grey matter of elderly subjects. *British Journal of Psychology, 114*(512), 797–811.

Boss, P., Wayne, C., Horbal, J., & Mortimer, J. (1990). Predictions of depression in caregivers in dementia patients: Boundary ambiguity and mastery. *Family Process, 29*(3), 245–254.

Bradburn, N. (1969). *Structure of psychological well-being.* Chicago: Aldine.

Brody, E. M. (1989). The family at risk. In E. Light & B. D. Lebowitz (Eds.), *Alzheimer's disease treatment and family stress: Directions for research* (pp. 135–156). Washington, DC: National Institute of Mental Health.

Campbell, T. L. (1986). Family's impact on health: A critical review. *Family Systems Medicine, 4*, 135–328.

Cohler, B. J., Groves, L., & Lazarus, L. (1989). Caring for family members with Alzheimer's disease. In E. Light & B. D. Liebowitz (Eds.), *Alzheimer's disease treatment and family stress: Directions for research* (pp. 50–105). Rockville, MD: U.S. Department of Health and Human Services.

Coyne, J. C. (1987). Some issues in the assessment of family patterns. *Journal of Family Psychology, 1*, 51–57.

Coyne, J. C., & Smith, D. A. (1991). Couples coping with a myocardial infarction: A contextual perspective on wives' distress. *Journal of Personality and Social Psychology, 61*, 404–412.

Doane, J. A., & Diamond, D. (1985). *Affect and attachment in the family: A family-based treatment of major psychiatric disorder.* New York: Basic Books.

Drotar, D. (1992). Integrating theory and practice in psychological intervention with families of children with chronic illness. In T. J. Akamatsu, A. P. Stephens, S. E. Hobfoll, & J. H. Crowther (Eds.), *Family health psychology* (pp. 18–23). Washington, DC: Hemisphere.

Epstein, N., Baldwin, L. M., & Bishop, D. S. (1983). The McMaster family assessment device. *Journal of Marriage and Family Therapy, 9*, 171–180.

Falloon, I., Boyd, J. L., McGill, C., Razoni, J., Moss, H. B., & Gilderman, H. M. (1982). Family management in the prevention of exacerbations of schizophrenia. *New England Journal of Medicine, 306*, 1437–1440.

Falloon, I., Boyd, J., & McGill, C. (1984). Family care of schizophrenia. New York: Guilford.

Felton, B. J., Brown, P., Lehman, S., & Liberator, P. (1980). The coping function of sex-role attitudes during marital disruption. *Journal of Health and Social Behavior, 21*, 240–248.

Fisher, L., & Lieberman, M. A. (1994). Alzheimer's disease: The impact of family characteristics on spouses, offsprings, and in-laws. *Family Process, 33*, 305–325.

Fisher, L., Ransom, D. C., Terry, H. E., & Burge, S. (1992a). The California Family Health Project: IV. Family structure/organization and adult health. *Family Process, 31*, 399–419.

Fisher, L., Ransom, D. C., Terry, H. E., Lipkin, M., & Weiss, R. (1992b). The California Family Health Project: I. Introduction and a description of adult health. *Family Process, 31*, 231–250.

Folstein, M. F., Folstein, S. A., & McHough, P. R. (1975). Mini Mental States: A practical method for grading cognitive states of patients for the clinician. *Journal of Psychiatric Research, 12*, 189–198.

Frank, K., Heller, S., & Kornfield, D. (1979). Psychological intervention in coronary heart disease. *General Hospital Psychiatry, 19*(1), 18–23.

Frankfather, P. L., Smith, M. J., & Caro, F. G. (1981). *Family care of the elderly.* Lexington, MA: Lexington Books.

Gillis, C. L. (1989). Family research in nursing. In C. L. Gillis, B. L. Highly, B. M. Roberts, & I. M. Martinson (Eds.). *Towards a science of family nursing.* Menlo Park, CA: Addison-Wesley.

Hauser, S., Jacobson, A., Wertlieb, D., Brink, S., & Wentworth, S. (1985). The contributions of family environment to perceived competence and illness adjustment in diabetic and acutely ill adolescents. *Family Relations, 34,* 99–108.

Haussman, C. P. (1979). Short-term counseling groups for people with elderly parents. *Gerontologist, 19,* 102–107.

Hill, R. (1949). *Families under stress.* Westport, CT: Greenwood Press.

Horowitz, A. (1985). Sons and daughters as caregivers to older parents: Differences in role performance and consequences. *Gerontologist, 25,* 612–617.

Jacobs, J. (1992). Understanding family factors that shape the impact of chronic illness. In T. J. Akamatsu, A. P. Stephens, S. E. Hobfoll, & J. H. Crowther (Eds.), *Family health psychology* (pp. 111–127). Washington, DC: Hemisphere.

Leff, J. P., Kuipers, L., Berkowitz, R., & Sturgen, D. (1982). A controlled trial of social intervention in the families of schizophrenic patients: Two-year follow-up. *British Journal of Psychiatry, 146,* 594–600.

Lidz, T., Fleck, S., & Cornelison, A. R. (1965). *Schizophrenia and the family.* New York: International Universities Press.

Lieberman, M. A., & Fisher, L. (1993). Predicting institutionalization of patients with dementia: The impact of disease severity, care setting and use of community services. *Facts and Research in Gerontology.*

Lieberman, M. A., & Fisher, L. (1995). The impact of chronic illness on the health and well-being of family members. *Gerontologist, 35*(4), 94–102.

Lieberman, M. A., & Fisher, L. (1995). The impact of a parent's dementia on adult children and their spouses: The contribution of family characteristics. *Gerontologist, 35,* 94–102.

Lieberman, M. A., & Kramer, J. (1992). Factors affecting decisions to institutionalize demented elderly. *Gerontologist, 31*(3), 371–374.

MacFarlane, W. R. (1991). Family psychoeducational treatment. In A. S. Gurman & D. P. Kniskern (Eds.), *Handbook of family therapy* (Vol. 2, pp. 37–45). New York: Brunner/Mazel.

Matthews, S. H., & Rosner, T. T. (1988). Shared filial responsibility: The family as primary caregiver. *Journal of Marriage and the Family, 50,* 185–195.

Medalie, J. H., & Goldbourt, U. (1976). Psychosocial and other risk factors as evidenced by a multivariate analysis of a five-year incidence study. *American Journal of Medicine, 60,* 910–921.

Menaghen, B., & Lieberman, M. A. (1986). Changes in depression following divorce. *Journal of Marriage and the Family, 48,* 319–328.

Mullan, J. (1981). *Parental distress and marital happiness: The transition to the empty nest.* Ph.D. dissertation, University of Chicago, Chicago, IL.

Niederehe, G., & Fruge, E. (1984). Dementia and family dynamics: Clinical research issues. *Journal of Geriatric Psychiatry, 10,* 21–56.

Olson, D. H., Russell, C. S., & Sprenkle, D. H. (1983). Circumplex model of marital and family systems: Theoretical update. *Family Process, 22,* 69–84.

Pearlin, L. I., Lieberman, M. A., Menaghan, E. G., & Mullan, J. T. (1981). The stress of process. *Journal of Health and Social Behavior, 22,* 333–356.

Pearlin, L. I., Mullan, J. T., Semple, S. J., & Skaff, M. M. (1990). Caregiving and the stress process: An overview of concepts and their measures. *Gerontologist, 30*(5), 583–594.

Ransom, D. C. (1981). The rise of family medicine: New roles for behavioral science. *Marriage and Family Review, 4,* 31–72.

Ransom, D. C., Fisher, L., & Terry, H. E. (1992). The California Family Health Project: II. Family worldview and adult health. *Family Process, 31,* 251–267.

Reiss, D. (1989). Families and their paradigms: An ecological approach to understanding the family and its social world. In C. N. Ramsey (Ed.), *Family systems* (pp. 119–134). New York: Guilford.

Reiss, D., & Oliveri, M. E. (1980). Family paradigm and family coping: A proposal for linking the family's intrinsic adaptive capacities to its responses to stress. *Family Relations, 29,* 431–444.

Rissman, R., & Rissman, B. Z. (1987). Compliance: A review. *Family Systems Medicine, 5,* 446–467.

Rogers, W. H., Donald, C. A., & Johnston, S. A. (1984). *Conceptualization and measurement of health for adults in the health insurance study: Vol. I. Model of health and methodology* No. R:1987/1-HEW. Rand Corporation.

Rolland, J. S. (1987). Chronic illness and the life cycle: A conceptual framework. *Family Process, 26,* 203–221.

Rolland, J. S. (1994). *Families, illness, and disability.* New York: Basic Books.

Schor, E., Starfield, B., Stidley, C., & Hanks, J. (1987). Family health: Utilization and the effects of family membership. *Medical Care, 25,* 616–626.

Schultz, R., Visintainer, P., & Williamson, G. (1990). Psychiatric and physical morbidity effects of caregiving. *Journal of Gerontology, 45,* 185–191.

Shanas, E. (1979). The family as a social support system in old age. *Gerontologist, 19,* 169–174.

Shields, C. G. (1992). Family interaction and caregivers of Alzheimer's disease patients: Correlates of depression. *Family Process, 31,* 19–33.

Smith, G. C, Smith, M. F., & Toseland, R. W. (1991). Problems identified by family caregivers in counseling. *Gerontologist, 31,* 15–22.

Soccorsi, S., Lombardi, F., & Paglia, P. R. (1987). Capturing death: Families of children recovering from oncological disease. *Family Systems Medicine, 5,* 191–205.

Steinglass, P., Gonzalez, S., Dosovitz, I., & Reiss, D. (1982). Discussion groups for chronic hemodialysis patients and their families. *General Hospital Psychiatry, 4,* 7–14.

Strawbridge, W. L., & Wallhagen, M. (1991). Impact of family conflict on adult caregivers. *Gerontologist, 31,* 770–778.

Stone, R., Cafferata, G. L., & Sangl, J. (1987). *Caregivers of the frail elderly: A national profile. Gerontologist, 27*(5), 616–625.

Stuifburgen, A. K. (1990). Patterns of functioning with chronically ill patients: An exploratory study. *Research in Nursing and Health, 13,* 35–44.

Walsh, F. (1982). Conceptualizations of normal family functioning. In F. Walsh (Ed.), *Normal family processes* (pp. 192–205). New York: Guilford.

Ware, J., Brook, R. H., Davies-Avery, A., Williams, K. N., Stewart, A. L., Rogers, W. H., Donald, C. A., & Johnston, S. A. (1984). *Conceptualization and measurement of health for adults in the health insurance study: Vol. I. Model of health and methodology* No. R:1987/1-HEW. Rand Corporation.

Zarit, S. (1990). Interventions with frail elders and their families: Are they effective and why? In M. A. Stephens, J. H. Crowther, S. E. Hobfoll, & D. L. Tennedbaum (Eds.), *Stress and coping in later life families* (pp. 241–265). Washington, DC: Hemisphere.

Zarit, S. H., Anthony, C. R., & Boutselis, M. (1987). Interventions with caregivers of dementia patients: Comparison of two approaches. *Psychology and Aging, 2,* 225–232.

Zarit, S. H., Reever, K. E., & Bach-Peterson, J. (1980). Relatives of the impaired elderly. *Gerontologist, 20,* 649–655.

CHAPTER 17

Cross-Cultural Perspective on Attitudes toward Family Responsibility and Well-Being in Later Years

Catherine B. Silver

INTRODUCTION

In this chapter, we used cross-national surveys from Japan and the United States to look at the perceptions of responsibility of children toward elderly parents, desirable ways of living in old age, and well-being in later years. By comparing Japan and the United States, we want to contribute to the analysis of the role of culture in mediating between values and age structures (Foner, 1984; Riley, Kahn, & Foner, 1994). The analysis of selected questions from these surveys, referred to as the Generations project,* is used to raise theoretical issues about shared attitudes toward aging and well-being, and the emergence of a trans-cultural sense of self among older people. By comparing age groups and looking at the discrepancies between younger adults' and older persons' perceptions of aging and normative expectations, we hope to throw some light on the discourse of aging in postmodern society. We further want to explore how the family provides a context that protects and isolates, helps and controls older people,

---

*The Generations project refers to national surveys carried out in Japan and the United States in 1993 under the sponsorship of the International Longevity Center in Tokyo, in cooperation with the Ministry of Health and Welfare (Koseisho). A joint report summarizing the key findings, The Generations Report (Muller & Silver, 1995), was jointly published by the International Longevity Centers (ILC–US and ILC–Japan).

CATHERINE B. SILVER • Brooklyn College and the Graduate Center of the City University of New York, 33 West 42nd Street, New York, New York 10036-8099.

Handbook of Aging and Mental Health: An Integrative Approach, edited by Jacob Lomranz. Plenum Press, New York, 1998.

creating tensions between emotional caring in the family and social isolation in the larger community, what we describe as paradoxes of attachment. Such an analysis requires that family relations be understood within the larger cultural framework of rights and obligations in each country.

It has been suggested that in postindustrial societies, age boundaries are becoming more flexible and open. Age is no longer a strong social marker (Giddens, 1991). Despite high levels of economic and technological development in Japan and the United States, there are still clear cultural differences in the way selfhood is defined (Lock, 1993; Roland, 1988), and in the way age influences social values (Silver & Muller, 1997). Talking about the self of older persons assumes that they have distinct attitudes and values from those of younger adults. In this chapter, we want to show how age groups are differentially affected by cultural norms and social prescriptions. We suggest that the older person's sense of self and feeling of well-being reflect cultural values as well as being shaped by his or her position of economic marginalization and psychological isolation from younger age groups. Similar structural positions reinforce rigid age boundaries between adults and elderly populations, and are likely to encourage the emergence, across cultures, of common values and attitudes toward aging. By contrasting patterns of age structures in Japan and the United States, and exploring cross-cultural differences and similarities in values, we want to contribute to an understanding of the many, sometimes contradictory, ways in which aging is defined and well-being is experienced.

In our analysis, we first describe normative expectations in the two societies by presenting standardized means and means differences, followed by an analysis of norms across age groups to assess variations in their internalization. In our study, we have conceptualized age groups around the following categories: 18–29 years (younger adults); 30–49 and 50–64 years (middle-aged adults); over 64 years (older persons).* These age groups correspond loosely to the different stages of the life cycle, reflecting roughly similar social and economic situations, but we do not assume that they reflect a linear process of human development. Older people are not a homogeneous group. There are differences due to a variety of economic, demographic, and social factors. However, in this overview chapter, we only focus on analyzing country and age effects, as they shape the perception of responsibility toward elderly parents, attitudes toward aging, and feelings of well-being.

The aforementioned theoretical issues cannot be analyzed unless we also look at the underlying assumptions and ideological premises embedded in doing cross-national survey research. There is a tradition of cross-national survey research on values and national identity (Inglehart, 1990), and there have been numerous criticisms of the concept of national character, especially as it was used in the 1950s and 1960s.† Among the criticism, it was suggested that the

---

*The age distribution ranges from 18 to 92 years. However, there were too few individuals among the oldest-old (85 years and over) to create a distinct category.
†For a review and critique of studies of National Character, see, for example, Inkeles (1997) and Johnson (1993).

approach led to unwarranted generalizations about a society and to stereotyping of different cultures. While this has happened, cross-national research does not have to achieve such negative results. We agree with Befu (1986) when he suggests:

> It may be impossible to eliminate stereotyping altogether even from scientific discourse. The question is, therefore, how to use stereotypes and how to interpret them when used by others. That Americans believe in free will, for example, does not mean that they will exercise it all the time or that their actions are based exclusively on it. Similarly, the truism that the Japanese are group oriented does not mean that all Japanese are, or that group orientation is the only form of relating Japanese recognized. (p. 13)

Survey methods have to be used with caution in cross-national research. However, when combined with cultural analysis, they can provide theoretical insights and a framework to compare systematically the interplay between culture and social structure* in ways that would be impossible using only in-depth interviews. A systematic study of the interplay of culture and social structures requires working with large random samples and the use of statistical models. Such analyses, far from creating stereotypes, can help disentangle the impact of country effects from other social factors, such as gender, class, and age, and to compare their interaction.† It is nonetheless essential to rely on multiple sources of information in order to uncover and understand the contradictions between social meaning and individual behavior, internalized ideologies and lived experiences, and symbolic order and social order. This is especially important when studying groups such as older people, who tend to be marginalized, vulnerable, and isolated. The lack of in-depth interviews in the Generations project led us to use available qualitative data and clinical accounts to provide deeper interpretations of our survey findings.

The Generations data reported here were collected through interviews using national random samples of men and women 18 years and older ($N = 1,764$ in Japan and $N = 1,497$ in the United States).‡ The original survey covered large areas of inquiry around values and their transmission in the family as well as a subset of questions about aging. In this chapter, we only use a few questions about family responsibility, desirable ways of living in old age, and general issues of well-being in order to analyze the tension between emotional caring and social isolation, and to understand the different, sometimes contradictory images of aging and well-being.

Doing cross-cultural research requires a constant flow, back and forth, of ideas between cultural frames that guide conceptualization, the creation of a research instrument, and the interpretation of findings. The dangers of projecting one's frame of reference onto the "other" culture is present in all research, including survey research, despite its formal and standardized format that

---

*Two edited volumes provide an array of excellent articles on key theoretical and methodological issues of doing comparative cross-cultural research of old age (Albert & Cattell, 1994; Maddox & Lawton, 1993).

†In this overview chapter, we are not using regression models. We are only looking at crosstabs.

‡Institutionalized populations were not included in the surveys.

supposedly enhances "objectivity." It was the unquestioned theoretical assumptions regarding the self that account for Ruth Benedict's (1946) depiction of Japanese society as being based on shame, compared to Western societies being based on guilt. This distinction has been seen by Japanese experts as misleading and simplistic (Doi, 1973; Johnson, 1993). It has been suggested that Benedict's classic work might perhaps be better read "less as an objective report on Japanese society than as a mirror of the author's underlying definition of the 'self,' that is, how a scholar born and educated in the West unconsciously projected her own culturally-constructed notion of the self onto Japanese" (Ikegami, 1995, p. 373).

The Generations survey, using researchers from both societies,* provides an arena to uncover shared theoretical presuppositions and biases. Despite our caution in writing a "neutral" questionnaire, the American emphasis was on issues of individual rights, autonomy, and gender, whereas the Japanese emphasis was on responsibility and mutual obligations of family members. The end product (i.e., the Generations questionnaire) reflects the many compromises and miscommunication that developed during the research process. Despite our efforts to create a questionnaire that was culturally contextualized, we faced obstacles in creating a comparable research instrument. The numerous meanings of similar words and the different ways of using language in formulating and interpreting survey questions made comparing societies often treacherous.† But these difficulties sensitized us to the role of language and the use of categorizations in the way aging is defined. In Japan, the emphasis is on fulfilling dependency needs and social guarantees, whereas in the United States, it is on autonomy and individual rights. These different conceptualizations are reflected in the ways governments define aging. Hashimoto (1996) makes an interesting case when she points out that in Japan, welfare guidelines are referred to as the responsibility of the State, not as the rights of individuals: "The Japanese declaration concerns itself with the notion of guarantee, whereas the American counterpart is geared to the entitlement to independent life" (pp. 38–39).

In this overview chapter, we draw upon a variety of sociological, cultural, and psychological conceptualizations to show general cultural patterns rather than test specific hypotheses. We explore (1) how the self of older persons is culturally organized through prescriptive norms and language categorizations; (2) how the structural position of older persons, namely their distance from the economic pressures to achieve and their social isolation, shapes the self; (3) how the links between methodological assumptions and theoretical questions affect the meaning and scope of the research findings. As an introduction, we wish to present an overall picture of some sociodemographic characteristics of older individuals in order to put the Generations study in a broader social framework.

---

*Charlotte Muller, an economist, and Catherine Silver, a sociologist, were the members of the American team. The Japanese team was also made up of sociologists and economists.
†The questionnaire was translated from English into Japanese and back into English by two independent Japanese students. Their translations were then compared. Any disagreement was discussed and led to a clarification of the cultural meaning of the questions.

Sociodemographic Features of Aging in Japan and the United States

Modern industrial societies have experienced drastic demographic and social changes over the years that have led to State intervention in responding to the social and economic needs of elderly populations (Campbell, 1992; Kinsella, 1995). Recent demographic changes in the past decade, such as the sharp increase in the population of the very old (85 years and over), the decrease in birthrates, the increase in longevity of men and women, and the coming of age of the baby-boomer generation, have created new pressures on governments (Cantor, 1983; Maeda, 1983). While the governments in Japan and the United States continue to play key roles in creating programs and policies to address these issues, such as the Golden Plan in Japan, the demographics of a post-industrial society have led to questioning the responsibilities of the State in providing resources and care in the later years (Soldo & Freedman, 1994). Japan and the United States have comparable levels of economic and technological development, but different systems of pensions, retirement plans, health benefits, and forms of governmental intervention at the community level (Campbell, 1992). It is not our intention to discuss any of these features in detail, but merely to give a simplified overview of key issues as a background to the analysis of our data.

What some have called industrialization's "gift of mass longevity"* has created an array of new social challenges for postindustrial nations, but nowhere has the impact of an aging population been more dramatic than in Japan (Kinoshita & Keifer, 1992; Plath, 1980). The "graying" of the Japanese population has been more accelerated than among Western nations, and this pace is expected to continue through the first two decades of the next century. One can observe in Japan, the United States, and many Western countries a gradual shift in the provision of care in the later years, particularly to the disabled elderly, from the government to individual families. This shift toward the responsibility of families has important social implications, especially regarding the expected role of women as caregivers (Bubeck, 1995).†) In the United States, aging has become the next frontier of the Women's Movement (Friedan, 1993). In Japan, the government asserts that the responsibility for the welfare of the aged belongs to the household, urging that the elderly can best be cared for in the home, and suggesting that women be the primary source of care (Lock, 1993, pp. 118–119). This position is increasingly becoming a critical issue for women in Japan (White, 1992).

In both Japan and the United States, survey analysis has taken on a key role in shaping and organizing values through the creation of standards of behavior. The Japanese Government provides yearly surveys of values that seem

---

*Life expectancy in the United States, as of 1990, was 73 years and 79 years for men and women, respectively. In Japan, the life expectancy was 76 years and 83 years for men and women, respectively, the highest life expectancies in the world (Muller, 1996).

†Gender plays a crucial role in caregiving. In this overview chapter, however, the focus is not on the role of gender. Such an analysis will be provided in a subsequent paper.

to play as much a descriptive as a prescriptive role.* As Lock commented, "Contemporary Japan is a number-cruncher's paradise: the dissemination of national surveys results and commentary is an integral part of the apparatus that promotes the postwar moral and behavioral order" (1993, p. 136). This tendency to use surveys to set moral standards that monitor behavior has influenced the use of social science as an instrument of social control. The use of surveys when studying aging issues is especially problematic, because older persons are vulnerable to labeling, stigmatization, and control, and because the government, under increasing social and economic pressures, is trying to legitimate the shift of caring for older persons, as mentioned earlier. The survey results presented here provide a normative view of attitudes toward aging, rather than being the expression of older individuals' points of view, spoken in their own words. However, we have tried to assess critically these views by comparing different age groups and exploring the different images of aging that they portray. We also relied, as much as possible, on available material from studies that recorded older persons' life stories and/or personal feelings about aging.

GENERAL FRAMEWORK:
FAMILY OBLIGATIONS AND THE SELF
IN JAPAN AND THE UNITED STATES

In this section, we first discuss the links between autonomy and (inter)dependence, caring and isolation, in looking after elderly parents within a general framework of social relations in Japan and the United States. This is followed by an analysis of the Generations data about adult children's perceived responsibility for parents with physical and financial needs, and about lifelong friendships. We propose an analysis of these issues that combines cultural and sociopsychological frameworks.

Contextualizing Family Relations

Familial Contexts.   In contrast to the United States, most Japanese elderly live with their children (over 60% compared with 20% or less in the West).† Although Japan (along with South Korea) continues to have the highest rate of three-generation households—Japan's Management and Coordination Agency reports that 79% of young adults live with their parents—the prevalence of three-generation households is expected to decline slowly (Kinoshita & Keifer, 1992). Multigenerational households reduce the financial and social burden of

---

*Government surveys by the National Character Research Committee for the Study of the Japanese National Character (Nipponjin No Kokuminsei, 1992). Other public surveys investigate all aspects of social life in publications labeled *White Papers*, such as the Japanese Ministry of Foreign Affairs (1994).

†Although this proportion has steadily dropped, the decrease has only been at a rate of about 1% per year (Koseisho, 1991).

taking care of the elderly. However, in urban settings, dwellings are often over-crowded, with a lack of privacy that can give rise to conflicts, jealousy, and mistreatment of the elderly despite an ideology of respect (Tomita, 1994). At present, the majority of Japanese aged 64 and over prefer to be looked after by their children. In one five-country study, 58% of the older Japanese stated that they would like to live with their children, whereas only 3% of older Americans responded the same way. Should they become physically ill, 95% of Japanese aged 64 and over would like family members to care for them and designate as preferred caregivers almost exclusively wives, daughters-in-law, or daughters (Lock, 1993, p. 121).

The rate of institutionalization is relatively low in Japan and the United States, about 5% in each country. However, the prevalence of extended family households—called the *ie* in Japanese—and the tradition of the oldest male child inheriting the house and the land (primogeniture) in exchange for the care of his elderly parents,* presents a striking contrast with the United States. Studies in the United States have shown that the disabled elderly also reported that they would like to be taken care of by family members as a first choice. But in the United States, 40% of elderly, who are currently living with children, expressed a desire to live alone in the future. Nonetheless, they would prefer to continue to live in close physical proximity to their children (Moody, 1994).†

Household structure has a strong impact on the values placed on the family as a source of economic sharing and psychological caring. In rural societies, the extended family has traditionally provided economic security and social protection to its members against public demands and the intrusion of the State (Banfield, 1958). The isolation of the extended family, its distance, and its hostility toward nonfamilial groups often made the emergence of trust and cooperation difficult (Fukuyama, 1995). In Japan, however, the isolation of the family is not the product of distrust of the Government or lack of cooperation with public institutions; rather, it stems from the complex system of social obligations and the organization of society around the categorization of "inside and outside" (*uchi/soto*), that orders social relations throughout society and provides both protection and isolation to older persons. Familism, as an ethos, also character-izes extended forms of family organization. It is defined by a set of values that link family members together economically and psychologically, making the family the primary center of their emotional attachment and social commitment. Familism is sustained by strong hierarchical systems of power and authority based on age and gender stratification. It can be a source of family cohesiveness, but it can also be an obstacle to change and adaptation, especially among younger generations, who feel stifled by this system of social relations (Hashi-moto, 1996; White, 1993). Furthermore, the value of family privacy and the shame of being exposed to public scrutiny constrain the use of outsiders such

---

*Despite the fact that Japanese law now requires equal distribution among the heirs, the tradition of favoring the oldest son is still widespread.
†Although the United States does not have a system of primogeniture and the importance of the traditional extended family has declined, the emergence of a modified extended family based on social and emotional support rather than physical contiguity is widespread.

as nurses or family helpers, increasing the isolation of the family, and espe-cially of older persons (Lock, 1993, p. 112). Thus, as far as the elderly are concerned, we must consider that the ideology of familism does not necessarily translate into caring behavior (Nydegger, 1983).

In the West, the emergence of the nuclear bourgeois family during the period of early industrialization introduced new concerns for greater privacy and a view of the family as providing a refuge from the cold and competitive world of the market (Aries, 1962).* The United States is characterized by a multiplicity of family forms. Some writers have argued that the weakening of the traditional family stems from the demise of community life, the loss of paternal authority, a decrease in moral responsibility, combined with a focus on personal needs and individual rights. It is argued that these features of American society have created an emotional vacuum, rather than a sense of intimacy based on bonds of attachment (Bellah, Sullivan, Swidler, & Tipton, 1985), and have helped develop the narcissistic personality of our time (Lasch, 1984). Feminists' critiques have further challenged the security and protection provided by the modern nuclear family to its members. They have pointed out that the modern family, ever more hidden behind the walls of privacy, has become a place of struggle, control, and violence especially directed toward children, women, and the elderly (Fineman & Mykitiuk, 1994). The debate over the decline of the American family does not concern us here; we only wanted to contrast the image of the family as a source of support and stability in Japan to that of vulnerability and deterioration in the United States. Such images influence the ways older persons are defined and treated. In both societies, older persons are socially and emotionally isolated from the broader social structure, but the isolation has a different cultural mean-ing and is expressed in different social contexts, as we discuss later.

Family Identity and Caring for Elderly Parents.   Caring for elderly par-ents reflects the different levels of resources available in Japan and the United States,† as well as deeper psychocultural factors. Family responsibility, partic-ularly the responsibility of adult children toward elderly parents, needs to be understood within the larger framework of social identity. In a previous paper, we analyzed and compared *familial identity*, *work identity*, *social identity*, and *cultural identity* using the Generations data (Silver & Muller, 1997). In the present chapter, we summarize the key components of familial identity as a backdrop to the analysis of caring for elderly parents. Familial identity among Japanese respondents combines concerns for generational linkages, identifica-tion with family history, ancestor worship, and a sense of national identity. Thus, Japanese familial identity incorporates historical as well as a national and religious dimensions (Lock, 1993, p. 88). It is located in an ongoing space–time

---

*This view of the family as a place of protection, renewal, and caring represents an idealized view of a type of family based on traditional/patriarchal principles of age and gender organization (Par-sons, 1964).

†With a sophisticated set of social services, including a two-tiered pension program and national health insurance, the elderly in Japan are economically less vulnerable than elderly in the United States (Campbell, 1992; Kinoshita & Kiefer, 1992; Takayama, 1992).

mutually reinforcing dynamic that interacts with the social order over time (Bachnik & Quinn, 1994, p. 145).* In this context, the image of the older person is imbued with respect and honor because it simultaneously symbolizes the past, present, and future of the family line. Furthermore, a rigid age stratification in Japan also strengthens the basis of intergenerational linkages in the family. In the United States, familial identity focuses on generational links, but without reference to historical or national identity. Educational achievement, rather than age, affects the acquisition and transmission of values (Silver & Muller, 1997).

From a psychological point of view, the Japanese familial self is anchored in strong achievement motivations to enhance familial honor and a sense of a "we-self." It is based on the internalization and fulfillment of maternal expectations for achievement as a repayment for her total devotion, combined with a constant fear of failure (Roland, 1988). The focus on achievement—in school and in the workplace—for the sake of the family's name creates constant pressure for high performance in order to avoid self-blame and family dishonor. In such a system, it is not surprising to find ambivalent feelings toward the elderly, who are no longer productive but still have to be honored and respected (Palmore & Maeda, 1985). The sense of familial identity affects the nature of social relations in caring for elderly parents, as we discuss in the next section.

Social Relations and Caring for Elderly Parents.
The Japanese view of social relations, based on intricate sets of reciprocal obligations, has been widely discussed in literature on the Japanese character (Doi, 1973; Lock, 1993; Plath, 1980). Unlike the United States, however, it is (inter)dependence, rather than dependence, that characterizes Japanese relationships at all levels of the social system. Hence, there is a reluctance to create embarrassing nonreciprocal relationships, even in the most intimate sphere of the family. The feelings of obligation that tie family members together are not based on general principles and abstract notions of individual rights. They reflect a sense of emotional dependency that is expressed in daily life, through what Japanese call *amae*.

Amae, translated as indulgent dependency, constitutes a combined verbal and nonverbal request for cherishment and security, a passive yearning for support and love in the image of a mother–infant relationship (Johnson, 1993, p. 85).† Dependence in Japan does not have a negative connotation; it is experienced at all ages throughout the life course, not just by infants and the very young. Indeed, it has been argued that unless this need for special, self-indulgent caring were met, the fabric of Japanese society would break apart (Smith, 1983). This passive demandingness among adults, however, often turns into resentment and rage when not fulfilled, as clinical accounts with Japanese patients

---

*The need for linking the past to daily life can be illustrated in the case of rural Japanese who keep an ongoing communication with dead family members, who continue to give them help and advice (Kristof, 1996).

†Intrapsychically, *amae* is present as "a motive, a drive, or a desire that becomes expressed as a yearning and expectation to be held, fed, bathed, made safe, kept warm, comforted emotionally and given special cherishment." (Johnson, 1993, p. 85)

reveal (Roland, 1988, pp. 274–310).* (Inter)dependence, as a principle of social organization in Japan, gives support and legitimacy to older persons' orientation toward greater familial identification, expectation of being cared for, interiority, and social withdrawal. From a Western point of view, we may see such processes as a way to marginalize and infantilize older persons by isolating them from other sources of sociability and well-being. While this may be objectively the case, one would need to understand the inner experience of older persons. The sense of selfhood, based on (inter)dependence, reflects social sharing and active inner involvement. Unlike the concept of dependence, (inter)dependence refers to an active involvement with others, and with oneself, that underscores different social and emotional mechanisms.

In the United States, the psychological meaning of dependency stresses that infants, born in a state of total dependency (symbiosis), have to strive through several stages of individuation toward autonomy and the creation of an "autonomous self" (Mahler, Pine, & Bergman, 1975). The maintenance of an autonomous self is seen as a lifelong goal. Seen through gross historical lenses, the autonomous self is the product of enlightenment philosophy and a free market economy in the West. In postindustrial societies, it is further argued, the self is characterized by a sense of emptiness and narcissistic injury (Lasch, 1979). This "empty self," the product of a consumer society and its advertising empire, needs to be constantly filled with consumer products. Thus, the "empty self" supports the dynamics of a market economy and benefits professionals, especially mental health professionals, in their unending attempts to help fill the void that is constantly recreated (Cushman, 1995). Individuals with empty selves are more vulnerable and thus more easily manipulated and controlled.

We would like to suggest that older persons are likely to feel less empty because, being removed from the pressures to achieve and consume in a market economy, they are more willing to rely on their own inner resources and enjoy greater "interiority." If so, we can expect older persons to be more satisfied than younger ones with their present lives, a point to which we shall return later in the analysis. We now illustrate these ideas by looking at the attitudes of adult children toward elderly parents using questions from the Generations survey.

Family Responsibility Seen through the Generations Survey

Family Responsibility for Disabled Parents. The Generations questionnaire asked several normative questions regarding attitudes toward the care of elderly parents. Separate questions were asked about parents with disabilities and parents with financial needs. For each question, three options were presented, reflecting different models of responsibility toward elderly parents.† The

*Takeo Doi, a Japanese psychoanalyst, goes as far as talking about an instinctual need for dependence that shapes the self, together with sexual and aggressive drives.
†In order to minimize the cultural difference in the propensity to agree with normative statements, we have standardized the means in the statistical tables. The sum of the Japanese means was set equal to the sum of the American means, to adjust for the differences between the two societies in the tendency for respondents to agree with an interviewer's statement.

Table 17-1. Norms of Responsibility toward Elderly Parents with Physical or Mental Disability

Type of responsibility	American means (N = 1,497)	Japanese means* (N = 1,764)	Means difference Japan–United States
Children have own responsibilities, no need to look after parents	0.02	0.06	0.04**
Children should look after parents as long as burden not too great	0.43	0.68	0.25**
Children should look after parents even if they have to make sacrifices	0.53	0.23	−0.30**
Average	0.32	0.32	0.0

*Japanese means adjusted so that sum of Japanese means equals sum of American means.
Based on U.S. Question No. 19 <1–3>, Japanese Question No. 14.
Level of significance: $*p < .05$; $**p < .01$

results show that both American and Japanese respondents were reluctant to disavow all responsibility for disabled aging parents, with low mean responses of .06 (Japan) and .02 (United States). Thus, Japanese respondents are less likely to put their personal needs first.

What is striking in Table 17–1 is the significant difference in the answers to the other two options. In one option, "Children should look after their disabled parents even if it means making sacrifices," Japanese have a mean of .23 compared to American respondents, with a mean of .53, and a highly significant mean difference of −0.30. The Japanese are less likely to support the abstract idea of sacrifice. The third option, "Children should look after their parents as long as the burden does not become too great," was more acceptable to the Japanese than to American respondents: Japanese show a mean of .68 compared to .43 for the American respondents, with a mean difference of 0.25. The Japanese are more likely to support the idea of mutuality. The norms of family responsibility are clearly different in the two countries.

In order to give meaning to these differences, we need to expand on our previous discussion of social relations. In Japanese society, norms regarding social and familial obligations are complex, shaped by the status of the person to whom one feels obligated. There are several words with many nuances that refer to social obligations (Benedict, 1946, p. 116). One meaning of "obligation" (what is called the *on*) is based on the Confucian moral precept commanding filial piety. It supposes a great emotional debt and indebtedness. Such sense of obligation creates an imbalance that needs to be corrected: "In order to minimize the potential indebtedness of the "on,"* Japanese strive to reduce obligations by rebalancing indebtedness through returning the "on" or reducing the obligatedness through a calibrated payoff of prior indebtedness" (Johnson, 1993, p. 81).

---

*The *on*, the term used to refer to filial obligations, is to be contrasted with *giri*, a Japanese term that refers to obligations outside the family that require some form of equalization. The *giri* relationships "constitute a potential license for the imposition of demands for reciprocity" (Lebra, 1976, p. 93).

The statistical results described show a preference in Japan for a normative situation in which the relationships between the children and the elderly parents are not overly one-sided, stressing instead a sense of "we-self." Thus, our findings should be understood within the framework of the dynamics of mutuality and reciprocity that characterize norms of family life in Japan.

American respondents, on average, were more likely to say that they would make sacrifices to help elderly parents. The structure of American families, no longer based on rigid age and gender stratification, supports an ideology of equality and individualism that often conflicts with the needs of the family as a whole (Bellah et al., 1985). In the United States, family life is organized around abstract principles and moral precepts rather than concrete rules of behavior, an observation made more than a century ago by Alexis de Tocqueville in his American tour (1840/1969). Thus, American respondents' answers to questions about the care of elderly parents have to be understood within a framework of moral principles and abstract concepts of responsibility. Engaging in some form of "bargaining" around how much care to give elderly parents is experienced as less moral than supporting the abstract idea of "sacrifice." We would like to suggest that the recourse to abstract thinking denotes the existence of coping mechanisms (intellectualization and idealization as defenses), used to distance oneself from painful social realities in a youth-oriented culture such as the United States when aging and the fear of death stay hidden and repressed (Silver, 1992).

When the Generations questionnaire was created, the Japanese and United States teams tried to contextualize the questions about responsibility to incorporate the different meanings of selfhood. However, we did not realize that the term *sacrifice* would have strikingly different meanings in the two cultures. After the data were collected, the findings about sacrificing for elderly parents surprised us, and we decided to interview three students from Japan doing graduate work in the United States. It became clear that *sacrifice* had a different meaning for Japanese and American respondents. The Japanese, whose sense of self is formulated in relation to the group, are so attuned to the needs of the others that they are not likely to experience "sacrifice" the way Westerners do (Smith, 1983, pp. 128–129). Americans, who are highly attuned to individual rights and needs, experience themselves as making sacrifices for the group in a variety of circumstances. If a Japanese person is asked to make a sacrifice on behalf of an elderly parent, the magnitude of the sacrifice may be understood as considerably greater than in the United States. A similar issue arose when analyzing the relationship between parents and their younger children. In Japan, giving-up one's time and career to help in the education of one's children is not perceived as a sacrifice; rather, it is a most important virtue (White, 1992). Sacrificing is part of a cluster of idealized features around endurance and suffering. In everyday life, sacrificing is idealized, especially in regard to mothers sacrificing for their young children, or elderly for the sake of younger generations.

The qualities of sacrifice and endurance for Japanese, and of autonomy and self-help for Americans, tap into deep layers of the self. However, it would be misleading to assume that these normative statements apply equally to all age groups. Indeed, despite the different cultural expectations regarding models of responsibility, our analysis of age groups shows how older persons in both countries have similar attitudes toward family responsibility and how different they are from younger age groups. In popular literature, the elderly are often seen as emotionally demanding and unrealistic, whereas younger people are seen as pragmatic and in control. Our results present a different image. In both countries, the older age group is more realistic, less likely to believe that children should make sacrifices for their parents, and more likely to think that children should provide care only if the burden is not too great. Looking at each country separately, we see significant age differences between the younger adults and older persons. In the United States, 60.5% of younger adults compared to 35% of older persons believe that children should make sacrifices for parents, while 60% of older compared to 36% of younger respondents believe that children should help as long as the burden is not too great. In Japan, we find a similar general pattern, but of a lesser magnitude. Younger adults are more likely to want to make sacrifices for their parents than older persons (34.5% and 21.3%, respectively).

How can we make sense of these findings? There are several overlapping theoretical interpretations: Younger adults have more recently undergone socialization processes and internalized social prescriptions. Their lack of experience in caring for elderly parents is more likely to make them rely on abstract moral principles. Another interpretation rests on the fact that younger adults are more likely than older persons to experience fears and anxieties about aging and old age. One way of coping with the anxiety is to become more idealistic and more emotionally removed. By contrast, older persons seem more realistic and less likely to idealize filial responsibility as a form of sacrifice. They have lowered their expectations about children's help and put greater emphasis on concrete human relations rather than on upholding abstract moral principles (Vaillant, 1993). Thus, despite clear differences in norms of responsibility, and despite different conception of selfhood, older people in both countries show similarities in their views of the importance of mutuality and their desire of not being fully dependent on their children.

Economic Responsibility of Children toward Elderly Parents in Need. Attitudes toward helping elderly parents in financial need was another way of understanding norms of family responsibility. In the Generations questionnaire, the following question was asked: "To what extent do you think that children should help their elderly parents economically when the parents have financial problems?" The same three options, used in the analysis of responsibility toward helping disabled parents, were used. The answers show a pattern similar to that in the previous question.

Table 17–2 shows that in Japan and the United States, only a very small percentage of respondents believe that children do not have to help their parents economically. Abnegating responsibility for one's parents is not looked on favorably in either society but the Japanese, again, show greater concern for putting their family's needs first. However, there are striking differences in the two other

Table 17-2. Norms of Responsibility toward Elderly Parents with Financial Needs

Type of responsibility	American means (N = 1,497)	Japanese means* (N = 1,764)	Means difference Japan–United States
Children have own responsibilities, no need to look after parents	0.03	0.07	0.04**
Children should look after parents as long as burden not too great	0.45	0.70	0.25**
Children should look after parents even if they have to make sacrifices	0.51	0.22	−0.29**
Average	0.33	0.33	0.0

*Japanese means adjusted so that sum of Japanese means equals sum of American means.
Based on U.S. Question No. 20 <1–3>, Japanese Question No. 15.
Level of significance: $*p < .05$; $**p < .01$

options. To the answer "Children should support their parents economically, even if they have to make sacrifices," the mean for Japanese is .22 compared to .51 for American respondents, with a highly significant mean difference of −0.29. In other words, American respondents are significantly more likely to believe in making sacrifices. In the third option, "Children should support their parents economically as long as the burden does not get too great," the mean is .70 for Japanese compared to .45 for American respondents, with a significant mean difference of 0.25. Thus, Japanese were less likely to want to make sacrifices but more likely to want to look after their parents as long as the economic burden was not too great. There are clear normative differences in the two countries that support our previous findings.*

Having found different cultural norms of responsibility toward parents in financial need, we now examine the perception of these norms in different age groups. In Japan and the United States, younger adults and older persons show significant differences in the way norms of responsibility are perceived. Younger adults are more likely than older persons to believe that children should sacrifice for their parents, whereas older persons are more likely to believe that children should help as long as the burden is not too great. In both countries, younger adults tend to be more idealistic (i.e., more willing to make economic sacrifices for the sake of elderly parents) than older persons, who tend to be more grounded in reality, concerned with reciprocal obligations. Thus, despite different norms of responsibility in Japan and the United States, older persons across cultures share attitudes toward family responsibility that stress mutuality while rejecting

*The full interpretation of these results would necessitate having information about family income, social class, and family size, and using multivariate analysis. In the present overview, however, we are only looking at general patterns of responsibility and their variations by age groups. We can report that in the United States, income did not make a difference regarding attitudes toward helping disabled parents. However, it did make a difference regarding economic help. Respondents with the highest income were more likely to believe that they had to make sacrifices for parents.

forms of idealization of family relations. In the next section, we pursue our analysis of family obligations by contrasting them with lifelong friendships in order to discuss the paradoxes of attachment.

Situated Meaning: Family Obligations and Lifelong Friendships. The analysis of lifelong friendships provides another avenue for understanding the role of the family in creating an arena for social and emotional support and, at the same time, restricting and isolating older family members from other forms of sociability. Doi (1985) has analyzed how the categorization of "inside–outside" (*uchi–soto*), structures all social relationships. Such categorization is a major organizational focus for self, social life, and language in Japan. The conceptual contrasts of *uchi* versus *soto* are too complex to be discussed here at length. We only need to mention that they cover a wide array of contrasts, such as self–other, included–excluded, us–them, known–unknown, and engaged–detached, to name a few.

As applied to the household (the *ie*), "inside" refers to an inner circle of family members and close relatives who share asymmetrical intimacy and passive acceptance of endearment (*amae*), as we have seen before. These experiences occur within hierarchical relationships whose boundaries are flexible through a system of reciprocal obligations. "Outside" refers to all other social relationships where emotional distance (*enryo*) is expected. The category "inside–outside–needs to be analyzed in relation to the concept of *freedom* in order to understand its full impact on older individuals' identification with the family. In Japan, unlike in the United States, freedom does not refer to abstract individual entitlements; rather, it refers to an individual's ability to join social groups outside of one's own family. Such freedom in Japan is not encouraged. Furthermore, obligations based on reciprocal interchange (*on*), as was discussed before, limit involvement outside the family for fear of incurring indebtedness. The ethos of family privacy, combined with the categorization of "inside–outside," blocks, for older persons, most other avenues of sociability. Friends are part of the "outside" social arena, unless they are recoded as belonging to the intimate circle of family relations.

The Generations survey provides data that can be used to illustrate the tension between involvement in the family and social isolation outside the family. Respondents were asked, "Do you have lifelong friends?" and "In what way did you get acquainted with them?" Japanese and American respondents report similar levels of involvement with lifelong friendships.

Table 17–3 shows distinctive patterns of friendship between the two countries. Japanese were more likely to have made lifelong friendships through childhood friends (mean difference 0.13), the armed forces (mean difference 0.09), and work colleagues (mean difference 0.04). These are the three major arenas of loyalty and identification outside the family. The largest difference is with "childhood friends," who are defined as an extension of the family, developed in childhood when the prescribed circles of intimacy and appropriateness were less rigidly defined (Kinoshita & Keifer, 1992). As for friends from the army

Table 17-3. Sources of Lifelong Friendship among U.S. and Japanese Respondents

Sources of Lifelong Friendship	American means (N = 1,497)	Japanese means* (N = 1,764)	Means difference Japan–United States
1. Childhood friends	0.58	0.71	0.13**
2. Friends from work	0.52	0.56	0.04*
3. Neighborhoods and the community	0.43	0.46	−0.03
4. Friends through hobbies, sports, study	0.33	0.30	−0.03
5. Friends through social activities	0.23	0.14	−0.09**
6. Friends through religious or political activities	0.27	0.11	−0.16**
7. Friends through family or relatives	0.37	0.27	−0.10**
8. Friends from the army	0.07	0.16	0.09**
Average	0.36	0.36	0.00

*Japanese means adjusted so that sum of Japanese means equals sum of American means.
Based on U.S. Question No. 25 <1–3>, Japanese Question No. 19.
Level of significance: *$p < .05$; **$p < .01$

and the workplace, Japanese invest a great deal of their loyalty and self-identification in these social spheres.*

Japanese respondents were less likely to report establishing lifelong friendships with neighbors (mean difference −0.03), with persons met through leisure activities (mean difference −0.03), through religious and political groups (mean difference −0.16), through friends of the family (mean difference −0.10), and through social activities (mean difference −0.09). In the logic of reciprocal obligations and indebtedness, it makes sense that families in Japan would want to restrict access to new acquaintances that enlarge the circle of obligations. The sources of friendship are very different in the United States, where numerous forms of sociability are encouraged. For older persons, friendship becomes a source of emotional support and social recognition, often becoming more important than family relations (Maddox & Lawton, 1993).

These patterns of friendship illustrate the different symbolic meanings of social relations in the two societies. The multiple obligations of reciprocity, through gifts and remembrances, show the familial paradox of attachment in Japan whereby solidarity enhances intimacy but at the same time isolates family members—especially older persons—from alternative sources of social and emotional support. In Japan, familial intimacy and support lead to greater social isolation for older persons and potential conflicts in family relations, especially between daughters-in-law and elderly parents. Furthermore, the characteristics of family obligations prevent the development of alternative systems of caring, such as nursing homes, retirement communities, or other group-living situations. This pattern, however, is changing as young generations born after World

*To a question regarding whether priority should be given to work obligations over family obligations, the Japanese were significantly more likely to agree with this statement than U.S. respondents (Muller & Silver, 1995, p. 168).

War II—particularly the women—are beginning to express some reluctance to sacrifice themselves for the elderly. Among older parents, there are also new signs of ambivalence and reticence about living with their children, as was described in the in-depth interviews with older persons (Hashimoto, 1996).*) In the United States, the paradox of attachment revolves around the tension between weaker norms of family solidarity and a tradition of active participation and involvement outside the family. These features of the social organization, combined with social and geographical mobility, induce older persons and their families to rely on friends and community, and to support alternative systems of caring. Having discussed the different meanings of family responsibility and the tensions between family support and social isolation, we now turn our attention to an analysis of the different definitions and experiences of well-being.

A COMPARATIVE ANALYSIS OF WELL-BEING IN JAPAN AND THE UNITED STATES

Emergence of a Transcultural Sense of Well-Being among Older Persons

Satisfaction with Present Life.   A popular image of older persons in the United States is that they are unhappy and depressed, whereas in Japan they are more likely to be satisfied and adjusted. Our findings present a somewhat different image. To the question, "To what extent are you satisfied with your present life?" a surprisingly high percentage of Americans—42%—answered that they were very satisfied with their present life, compared to only 22% among the Japanese respondents†—a significant difference. While the full interpretation of these findings requires data on economic and social variables, an analysis not undertaken here, the difference reflects cultural definitions of what is acceptable to feel and to express in each country. As was mentioned before, sacrifice, suffering, and endurance are seen as core values that define the Japanese "(inter)dependent self." In the United States, however, we judge ourselves by how "happy" we are, how "good" we feel, and how much we smile—all a reflection of our ability to satisfy our narcissistic needs and enhance our "autonomous self." How do these general views about satisfaction with present life differ by age groups?

We saw previously that age introduces significant variations between younger adults and older persons regarding norms of responsibility in caring for elderly parents. We also saw that older persons across countries show sim-

*Age differences are not introduced in this analysis, because respondents' positions in the life cycle make their life experiences noncomparable. For example, many younger adults have not yet been inserted into the workforce, the army, or the local community.

†The full distributions are as follows: *Very satisfied*—22% (Japan) and 42% (United States); *Satisfied*—57% (Japan) and 46% (United States); *More or less satisfied*—12% (Japan) and 6% (United States); *Dissatisfied*—7% (Japan) and 4% (United States); *Very dissatisfied*—2% (Japan) and 1% (United States).

ilarities in their emphasis on reciprocity. We expect age to have an equally important impact on perceptions of well-being.

Despite the tensions between caring in the family and social isolation discussed earlier, we find the highest percentages of very satisfied individuals among older respondents. When looking at Figures 17–1 and 17–2 separately, we see that there is a clear effect of age on satisfaction with present life. In each country, the older the age group, the more likely that respondents are very satisfied with their present life. In Figure 17–1, we see a linear increase of the percentage of U.S. respondents who are very satisfied with their present lives: 34% (18–29 age group), 39% (30–49 age group), 49% (50–64 age group) and 54% (over 64 age group). In Figure 17–2, we see that in Japan, the increase is not as great but the linear effect is equally clear: 18% (18–29 age group), 18% (30–49 age group), 23% (50–64 age group) and 33% (over 64 age group), are very satisfied with their present life. Across countries, the older age groups are significantly more likely to be very satisfied with their present lives than younger ones.

How can we make sense of these findings? We expected that older persons' position of marginalization and isolation would make them less satisfied with their present lives. However, our findings tell a different story. Despite, or be-

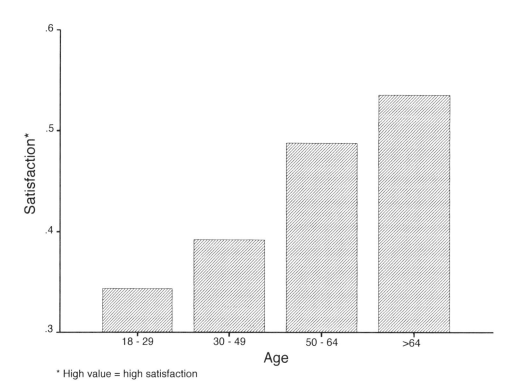

* High value = high satisfaction

Figure 17–1. Satisfaction with present life by age—United States.

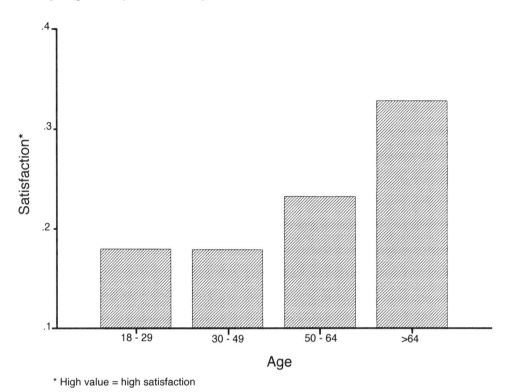

* High value = high satisfaction

Figure 17–2. Satisfaction with present life by age—Japan.

cause, of their structural position in society, older persons have created their own world, distinct and separate from that of younger people. Satisfaction with present life is an indicator of inner contentment, and a form of personal achievement. We suggest that older individuals are able to distance themselves emotionally from normative constraints and create a world of their own, a "limbo state" to use Hazan's (1980) formulation, protected from past and future social and emotional demands. Our research supports the existence of commonalities—such as a present orientation, weaker normative expectations, an ability for self-expression, and a sense of interiority (Erikson, Erikson, & Kivnick, 1986; Gutmann, 1964; Vaillant, 1993)—that characterize the transcultural self of older persons. While satisfaction with present life represents an indicator of personal well-being, we now turn to an examination of satisfaction with society that represents an indicator of social well-being.

Satisfaction with Society. Satisfaction with society, a less personal expression of well-being, is more likely to be shaped by cultural prescriptions. Thus, we expect to find clear differences between the two countries. Japanese respondents are more satisfied with society than American respondents (42%

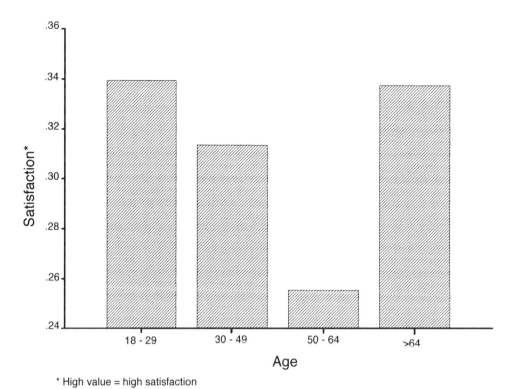

* High value = high satisfaction

Figure 17–3. Satisfaction with society by age—United States.

and 29%, respectively), the reverse pattern from the answers to satisfaction with present life.* These findings can be explained by a combination of factors: There is a greater tendency among Japanese to approve social arrangements and not to verbalize their dissatisfaction, whereas Americans are more likely to be direct and critical of the social order; Japanese society is more likely to provide greater economic resources in the form of social safety nets, especially for older persons; Japanese are more likely to identify with the country's history and to exhibit a sense of social and national loyalty, as we discussed earlier.

We saw that age introduced significant variations regarding satisfaction with present life, older persons having a higher likelihood of being very satisfied. We now explore age variations in respondents' level of social well-being.

Unlike respondents' satisfaction with present life, we do not find comparable age patterns in the two countries. Figure 17–3 shows that in the United States, the younger adults and the older persons have equally high levels of

---

*The full distributions are as follows: *Very satisfied*—3.5% (Japan) and 3% (United States); *Satisfied*—38% (Japan) and 26% (United States); *More or less satisfied*—27% (Japan) and 12% (United States); *Dissatisfied*—24% (Japan) and 34% (United States); *Very dissatisfied*—6% (Japan) and 24% (United States). In the analysis of satisfaction with society, we have combined *Very satisfied* and *Satisfied* answers.

satisfaction with society (33.9% and 33.8%, respectively), compared to middle-aged groups (30–49 and 50–64 years), with 31.4% and 25.6%, respectively, suggesting a cohort effect rather than an age effect. The 50–64 age group has the lowest level of satisfaction with society, representing a cohort faced with the combined pressures of retirement and caring for elderly parents. The higher level of satisfaction with society among the younger and older age groups may point to similarities of values compared to the middle-aged adults. Additional research needs to be undertaken to specify these common values. However, Figure 17–4 shows that in Japan, there is a clear linear effect of age on satisfaction with society. The older the age group, the more likely respondents are to be satisfied with society: 35% (18–29 age group), 36% (30–49 age group), 46% (50–64 age group) and 56% (over 64 age group). These results show the continuous impact of age norms in Japan based on the expectations of caring, (inter)dependency, and social entitlement in later years.

In both countries, older respondents have among the highest levels of satisfaction with society, despite ageism and marginalization. Different theoretical explanations could be suggested: Older individuals reframe social encounters by giving them a more positive light as a form of self protection (Silver, 1992); older people are likely to have lowered their expectations and become more

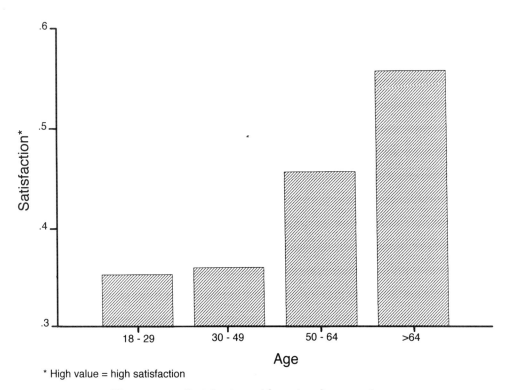

* High value = high satisfaction

Figure 17–4. Satisfaction with society by age—Japan.

disengaged and socially detached (Cumming & Henri, 1961); older persons are sheltered from the pressures of economic competition and social performance (Mouer & Sugimoto, 1986). Thus, despite cultural differences, the structural position of older persons induces common attitudes regarding general feelings of well-being. The extent to which this general feeling of well-being translates into desirable ways of living in old age is the subject of our next section.

Controlling the Discourse of Aging: Desirable Ways of Living in Old Age

When studying older persons' well-being, it is essential to look at both their general satisfaction with life and concrete, desirable ways of living in later years. Respondents were asked what activities they would like to be engaged in during their old age. A battery of 12 items, around "Desirable ways of living in old age," provides an image of how respondents would envision their lives in these later years.

Table 17–4 shows three patterns of results. In the first pattern, Japanese are less likely to want to get involved in voluntary associations (mean difference − 0.12), teach children in school (−0.13); take on leadership responsibilities in the community (0.06); stay involved in political activities (−0.07); enjoy the company of friends and colleagues (−0.12); and say that they would enjoy living

Table 17-4. Desirable Ways of Living in Old Age among U.S. and Japanese Respondents

Desirable ways of living in old age	American means (N = 1,497)	Japanese means* (N = 1,764)	Means difference Japan–United States
1. Contributing through volunteer activities	0.57	0.45	−0.12**
2. Teaching school subjects to children	0.40	0.27	−0.13**
3. Taking leadership in social development	0.28	0.22	−0.06**
4. Detaching from social, political, and job	0.38	0.31	−0.07**
5. Enjoying traveling, hobbies or sports	0.64	0.85	0.21**
6. Enjoying learning	0.50	0.50	0.00
7. Continuing career as long as possible	0.30	0.52	0.22**
8. Taking up new business or occupation	0.23	0.27	0.04
9. Living peacefully with offspring	0.52	0.62	0.10**
10. Living in harmony with husband/wife	0.73	0.65	−0.08**
11. Enjoying living alone	0.26	0.26	0.00
12. Enjoying company of friends and colleagues	0.73	0.61	−0.12**
Average	0.46	0.46	0.00

*Japanese means adjusted so that sum of Japanese means equals sum of American means.
Based on U.S. Question No. 17 <1–3>, Japanese Question No. 12 <55, 56>.
Level of significance: *$p < .05$; **$p < .01$

in harmony with their spouse (−0.08). All the items, with the exception of the last one, fit into our previous theoretical discussion, in as such as the image of aging in Japan that is depicted stresses greater family (inter)dependence, lesser active involvement in the community, and participation in voluntary associations. These findings seem to support an image of aging based on withdrawal into family life combined with a reluctance to reach out for the company of friends in the community.

However, it would be a mistake to conclude that older people in Japan are disengaged. Such a conclusion uses United States values as standards of comparison that reflect normative statements that may be strikingly different from the norms of other societies such as Japan. Indeed, the battery of questions used in defining desirable ways of living in old age emphasizes activities rather than contemplative inner states, and does not provide questions about what Roland calls the "spiritual self" (1988, p. 307). An emphasis on activities introduces a bias in the direction of a cultural image of "productive aging" (Butler, 1975), often with little room for reflexivity and interiority. This image is especially strong in a consumer-driven culture such as the United States, which has a weak tradition of reliance on spiritual inner-self as a source of intrapsychic autonomy (Featherstone & Wernick, 1995).

In the second pattern of findings, we see that Japanese respondents are more likely to desire continuing a career as long as possible (mean difference 0.20); enjoying traveling, hobbies, and sports (mean difference 0.21); desiring to live peacefully with offspring (0.10); and taking up a new occupation (0.04). Paradoxically, these items give an image of elderly persons in Japan as more active and involved in work and leisure activities compared to their American counterparts. How can we make sense of these findings? The interest in continuing one's career in Japan can be partly explained by socioeconomic factors: Mandatory retirement ages have been quite low (between 55 and 60 years at major private companies), and the Japanese government continues to seek higher retirement ages by providing incentives and organizational support for retirees who want to continue to work (Campbell, 1992, pp. 263–281; Palmore & Maeda, 1985). The desire to continue a career as long as possible is also based on psychocultural factors. In Japan, work means an attachment to an institution that requires strong links of loyalty and identification. Metaphorically, the workplace has become a family outside the family. Retirement from the work arena creates psychological stress for Japanese that can ignite a deep sense of loss of their own social identity. With few alternative sources of emotional identification outside the family, this shift to retirement is momentous (Hashimoto, 1996; Johnson, 1993). In the United States, there is also, among retirees, a desire to continue to work, if only part time, but the identification with the workplace is weaker. Furthermore, the lack of fit in the United States between older individuals' fast-changing life patterns and actual organizational arrangements has created new social problems for older persons (Riley et al., 1994).

The interest in hobbies and other leisure activities reflects the Japanese passion for using hobbies as a means of asserting individual identity, as well as the notion that old age is a time for relative liberation from the demands of work and the responsibilities of family life (Reischauer, 1977). In the Confucian tradition, daily life comprised duties and mutual obligations until, at the age of 70, following the example of Confucius, individuals could for the first time "follow their hearts' desire" without violating social expectations (Lock, 1993, p. 205). In the United States, leisure activities among older persons are also used to express individuality, but above all, to reinforce support systems and enhance sociability outside the family during later years (Mancini & Sandifer, 1994).

The last pattern of findings refers to two items that show no significant difference between Japan and the United States: "Enjoying learning things that you did not have time for before" and "Enjoying living alone." The lack of differences between the countries is the interesting finding here. What this may suggest is the existence of transcultural views about desire to learn, to be intellectually active, and to live alone. Indeed, the joy of "pure" (i.e., nonapplied) learning is a central thrust among the older persons in the University of the Third Age studied by Hazan (1996). Among older persons, learning is no longer an investment in the future but becomes an enjoyable expression of the self in the present. We were surprised to find no difference between countries about "Enjoying living alone" in view of the group orientation of the Japanese discussed previously. This finding illustrates another transcultural image of aging, as a time freer of familial obligations and social constraints. The statistical means discussed earlier provide a general view of normative expectations. But the internalization of norms varies as a function of age. As we saw before, Japan has stronger age norms than the United States. We also observed that the older age groups in both countries have strikingly high levels of satisfaction with life and society. Are similar patterns reproduced in respondents' projected desired ways of living in later years?

There are clear differences in the way the older age groups define aging in later years. In Japan, the image of aging among the older age group reflects a vision that includes a desire for spiritual leadership and a sense of honor and recognition, combined with the joys of family life. This image of aging is richer than that of the United States, where, despite the emphasis on active aging, it is more narrowly defined around the wish to live peacefully with children and grandchildren, enjoying the company of friends or colleagues, but without the image of honor and public recognition. In both countries, older age groups share common views—views that for many of them have become reality—showing a weaker desire for social activities, including learning, and a stronger wish to enjoy the company of family and friends, as well as living alone.

In Japan and the United States, the younger age groups are more likely to have an active image of old age, organized around hobbies, sports, traveling, the continuation of a career, the challenge of a new business enterprise, and taking the lead in social development. In both countries, the views of old age are projections of present interests and needs. Such an image of active aging, however, does not correspond to the image of older persons themselves. Among the older age groups, there seem to be a qualitative shift toward emotional involvement with friends/colleagues and a desire for interiority, rather than active participation in social activities. This view of "productive aging" represents the image of younger adults rather than those of older persons themselves. The contrast between these images is disquieting because this view of productive aging in a youth-oriented culture, like the United States, takes on a universal meaning that implies a natural link between productive aging and mental health. However, what we see in the Generations survey are the many, sometimes contradictory, images of aging across cultures and age groups. Our findings seem to suggest that younger adults are in a position to enhance their own interests and keep their fears of aging at bay by controlling the discourse of aging. These observations raise the question of appropriateness of the categorizations used to describe older persons as either active or passive, involved or isolated, (inter)dependent or autonomous, and withdrawn or self-attuned.

CONCLUSION: THEORETICAL AND METHODOLOGICAL IMPLICATIONS

Cross-cultural research is a powerful and humbling experience that has raised many theoretical and methodological questions in my mind. As a conclusion, I would like to briefly discuss some of the theoretical implications of our findings and address a few themes that emerged in the research process.

A first theoretical implication has to do with the importance of culture in defining feelings of responsibility toward elderly parents and desirable ways of living in old age. Our research demonstrates the role of cultural norms in the way they shape perceptions and values about aging. It also shows the importance of contextualizing answers by relating them to conceptions of social obligations and definitions of selfhood in each society. Equally important, our findings point to clear differences in the way age groups internalize norms, challenging some of the stereotypical views of older persons in each society. But, despite cultural differences, older persons, across countries, report higher levels of satisfaction with their present lives and with society. Older age groups are less likely than younger ones to idealize, more likely to have lower expectations about children's obligation to sacrifice themselves, and less likely to emphasize active participation in the community. While these findings reflect a tendency toward conformity, they may suggest that older people create a sphere of their own, insulated from the pressures and ageism of the social environment. Thus, satisfaction with present life reflects a feeling of contentment that simultaneously protects and insulates older persons.

We suggest that older persons' marginalization from productive spheres and their psychological isolation lead to a social and emotional withdrawal from the world of middle-aged and younger adults. The high levels of satisfaction and shared values across countries point toward an emergent transcultural sense of self. We need to understand how this sense of inner well-being emerges and is sustained through the creation of distinctive language(s), symbolization, images, and spiritual experiences around permeable boundaries between self and others. However, in view of the pervasive ageism of both societies, inner contentment and satisfaction with self and society may well protect older persons, but, at the same time, sustain images of aging that fit younger adults' social and psychological needs, and reinforce their control over the discourse of aging. The social and political implications of these observations are far-reaching at a time when the growth of elderly populations has created new economic pressures and greater social obligations toward the elderly, a situation likely to strengthen the need to control the discourse of aging.

A second theoretical implication has to do with the meaning of concepts such as individuality, autonomy, and (inter)dependence. We need to explore theoretical models that contextualize these concepts and look at their reciprocal influence in order to understand their linkages rather than seeing them as opposite formulations. For example, Cohler's (1983) contention that (inter)-dependence in the family is the basis for the emergence of a sense of individuality provides such a model. The ability to be (inter)dependent, based on sharing and mutuality, is likely to promote a sense of autonomy and individuality. Comparative analysis, by eliciting new theoretical questions and conceptual linkages, facilitates the creation of alternative aging models. The study of aging has traditionally emphasized the values of dependence in Japan and autonomy in the United States, providing a distorted and simplified image of social reality. Theoretical models of the role of autonomy and individuality in the family reflect historical circumstances, ideologies, and cultural prescriptions. The focus on these features of the self delegitimizes the expression of needs for connectedness and interiority. The need for passive caring, interiority, and self-indulgent behavior should be explored in Western models of human development. The suppression of these features in theories of aging needs to be understood through a critical analysis of the sociocultural and ideological factors that privilege concepts of activity, productivity, consumption, and independence as the main constituents of the modern American self (Cushman, 1995). In Japan, the use of models that underplay autonomy and individuality should undergo the same critical analysis (Mouer & Sugimoto, 1986).

A third theoretical implication refers to the distorted image of older people as conforming to normative expectations. Underneath the conformity, there is a layer of needs and feelings that seem to go counter to, or coexist with, existing social norms. The value placed on group orientation in Japan and individuality in the United States are among the most accessible and acceptable features of the self, those that get easily identified in surveys. However, there are deeper layers of needs and wishes that challenge these characteristics of the self. In our research, the expression of individuality and the yearning for individual recognition, education, and independence was visible among Japanese elderly, despite the expected social norms of conformity to group needs. Among older Americans, the yearning for passive emotional caring and cherishment was tentatively expressed, despite the norms of autonomy and active aging. These observations are supported by the in-depth interviews of older persons, undertaken by Margaret Lock (1993), that clearly show attitudes and values that do not fit the modal self. We need theoretical and methodological tools that can reach underneath social conformity and self-deception to express the contradictory or ambivalent feelings, needs, and thoughts that reflect older persons' sense of self as captured, for example, through the concept of *aintegration* developed by Lomranz (1997).

A fourth theoretical implications refers to the fact that most models of aging are based on views of aging that fit the ideas and needs of the nonelderly, creating knowledge about older persons that can be used as tools for controlling the definition of the aging process (Mouer & Sugimoto, 1986). As we saw earlier, there are important differences between age groups in their views of family responsibility, sense of well-being, and desirable ways of living in old age. With increasing life expectancy, the meaning and definition of aging are changing. The reference point of the aging process seems to have moved toward a greater identification with younger adults, demonstrating the increasing role of middle-aged values and lifestyles. Thus, we need to compare the views and attitudes of middle-aged groups to those of younger adults and older persons. Our data shows that in the United States, middle-aged respondents (the 50–64 age group, traditionally referred to as "young elderly"), are closer in their values and attitudes to the younger middle-aged groups (30–49 years) than to the older age group (over 64), reinforcing the already rigid boundaries between adults and elderly. In Japan, however, this pattern of the relationship between age groups shows greater continuity and less cleavages than in the United States.

While these theoretical implications are important, we also need to assess the challenges and limitations of doing cross-national research in the study of aging. As part of the research process, we struggled with several issues. We attempted, with only partial success, to write a questionnaire that was culturally contextualized. Our difficulty stemmed from the differences in language, communication patterns, and social expectations used by the two research teams. Not only did the same words mean different things in the two countries, but in Japan, a word can take on a variety of meanings, depending on the context in which it is used. As explained before, it was after being confronted by some surprising findings that we went back to analyze the formulation of questions. These difficulties sensitized us to the use of categorizations to describe the self and the social order, providing an entry into the complex patterns of social relations and the paradoxes of attachment.

The danger of stereotyping the "other" culture in cross-national research is real, but the unchallenged assumptions about one's own culture and a lack of critical thinking about its ideological underpinnings are equally problematic. Indeed, it was easier to see cultural distinctiveness and ideological premises as they characterize the "other" country than to see one's own theoretical presuppositions. Critical analysis is especially needed with large-scale social surveys—especially State-sponsored surveys—studying elderly populations, because they are used to monitor a country's process of change or "modernization," creating an unacknowledged collusion between researchers' agendas and policy demands that tend to misrepresent older persons. This issue is compounded by the fact that Japanese researchers often replicate American models of research, incorporating uncritically parameters of social reality in the study of their own social structures. Thus, an important implication of these observations about the research process is the need to analyze questionnaires as a "text" to uncover the different theoretical presuppositions and ideological agendas encoded in them. Furthermore, the unchecked tendency of researchers to project their own fears and anxieties about aging and death onto their visions of older persons should not be underestimated. These tendencies create another potential for collusion between the researchers' own agendas, the normative image of aging, and official ideologies reinforcing what Hazan (1980) called "knowledge traps." The challenge for gerontologists is how to get beneath the conscious and unconscious compliance to detect anxieties, tensions, conflicts, and splits that go into the research process, as well as into respondents' answers. Cross-national research provides an arena to reflect on these unchecked tendencies in ways that can help deconstruct the experience of aging.

These implications, stemming from an analysis of the Generations survey, are important for understanding the well-being of older people. Cross-cultural analysis can challenge the definition of aging as a linear process of deterioration, loss, and depression, as well as the idealization of aging as a time of peace, honor, productivity, and self-discovery. It can provide an arena for comparing mechanisms of social and emotional control that keep older persons in their place. Finally, the tendency of older persons to be submerged in the societal needs and values of adult populations makes discovering and hearing their separate voice across nations an ever more meaningful task for sociologists. Indeed, despite the growing proportion of older persons in advanced industrial societies, they have yet to contribute to defining the discourse of aging through their own vision and in their own terms.

ACKNOWLEDGMENTS.   I would like to acknowledge the colleagues, friends, and students who have given me feedback and editorial help: Michele Allison, Loren McDonald, Micki McGee, Pat Lander, Jack Lomranz, Aruko Noguchi, Charlotte Muller, and Seymour Spilerman. I would also like to thank Robert Butler and the International Longevity Center for providing access and help in the analysis of the Generations Data, as well as Jack Habib for inviting me as a visiting scholar to the JDC-Brookdale Institute (Jerusalem), during which time the first draft of this paper was written. Finally, I would like to acknowledge the PSC–CUNY Research Foundation for providing me with a grant (No. 6-65482) to carry out this research.

REFERENCES

Albert, S. M., & Cattell, M. (1994). *Old age in a global perspective: Cross cultural and cross national views*. New York: G. K. Hall.
Aries, P. (1962). *Centuries of childhood*. (R. Balldick, Trans.). New York: Vintage.
Bachnik, J. M., & Quinn, C. (1994). *Situated meaning: Inside and outside in Japanese self, society and language*. Princeton, NJ: Princeton University Press.
Banfield, E. (1958). *The moral basis of a backward society*. Glencoe, IL: Free Press.
Befu, H. (1986). The social and cultural background of child development in Japan and the U.S. In H. Stevenson, H. Azuma, & K. Hakuta (Eds.), (pp. 13–27). *Child development and education in Japan*. New York: Freeman.
Bellah, R. N., Sullivan, Swidler, & Tipton. (1985). *Habits of the heart: Individualism and commitment in American life*. Berkeley: University of California Press.
Benedict, R. (1946). *The chrysanthemum and the sword: Patterns of Japanese culture*. Boston: Houghton Mifflin.

Bubeck, E. D. (1995). *Care, gender and justice*. Oxford, UK: Clarendon Press.

Butler, R. N. (1975). *Why survive? Being old in America*. New York: Harper & Row.

Campbell, J. C. (1992). *How policies change: The Japanese government and the aging society*. Princeton, NJ: Princeton University Press.

Cantor, M. H. (1983). Strain among caregivers: A study of experience in the United States [Special issue: Family support of the elderly: A cross national perspective.] *Gerontologist, 23*, 507–604.

Cohler, B. (1983). Autonomy and interdependence in the family of adulthood: A psychological perspective. *Gerontologist, 23*, 33–39.

Cumming, E., & Henri, W. (1961). *Growing old: The prospect of disengagement*. New York: Basic Books.

Cushman, P. (1995). *Constructing the self, constructing America: A cultural history of psychotherapy*. New York: Addison-Wesley.

Doi, T. (1973). *The anatomy of dependence*. Tokyo: Kodansha International.

Doi, T. (1985). *The anatomy of self*. Tokyo: Kodansha International.

Erikson, E. H., Erikson, J. M., & Kivnick, H. Q. (1986). *Vital involvement in old age*. New York: Norton.

Featherstone, M., & Wernick, A. (Eds.). (1995). *Images of aging: Cultural representations of later life*. New York: Routledge.

Fineman, M. A., & Mykitiuk, R. (Eds.). (1994). *The public nature of private violence: The discovery of domestic abuse*. New York: Routledge.

Foner, A. (1984). *Ages in conflict: A cross cultural perspective on inequality between old and young*. New York: Columbia University Press.

Firedan, B. (1993). *The fountain of age*. New York: Simon & Schuster.

Fukuyama, F. (1995). *Trust: The social virtues and the creation of prosperity*. New York: Free Press.

Giddens, A. (1991). *Modernity and self-identity: Self and society in late modern age*. Stanford, CA: Stanford University Press.

Gutmann, D. L. (1964). An examination of ego configuration in middle and later life. In B. Neugarten & Associates (Eds.), *Personality in middle and late life* (pp. 114–148). New York: Atherton Press.

Hashimoto, A. (1996). *The gift of generations: Japanese and American perspectives on aging and the social contract*. Cambridge, UK: Cambridge University Press.

Hazan, H. (1980). *The limbo people: A study of the constitution of the time universe among the aged*. London: Routledge & Kegan Paul.

Hazan, H. (1996). *From first principles: An experiment in aging*. Westport, CT: Bergin & Garvey.

Ikegami, E. (1995). *The taming of the Samurai: Honorific individualism and the making of modern Japan*. Cambridge, MA: Harvard University Press.

Inglehart, R. (1990). *Cultural shift in advanced industrial societies*. Princeton, NJ: Princeton University Press.

Inkeles, A. (1997). *National character: A psycho-social perspective*. New Brunswick, NJ: Transaction.

Japanese Ministry of Foreign Affairs. (1994). The lives of elderly people: An international comparison. Informational Bulletin from *White Paper on the Life of the Nation*, Tokyo, Japan.

Johnson, F. (1993). *Dependence and Japanese socialization: Psychoanalytic and anthropological investigations into Amae*. New York: New York University Press.

Kinoshita, Y., & Kiefer, C. W. (1992). *Refuge of the honored: Social organization in a Japanese retirement community*. Berkeley: University of California Press.

Kinsella, K. G. (1995). *Older workers, retirement, and pensions: A comparative international chart book*. Washington, DC: U.S. Department of Commerce, Economics and Statistics, Administration Bureau of the Census.

Koseisho. (1991). Populations Trends. *Basic Survey of National Life*. Tokyo, Japan.

Kristof, N. (1996, September 29). For rural Japanese, death doesn't break family ties. *New York Times* 1, p. 10.

Lasch, C. (1979). *The culture of narcissism*. New York: Warner.

Lasch, C. (1984). *The minimal self: Psychic survival in troubled times*. New York: Norton.

Lebra, T. S. (1976). *Japanese patterns of behavior*. Honolulu: University of Hawaii Press.

Lock, M. M. (1993). *Encounters with aging: Mythologies of menopause in Japan and North America*. Berkeley: University of California Press.

Maddox, G. L., & Lawton, P. M. (Eds.). (1993). *Annual review of gerontology and geriatrics: Focus on kinship, aging and social change*. New York: Springer.

Maeda, D. (1983). Family care in Japan [Special issue: Family support of the elderly: A cross national perspective]. *Gerontologist, 23*, 579–583.

Mahler, M., Pine, F., & Bergman, A. (1975). *The psychological birth of the human infant: Symbiosis and individuation*. New York: Basic Books.

Mancini, J. A., & Sandifer, D. M. (1994). Family dynamics and the leisure experiences of older adults: Theoretical view points. In R. Blieszner & V. Bedford (Eds.), *Aging and the family* (pp. 132–148). Westport, CT: Praeger.

Moody, H. R. (1994). *Aging: Concepts and controversies*. Thousand Oaks, CA: Pine Forge Press.

Mouer, R., & Sugimoto, Y. (1986). *Images of Japanese society: A study in the social construction of reality*. London: Kegan Paul International.

Muller, C. (1996). *New almanac on longevity and society: An international comparison*. New York: International Longevity Center, Mt. Sinai School of Medicine and the United Nations.

Muller, C., & Silver, C. (1995). *The Generations report*. New York: International Longevity Center, Mount Sinai School of Medicine.

Nipponjin No Kokuminsei. (1992). *A study of the Japanese national character: Vol. 5*. Research Committee for the Study of the Japanese National Character. Tokyo: Idemitsu Shoten.

Nydegger, C. N. (1983). Family ties of the aged in cross-cultural perspective. *Gerontologist, 23*, 27–32.

Palmore, E. B., & Maeda, D. (1985). *The honorable elders revisited: A revised cross-cultural analysis of aging in Japan*. Durham, NC: Duke University Press.

Parsons, T. (1964). *The social system*. New York: Free Press.

Plath, D. W. (1980). *Long engagements: Maturity in modern Japan*. Stanford, CA: Stanford University Press.

Reischauer, E. O. (1977). *The Japanese*. Cambridge, MA: Harvard/Belknap Press.

Riley, M. W., Kahn, R. L., & Foner, A. (Eds.). (1994). *Age and structural lag: Society's failure to provide meaningful opportunities in work, family, and leisure*. New York: Wiley.

Roland, A. (1988). *In search of self in India and Japan: Toward a cross-cultural psychology*. Princeton, NJ: Princeton University Press.

Silver, C. (1992). Personality structure and aging style. *Journal of Aging Studies, 6*, 333–350.

Silver, C., & Muller, C. (1997). Effect of ascribed and achieved characteristics on social values in Japan and the U.S. *Research in Social Stratification and Mobility, 15*, 153–176.

Smith, R. J. (1983). *Japanese society: Tradition, self, and social order*. Cambridge, UK: Cambridge University Press.

Soldo, B. J., & Freedman, V. A. (1994). Care of the elderly: Division of labor among the family, market, and the state. In Martin & Preston (Eds.), *Demography of aging* (pp. 195–216). Washington, DC: National Academy Press.

Takayama, N. (1992). *The greying of Japan: An economic perspective on public pensions*. Tokyo & New York: Kinokuniya. (Distributed outside Japan by Oxford University Press).

Tocqueville, A. de (1969). *Democracy in America* George Lawrence, Trans., J. P. Mayer (Ed.). Garden City: Doubleday, Anchor Books. (Original published 1840)

Tomita, S. K. (1994). The consideration of cultural factors in the research of elder mistreatment with an in-depth look at the Japanese. *Journal of Cross-Cultural Gerontology, 9*, 39–51.

Vaillant, G. (1993). *The wisdom of the ego*. Cambridge, MA: Harvard University Press.

White, M. (1992). Home truths: Women and social change in Japan. *Daedalus, 121*, 61–82.

White, M. (1993). *The material child: Coming of age in Japan and America*. New York: Free Press.

PART VI

Memory and Dementia

Perhaps in no other area are we as aware of mind–body, physical–mental issues as in the areas of cognition, memory, and dementia. While we hope for a sound mind and a sound body, we feel greater despair when the former fails us. "My mind to me a kingdom is," wrote the English poet Edward Dyer, and that may be what many human beings believe, feeling that only the mind distinguishes them from animals. It is no wonder then that in old age, as we enjoy increased longevity but are discontented with its quality, we expect to have achieved wisdom but are terrified by possible memory decline. In studies of dementia in various countries, prevalence rates for those over age 65 have ranged from 2.5% to 24.6% (Ineichen, 1987), with variability between studies probably reflecting methodological differences. Dementia prevalence doubles approximately every 5 years after age 65 (Jorm, 1990). Although it is clinically important to be on the alert for potentially reversible causes of dementia, Alzheimer's disease—a presently irreversible degenerative disease of the brain—and vascular dementia account for the largest proportion of all causes of dementia. The chapters in Part VI cover cogent issues ranging from memory complaints to dementia.

Niederehe (Chapter 18) undertakes to fathom the phenomenon of memory complaints, knowledge about which is very limited. The author asks about the meaning and significance of memory complaints. Are they precursors of dementia? How can they be clinically interpreted? In what theoretical and methodological frameworks can they best be understood? Niederehe reviews conceptions and findings in the field and analyzes the incongruence between memory complaint and memory performance and the validity of self-reports. He identifies areas ripe for future research, demonstrates how we need to reevaluate our approach to the topic, and presents new ways of conceptualizing and testing this phenomenon. The author develops his argument that research here has been too cognitive in its orientation and has overemphasized the accuracy question to the neglect of other issues. Niederehe demonstrates the theoretical relevance and provides methodological suggestions for such issues as the complainer's self-concept, personality, affect (especially depression), attitudes, beliefs, interpersonal relationships, and social norms and functions, all of which may influence complaint behavior and be equally important in affording an understanding of memory complaints. The author relates experimental, cognitive, behavioral, and psychodynamic perspectives in his attempt to provide a differentiated conceptual framework. Niederehe criticizes the prevailing assessment technology in cognitive psychology and neuropsychology that focuses on quantifying memory performance in an "objective" manner. He alerts us to measurement artifacts and suggests improved self-report and self-appraisal measures, as well as clinical approaches, all of which make his suggested hypotheses more easily testable. Niederehe's clinically differentiated model of memory complaints (Schema C) carries a high integrative potential. It provides an intriguing, encompassing model, which may organize the existing research on memory complaints in a different light, suggests an innovative direction for future research, and enriches our comprehension of this important phenomenon.

Reischies (Chapter 19) provides us with an extensive conceptual analysis of the relationship between age-related cognitive decline (ARCD) and dementia, and of problems in the diagnosis of dementia as a breakdown of cognitive performance. Differentiation is the hallmark of Reischies's investigations. He emphasizes the distinction between nonspecific age effects and the effects of dementia disease on cognition. Separating definitions, types, and concepts of dementia and notions of thresholds, and clarifying that ARCD is different for the various concepts of dementia, Reischies argues that a slowly progressing type of senile dementia can be explained by normal cognitive aging. The author distinguishes between different levels of syndrome formation, between dementia syndromes as complex and narrow (see Korczyn, Kahana, & Friedland, Chapter 20). He also explains how accepting mainly the rapidly progressing senile dementia type can result in the overestimation of the prevalence of dementia. One has to analyze dementia thresholds in order to comprehend how normal cognitive aging can misleadingly be classified as a dementia syndrome. Since dementia is a multiple-threshold diagnosis, the various thresholds, including clinical thresholds and their relationships to various state and trait markers, have to be defined separately. The additivity of dementia and ARCD has to be clarified, and since unspecific age-related effects on test performance are apparent, age corrections should be made in the testing and diagnosis of dementia. Reischies's model shows that a dementia threshold is passed if the adult cognitive level is so diminished by ARCD and dementia-related decline that the present cognitive level is below a certain age-related limit, resulting in an oblique threshold. The author also elaborates the importance and complexity of thresholds in behavioral areas that reflect impairment of daily activities. Reischies enriches our knowledge by clarifying the relationship of normal aging to dementia processes. His conceptual analysis has crucial implications for the future research of dementia as well as for modes of diagnosis, the age factor, treatment, and policymaking in the field.

Korczyn et al. (Chapter 20) explores the relationship between education and dementia of the Alzheimer's type (DAT). The authors, who tend to approach DAT as a syndrome rather than as a disease with a single etiology and process, emphasize the need for differentiation (e.g., between risk factors and risk indicators, or between factors triggering or accelerating the disease, or between epidemiological counts of prevalence or incidence) as they investigate the causes and risk factors of DAT. The authors, examining the idea that education may be a guard against dementia, discuss the variability of the educational component, its function as a protective factor, as well as its position as a surrogate for other variables (e.g., socioeconomic level) and as a confounding factor (e.g., smoking). Possible important relationships between biological mechanisms, education, and the appearance of dementia are explicated. This chapter deals with methodological issues relating to the epidemiology of DAT, defines the limitations of data collection and the interpretation of research results, and suggests hypotheses testing as well as directions for future research in the field.

REFERENCES

Ineichen, B. (1987). Measuring the rising tide: How many dementia cases will there be by 2001? *British Journal of Psychiatry, 150,* 193–200.

Jorm, A. (1990). *The epidemiology of Alzheimer's disease and related disorders.* London: Chapman & Hall.

CHAPTER 18

The Significance of Memory Complaints in Later Life

Methodological and Theoretical Considerations

GEORGE NIEDEREHE

INTRODUCTION

In their seminal study of 1,134 elderly San Franciscans, Lowenthal, Berkman, and their associates (1967) found complaints of failing memory so frequently that they termed them (alongside reports of decreased energy) "stereotypes of aging." Declining memory was reported by nearly half the community residents and by even higher percentages of those evidencing psychiatric symptoms, whether hospitalized or living in the community. Though self-reports of memory decline increased with age, this pattern was not substantiated by scores on objective cognitive tests, which remained stable with age. These findings were consistent with some other reports mentioning discrepancies between patients' performance on objective tests or measures of function and the levels of impairment that clinicians had expected to find, based on patients' self-reports (e.g., Friedman, 1964).

These early gerontological studies raised many questions about what it represents when an older person presents a concern about memory decline or difficulty, and encapsulated most of the themes that have since then preoccupied researchers on memory complaints. In particular, it is unclear what kind of information such complaints provide and how they should be interpreted clinically. These issues have perplexed many gerontologists and drawn their fair share of research attention over the past 20 years. The objectives of this chapter are to review several different conceptual frameworks for late-life memory

GEORGE NIEDEREHE • Adult and Geriatric Treatment and Preventive Intervention, Research Branch, National Institute of Mental Health, Rockville, Maryland 20857.

Handbook of Aging and Mental Health: An Integrative Approach, edited by Jacob Lomranz. Plenum Press, New York, 1998.

complaint, with an emphasis on publications within the past 10 years, and to identify areas ripe for further research.

IMPLICIT MODELS OF MEMORY COMPLAINT

According to a man on the street's commonsensical view, an individual who perceives/reports a memory problem is simply operating as a neutral observer and reporting objectively on experienced events. The presumption is that self-report is isomorphic with functioning, and that complaints simply reflect a prior objective reality (i.e., memory impairment); in turn, because of common cultural expectations that memory deteriorates with age, the latter is considered an inevitable part of "aging." This implicit model (see Figure 18–1, Schema A) predicts increased memory complaints with aging.

A medical or neuropsychological variant of this stereotypic model (Figure 18–1, Schema B) simply inserts neurobiological changes (e.g., changes in brain structure) as the proximal antecedent of memory impairment, while retaining the assumptions of isomorphism between complaint and impairment, and of increased impairment with aging. In line with this type of viewpoint, it is fairly traditional in medical fields, such as neurology, to take subjective memory complaints at face value as evidence that memory changes are occurring, even if too subtly to be clinically detected. Though the aging effect is assumed to be mediated largely by age-related neurobiological changes, this model allows for the fact that impairment may occur at any age due to other physiological causes.

The studies of Lowenthal et al. (1967) and others, however, suggest a dissociation between memory complaint and memory performance. Though they may share some degree of relationship, these two domains have distinct patterns of correlates and must be assumed to be separate variables. Recognition of this dissociation led to a more differentiated implicit model of memory complaints (see Figure 18–1, Schema C) in which additional factors (to be discussed later) could be explored as influences on either actual memory functioning or on complaints about it. With these implicit models as background, we proceed to examine several conceptual frameworks for memory complaints and the research associated with them.

ACCURACY OR VALIDITY
OF SELF-REPORTS ABOUT MEMORY

The research conducted over the past 20–30 years in this area has focused predominantly on Relationship h in Schema C, the congruence or lack thereof between self-reports and objective test data, gauging the match in terms of difference scores, correlation or regression coefficients, or other measures of association (e.g., factor loadings). Diverse methods have been used to assess each domain, and studies have varied greatly with respect to subject sampling. The focal question has generally been whether memory self-reports are "accurate" or

a. Stereotypic Model

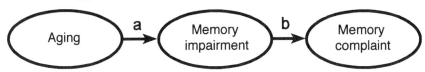

b. Simple Medical/Neuropsychological Model

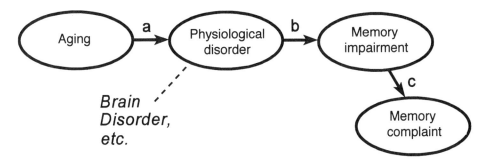

C. Clinically Differentiated Model

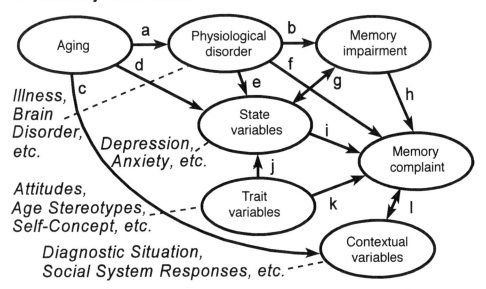

Figure 18–1. Schematics depicting tacit models of memory complaint.

"valid" indices of actual memory functioning. This conceptual framework or perspective thus focuses on a concurrent validity question, the "objective reference" or accuracy of complaints, and the associated research tends to be fundamentally of a cognitive or neuropsychological sort, whether conducted in the context of large-scale surveys or smaller, laboratory-based studies.

The questions that are emphasized within the accuracy framework have a good deal of real-world importance. When older adults report that they are experiencing (increased) memory difficulties, others often consider this indicative of cognitive decline, perhaps the first signs of an incipient dementing process. Of course, it is also the case that many older persons experience memory changes that appear to plateau rather than progress into dementia syndromes, as described in such constructs as "benign senescent forgetfulness" (Kral, 1962), "age-associated memory impairment" (AAMI; Crook et al., 1986), the DSM-IV syndrome of "age-related cognitive decline" (ARCD; American Psychiatric Association, 1994), and the ICD-9 category of "slight cognitive failure."

Given that, logically speaking, the individual should be in the best position to pick up on cognitive changes while they are still subtle, there has been considerable interest in whether self-reports about memory can be used effectively in screening for dementia, or as a stand-in for objective testing in large-scale surveys of the elderly. Indeed, self-reported concerns about memory are among the criteria for diagnosing the AAMI, ARCD, and ICD-9 constructs, effectively requiring that diagnosable changes be detected by the individual as well as documented by subpar performance on standardized memory or other cognitive tests.

However, at the population level, various surveys have indicated that memory complaints tend to be far more prevalent among older persons (25–88% of respondents) than are diagnosable memory disorders (e.g., Bassett & Folstein, 1993; Bolla, Lindgren, Bonnacorsy, & Bleecker, 1991; Livingston, Hawkins, Graham, Blizard, & Mann, 1990). There have also been reports that the memory clinics that have proliferated in recent years are being frequented by many elderly who do not seem to be experiencing any serious cognitive difficulties upon neuropsychological evaluation, and who should be numbered among the "worried well" (Dawe, Procter, & Philpot, 1992). Based on such observations, a reasonable expectation has been that many complaints presented by older persons turn out to be unverifiable and unreliable as signposts for the identification of memory dysfunction.

When subjects have been asked to report about their typical *everyday* memory, psychological studies have produced very mixed findings. At least seven studies with normal elderly samples have shown moderate relationships, such that performance can be said to contribute significantly to variance in self-reports (e.g., Larrabee, West, & Crook, 1991). However, the relationships demonstrated tend to be weak, the pattern of findings not predicted a priori, and the overall results inconsistent from study to study. An equal number of other studies have indicated poor or no correspondence between self-reports and objective test data (e.g., O'Boyle, Amadeo, & Self, 1990).

From a cognitive psychology perspective, memory self-reports are based in the domain of cognitive skills known as metamemory. This subsystem of the general memory system involves knowledge about memory in general, monitoring and awareness of one's own memorial activity, selection and use of mnemonic strategies, and the like. Over recent years, considerable progress has occurred in developing and psychometrically refining questionnaires that quantify subjects' memory self-perceptions in increasingly detailed and differentiated ways linked with metamemory constructs, and that are better validated as measures (see several reviews of 10 measures by Gilewski & Zelinski, 1986; Zelinski & Gilewski, 1988). Factor-analytic work with these instruments has assisted in mapping out the dimensions of metamemory that can be reliably assessed via a self-report questionnaire; some primary domains appear to be knowledge about memory and about one's own performance ability, use of mnemonic strategies, expectations regarding age-related cognitive change, sense of memorial self-efficacy, and memory-related affect (Hertzog, Hultsch, & Dixon, 1989).

As opposed to focusing on self-perceptions about one's *typical* functioning (performance), other research using a memory prediction paradigm has examined whether people *have the ability to* perceive and judge their functioning accurately (competence). These studies typically require subjects to make predictions (and/or posttask judgments) in terms of specific experimental laboratory tasks. In such studies, much appears to depend on the nature and familiarity of the tasks, how much contextual information is actually made available to subjects, and so on. Whereas no clear age-related trends have emerged, in research by Bieman-Copland and Charness (1994), there has been some suggestion that older subjects tend to monitor and self-correct their memory performance in a less fine-grained manner than younger subjects. These investigators have speculated that older individuals' global complaints about memory may stem from this form of metamemorial inability.

Dementia Diagnosis and Prognosis

Yet another subcategory of cognitive/accuracy studies has looked at self-reports about memory for their value as a marker or screening variable in early diagnosis of dementia or other physical deterioration, thereby addressing the time lag between first appearance of complaints and eventual clear-cut validation of the deteriorative condition (a predictive validity question). This literature often examines differences between older individuals' self-reports and reports given by family informants, generally finding informant reports a better predictor of objective performance on cognitive measures (e.g., McGlone et al., 1990; Wilder et al., 1994). In examining these issues, longitudinal or prognostic studies are useful.

For example, O'Brien et al. (1992) followed up 68 memory clinic patients whose complaints had been determined to represent either benign senescent forgetfulness or no disorder. After an average of 3 years, only 9% had developed dementia. Though memory complaints thus represented approximately a twofold increase in dementia risk over this period, the vast majority of cases remained cognitively normal and neither the complaints nor other clinical factors studied predicted the development of dementia. In another recent study, memory complaints showed little sensitivity in identifying persons who developed cognitive impairment over an interval averaging 3.7 years (Smith, Petersen, Ivnik, Malec, & Tangalos, 1996). Taken together, these recent longitudinal studies demonstrate little predictive value for cognitive complaints as a means of identifying individuals who go on to develop clear-cut cognitive decline or dementia after an interval of several years.

Conclusions about the Accuracy Framework

Overall, then, in most studies, the correspondence between memory performance and memory self-reports has been at best weak, if not altogether lacking. This implies that, at the individual level, memory self-reports cannot be considered reliable indices of the individual's functional status in everyday life. A logical pitfall to guard against, however, is the unwarranted conclusion that complaints never indicate a real cognitive problem. Even if complaints' correlation with cognitive testing results is taken to be $r = .00$, this does not mean that complaints are invariably inaccurate or should be routinely discounted. Rather, over a series of patients with memory complaints, the nonsignificant correlation might be thought of as leaving a 50:50 chance that an actual memory problem might be found. An appropriate conclusion would be that, when questions arise about them, cognitive abilities need to be assessed directly.

Methodological limitations may account for a good deal of the mixed or negative findings regarding the accuracy of memory complaints. As a primary shortcoming, in many studies, the memory tests used may not be sensitive to the sorts of memory changes that subjects notice and complain about, such as the subtle decrements seen in early dementia. Or they may be poor indices of the everyday memory of which subjects speak; in fact, the correspondence with self-reports is improved when researchers use representative, everyday memory tasks rather than laboratory memory tests (Zelinski & Gilewski, 1988). Even aside from these problems, it is difficult to assure that self-reports and tests are actually tapping the same subdomains of memory and/or are pegged at the same levels of generality (e.g., Rabbitt & Abson, 1990).

Another possible methodological reason for poor correspondence between complaint and performance could be that the measures used to gather self-appraisals may be too rough or global to reflect what the subjects actually know or perceive about their memory. Although significant progress has been made in refining self-report measures, researchers have probably not yet reached the limits of the information to be gained by probing subjects' memory self-perceptions in greater detail or in more sophisticated ways. Subjects may be able to make relatively veridical self-observations of their memory functioning if the right questions are asked about particular areas of the memory domain. Some observers have suggested that subjects are not capable of judging their memory in absolute terms, but only relative to what they consider typical for others their same age (Sunderland, Watts, Baddeley, & Harris, 1986). Christensen (1991), indeed, reported that certain patterns of self-report corresponded better with memory performance (describing deficits as recently acquired and worse than those of peers), particularly if IQ was taken into account in terms of expected levels of performance. Interestingly, in several recent regional brain imaging studies using positron emission tomography (PET) to examine the presumed neural substrate for memory deficits, a seemingly indirect index of memory difficulties (mnemonics usage) was the self-report variable that showed a consistent relationship to glucose hypometabolism in the frontal cortex (Small, Komo, LaRue, Kaplan, & Mandelkern, 1995; Small et al., 1994). In any case, improved self-report measures may help to demonstrate that subjects have somewhat more accurate self-knowledge about their memory than research has thus far tended to indicate.

An educated guess, however, is that advances in this particular regard are likely to be marginal. We might be more hopeful that certain aspects of self-report can be identified as having "sign value" for pointing toward the various influences that may be present in the individual case and contributing to memory complaints. For example, some patterns of self-report may have a high probability of reflecting dementing changes, others a greater likelihood of being associated with depression, and so forth. Useful indices might also emerge from comparisons among multiple self reports. Determining such informative self-report "patterns" will require descriptive and correlational studies similar to those that have been conducted in developing various Minnesota Multiphasic Personality Inventory (MMPI) scales and indices.

Measurement artifacts have rarely been taken into account in memory self-report accuracy research. For simplicity, one may think of measured "accuracy" as being a difference score (or some similar statistic) calculated between self-reports and objective measures of a particular construct. Given that self-reports on stereotypical constructs such as memory tend not to vary much, either between subjects or within subjects over time, it follows that variance in measured accuracy tends to be mostly an artifactual reflection of naturalistic variability in the objective measure. For example, subjects whose actual memory function happens to fall into the stereotypical range will be credited for greater accuracy, not because they discriminate their individual positioning with any more sensitivity than others but merely accidentally. This particular problem, known as "stereotype accuracy" (Cronbach, 1955; Gage & Cronbach, 1955), creates statistical artifacts in accuracy measures that need to be controlled for but usually are not.

Given the research results, we should take stock of the assumptions that have commonly been made regarding the ability of people in general to describe their memory abilities with precision. Viewing memory self-reports from an accuracy perspective, it appears that some degree of discrepancy between self-report/complaint and performance is the general rule in self-perception rather than an oddity. With many personal attributes, normal people do not show a great deal of skill at discriminating their unique attributes or status, but rather tend to view themselves as positioned relative to normative concepts of the "generalized other," that is, cultural stereotypes; most typically, they describe themselves as being average or similar to peers. Self-perception, then, does not routinely operate according to an accuracy metric, and our research should reflect an awareness of this reality.

The following three sections discuss several other foci and lines of research that deserve attention as potential avenues toward gaining greater understanding of memory complaints, namely, (1) the role of affect, (2) attitudes and self-concept, and (3) interpersonal relationships, and the possible social functions of memory complaints. Such foci imply an underlying conceptual framework that recognizes that other factors than memory performance or ability itself may influence the self-reports given about it. Relative to Figure 18–1, the three considerations mentioned roughly correspond to expanding Schema C so as not only to differentiate complaint from performance (as in the accuracy focus), but also to take into account the potential influences on complaint behavior of state, trait, and contextual variables, respectively.

AFFECTIVE STATE VIS-À-VIS MEMORY COMPLAINT AND PERFORMANCE

As a further specification of earlier findings that appeared to associate psychiatric status with inaccuracy in memory self-reports, Kahn, Zarit, Hilbert, and Niederehe (1975) reported that, in a clinical sample, memory complaint correlated with patients' depression levels but not with their tested memory performance, whereas actual performance was linked with measures that screen for the presence of dementing changes and not with depression. Similar findings have subsequently been reported by many other investigators, including studies in other cultures (Grut et al., 1993; O'Connor, Pollitt, Roth, Brook, & Reiss, 1990). In the previously cited McGlone et al. (1990) study, older adults' self-reports were associated with depression but not with their objective cognitive performance, whereas the pattern of associations was the opposite for relatives' reports. Many consider the linkage between memory complaint and depression to be a by-product of the fact that depression itself may in some instances be an early marker of incipient dementia that will become fully evident only later, at more advanced stages. In severe dementia, both depression and self-awareness tend to become less common. There is some evidence that complaint and depression both decrease at more severe stages of dementia, whereas denial increases (O'Connor et al., 1990; Sevush & Leve, 1993). However, in most studies, increased memory complaint has consistently been found to relate to greater depression, both in cognitively normal elders and in those with actually compromised cognitive status (e.g., O'Boyle et al., 1990).

According to Gilewski and Zelinski (1986), essentially all studies up until the mid-1980s that had examined affective status as a variable had replicated the finding that memory self-reports tend to be associated more strongly with depression (Relationship i in Figure 18–1, Schema C) than with measured memory performance (Relationship h), and this trend has continued across at least eight more recent studies (e.g., Barker, Prior, & Jones, 1995; Bolla et al., 1991; O'Connor et al., 1990). The same pattern has been reported relative to the range of depressive symptoms found both in community samples, and in samples specifically with clinical depression. In one study, complaints were elevated equally in those with depressive symptoms only and those who met diagnostic criteria for major depression (O'Hara, Hinrichs, Kohout, Wallace, & Lemke, 1986).

The association of memory complaints with depression is not assured or invariable, however. In the community survey by Livingston et al. (1990), only 26% of those with memory complaints had diagnosable depression. Likewise, studies of subjects who self-refer to memory clinics or volunteer for memory training programs have not always found depression to be a significant contributing factor (Scogin, Storandt, & Lott, 1985). Moreover, the theoretical role of depression in producing memory complaints that are not associated with objective cognitive impairment is far from clear. One possibility is that depression may simply entail a negativistic bias that colors many aspects of self-regard and is expressed in many types of complaints (Williams, Little, Scates, & Blockman, 1987).

Older individuals' tendency toward memory complaint may also be influenced by other comorbid conditions instead of, or in addition to, depressive states. For instance, in one study, life satisfaction and anxiety were more strongly related to complaints than was depression (West, Boatwright, & Schleser, 1984). To date, research on memory self-reports in other affective states such as anxiety, and in various health conditions, has not produced consistent results to indicate whether these comorbid conditions play a role prior to or more prominent than depression. However, complaint patterns may differ across various physical diseases.

The role of depression may be more complex than simply influencing self-reports, and its intervening effects on memory performance per se may also need to be taken into account. Even though studies of this latter relationship have yielded quite mixed findings (Niederehe, 1986), according to a recent meta-analysis, the research literature does indicate a modest but consistent association between depression and memory impairment (Burt, Zembar, & Niederehe, 1995). The association appears to be stronger in studies of depressed inpatients versus outpatients and, counterintuitively, in samples with younger rather than older mean ages, but not to differ consistently by such other potential moderator variables as unipolar versus bipolar subtype, patients' medication status, immediate versus delayed retention intervals, or verbal versus visual memory.

Though the meta-analysis shows an association between depressed status and memory impairment, it provides little clue to the causal factors involved. Depressed affect may or may not be the critical influence. For example, since late-life depression is often associated with other medical diseases, memory could be impaired by the physical comorbidity rather than by depression itself, or by neurobiological changes that occur in depression (see Chapter 21 by Katz, this volume). Interestingly, studies that have controlled rigorously for physical

health tend not to show significant depression–memory impairment relationships. However, such studies may simultaneously tend to feature outpatient
samples and less-than-severe forms of depression. No path analysis or structural
modeling studies appropriate to check out whether the effect of depression on
self-report is partially mediated through intervening effects on actual memory
functioning have yet been done.

In practical terms, memory complaints are frequently influenced by subjects' depression and possibly by other aspects of their clinical state. The presence of complaints should trigger clinical assessments screening for these conditions via independent diagnostic procedures.

TRAIT AND SELF-CONCEPT VARIABLES
AND MEMORY COMPLAINTS

An approach focusing on trait variables attempts to understand memory
complaints in terms of enduring individual differences, such as personality
characteristics or attitudes, rather than temporary fluctuations in affect (Relationship k in Figure 18–1, Schema C). A growing list of studies has linked
memory complaints with subjects' personalities or specific traits, and has suggested that the tendency to make complaints may be less variable than subjects'
affective state. Both Zonderman, Costa and Kawas (1989) and Hanninen et al.
(1994) have reported generalized tendencies toward somatic complaining in
those with memory complaints. Other studies suggest that complainers show
greater neuroticism and trait anxiety, and a tendency to experience greater
distress in response to the same changes (Barker et al., 1995; Vermuelen, Aldenkamp, & Alpherts, 1993).

Many observers suspect that negative beliefs about age changes in memory
are a predisposing factor. For example, older adults with such beliefs may
generate corresponding personal expectations and interpret isolated instances of
memory failure as indicative of a general problem. This predisposition may be
strengthened if they also have concerns or anticipatory worry about developing
dementia. A number of the questionnaires used to assess memory complaints
include subscales that attempt to capture such beliefs and attitudes. Kahn et al.
(1975) speculated that a tendency to think and express oneself in stereotyped
ways may be part of memory complaint in old age. Indeed, Derouesne et al.
(1989) found more severe memory complaints among those who hold negative
stereotypes about aging.

The stability of memory complaints over time has been investigated via
naturalistic follow-ups of individuals with concerns about their memory and in
outcome studies on memory training programs and other treatments. Such
studies have produced extremely variable results that do not allow for any firm
conclusions. In a follow-up of the subjects studied by Kahn et al. (1975), despite
significant changes in depression for a number of subjects, there did not tend
to be associated changes in either memory performance or complaint (Niederehe, 1976). However, in other research, older patients successfully treated for

depression with either antidepressant medications or group psychotherapy have manifested corresponding reductions in memory complaint (Plotkin, Mintz, & Jarvik, 1985; Popkin, Gallagher, Thompson, & Moore, 1982). In some intervention studies, elderly subjects who were given memory training have not manifested changes in depression or memory complaints (Scogin & Bienas, 1988; Scogin et al., 1985), whereas in others, reductions in memory concerns have been reported, even though posttraining self-reports appear to remain correlated with depression levels rather than with performance (e.g., Zarit, Gallagher, & Kramer, 1981).

One alternate way to approach memory complaints may be to study their role in older adults' self-conceptions. It may be impossible to understand what memory complaints "mean" without reference to how the older individual thinks about him- or herself more broadly (see Cavanaugh, 1989). In making this point, I do not mean to advance any particular theory of the self. Various theories in clinical psychology, social psychology (see conservation of resources viewpoint in Chapter 5 by Hobfoll and Wells, this volume), psychoanalysis, or other fields provide useful conceptual frameworks within which to delineate ways that memory complaints may reflect older adults' conceptions of themselves or arise at transition points in self-understanding. It is worth noting that little research has been done relating memory complaints to life-course transitions or events (see discussion of "trigger events" in Chapter 12 by Gutmann, this volume).

Self-efficacy concepts represent one example of a specific framework that has already been applied to memory self-reports to some degree (e.g., Berry, West, & Dennehey, 1989). Hertzog et al. (1989) found a self-efficacy factor in several of the most used metamemory questionnaires. Seligman's learned helplessness–learned optimism theory (see Chapter 4 by Gatz, this volume) suggests various ways of bringing social learning perspectives and motivational variables into the picture. Certainly, the attributional styles detailed in the "reformulated" version of the learned helplessness paradigm (Abramson, Seligman, & Teasdale, 1978) might be useful in understanding how tendencies to think in global, static, and self-referential terms could lead certain individuals to formulate memory complaints by interpreting their experiences in terms of general stereotypes about the aging process.

Such theories about self processes may yield additional testable hypotheses about how depression bears upon memory complaints. A purely cognitive–accuracy perspective is inadequate to handle the paradoxical finding that depressed individuals may show seemingly greater accuracy than others in interpersonal and self-perception situations (Edison & Adams, 1992; Lewinsohn, Mischel, Chaplin, & Barton, 1980), demonstrating what has sometimes been termed a "depressive realism." What is needed is a conceptual framework that recognizes that social perceptions and judgments are made relative to various social norms and stereotypes, rather than to a criterion of logical precision. In my own research, the change in self-perception that occurs with depression appears to be an overall shift or bias toward seeing oneself more negatively than is typical, relative to these social norms. In the case of memory, as with other diffuse personal attributes such as social competence, people normally tend to overestimate their abilities. Under these conditions, the effect of depression is to reduce the typical tendency to overestimate (Lewinsohn et al., 1980; Niederehe, 1976). The greater "accuracy" of the depressed individuals, however, is an accidental by-product of the stereotype accuracy phenomenon discussed earlier, rather than of superior perceptual sensitivity or "differential accuracy."

It may be useful to take certain lessons from the research literature on somatic complaints/hypochondriasis and self-perceptions of health and, paradoxically, to deal with memory in a *less detailed* way than is typical in cognitive psychology or neuropsychology. In thinking about self-perceptions of "health," it is easier to recognize that neither the older individual nor her or his physician, nor the researcher has a superior capacity to define the overarching construct (i.e., there is no consensually agreed-upon "gold standard" of health). We would do well to show a greater awareness that much the same is true of memory. Despite our ability to devise tests of various skills that go into "memory," ultimately, we cannot precisely define this global term, and we certainly have not been looking at how our older subjects understand it. Simply summating multiple discrete tests and calling that the objective criterion of overall memory begs the question. To demonstrate that subjects' self-reports fail to correspond to this kind of criterion does not ultimately invalidate them as behavioral data; it simply establishes that the self-reports are not useful markers to indicate the kinds of impairment of interest to those who adopt a cognitive or neuropsychological slant on memory.

Psychodynamic Perspectives

Very little research involving memory complaint has been done to look into the psychodynamic meanings of perceiving oneself as having altered memory. Admittedly, it has been notoriously difficult to articulate testable theories of such private meanings in any area of behavior, and to devise operational methods that meet with broad acceptance as being of adequate scientific rigor. At the heart of the problem is the difficulty of dealing with "personal meaning" in a generalizable way. Unless generalizable standards of, or ways of assessing, meaningfulness can be defined, independently of outcomes such as symptom course, the theories adduced to explain the symptoms tend to be circular and not open to disproof. If meaning is regarded as idiosyncratic to each individual, it can hardly be studied scientifically, for any failures to prove the hypotheses can always be rationalized as due to flawed methods that have inadequately ascertained the "true meaning" for the individual.

However, there are broader regularities and social structures associated with "meaning making" (see Chapters 9 and 10 by Kegan and Lomranz, respectively, this volume). Useful research should be possible in this vein and clearly could contribute importantly to advancing our clinical understanding of memory complaints. For example, descriptive research linking clinical complaint with self-perception would be helpful. Perhaps hermeneutic methods or content analysis of older persons' descriptions of their self-conceptions regarding memory can provide insights into broadly shared patterns of personal meaning. Likewise, assessments of complainers versus noncomplainers might focus on their attitudes toward aging and related cognitive changes, or on other personal attributes that might predispose toward both complaining and focusing on memory. An alternate research strategy would be to identify subgroups of older persons inclined to offer particularly negative self-appraisals of memory in response to cognitive failures or other stresses, and then probe the bases for this sensitivity (e.g., subjects' degree of everyday reliance on memory, prominence of memory skills within their self-concept, anticipatory fears of memory decline— see discussion of the sense of an endangered self in Cohler, Chapter 11, this volume).

In terms of examining such sensitivities, researchers have done little to link memory complaints to other theories about memory that emphasize the *non-cognitive functions of memory activity* rather than the information-processing skills involved. Almost no linkage has been made to the extensive literature on reminiscing, in which memory activity is conceptualized relative to such functions as reviewing failures to master life tasks, resolving problems of meaning, maintaining socialization, and helping to achieve ego integrity in the sense of Erikson's developmental stage model (Butler, 1963). Using the reminiscence variable as an indirect gauge of the meaning or functional importance of memory activity to the individual, one might investigate, for example, whether memory complaints are increased in individuals who tend to be reminiscers when that activity is impeded or threatened. Analogously, the ego-defensive functions of memory complaint have not received much research attention (Cavanaugh, 1989).

In summary, memory complaints may be influenced by personality factors and/or other general cognitive traits and beliefs (e.g., self-efficacy), or may represent just an arbitrary focus within a more generalized phenomenon of negative self-perception/self-concept. Such features should be evaluated and targeted as part of a comprehensive treatment approach.

THE INTERPERSONAL
CONTEXT AND COMPLAINT

Very little research has been done to study memory complaints as a form of operant behavior in terms of their interpersonal functions and consequences. This neglect of how complaints relate to their social context is a particularly serious oversight (see further discussion of contextual factors in Mostofsky (Chapter 23, this volume). The cognitive approach looks only at antecedents of self-perception, hardly at all at their motivational dimensions or situational consequences (represented as a bidirectional Relationship 1 in Figure 18–1, Schema C). Clearly, there is an interpersonal aspect to complaining about anything; to complain is to present remarks to someone else. Generally, this occurs within the context of an expectation that the recipient of the complaint should do something about it, or at least respond in some fashion. However, we have essentially no empirical data on the interpersonal contexts in which memory complaints initially arise, how they are responded to, what functional contingencies may contribute to their genesis and maintenance, or the like. Researchers have not clearly differentiated—either conceptually or methodologically—these interpersonal dimensions from the purely cognitive (e.g., self-perceptual and self-evaluative) aspects of memory self-reports. We have tended to take the responses to the items in memory questionnaires and simply label any and all of them "memory complaints." From a clinical perspective, this is foolhardy and potentially misleading.

For example, in understanding how memory complaints are associated with depression, it may be critical to distinguish simply having a privately pessimistic opinion of one's abilities from actively presenting that view to someone responsible for dealing with such problems (Niederehe & Yoder, 1989). According to an interpersonal systems perspective, patients and their doctors engage in a mutual process of negotiating the matters that will be deemed symptoms and defining the problems about which the doctor can perhaps do something (Balint, 1964). Depressed behavior constitutes a communicative (possibly "help-seeking") activity within such interpersonal situations, and contributes to the doctor–patient negotiating process. Coyne (1976), Bonime (1966), and others have provided theoretical frameworks for conceptualizing the interpersonal influences of depressive symptoms that may offer useful templates for exploring the degree to which memory complaints have similar functions. Likewise, family systems theories and paradigms for studying interpersonal behavior can suggest models for researching such behaviors in the home environment as well as in professional clinical settings.

Social desirability is another methodological concern that has received little attention in memory complaint research. Clearly, there is the potential for older subjects to preferentially view or report themselves as experiencing memory problems rather than other difficulties, simply because these are so socially expected and nonstigmatizing.

It is not entirely clear how self-report questionnaires can be structured to build in ways of assessing the interpersonal functions of memory complaints or, indeed, whether it is even feasible to capture such realities via self-report. However, it would probably be useful to probe at least what elderly subjects have *done* relative to their self-perceptions of changed or deficient memory (e.g., talking to others, seeking professional help, using mnemonic or other self-help strategies, etc.). Collecting such data may require assessments via interview, rather than merely by self-report questionnaires. For example, rather than simply quantifying the degree of negativity of the response when structured questions are asked about memory, it may be important to differentiate whether complaints about memory are spontaneously generated by patients or presented in response to general clinical probes (e.g., What brings you here today?). This sort of dimension was part of the coding scheme for memory complaints used by Kahn et al. (1975).

Some skepticism and scrutiny are also needed regarding what we are actually measuring and labeling as "memory complaints" in the research literature.

Often, definitions and measurements of memory complaint have not limited the focal domain of behavior exclusively to either memory or complaining. A more neutral and descriptive phrase for the central variable in many studies would probably be something like "self-reports about cognitive functioning." It would help bring clarity to this area if the phrase *memory complaint* were reserved exclusively for proactively communicative sorts of complaining behavior, and some alternate terminology used in referring to the content of self-perceptions expressed in response to questions about memory (e.g., "opinions about memory"). A theoretical prediction would be that age differences will relate only to the self-perceptual aspects of self-reports about memory, not to an increase in complaining, whereas depression will likely be associated with both aspects.

Analogously, Sunderland et al. (1986) criticized researchers' failure to differentiate between the mere "awareness of memory decline and the perception of memory failures as a handicap" (p. 383). These investigators found that many older subjects perceived decline in their memory, but few felt this to be more than a slight nuisance. Thus, the functional importance or interference attributed to memory changes, as well as what actions the individual is compelled to take relative to the problem, may be keys to the significance of the reported difficulties. In another study, younger and older subjects were asked to judge the relative significance of various personal attributes vulnerable to age changes, including the prospect of experiencing impaired memory. Most subjects considered having a good memory to be only of intermediate significance—and less important than maintaining good sensory acuity, physical health, mobility, and family relationships (Niederehe & Yoder, 1989).

It may often be tricky to ascertain whether self-reports given in response to questions constitute help-seeking or other interpersonally motivated behavior, or have a sense of urgency attached, rather than representing merely the experimenter's elicitation of subjects' privately held opinions. This distinction may depend on the context within which the questionnaire or interview is administered. If it is clear to subjects that the data are being collected as part of an overall clinical assessment process, then even questionnaire responses may qualify as complaining communications in the sense described here. However, if the context is clearly a research one and subjects are simply normal volunteers, then this aspect of self-reporting may rarely occur, even in interview situations. Nonetheless, it may be essential to make these sorts of distinctions to advance toward a better understanding of memory complaints in older adults.

NEW DIRECTIONS
IN RESEARCH AND THEORY

On the whole, despite the past several decades of research, our understanding of memory complaints as clinical phenomena remains limited. We need to reevaluate our approach to the topic and consider possible new ways of conceptualizing and studying memory complaints. A primary observation is that the research has been too exclusively cognitive in orientation, and has over-emphasized the accuracy question to the neglect of other issues related to memory complaints that may be of equivalent clinical importance. Perhaps we automatically (but mistakenly) assume that issues of memory are wholly cognitive in nature. Or perhaps the field has been seduced by the assessment technology available in neuropsychology and cognitive psychology, and the apparent ease of quantifying memory performance in an "objective" and fine-grained manner. However, for most people self-perception does not seem to operate along logical lines or to yield percepts that fall into readily quantified categories; I suspect this is true with respect to self-perceptions about memory, as well as other personal attributes. Our research efforts aimed at understanding what is happening when older adults present memory complaints might benefit if more weight were given to certain other perspectives traditional in clinical psychology, which would lead toward focusing on somewhat different dimensions of self-perception than accuracy and factoring in other elements of the situation and the individual's life context. I have suggested, in particular, greater attention to complainers' affect, attitudes, self-concepts, and interpersonal relationships, and possible social functions of memory complaints.

REFERENCES

Abramson, L. Y., Seligman, M. E. P., & Teasdale, J. (1978). Learned helplessness in humans: Critique and reformulation. *Journal of Abnormal Psychology, 87*, 49–74.
American Psychiatric Association. (1994). *Diagnostic and statistical manual of mental disorders (4th ed.)*. Washington, DC: American Psychiatric Press.
Balint, M. (1964). *The doctor, his patient and the illness* (rev. ed.). New York: International Universities Press.
Barker, A., Prior, J., & Jones, R. (1995). Memory complaint in attenders at a self-referral memory clinic: The role of cognitive factors, affective symptoms and personality. *International Journal of Geriatric Psychiatry, 10*, 777–781.
Bassett, S. S., & Folstein, M. F. (1993). Memory complaint, memory performance, and psychiatric diagnosis: A community study. *Journal of Geriatric Psychiatry and Neurology, 6*, 105–111.
Berry, J. M., West, R. L., & Dennehey, D. M. (1989). Reliability and validity of the memory self-efficacy questionnaire (MSEQ). *Developmental Psychology, 25*, 701–713.
Bieman-Copland, S., & Charness, N. (1994). Memory knowledge and memory monitoring in adulthood. *Psychology and Aging, 9*, 287–302.
Bolla, K. I., Lindgren, K. N., Bonnacorsy, C., & Bleecker, M. L. (1991). Memory complaints in older adults. *Archives of Neurology, 48*, 61–64.
Bonime, W. (1966). The psychodynamics of neurotic depression. In S. Arieti (Ed.), *American handbook of psychiatry* (Vol. 3). New York: Basic Books.
Burt, D. B., Zembar, M. J., & Niederehe, G. (1995). Depression and memory impairment: A meta-analysis of the association, its pattern, and specificity. *Psychological Bulletin, 117*, 285–305.
Butler, R. N. (1963). The life review: An interpretation of reminiscence in the aged. *Psychiatry, 26*, 65–76.
Cavanaugh, J. C. (1989). I have this feeling about everyday memory aging ... *Educational Gerontology, 15*, 597–605.
Christensen, H. (1991). The validity of memory complaints by elderly people. *International Journal of Geriatric Psychiatry, 6*, 307–312.
Coyne, J. C. (1976). Toward an interactional description of depression. *Psychiatry, 39*, 28–40.

Cronbach, L. J. (1955). Processes affecting scores on "understanding of others" and "assumed similarity." *Psychological Bulletin, 52*, 177–193.

Crook, T., Bartus, R., Ferris, S., Whitehouse, P., Cohen, G., & Gershon, S. (1986). Age-associated memory impairment: Proposed diagnostic criteria and measures of clinical change—Report of a National Institute of Mental Health work group. *Developmental Neuropsychology, 2*, 261–276.

Dawe, B., Procter, A., & Philpot, M. (1992). Concepts of mild memory impairment in the elderly and their relationship to dementia: A review. *International Journal of Geriatric Psychiatry, 7*, 473–479.

Derouesne, C., Alperovitch, A., Arvay, N., Migeon, P., Moulin, F., Vollant, M., Rapin, J. R., & Le Poncin, M. (1989). Memory complaints in the elderly: A study of 367 community-dwelling individuals from 50 to 80 years old. *Archives of Gerontology and Geriatrics, 1*(Suppl. 1), 151–164.

Edison, J. D., & Adams, H. E. (1992). Depression, self-focus, and social interaction. *Journal of Psychopathology and Behavioral Assessment, 14*, 1–19.

Friedman, A. S. (1964). Minimal effects of severe depression on cognitive functioning. *Journal of Abnormal and Social Psychology, 69*, 237–243.

Gage, N. L., & Cronbach, L. J. (1955). Conceptual and methodological problems in interpersonal perception. *Psychological Review, 62*, 411–422.

Gilewski, M. J., & Zelinski, E. M. (1986). Questionnaire assessment of memory complaints. In L. W. Poon, T. Crook, K. L. Davis, C. Eisdorfer, B. J. Gurland, A. W. Kaszniak, & L. W. Thompson (Eds.), *Handbook for clinical memory assessment of older adults* (pp. 93–107). Washington, DC: American Psychological Association.

Grut, M., Jorm, A. F., Fratiglioni, L., Forsell, Y., Viitanen, M., & Winblad, B. (1993). Memory complaints of elderly people in a population survey: Variation according to dementia stage and depression. *Journal of the American Geriatrics Society, 41*, 1295–1300.

Hanninen, T., Reinikaiene, K. J., Helkala, E.-L., Koivisto, K., Mykkanen, L., Laakso, M., Pyorala, K., & Riekkinen, P. J. (1994). Subjective memory complaints and personality traits in normal elderly subjects. *Journal of the American Geriatrics Society, 42*, 1–4.

Hertzog, C., Hultsch, D. F., & Dixon, R. A. (1989). Evidence for the convergent validity of two self-report metamemory questionnaires. *Developmental Psychology, 25*, 687–700.

Kahn, R. L., Zarit, S. H., Hilbert, N. M., & Niederehe, G. (1975). Memory complaint and impairment in the aged: The effect of depression and altered brain function. *Archives of General Psychiatry, 32*, 1569–1573.

Kral, V. A. (1962). Senescent forgetfulness: Benign or malignant. *Canadian Medical Association Journal, 86*, 257–260.

Larrabee, G. J., West, R. L., & Crook, T. H. (1991). The association of memory complaint with computer-simulated everyday memory performance. *Journal of Clinical and Experimental Neuropsychology, 13*, 466–478.

Lewsinsohn, P. M., Mischel, W., Chaplin, W., & Barton, R. (1980). Social competence and depression: The role of illusionary self-perceptions? *Journal of Abnormal Psychology, 89*, 203–212.

Livingston, G., Hawkins, A., Graham, N., Blizard, B., & Mann, A. (1990). The Gospel Oak study: Prevalence rates of dementia, depression and activity limitation among elderly residents in inner London. *Psychological Medicine, 20*, 137–146.

Lowenthal, M. F., Berkman, P. L., & Associates. (1967). *Aging and mental disorder in San Francisco: A social psychiatric study*. San Francisco: Jossey-Bass.

McGlone, J., Gupta, S., Humphrey, C., Oppenheimer, S., Mirsen, T., & Evans, D. R. (1990). Screening for early dementia using memory complaints from patients and relatives. *Archives of Neurology, 47*, 1189–1193.

Niederehe, G. (1976). Self-appraisal of memory in depressions of later life. Doctoral dissertation, University of Chicago. *Dissertation Abstracts International, 37*(4-B), 1921.

Niederehe, G. (1986). Depression and memory impairment in the aged. In L. W. Poon, T. Crook, K. L. Davis, C. Eisdorfer, B. J. Gurland, A. W. Kaszniak, & L. W. Thompson (Eds.), *Handbook for clinical memory assessment of older adults* (pp. 226–237). Washington, DC: American Psychological Association.

Niederehe, G., & Yoder, C. (1989). Metamemory perceptions in depression of young and older adults. *Journal of Nervous and Mental Disease, 177*, 4–14.

O'Boyle, M., Amadeo, M., & Self, D. (1990). Cognitive complaints in elderly depressed and pseudo-demented patients. *Psychology and Aging*, 5, 467–468.

O'Brien, J. T., Beats, B., Hill, K., Howard, R., Sahakian, B., & Levy, R. (1992). Do subjective memory complaints precede dementia? A three-year follow-up of patients with supposed "benign senescent forgetfulness." *International Journal of Geriatric Psychiatry*, 7, 481–486.

O'Connor, D. W., Pollitt, P. A., Roth, M., Brook, P. B., & Reiss, B. B. (1990). Memory complaints and impairment in normal, depressed, and demented elderly persons identified in a community survey. *Archives of General Psychiatry*, 47, 224–227.

O'Hara, M. W., Hinrichs, J. V., Kohout, F. J., Wallace, R. B., & Lemke, J. H. (1986). Memory complaint and memory performance in the depressed elderly. *Psychology and Aging*, 1, 208–214.

Plotkin, D. A., Mintz, J., & Jarvik, L. F. (1985). Subjective memory complaints in geriatric depression. *American Journal of Psychiatry*, 142, 1103–1105.

Popkin, S. J., Gallagher, D., Thompson, L. W., & Moore, M. (1982). Memory complaint and performance in normal and depressed older adults. *Experimental Aging Research*, 8, 141–145.

Rabbitt, P., & Abson, V. (1990). "Lost and found": Some logical and methodological limitations of self-report questionnaires as tools to study cognitive ageing. *British Journal of Psychology*, 81, 1–16.

Scogin, F., & Bienas, J. L. (1988). A three-year follow-up of older adult participants in a memory-skills training program. *Psychology and Aging*, 3, 334–337.

Scogin, F., Storandt, M., & Lott, L. (1985). Memory skills training, memory complaints, and depression in older adults. *Journal of Gerontology*, 40, 562–568.

Sevush, S., & Leve, N. (1993). Denial of memory deficit in Alzheimer's disease. *American Journal of Psychiatry*, 150, 748–751.

Small, G. W., Komo, S., LaRue, A., Kaplan, A., & Mandelkern, M. A. (1995). Memory self-appraisal and cerebral glucose metabolism in age-associated memory impairment. *American Journal of Geriatric Psychiatry*, 3, 132–143.

Small, G. W., Okonek, A., Mandelkern, M. A., LaRue, A., Chang, L., Khonsary, A., Ropchan, J. R., & Blahd, W. H. (1994). Age-associated memory loss: Initial neuropsychological and cerebral metabolic findings of a longitudinal study. *International Psychogeriatrics*, 6, 23–44.

Smith, G. E., Petersen, R. C, Ivnik, R. J., Malec, J., & Tangalos, E. G. (1996). Subjective memory complaints, psychological distress, and longitudinal change in objective memory performance. *Psychology and Aging*, 11, 272–279.

Sunderland, A., Watts, K., Baddeley, A. D., & Harris, J. E. (1986). Subjective memory assessment and test performance in elderly adults. *Journal of Gerontology*, 41, 376–384.

Vermuelen, J., Aldenkamp, A. P., & Alpherts, W. C. (1993). Memory complaints in epilepsy: Correlations with cognitive performance and neuroticism. *Epilepsy Research*, 15(2), 157–170.

West, R. L., Boatwright, L. K., & Schleser, R. (1984). The link between memory performance, self-assessment, and affective status. *Experimental Aging Research*, 10, 197–200.

Wilder, D. E., Gurland, B. J., Chen, J., Lantigua, R. A., Killeffer, E. H. P., Katz, S., & Encarnacion, P. (1994). Interpreting subject and informant reports of function in screening for dementia. *International Journal of Geriatric Psychiatry*, 9, 887–896.

Williams, J. M., Little, M. M., Scates, S., & Blockman, N. (1987). Memory complaints and abilities among depressed older adults. *Journal of Consulting and Clinical Psychology*, 55, 595–598.

Zarit, S. H., Gallagher, D., & Kramer, N. (1981). Memory training in the community aged: Effects on depression, memory complaint and memory performance. *Educational Gerontology*, 6, 11–27.

Zelinski, E. M., & Gilewski, M. J. (1988). Assessment of memory complaints by rating scales and questionnaires. *Psychopharmacology Bulletin*, 24, 523–529.

Zonderman, A., Costa, P., & Kawas, C. (1989). Personality predicts complaints of benign memory loss. *Neurology*, 39(Suppl. 1), 194.

CHAPTER 19

Age-Related Cognitive Decline and the Dementia Threshold

Friedel M. Reischies

INTRODUCTION

There is unanimous evidence that increased age is associated with lower cognitive functioning. Almost everyone knows older persons who are slow and forgetful. The term *age-related cognitive decline* (ARCD) has been coined for this, but several other names are established (for diagnostic issues, see Blackford & La Rue, 1989). And because in old age the prevalence of dementia also increases steeply (Jorm, Korten, & Henderson, 1987; Wernicke & Reischies, 1994), it is tempting to speculate about an intimate, if not a causal, relationship between the two.

It has been proposed (Sourander & Sjörgren, 1970) that there is a heterogeneity in dementia of old age, one type being rapidly progressing dementia, dementia of the Alzheimer type (DAT) and a second, milder form, representing a special senile dementia.

The purpose of this chapter is to argue that a slowly progressing type of senile dementia can be explained by normal cognitive aging. There are some important consequences of the distinction between slowly and rapidly progressing senile dementia:

1. If one accepts only the rapidly progressing type as true dementia, the conventional diagnostic procedure will result in an overestimation of dementia prevalence in very old age. This would be the case because there are many slowly progressing dementia cases in old age.
2. The second consequence is discussed at the end of this chapter, namely, that the care of those slowly progressing dementia patients is prolonged, with significant economic consequences.

FRIEDEL M. REISCHIES • Psychiatric Clinic, Freie Universität, 14050, Berlin, Germany

Handbook of Aging and Mental Health: An Integrative Approach, edited by Jacob Lomranz. Plenum Press, New York, 1998.

In order to demonstrate that normal cognitive aging can result in a state that may be classified as a dementia syndrome, a close look should be taken at the conventional diagnostic procedure for dementia and especially the dementia threshold.

Because there are unspecific, age-related effects on test performance, arguments will be presented that the effect of a dementia disease is additive to unspecific, age-related cognitive deterioration. Therefore, an age correction of the threshold should be made for the diagnosis of dementia in case of an investigation without repeated measurement of the progression of the disease.

CONCEPTS OF DEMENTIA

First, the current types of dementia concepts will be set forth, including a brief description of some of their problems. The aim of this section, however, is not to justify preference for one or the other of these dementia concepts, but rather to clarify the impact of age-related cognitive decline on some of the dementia concepts.

Two main concepts of dementia are currently in use, namely, dementia as a clinical syndrome (with several definitions), and dementia as a dementia disease, of which many distinct entities are known.

Dementia Syndrome

A syndrome usually signifies the clinical finding of a common combination of symptoms or signs belonging to different physiological systems. Fever, for example, is manifested in high temperature but also in flush, palpitations, and sometimes—in subjects with a special disposition—seizures. It is possible to differentiate at least two forms of symptom co-occurrence: the symptom complex and the syndrome with an inherent interrelation of symptoms.

The *symptom complex* type of the concept dementia defines dementia by a number of unrelated symptoms often occurring together but not necessarily sharing a common pathophysiological mechanism. The criteria given by the American Psychiatric Association (DSM-III and -IV) are dementia syndrome definitions for the purpose of diagnosing dementia in a one-step investigation. Several cerebrovascular infarcts in a young man may produce a clinical picture of memory disturbance, slowness, some memory and naming difficulties, and impaired abstract thinking due to lesions of the specific areas of the brain. A similar picture can be found in Alzheimer's disease in the case of an old man with some slowing, which can be related to normal aging, and with difficulties in memory and naming, which are early manifestations of the specific dementia disease. Both individuals are diagnosed as suffering from a dementia syndrome, although quite different brain lesions underlie their clinical syndrome.

The dementia syndrome can also be defined in a more strict sense of the term *syndrome*. In this sense, a common pathophysiological mechanism should be at work to precipitate the various symptoms. This pathophysiological mechanism may be etiologically unspecific: It may function as the final common pathway in several different diseases. In the case of dementia, different levels of syndrome formation can be conceived of and will be described in the paragraphs below.

The first level of syndrome formation is related to the neighborhood of cortical areas with different functions. These lesions correspond to the usual neuropsychological syndromes that have long been observed in the investigation of localized brain injuries (e.g., Hécaen & Albert, 1978). Apraxia and aphasia are the examples for parietotemporal lobe syndromes, which may occur together because of a large parietotemporal lesion. It has been proposed that the usual sequence of clinical symptoms of Alzheimer's dementia can be explained by an enlarging area of degeneration starting from mediotemporal regions and proceeding to the temporal and parietal lobes (Braak & Braak, 1991).

A second pathophysiological level represents biochemical or metabolic subsystems (e.g., regarding the symptoms that appear if the physiological system of the transmitter acetylcholine is chemically or biologically impaired). Other pathophysiological factors may also be mentioned, such as disturbances at the cellular level (e.g., a disorder of dendritic plasticity at the neuronal level).

A third level of common pathophysiological factors for dementia syndrome is considered less often. A breakdown of cognitive performance can be expected if an individual suffers from failures in critical, indispensable cognitive functions. This happens because these functions are interrelated and dependent on each other, just as complex reasoning within a card game depends on working memory. Many intelligence tests require some working memory.

One problem is that if dementia syndrome is considered as a breakdown of a hierarchy of cognitive performances, this syndrome concept is applicable only for advanced and severe cases. Only in these cases is the impairment of basic cognitive functioning severe enough. Another problem with this kind of concept is that there are distinct mental functions that escape such a breakdown of function. The finding of largely intact reasoning functions in aphasic persons demonstrates this most clearly (e.g., Hécaen & Albert, 1978). Elementary motor functions, perceptual functions, and behavior control functions may be relatively intact even in a subject unable to understand a task or keep elements of an action in mind while performing the first part of a complex action.

Irrespective of the concepts with regard to the syndrome or symptom complex, there are conventional definitions of the dementia syndrome. Most include acquired chronic dysfunctions in multiple cognitive domains appearing in clear consciousness. Additionally, according to most criteria, memory should be included as one domain, and the severity of the symptoms should be such that everyday activities are impaired (DSM-IV, ICD-10).

Progressive Dementia Syndrome

Psychiatric diagnoses can be understood as constructs that are used because the etiology underlying the clinical signs is unknown or a common pathophysiology is not observable. A very common type of definition of psychiatric diseases is the combination of characteristics of the state and the time course of the symptoms. A longitudinal type of feature is included in the definition of the International Classification of Diseases (ICD-10): rapid progression, at least a decrease of functional level from a previously higher level. The progression should be more rapid than the age-related cognitive decline, either continuously or in a stepwise manner. Sometimes, however, a plateau of dementia progression occurs. Anamnesic information can clarify whether there was in fact a period of progression to a now stable cross-sectional dementia syndrome. But anamnesic information from the patient is not always reliable, and it is not always available from closely related persons (Henderson et al., 1994).

In most cases, the presentation of Alzheimer's disease comprises memory problems before other cognitive domains are affected (e.g., Almkvist & Bäckman, 1993); often a sequential occurrence of symptoms is part of the definition. Again, trustworthy anamnesic information for the identification of such a time course may be not readily available. An additional problem with this definition is that syndromes may be excluded in which the disease is presented primarily or exclusively as involving pronounced slowing or personality changes. Pick's disease, a lobar atrophy primarily involving the frontal lobe, is usually manifested not in memory deficits but in behavioral abnormalities and personality deviation.

Dementia Diseases

The second principal conception of dementia is a distinct brain disease ultimately leading to the dementia syndrome. Many diseases can cause a dementia syndrome; some authors have named over 60 nosological entities (Cummings, 1985). Not only primary brain diseases but extracerebral, general medical conditions such as metabolic disorders may also lead to a dementia syndrome, irreversible or reversible in its time course. With regard to specific therapies, of course, a dementia diagnosis that identifies the etiological or nosological type is preferable. But very often, the diagnosis of the disease cannot be clinically ascertained.

In most cases of a dementia syndrome, Alzheimer's disease or one of the vascular dementias (or a combination of both) are causes of the cognitive deterioration. But the *intra vitam* investigation is not conclusive with respect to the differential diagnosis. This would lead to a long list of possible diseases that cannot be decided upon in every individual dementia case—unacceptable in the clinical situation.

The age relationship differs for the various dementia diseases. As far as we know, to date, an early age peak of incidence exists for presenile genetic forms of DAT or possibly for forms of vascular dementia. In old age, the spectrum of diagnosed dementia etiologies seems to be more restricted to DAT, vascular dementia, and the many combined forms (Tomlinson, Blessed, & Roth, 1970). Therefore, age-related cognitive dementia is of relevance only in some of these dementia concepts. It is certainly irrelevant for presenile dementias, especially for the genetically determined forms of DAT that occur early.

THRESHOLDS

Diagnosis Threshold

Clinical Diagnosis.   The diagnosis threshold exists at both the clinical and neuropathological level (Kirkwood, 1994). At the clinical level, psychopathological or neuropsychological symptoms and brain-imaging findings represent continuous parameters.

Also, if one investigates the time course, a discrete dementing event in most cases does not occur: A development over time should be observed in the individual case (Berg et al., 1990) and a continuum of deterioration speed must be analyzed. Beginning from the individual's normal cognitive state, the deterioration progresses to the point of severe dementia and must be compared with the population norm with regard to the speed of age-related cognitive decline.

Therefore, a threshold is necessary for the application of the term *dementia*. In dementia research, much can be learned from arterial hypertension, in which blood pressure as a continuous variable must be analyzed in indicating caseness. These persons suffer from one of several pathophysiologically distinct diseases that may in the near future or after a latent period lead to serious consequences and death. In dementia, however, in contrast to hypertension, no single parameter, and accordingly, no single threshold is sufficient for the diagnosis of dementia.

If one looks at the conventional definitions of the dementia syndrome such as that of DSM-IV, several thresholds must be defined, one for each of the different domains included in the definition: a threshold for amnesia, aphasia, apraxia, and so on. There is no single distinctive feature for dementia for which only one threshold is needed. Otherwise, that one threshold could be looked for by a task force in order to solve all diagnostic problems. Dementia, like many psychiatric diseases, is a multiple-threshold diagnosis. ICD-10 in principle adds even one more: the threshold for the time course of deterioration. The critical speed of cognitive decline must be known in order to distinguish dementia from normal aging. The reason for this is shown in Figure 19–1.

Diagnostic Profiles and Biological Markers.   It has been stressed by several authors that there are not only quantitative differences between senile and presenile dementia but also qualitative differences as well. One example is the occurrence of apraxia and aphasia. Controversial data exist as to whether these tend to occur primarily in presenile dementia.

If biological markers for a disease are investigated, state and trait markers must first be differentiated. For most state and trait markers, a threshold must also be determined. On the one hand, biological markers can be found most probably only for specific dementia diseases. There is an intensive research for biological markers for DAT. On the other hand, even DAT is genetically heterogeneous. It is plausible that only state markers can be found for pathophysiologically common final pathways in the different forms of DAT, and possibly other dementia diseases. Some of the unspecific markers will indicate neuronal death, neuronal damage, and so on.

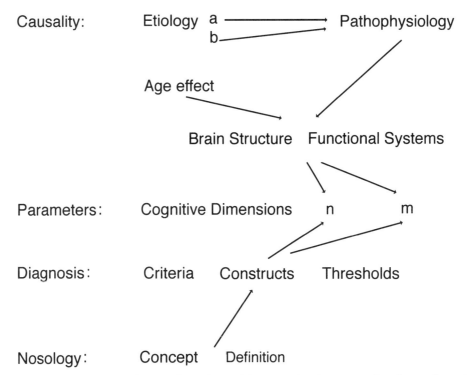

Figure 19–1. Etiology and pathophysiology of dementia (top) contrasted with nosological and diagnostic efforts (bottom) for clinical investigation. Several etiologies (a and b as examples) with possibly common pathophysiological steps precipitate cognitive symptoms by disturbing brain structure or function. Dementia concepts lead to constructs for which thresholds of cognitive dimensions (n and m as examples) must be found. Behavioral symptoms are excluded for reasons of simplicity. There may be an interaction between age-effect and dementia-pathophysiology.

The recent finding of a possibly relevant factor has received much attention, apolipoprotein E4 (APOE-4) (Geßner et al., 1997; Roses, 1995), which may be intimately involved in the pathophysiology of dementia. APOE-4 is a protein for fat metabolism. This finding confronts us with the problem as to what to do with a positive result in a subject who is not demented at that point in time. There is some uncertainty as to whether this person will in fact get the disease. Even in a homozygous case, we still need a diagnosis criterion for the clinical onset of the disease. Even if more potent trait markers are found in the future, clinical thresholds will still be necessary to determine onset of the disease.

For the reasons described earlier, the clinical dementia diagnosis threshold will most probably be of great importance in the future. This is true especially for indicating early treatment in dementia cases.

Neuropathological Diagnosis.   The neuropathologist also has criteria for diagnosing DAT, applying thresholds for counts of the nonspecific features of the disease, namely, senile plaques and neurofibrillary tangles. It has been shown that senile plaques—and to a lesser extent, neurofibrillary tangles—are also ubiquitously found in normal aging. In this case, an age-related correction of the threshold must be considered, as in the case of age-related cognitive decline. In this context, it should be mentioned that Mountjoy, Roth, Evans, and Evans (1983) found no difference in cell counts between very old demented patients and matched controls; and in simple dementia of the very old, no significant deficiency has been detected in the neurons of the *nucleus basalis* of Meynert, the source of cholinergic innervation (Tagliavini & Pilleri, 1983). The same pattern of results can be found in the cranial computer tomogram, that is, no difference between normal and demented persons over 90 years old (Reischies, Rossius, & Felsenberg, submitted). These empirical data point to problems in the diagnosis of dementia in very old age.

Threshold for the Impairment of Activities of Daily Living: The Dementia Case

The conventional definitions of dementia syndrome contain a case definition that requires sufficient severity of the syndrome in order to be labeled as a diagnostic category. Consequently, a person is diagnosed as demented only when cognitive difficulties reach such a level that everyday activities are impaired. In one sense, a threshold of the activities of daily living (ADL) belongs directly to the previous section. Impairment in the field of ADL is determined largely by cognitive deficits in dementia cases. The difference lies in the nature of the test, the objective, highly standardized test contrasting with the probe of everyday function.

This threshold is problematic for many reasons. The demands of individual, everyday activities are highly variable and adaptive, intraindividually and interindividually. Persons with mental retardation can live in the community at a very low IQ level (Edgerton, 1988). Furthermore, development is discontinuous at the point of job retirement or at the point an individual moves into a sheltered living situation. There is therefore a striking relation between age and demands of everyday activities.

The threshold for defining a dementia case by virtue of impairment in daily living is extremely difficult to determine with any precision. Age effects and the influence of social status and income, particularly the degree of adaptation to a surrounding, come into play. And professional help may be much more readily available for persons with high incomes.

In summary, several concepts exist for clinical diagnosis of dementia, each with its own purpose. Nosological concepts lead at the diagnostic level to the formulation of special thresholds. Age-related cognitive decline will affect these in general ways, to be considered next.

AGE-RELATED COGNITIVE
DECLINE AND DEMENTIA

Age-Related Cognitive Decline

Age-related cognitive decline cannot be described in detail in this chapter (for reviews, see, e.g., Crum, Anthony, Basset, & Folstein, 1993; Salthouse, 1991; Schaie, 1994). In short, practically all areas of cognitive function are impaired in old age to a greater or lesser extent. Unspecific, age-related cognitive decline can be found not only in intelligence and memory tests but also in tests designed to measure dementia effects, for example, the Mini-Mental State Test (Crum et al., 1993; Reischies & Lindenberger, 1996; Reischies, Schaub, & Schlattmann, 1996). Age-related cognitive decline has long been investigated in the perspective of the differential diagnosis of dementia (Dorken, 1958). The position has been generally held that differences between age-related cognitive decline and dementia indeed exist, and that dementia does not merely represent accelerated aging.

In the last few years, data have accumulated on the cognitive performance of very old subjects, over 90 years of age. These data have revealed that a marked decline of cognitive function takes place up to this age in nondemented subjects. Several investigators have stressed lowered speed functions as characteristic of normal old age (Salthouse, 1991). We were able to confirm this in a comparison of younger and older persons with high level of cognitive functioning (70–84 years vs. ⩾ 85 years; Reischies & Lindenberger, 1995). In the same study, however, it could be shown that those older persons with subnormal cognitive functioning differ from mildly demented subjects not in the dimension of speed but in the dimension of memory and, to a lesser extent, in verbal fluency. The demented subjects are not simply the ones who are even slower. Therefore, it can be assumed that the dimensions of change by age differ from the dimensions of change by dementia. Age effect and dementia effect on cognition can be differentiated. Some of the additional data on ARCD are discussed under the headings that follow.

Dementia Effect and Age Effect on Cognition: Additivity. Dementia diseases exert their effect on brain function and therefore on cognitive test performance. Age also affects cognition, but in a somewhat different pattern, as has been mentioned. In Figure 19–2, unspecific age effects on cognition are shown on input components (e.g., vision), output components (e.g., muscle force), or general speed of mental processes.

Age-related cognitive changes or processes of age-related cognitive decline are explained in several ways. First, an accumulation of unspecific lesioning is postulated; it affects the cell function of the brain and depends on the factor of time. This lesioning affects everyone, with possible variation due to individual disposition to certain factors. Second, there are time-related internal cellular processes that lead to cell death after a certain lifespan (e.g., programmed cell death). And a last group of factors involves nonbrain structures on which the

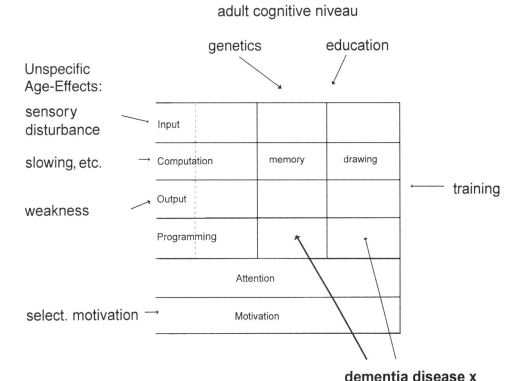

Figure 19–2. The cognitive system and different positive and negative additive factors. As examples, memory and drawing functions are shown with input, computational, output, and programming levels. Attention and motivational functions are mentioned here as examples of performance factors. The adult cognitive level is dependent, for example, on genetic and educational factors. The amount of training of the functions influences maintenance and also eventual decline. For nonspecific age effects, the examples are given of sensory loss, paresis, or weakness of muscles and general slowing. Selective motivational aspects for aging are important as well. The effect of one of the dementia diseases will be highest on memory: A cognitive dementia pattern results.

cognitive test performance relies (affecting the sensory system, e.g., the lens of the eye or muscular force, and so on).

If one accepts the distinction between dementia diseases and normal cognitive aging, then the additivity of both effects must be explained in the next step. An additional argument stems from unspecific plaque pathology in the brain, increasing with age, and the specific tangle pathology for Alzheimer dementia (Esiri, 1994), in which the plaque pathology of aging may be only one risk factor for the tangle pathology of Alzheimer's disease, explaining the age-related increase in incidence.

Diagnostic investigation in old-age psychiatry is interested in the amount of change in cognitive performance that can be attributed to the presumed dementia disease. The adult level of cognitive functioning and nonspecific, age-related cognitive decline must be taken into account first. A dementia threshold is passed if the adult cognitive level is diminished by age-related decline and dementia-related decline to such an extent that the present cognitive level is below a certain age-related limit; that is, the age-related decline results in an oblique threshold (see Figure 19–3).

This oblique, age-corrected dementia threshold is in contrast to models proposing that when a certain amount of degeneration in the brain has been reached, a clinical dementia syndrome would result, irrespective of the age of the person (Kirkwood, 1994).

A further aspect should be mentioned here. There may be nonadditive (multiplicative or even nonlinear) types of cognitive syndrome development. This can happen if an organic brain disease (or an intoxication) disturbs system

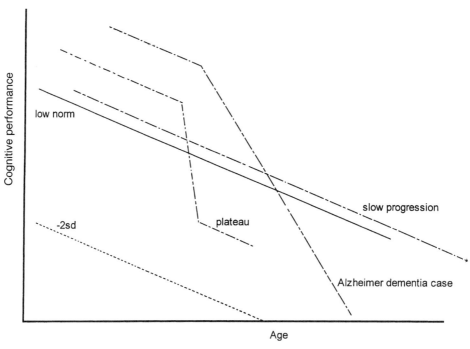

Figure 19–3. Age effect on performance in cognitive tests is considerable. From cross-sectional data a decline must be assumed of one to two standard deviations from 70 to approximately 100 years of age (compared to 70- to 74-year-old nondemented persons; Reischies et al., 1996), dependent on the cognitive demands of the test. Rapid progression syndrome will begin from the cognitive level determined by adult level and amount of unspecific age effect: An oblique threshold results. Subjects with a low adult cognitive level will not reach the threshold.

components, such as attention, that are central for cognitive functioning. A lesion of brain areas critical for attention is not the only cause of these symptoms. Often, rapid development of extensive cortical damage will result in temporary attention failures. In these cases, an impairment of consciousness is frequently observed, and an acute organic brain syndrome will be diagnosed. In such a case, the difference from extensive cortical failures in dementia lies in the time course. An assessment of rapid development of extensive cognitive deficit must include attentional symptoms and disorder of consciousness. In such cases, where the attentional system readapts and consciousness returns on a somewhat lower level, a dementia state has been reached.

Dementia Syndrome in Low Intelligence Persons with Age-Related Cognitive Decline

Age-related cognitive decline leads to an increasing percentage of persons with very low adult cognitive performance, who might be considered as suffering from a dementia syndrome if one does not accept the age-corrected threshold. These persons were always within the range of low IQ, but in old age, cognitive performance has declined considerably, not by virtue of a disease, but by virtue of normal aging. In the Berlin Aging Study (Baltes, Mayer, Helmchen, & Steinhagen-Thiessen, 1993), a long list of cognitive tests was compared to estimate the amount of cognitive decline. When the nondemented subjects in the age group 70–74 were compared to those of 95+ years, we found a decline of a magnitude of one to two standard deviations from the young sample (see Figure 19–3; Reischies & Lindenberger, 1996). Let us assume that an individual has an IQ of 85 during late adulthood (i.e., one standard deviation below the population mean). This individual will perform at the age of over 95 more than two standard deviations below the norms of most tests. For many clinicians, a mild dementia syndrome will be present. However, the definition of a progressive dementia syndrome, the strict criterion for accelerated decline according to ICD-10, will exclude this case as well as diagnosis under the assumption of an age-corrected threshold.

A few further comments should be made about this example. As indicated, the quantitative criterion of test performance might be met. What about everyday activities? We have stressed above that only a very approximate threshold can be established in this area. A very old person must often be cared for, and because of the multimorbidity of the oldest-old, it is very difficult to determine exactly to what extent somatic disturbances on one hand and mental deficiencies on the other determine the need for assistance. The investigator's subjective impression may be that the ADL threshold had been passed as well; the person is considered to be a dementia case.

The argument here is that many of the data on a mild form of DAT occurring in old age could be explained by the fact that within the sample, an admixture takes place of persons with DAT and persons suffering from low premorbid intelligence showing an age-related cognitive decline but no dementia disease. Thus, the difference from the Sourander position (Sourander et al., 1970) is that no special senile form of DAT must be postulated. If the focus is only on those individuals with progressive dementia syndrome, the inclusion of not-very-gifted individuals with a nonprogressive dementia syndrome and ARCD will also lead to an overestimation of the prevalence and incidence of dementia diseases.

The amount of overestimation of dementia diseases is difficult to estimate. The reason for this is that no firm assumptions can be made about mortality of subjects who perform between one and two standard deviations of cognitive functioning in late adulthood. These persons represent about 15% of the population. Subjects with slowly progressing dementia syndromes may, as we have seen, live for many years without exceeding normal age-related decline. Thus, the time during which these individuals require care will be even longer compared with rapidly progressing dementia cases. In this sense, these cases are even more relevant to economic aspects of the dementia syndrome and the burden that they pose to the caretaker within the family.

One statistical attempt to take into account covariates such as education, premorbid verbal intelligence, and depressive symptoms has been proposed by Jorm (1994). Had age been included in this kind of regression analysis, an age-correlated dementia parameter would result. In this case, only the amount of cognitive deficit that cannot be explained by age (or, additionally, adult intelligence level) would be scored for dementia detection.

Late Dementia Syndrome

The cognitive symptoms in dementia diseases are early symptoms of a general behavioral disorder. In most cases, other symptoms accrue later in the course of time. There will be loss of affective control, not only with crying spells but also outbursts of aggression. Patients run away partly because of spatial disorientation; at times, patients appear to suffer from extreme anxiety. The personality is profoundly changed. These syndromes have commonly been designated as "organic psychoses," because the subjects demonstrate dramatic alteration in their familiar pattern of experience and reaction, and also because they lose contact with reality. Paranoid ideas and hallucinations frequently compound the late dementia syndrome. Behavioral dementia symptoms and organic personality syndrome have been excluded from dementia criteria in DSM-IV. However, it must be borne in mind that diagnostic criteria are designed for early diagnosis, excluding all nonspecific symptoms. The additional features of a psychiatric disease that may only occur late in the course of time are omitted. Also omitted are symptoms that are not diagnostically specific but may even be life threatening and are very common.

In a subject with age-related cognitive decline and low adult intelligence, the cognitive state at the time of diagnosis might be at the level of mild dementia. The hypothesis is that in the distant future, late dementia syndrome will occur no more often than in the general population. If this turns out to be the case, it is a further argument that it may be appropriate to differentiate slowly and rapidly progressing dementia syndromes in nosological terms.

CONCLUSION

A distinction has been shown between the unspecific age effect and the effect of a dementia disease on cognition in old age. Those individuals of low adult intelligence who are 95 years and older are clinically regarded to have passed a conventional non-age-corrected dementia threshold by virtue of normal age-related cognitive decline. But these cases should not be considered to be demented in the sense of 70-year-old individuals with a typical 7-year development of dementia. We have shown that these low-IQ ARCD dementia subjects are diagnosed as demented following some of the dementia concepts and thresholds currently in use. This should be considered in the choice of dementia concepts for future research.

The distinction between slowly and rapidly progressing dementia syndromes in old age has considerable consequences in economic terms and with regard to the burden on the family providing patient care. The diagnostic distinction between the two progressing types can be achieved in principle by longitudinal follow-up investigations and, as has been shown here, by applying an age correction to the dementia threshold. Low premorbid IQ must be estimated with some precision, and the profile of the neuropsychological disorder can give hints as to the pathophysiology of the dementia syndrome.

The correction of cognitive dementia parameters for unspecific age effects and, in addition, for education (Crum et al., 1993; Jorm, 1994) and other variables will probably lead in the future to more precise descriptions of different dementia syndromes in very old age. And the validation of the different time course and outcome of the two progression types could contribute to the knowledge of the relation between normal aging and dementia processes.

REFERENCES

Almkvist, O., & Bäckman, L. (1993). Progression in Alzheimer's disease: Sequencing of neuropsychological decline. *International Journal of Geriatric Psychiatry, 8,* 755–763.

American Psychiatric Association. (1994). *Diagnostic and Statistical Manual of Mental Disorders* (4th ed.). Washington, DC: Author.

Baltes, P. B., Mayer, K. U., Helmchen, H., & Steinhagen-Thiessen, E. (1993). The Berlin Aging Study (BASE): Overview and design. *Ageing and Society, 13,* 483–515.

Berg, L., Coben, L. A., Smith, D. S., Morris, J. C., Miller, J. P., Rubin, E. H., & Storandt, M. (1990). Mild senile dementia of the Alzheimer type: 3. Longitudinal and cross-sectional assessment. *Annals of Neurology, 28,* 648–652.

Blackford, R. C., & La Rue, A. (1989). Criteria for diagnosing age-associated memory impairment: Proposed improvements from the field. *Developmental Neuropsychology, 5,* 295–306.

Braak, H., & Braak, E. (1991). Neuropathological staging of Alzheimer-related changes. *Acta Neuropathologica, 82,* 239–259.

Classification of Mental and Behavioural Disorders: ICD-10. (1994). Edinburgh, London, Melbourne, New York, Tokyo: World Health Organization/Churchill Livingstone.

Crum, R., Anthony, J. C., Bassett, S. S., & Folstein, M. F. (1993). Population-based norms for the Mini-Mental State Examination by age and educational level. *Journal of the American Medical Association*, *269*, 2386–2391.

Cummings, J. L. (1985). *Clinical neuropsychiatry*. Orlando, FL: Grune Stratton.

Dorken, H. (1958). Normal senescent decline and senile dementia: Their differentiation by psychological tests. *Medical Services Journal of Canada*, *14*, 18–23.

Edgerton, R. B. (1988). Aging in the community: A matter of choice. *American Journal of Mental Retardation*, *92*, 231–235.

Esiri, M. M. (1994). Dementia and normal aging: Neuropathology. In F. A. Huppert, C. Brayne, & D. W. O'Connor (Eds.), *Dementia and normal aging* (pp. 385–436). Cambridge, UK: Cambridge University Press.

Geßner, R., Reischies, F. M., Kage, A., Geiselmann, B., Borchelt, M., Steinhagen-Thiessen, E., & Köttgen, E. (1997). In an epidemiological sample the apolipoprotein E4 allele is associated with dementia and loss of memory only in the very old. *Neuroscience Letters*, *222*, 29–32.

Hécaen, H., & Albert, M. (1978). *Human neuropsychology*. New York: Wiley.

Henderson, A. S., Jorm, A. F., MacKinnon, A., Christensen, H., Scott, L. R., Korten, A. E., & Doyle, C. (1994). A survey of dementia in the Canberra population: Experience with ICD-10 and DSM-III-R criteria. *Psychological Medicine*, *24*, 473–482.

Jorm, A. F. (1994). A method for measuring dementia as a continuum in community survey. In F. A. Huppert, C. Brayne, & D. W. O'Connor (Eds.), *Dementia and normal aging* (pp. 244–253). Cambridge, UK: Cambridge University Press.

Jorm, A. F., Korten, A. E., & Henderson, A. S. (1987). The prevalence of dementia: A quantitative integration of the literature. *Acta Psychiatrica Scandinavica*, *76*, 465–479.

Kirkwood, T. L. B. (1994). How do risk factors for dementia relate to current theories on mechanisms of ageing. In F. A. Huppert, C. Brayne, & D. W. O'Connor (Eds.), *Dementia and normal aging* (pp. 230–243). Cambridge, UK: Cambridge University Press.

Mountjoy, C. Q., Roth, M., Evans, N. J. R., & Evans, H. M. (1983). Cortical neuron counts in normal elderly controls and demented patients. *Neurobiology of Aging*, *4*, 1–11.

Reischies, F. M., & Lindenberger, U. (1995). Discontinuity of dementia and age-related cognitive decline. In M. Bergener, J. C. Brocklehurst, & S. I. Finkel (Eds.), *Aging, health and healing* (pp. 204–211). New York: Springer.

Reischies, F. M. & Lindenberger, U. (1996). Grenzen und Potentiale kognitiver Leistungsfähigkeit im Alter. In K. V. Mayer & P. B. Baltes (Eds.), *Die Berliner Altersstudie* (pp. 351–377). Berlin: Akademie-Verlag.

Reischies, F. M. Rossius, W., & Felsenberg, D. (submitted). CT parameters of demented and non-demented subjects in a population-based sample of very old subjects.

Reischies, F. M., Schaub, R. T., Schlattmann, P. (1996). Normal ageing, impaired cognitive functioning and senile dementia—a mixture distribution analysis. *Psychological Medicine*, *26*, 785–790.

Salthouse, T. A. (1991). *Theoretical perspectives on cognitive aging*. Hillsdale, NJ: Erlbaum.

Schaie, K. W. (1994). The course of adult intellectual development. *American Psychologist*, *49*, 303–313.

Sourander, P., & Sjögren, H. (1970). The concept of Alzheimer's disease and its clinical implications. In G. E. W. Wolotenholme & M. O'Connor (Eds.), *Alzheimer's disease and related conditions*. London: J. A. Churchill.

Tagliavini, F., & Pilleri, G. (1983). Basal nucleus of Meynert: A neuropathological study in Alzheimer's disease, simple senile dementia, Pick's disease and Huntington's disease. *Neuroscience Letters*, *62*, 243–260.

Tomlinson, B. E., Blessed, G., & Roth, M. (1970). Observations on the brains of demented old people. *Journal of Neural Sciences*, *11*, 205–242.

Wernicke, T. F., & Reischies, F. M. (1994). Prevalence of dementia in old age—clinical diagnoses in subjects aged 95 years and over. *Neurology*, *44*, 250–253.

CHAPTER 20

Education and Dementia

A. D. Korczyn, Esther Kahana, and Robert P. Friedland

INTRODUCTION

The very high prevalence of Alzheimer's disease (AD) among the elderly is a cause of great concern. Unfortunately, there is still no unanimity concerning basic issues, going as far as even questioning whether AD is a single nosological entity. The clinical diagnosis entertains significance uncertainties (Korczyn, 1991), necessitating diagnostic criteria (American Psychiatric Association, 1995; McKhann et al., 1984). While these are of great importance in setting methodological unity, their validation against outside "gold standards" is difficult. The most commonly agreed upon criterion for validation of clinical criteria consists of a set of pathological changes that can be observed microscopically in the brains of deceased people (less frequently, biopsy material is available). These changes consist primarily of amyloid (senile) plaques (SP) and neurofibrillary tangles (NFT), although both can frequently be seen in other dementing diseases as well as in nondemented elderly people. Moreover, even among AD patients, there is only a poor correlation between the *degree* of dementia and the number of SP and NFT. It thus was suggested that SP are essentially tombstones, which result and accumulate during certain degenerative processes of the brain. Although obviously not all forms of brain degeneration lead to SP and NFT formation, there is at present no compelling reason to assume that the latter result from a highly specific process. Some data suggest that the cognitive decline in AD is more closely linked to loss of cortical synapses (Masliah, Miller, & Terry, 1993), although these changes are also not likely to be specific to AD.

A. D. Korczyn • Sieratzki Chair of Neurology, Sackler Faculty of Medicine, Tel Aviv Universit· 69978 Tel Aviv, Israel.   Esther Kahana • Department of Neurology, Barzilai Hospital, A kelon, Israel.   Robert P. Friedland • Department of Neurology, Case Western Reserve Ur sity, 10900 Euclid Avenue, Cleveland, Ohio 44106.

Handbook of Aging and Mental Health: An Integrative Approach, edited by Jacob Lomraɒ Press, New York, 1998.

Based on all these difficulties, it is conceivable that AD is not really a disease, with a single etiology and underlying process, but rather a syndrome, in the same sense that neither atherosclerosis nor cancer are unitary disorders. According to Kraepelin, Alois Alzheimer himself did not see his disease as a unitary process: "Alzheimer ... tended to regard the illness named after him not as a single disease, but rather as an "atypical" form of senile dementia, perhaps with a deviating spread of the disease process." In routine clinical practice, however, it is more appropriate to speak of dementia of the Alzheimer type (DAT) than of AD, and this is particularly so in epidemiological studies. Pathological comparisons with clinical diagnosis of DAT suggest that the latter are 80–90% accurate (Morris, McKeel, Fulling, Torak, & Berg, 1988).

CAUSES AND RISK FACTORS
OF ALZHEIMER'S DISEASE

All these uncertainties have not detracted from the formidable quest for the cause, or causes, of AD. A few conditions have been identified, some of which could conceivably be *risk factors*, while others could better be termed *risk indicators*. While risk factors are thought to be involved in triggering a cascade of events culminating as AD, risk indicators have a more tenuous relationship to the pathophysiological process and may be surrogates for the real causative factors.

Another important distinction should be made between factors that may trigger a disease, and factors that may accelerate its progression. Epidemiological field studies are the main tool in identifying risk factors as well as risk indicators, but they are rather poor tools in differentiating those factors associated with the initiation of a disease from those that accelerate the progression of the presymptomatic stage, since either will similarly alter prevalence rates. Nevertheless, factors that accelerate or slow down the progression of a disease may have a different effect if they act on the presymptomatic stage or the symptomatic phase. In AD, the presymptomatic phase is likely to extend for several years, possibly even decades in duration. While the frequency of causative or triggering factors will be higher among AD patients than among appropriate controls, this is not the case for factors associated *with the rate at which the disease progresses after it has started*. Factors that accelerate the disease process will be expected to have a *lower* frequency among AD patients than their true effect, since they tend to decrease survival. Of course, these same factors, when operating in the preclinical stage, may increase the incidence of the disease, so their net effect on the prevalence cannot be predicted. It is therefore important in epidemiological studies to examine not only the *prevalence* (i.e., the number of cases present in a population at one point in time), but also the *incidence* (i.e., the rate at which new cases occur in a defined population). The incidence figures can best indicate the existence of risk factors, while comparisons between prevalence and incidence may indicate factors that are responsible for changes in disease process.

The most significant risk factor for AD is age, although it is more useful to view age as a risk indicator, operating possibly through the deterioration in senescence of biological mechanisms (such as scavenging of free radicals). Other suggested risk factors are both genetic and environmental (e.g., traumatic brain injury).

In addition to risk factors, protective factors have also been proclaimed, including again genetic and environmental influences. The latter include smoking, presently the focus of much attention, as well as education and the use of estrogen replacement therapy (ERT) and nonsteroidal anti-inflammatory drugs (NSAIDs). Smoking, education, and use of ERT and NSAIDs are of great importance, since they may not only indicate disease processes but also suggest possible interventions to reduce the risk of developing AD. Nevertheless, the distinction between causative (or protective) factors and accelerating (or decelerating) processes was not specifically investigated for any of these factors.

The intriguing relationship of education to the development of AD is of particular interest. Several studies, conducted in both urban and rural communities on three continents, have supported this relationship (Kahana, Galper, & Korczyn, 1992; Katzman, 1993; Snowdon, Ostwald, & Kane, 1989). In other studies (Bear, Kokmen, Offord, & Kurland, 1992), the association between less education and the prevalence of dementia was not significant. It is remarkable that all these results were cross-sectional *prevalence* studies and, to date, there are no data on the influence of education (or lack of it) on the *incidence* of DAT.

THE ASHKELON STUDY

With these problems in mind, we attempted to determine demographic issues relating to AD in a well-defined population. The elderly population of Ashkelon is diverse in its genetic, cultural, and social background. The health facilities are readily available for everyone, thus allowing a substantial certainty about health care and data even prior to disease onset. Demographic data are available on the total population, and particularly regarding the elderly who benefit from the National Social Security old-age pensions. The size of the township is relatively small, allowing a home visit to each elderly subject. Finally, the population is cooperative, and refusal rate is extremely small. The first stage has dealt with data collection for prevalence study. The second stage, currently under way, attempts to verify incidence data as well as DNA samples for apoliproprotein E status. In the present chapter, mainly demographic data will be presented.

The prevalence study of DAT in Ashkelon, Israel, began in 1989. In that study, the total population over 75 years old, consisting of 1,720 people, was screened. Two evaluations were used, one based on an instrument developed by the Brookdale Institute in Jerusalem, the Brookdale Cognitive Screening Test (BCST; Davies, 1987), and the other consisted of a family evaluation. In the BCST, respondents had to answer simple questions, obtaining a maximum score of 26 points. The BCST was developed so as to be relatively independent of cultural influences. For example, it requires no knowledge of reading or writing. The *family evaluation* was supplied by the closest relative available or a caregiver and ranked the subject as (1) completely independent, requiring no assistance in everyday life; (2) having a mild memory loss, but still independent; (3) having more advanced memory difficulties and additional cognitive problems necessitating some assistance in activities of daily living; or (4) total dependence on others because of cognitive decline (Kahana et al., 1993). The latter two stages correspond to the definition of dementia in the DSM-IV. A high correlation existed between the two measures at each education level (Table 20–1).

EDUCATION AS A PROTECTIVE FACTOR AGAINST DEMENTIA

Previous studies of the relationship of education and AD have employed other instruments, such as the DSM-IV criteria for dementia (American Psychiatric Association, 1995) and the Mini-Mental State Examination (MMSE; Folstein, Folstein, & McHugh, 1995). These are similar to our criteria of family assessment and the BCST, respectively. One obvious criticism that has been leveled at these studies is that uneducated people are less likely to get the full score on neuropsychological tests (like the MMSE), thus artefactually increasing the prevalence rates of dementia in less educated subjects. For example, when we devised a Hebrew cognitive scale applicable to the Israeli population, we

Table 20–1. Correlation between Rates of Dementia by Clinical Evaluation and on BCST in Different Levels of Education and Gender

Level of education (years)	Percent with dementia		
	(A) Clinical evaluation	(B) BCST $\geqslant 9$	B/A
Male			
0	11.5	12.9	1.12
1–7	9.5	8.7	0.92
8–11	5.3	2.3	0.43
12+	3.7	0	0
Female			
0	18.4	25.2	1.37
1–7	9.1	10.6	1.16
8–11	8.0	6.8	0.85
12+	4.8	2.9	0.6
Total			
0	16.2	20.0	>9 1.23
1–7	9.3	9.4	>9 1.01
8–11	6.6	4.2	$\geqslant$10 1.64
12+	4.2	1.4	$\geqslant$11 0.33

found that scores decreased with age, and that subjects with higher education had consistently higher scores than those with lower number of years spent in school (Treves, Ragolski, Gelernter, & Korczyn, 1990). In order to correct for this education effect, a different cutoff score was used in the MMSE to indicate the existence of dementia, depending on the education level (Freidl et al., 1996). Obviously, this educational adjustment of the MMSE reduces the number of subjects assigned as demented. Whether—and to what extent—this corrects the assumed artifact is unknown. Neither has the cutoff score for each education level been validated. The BCST was designed as being "education free"; nevertheless, mean scores of people with fewer years of education are lower than those with higher education. In the Ashkelon study, we found that different cutoff scores of the BCST were required to optimally differentiate patients who were considered by their families to be cognitively intact (even if mildly forgetful) from those considered to be more severely affected, that is, demented (Table 20–2).

Although poor performance on cognitive tests may be expected from patients with fewer scholastic years, it is interesting that family assessment independently confirmed that poorly educated people had a higher frequency of dementia. As discussed later, education can delay the onset of dementia through several mechanisms. Nevertheless, it is prudent to stress that education may also serve as a surrogate (or risk indicator) for other factors, for example, socioeconomic level, diet, or drug use. People of low socioeconomic background are likely both to attain fewer years of education and to have had deficient nutrition during childhood. The latter is related to stunted cerebral growth (Morley & Lucas, 1994). The possibility that this may lead to lower intelligence has not yet been examined systematically and, for obvious reasons, is hard to study. One way to approach the question, however, is to look into the rate at which dementia develops in people of similar genetic and socioeconomic backgrounds who were separated at a young age and for whom life thereafter did not provide the same opportunities. For example, Jews who had fled Europe (e.g., to the United States) in the early part of the century could perhaps provide superior education to their children than was offered to their cousins who have remained in Europe or immigrated to Israel as refugees before or immediately after World War II. Comparing the incidence and prevalence of dementia between these two groups is now feasible and could throw more light into this issue.

Table 20–2. Distribution of BCST Scores in Persons Graded Clinically as Having Normal Cognition or Mild Forgetfulness, by Level of Education

Years of education	BCST scores (90% confidence limits)	Scores indicating dementia	Percent demented (BCST)	Percent demented (clinical evaluation)
0 ($n = 263$)	21.4–9.1	≤9	20.2	16.2
1–7 ($n = 260$)	24.4–11.5	≤12	16.5	9.3
8–11 ($n = 201$)	25.4–14.0	≤14	13.9	6.6
≥12 ($n = 142$)	25.7–16.9	≤17	10.8	4.2

SMOKING AS A PROTECTIVE
FACTOR AGAINST DEMENTIA

One confounding factor that should be discussed as being responsible for the correlation between education and dementia is smoking. Several studies have demonstrated an inverse relationship between smoking and the prevalence of AD (Brenner et al., 1993), and this was confirmed in our Ashkelon study (Table 20–3). In most developed countries, smoking is more frequent in lower socioeconomic classes. The higher prevalence of dementia among less educated groups is, therefore, the reverse of what would be expected. It is interesting to consider whether the differences in rates of dementia between highly and lowly educated groups would increase if the data were adjusted for smoking rates. Furthermore, the observed education effects might change if the control group did not contain subjects who have as yet preclinical AD. Morris and colleagues (1996) have recently shown that 9 out of 21 healthy subjects included as controls in a comprehensive prospective study of AD and studied postmortem had very high plaque densities in the neocortex. Thus, rather than relying on a single cognitive examination in epidemiological studies of dementia, it would be advantageous to separate those who have developed clinical DAT within a few years after prevalence day.

There are data suggesting that people belonging to higher social classes (usually those with more education), are more likely to have stopped smoking. Looking into early smoking might provide interesting information about the relationships among smoking, education, and DAT. If early, rather than late or lifetime smoking is the protective factor against future development of DAT, then it may in fact be demonstrated that education is a surrogate for early smoking. In order to test this hypothesis, early smoking, recent smoking, and education interactions with dementia should be explored. In Ashkelon, the protective effect of smoking and of education seemed to be independent (Table 20–4).

Other possible confounders are later-life factors, such as socioeconomic levels, income, profession, and hobbies (Friedland, 1993). Under normal circumstances, it is difficult to disentangle these from early education. However, given the special case of Holocaust survivors who have been exposed to extreme hardships in Europe during World War II, this may indeed be possible, since

Table 20–3. Frequency of Dementia and Smoking Status

		Percent with dementia	
		Clinical evaluation	BCST ≤ 9
Never smoked	1,160	7.2	12.4
Stopped smoking	200	3.0	5.6
Smoking	138	0.7	5.0

Table 20–4. Frequency of Dementia among Smokers and
Nonsmokers, Related to Education Level

Level of education (years)	Clinical evaluation		BCST ≤ 9	
	Smokers	Nonsmokers	Smokers	Nonsmokers
0	8.4	17.9	10.8	22.1
1–7	8.5	9.3	7.5	9.5
8–11	1.4	8.0	0	5.7
12+	1.5	5.4	0	2.0

these people did not always attain expected early education levels but may have nonetheless achieved appropriate socioeconomic status after the war.

As discussed earlier, available data on the relationship of education to dementia relate to prevalence rather than incidence. Since people of low socio-economic class have decreased survival (Greenwald, Pollisar, Borgatta, & Mc-Corkle, 1994), it is reasonable to assume that even higher discrepancy will be demonstrated if incidence, rather than prevalence rates, are compared for different rates of education (assuming that survival will in fact be different in demented people of different socioeconomic—and educational—levels). However, unexpectedly, Stern, Xi Tang, Denaro, and Mayeux (1995b) demonstrated diminished survival of demented people with higher education as compared to those with lower education. This observation has not been confirmed. In fact, in our Ashkelon study, preliminary data suggest that mortality is not related to educational grades (Table 20–5).

MECHANISMS RESPONSIBLE
FOR THE RELATIONSHIP
OF EDUCATION TO DEMENTIA

Although attempts are continuing to establish whether the protective effect of education is related to other factors (to which education is a surrogate), the possibility of a direct relationship should not be excluded. In this context, biological processes are important to consider. Several lines of evidence suggest that early environment influences brain development. A limited neonatal environment influences irreversibly the development of the visual system of kittens (Blakemore, 1991) and the same principle probably applies to humans as well. Critical periods exist for attainment of certain skills, such as vision, language, and musical aptitude. Although the exact changes occurring in the brain under these conditions are unknown, it is plausible that an enriched early environment acts through increasing the number of cortical synapses, thus creating a larger reserve. If, indeed, dementia results when a critical number of synapses remain (perhaps in a specific brain area such as the hippocampus), then enriching the environment (e.g., by early education) could provide the necessary reserve to

Table 20–5. Death Rate According to Educational
Levels and Presence of Dementia (Clinical Evaluation)

Level of education (years)	Persons with no dementia		Persons with dementia	
	N	Percent died, 1989–1995	N	Percent died, 1989–1995
0	438	(36.3)	54	(74.1)
1–7	430	(40.9)	20	(80.0)
8–11	324	(36.0)	10	(70.0)
≥12	210	(32.4)	3	(66.7)

delay the onset of dementia. It is therefore possible that education may create a reserve, which is reflected in delayed appearance of dementia. If this is so, greater pathology will be expected in more educated than in the less educated people for any given degree of dementia. Although pathological studies are not available relating to this issue, some support was lately advanced by Stern, Alexander, Prohovnik, and Mayeux (1992). In their study, the investigators measured the regional cerebral blood flow of AD patients and found the expected parietotemporal perfusion deficits. When matched for clinical severity of the dementia, greater deficits were observed in the more educated subjects. Furthermore, the enhanced neuronal activity provided by occupational and recreational mental activities, as well as education, is expected to increase cerebral blood flow, glucose metabolism, and favor molecular mechanisms leading to reduced amyloid beta protein production and aggregation (Friedland, 1993). It is not easy to distinguish between possible effects of education and later-life activities, since the two are highly interdependent. Nevertheless, recent studies have demonstrated that lifetime occupation is more strongly related to the risk of developing DAT than years of education, and that the two factors together had a still greater effects (Dartigues et al., 1992a, 1992b).

Although previous surveys studied the relationship of education to dementia of any cause, or specifically to DAT, it is important to find out whether patients with other types of dementia are similarly protected by early education or its several possible surrogates. Data on this point are meager. Education may also be protective against vascular dementia (perhaps the second most common cause of dementia) (Skoog, 1994).

CONCLUSIONS

This chapter deals with methodological issues relating to the epidemiology of DAT. Using published data, as well as our own, we have focused on the relationship of education to the future development of dementia. The limitations of data collection and of the interpretation of the results are discussed. Future studies should focus on incidence studies, since these are more likely to reflect the true relationship. Furthermore, other studies should be performed that are aimed to establish whether education may be a surrogate for other factors.

REFERENCES

American Psychiatric Association. (1987). *Diagnostic and statistical manual of mental disorders* (3rd ed., rev.). Washington, DC: Author.

American Psychiatric Association. (1994). *Diagnostic and statistical manual of mental disorders* (4th ed.). Washington, DC: Author.

Beard, C. M., Kokmen, E., Offord, K. P., & Kurland, L. T. (1992). Lack of association between Alzheimer's disease and education, occupation, marital status, or living arrangement. *Neurology*, *42*, 2063–2068.

Blakemore, C. (1991). Sensitive and vulnerable periods in the development of the visual system. *Ciba Foundation Symposium*, *156*, 129–147.

Bonaiuto, S., Rocca, W. A., Lippi, A., Giannandrea, E., Mele, M., Cavarzeran, F., & Amaducci, L. (1995). Education and occupation as risk factors for dementia: A population-based case-control study. *Neuroepidemiology*, *14*, 101–109.

Brayne, C., & Calloway, P. (1990). The association of education and socioeconomic status with the Mini-Mental State Examination and the clinical diagnosis of dementia in elderly people. *Age and Ageing*, *19*, 91–96.

Brenner, D. E., Kukull, W. A., van Belle, G., Bowen, J. D., McCormick, W. C., Teri, L., & Larson, E. B. (1993). Relationship between cigarette smoking and Alzheimer's disease in a population-based case-control study. *Neurology*, *43*, 293–300.

Dartigues, J. F., Gagnon, M., Mazaux, J. M., Barberger-Gateau, P., Commenges, D., Letenneur, L., & Orgogozo, J. M. (1992a). Occupation during life and memory performance in nondemented French elderly community residents. *Neurology*, *42*, 1697–1701.

Dartigues, J. F., Gagnon, M., Letenneur, L. Barberger-Gateau, P., Commenges, D., Evaldre, M., & Salamon, R. (1992b). Principal lifetime occupation and cognitive impairment in a French elderly cohort (Paquid). *American Journal of Epidemiology*, *135*, 981–988.

Davies, M. A. (1987). Epidemiology of senile dementia in Jerusalem: Design of a screening instrument for cognitive dysfunction in the elderly. *Brookdale Foundation Publications*, Jerusalem.

Fillenbaum, G. G., Hughes, D. C., Heyman, A., George, L. K., & Blazer, D. G. (1988). Relationship of health and demographic characteristics to Mini-Mental State Examination score among community residents. *Psychological Medicine*, *18*, 719–726.

Folstein, M. F., Folstein, S. E., & McHugh, P. R. (1975). Mini-mental state: A practical method for grading the mental state of patients for the clinician. *Journal of Psychiatric Research*, *12*, 189–198.

Fratiglioni, L. Grut, M., Forsell, Y., Viitanen, M., Grafstrom, M., Holmen, K., Ericsson, K., Backman, L., Ahlbom, A., & Winblad, B. (1991). Prevalence of Alzheimer's disease and other dementias in an elderly urban population: Relationship with age, sex and education. *Neurology*, *41*, 1886–1892.

Fratiglioni, L., Jorm, A. F., Grut, M., Viitanen, M., Holmen, K., Ahlbom, A., & Winblad, B. (1993). Predicting dementia from the Mini-Mental State Examination in an elderly population: The role of education. *Journal of Clinical Epidemiology*, *46*, 281–287.

Freidl, W., Schmidt, R., Stronegger, W. J., Irmler, A., Reinhart, B., & Koch, M. (1996). Mini-Mental State Examination: Influence of sociodemographic, environmental and behavioral factors and vascular risk factors. *Journal of Clinical Epidemiology*, *49*, 73–78.

Friedland, R. P. (1993). Epidemiology, education and the ecology of Alzheimer's disease. *Neurology*, *43*, 246–249.

Friedland, R. P. (1994). Epidemiology and neurobiology of the multiple determinants of Alzheimer's disease. *Neurobiology of Aging*, *15*, 239–241.

Greenwald, H. P., Polissar, N. L., Borgatta, E. F., & McCorkle, R. (1994). Detecting survival effects of socioeconomic status: Problems in the use of aggregate measures. *Journal of Clinical Epidemiology, 47,* 903–909.

Kahana, E., Galper, Y., & Korczyn, A. D. (1992). Dementia survey in the elderly in Ashkelon, Israel. *Gerontology, 56,* 19–25.

Katzman, R. (1976). The prevalence and malignancy of Alzheimer disease: A major killer. *Archive of Neurology, 33,* 217–218.

Katzman, R. (1993). Education and the prevalence of dementia and Alzheimer's disease. *Neurology, 43,* 13–20.

Korczyn, A. D. (1991). The clinical differential diagnosis of dementia: Concept and methodology. *Psychiatric Clinics of North America, 14,* 237–249.

Korczyn, A. D., Kahana, E., & Galper, Y. (1991). Epidemiology of dementia in Ashkelon, Israel. *Neuroepidemiology, 10,* 100.

Martyn, C. (1996). Blood pressure and dementia. *Lancet, 347,* 1130–1131.

Masliah, E., Miller, A., & Terry, R. D. (1993). The synaptic organization of the neocortex in Alzheimer's disease. *Medical Hypothesis, 41,* 334–340.

Morley, R., & Lucas, A. (1994). Influence of early diet on outcome in preterm infants. *Acta Paediatrica* (Suppl.), *405,* 123–126.

Morris, J. C., McKeel, D. W., Fulling, F., Torak, R. M., & Berg, L. (1988). Validation of clinical diagnostic criteria for Alzheimer's disease. *Annals of Neurology, 24,* 17–22.

Morris, J. C., Storandt, M., McKeel, D. W., Jr., Rubin, E. H., Price, J. L., Grant, E. A., & Berg, L. (1996). Cerebral amyloid deposition and diffuse plaques in "normal" aging. *Neurology, 46,* 707–719.

Nesse, R. M., & Williams, G. C. (1994). *Why we get sick: The new science of Darwinian medicine.* New York: Random House.

Plassman, B. L., Welsh, K. A., Helms, M., Brandt, J., Page, W. F., & Breitner, J. C. S. (1995). Intelligence and education as predictors of cognitive state in late life: A 50-year follow-up. *Neurology, 45,* 1446–1450.

Skoog, I. (1994). Risk factors for vascular dementia: A review. *Dementia, 5,* 137–144.

Skoog, I., Lernfelt, B., Landahl, S., Palmertz, B., Andreasson, L.-A., Nilsson, L., Persson, G., Oden, A., & Svanborg, A. (1996). Fifteen-year longitudinal study of blood pressure and dementia. *Lancet, 347,* 1141–1145.

Snowdon, D., Ostwald, S., & Kane, R. (1989). Education, survival and independence in elderly catholic sisters, 1936–88. *American Journal of Epidemiology, 130,* 999–1012.

Stern, Y., Alexander, G. E., Prohovnik, I., & Mayeux, R. (1992). Inverse relationship between education and parieto-temporal perfusion deficit in Alzheimer's disease. *Annals of Neurology, 32,* 371–375.

Stern, Y., Alexander, G. E., Prohovnik, I., Stricks, M. S., Link, L., Lennon, M. C., & Mayeux, R. (1995a). Relationship between lifetime occupation and parietal flow: Implications for a reserve against Alzheimer's disease pathology. *Neurology, 45,* 55–60.

Stern, Y., Gurland, B., Tatemichi, T. K., Tang, M. X., Wilder, D., & Mayeux, R. (1994). Influence of education and occupation on the incidence of Alzheimer's disease. *Journal of the American Medical Association, 271,* 1004–1010.

Stern, Y., Xi Tang, M., Denaro, J., & Mayeux, R. (1995b). Increased risk of mortality in Alzheimer's disease patients with more advanced educational and occupational attainment. *Annals of Neurology, 37,* 590–595.

Treves, T. A., Korczyn, A. D., Zilber, N., Kahana, E., Leibowitz, Y., Alter, M., & Schoenberg, B. S. (1986). Presenile dementia in Israel. *Archives of Neurology, 43,* 26–29.

Treves, T. A., Ragolski, M., Gelernter, I., & Korczyn, A. D. (1990). Evaluation of a Short Mental Test for the diagnosis of dementia. *Dementia, 1,* 102–108.

PART VII

Depression and Aging

In light of the tendency to view most mental health problems in old age as related to the different kinds of dementia, the question was asked, "Where have all the neuroses gone" in old age (Kral, 1990). While dementia constitutes a crucial issue, as reflected in Part VI, mental disorders in old age extend over a very wide spectrum, encompassing a great variety of disorders. In that spectrum, the affective disorders, mainly depression, constitute the majority. The National Institute of Health (Schneider, Reynolds, & Lebowitz, 1994) panel on depression noted the consequences of failure to diagnose and treat depression in elderly people adequately and described the grave consequences of severe strain, decreased happiness, costs, and reduced quality of living. The question is, how is depression best understood, diagnosed, and treated? The three chapters that follow deal with these questions.

While Katz (Chapter 21) cautions against overlooking social causes of depression in association with medical illness, the points of departure of his chapter are biological, and he basically presents an integrative conceptualization as he demonstrates how depression can play a pivotal role in secondary aging. The chapter sets forth the processes by which medical illnesses may accumulate as a correlate of increased aging and depression may result, among other factors, from disease-related changes in the brain and the cerebral environment. Katz provides conceptual orientations as he dwells on different biological mechanisms (specific and general) and explicates the implications of various structural brain diseases (atrophy, stroke, poststroke depression, subclinical and cerebrovascular disorders) and neural mechanisms. For instance, systemic illness can lead to the generation of peripheral signals that trigger neural and behavioral responses, which could either facilitate adaptation or cause depression, or the role of cytokines in central nervous system functioning and the adaptive quality of symptoms activated by cytokine in coping with acute illness. The author suggests focusing on the question of whether depressive symptoms are adaptive or maladaptive and considering pharmotherapy in that light. Katz also discusses the significance of multiple mechanisms and their implications for research. He illustrates how depression interacts with medical or neurological illness to modify the course of the disease and/or to amplify medical morbidity. He demonstrates this in the areas of disability, pain, drug side effects, malnutrition, health service use, and mortality, all indicating that the diagnosis and treatment of depression occurring in association with significant medical illness can have a major impact on patients' overall health. Regarding these areas, Katz indicates treatment approaches.

Katz provides knowledge of depression and medical–psychiatric comorbidity, which is crucial to understanding deterioration and disability in late life, in a manner that sheds light on the multiinteractive biopsychomedical modalities operating in these processes. He shows how interactions between medical illness and psychiatric symptoms are extensive, complex, and bidirectional, and that secondary aging is an interrelated medical, physical, and social phenomenon. This chapter integrates research findings, spans perspectives, suggests possible hypotheses, and future research directions.

The present conspicuous variability and diversity of depression in old age poses theoretical, methodological, clinical, and research problems. This variability clearly indicates the urgent need for an appropriate theoretical framework and its methodological derivative to comprehend, measure, and treat depression in old age. Meador and Blazer (Chapter 22) propose a narrative approach as an integrative concept to address these problems. Their review reveals that the variability of depression is pronounced in the realm of descriptive and diagnostic contradictory findings as found in the research on clinical, generational, and epidemiological, as well as interracial, differences in depression. Sociocultural particularity and contextual contents have also not been adequately considered (see Silver, Chapter 17). The authors further emphasize bereavement, physical frailty, and illness (see Katz, Chapter 21) as major contributing factors to the variability of depression and expose the limitations of reductionistically categorical models of depression in old age. Meador and Blazer claim that the different diagnostic tools in use are not differential or sensitive enough and do not seem to provide reliable measures of depression. They stress the need for an operational construct that provides a fluid yet substantive structure, along with diagnostic and clinical utility, while retaining a contextual and historical integrity that accommodates the heterogeneity of aging and facilitates adequate formulations of depression within the life course. The authors contest the idea that the multiple biopsychosocial dimensions, framed in a contextually and historically based narrative, constitute the central medium through which to comprehend the manifestations of depression in old age. A narrative construct (see Cohler, Chapter 11), they maintain, allows examination of personal, contextual, and historical contingencies enabling creativity and alternatives of adaptation. They place a particular emphasis on the communality inherent in a narrative, how "stories implicate knowledge," and that the "acceptability" of stories carries an underlying component of belonging to a community. Meador and Blazer convincingly proffer their specific version of a narrative model, embodied in biopsychosocial considerations, as containing psychodiagnostic and psychotherapeutic qualities while maintaining the diversity and variability of depression.

While depression serves as a "test case" premise on which Mostofsky (Chapter 23) attempts to integrate behavioral medicine and clinical gerontology, this chapter basically argues for an epistemological shift in the area of mental health in general and, specifically, that of mental health in old age. This chapter contains a wealth of ideas and conceptual differentiations (e.g., between "disorders," "diseases," "deficit," "dysregulation," "illness," and "sickness"). Mostofsky explicates how scientific approaches to clinical concepts are not holistic but fractionated, and argues for alternative, nonlinear models. He attempts to apply the approach of behavioral medicine to mental health in gerontology. His perspective is based on a model that formulates a triaxial distinction between the factors of disease, illness, and predicament, or their equivalents labeled as structure, function, and contextual systems. The model conceptualizes the separate dimensions of sickness (e.g., disease as a structure and illness as a function) and is in many ways a unique model conceptualizing mind–body relationships. The multidimensional elements of a sickness have different meanings when one considers them in light of the different triaxial dimensions. The axes themselves are interactive and relational. Mostofsky attempts to invest the biopsychosocial concept with new meaning as he views it in a differential perspective and in behavioral and functional terms. Thus, his multidimensional model, while integrative, allows for specificity, as in comprehending the treatment of depression (see Gatz and Katz, Chapters 4 and 21, respectively). It spans a variety of disciplines and addresses questions that range from the micromolecular properties of an organic entity to psychological and social forces that affect the course and severity of a disorder and engage the community, social agencies, and governmental policies—all of which have serious bearing on the status of the individual's health. Mostofsky maintains that aging and the nature of disorders are behavioral, and that pathology must not necessarily be understood in terms of impairments and deficits but can be comprehended as functional, enhancing survival (as in mourning), resiliency, and even promoting growth (see Ryff et al., Chapter 3). Treatment interventions should not be geared toward what we term *disease* conditions but should operate in the realm of salutary. This chapter elaborates the inherent interdisciplinary approach to mental disorders and presents new avenues by which to address mental health and aging. We should heed the implications of this chapter as relevant to theoretical formulations, clinical methodology, training, and policymaking.

REFERENCES

Kral, V. (1990). Where have all the neuroses gone? *Clinical Gerontologist, 31*, 10–18.
Schneider, L., Reynolds, C., & Lebowitz, B. (1994). *Diagnosis and treatment of depression in late life: Results of the NIH consensus development conference.* Washington, DC, American Psychiatric Press.

CHAPTER 21

Depression as a Pivotal Component in Secondary Aging

Opportunities for Research, Treatment, and Prevention

IRA R. KATZ

INTRODUCTION

There is increasing evidence that depression, together with related affective and behavior symptoms, can play a pivotal role in secondary aging, the process by which medical illnesses accumulate as a correlate of increasing age. In addition to mechanisms by which it can result from psychological mechanisms associated with the stress and losses of function associated with medical illness, depression can result from disease-related changes in the brain and the cerebral environment. Moreover, once depression occurs, it can affect the course of associated medical illness, amplifying distress, disability, morbidity, and, possibly, mortality. Thus, knowledge of depression and of medical–psychiatric comorbidity in late life can be critical to understanding the downward spiral of deterioration and disability that is frequent in late life.

From among the chapters in this volume, this may be the one that speaks most narrowly about the mental disorders of late life from a biomedical perspective. The research that I, together with an extraordinary group of colleagues including M. Powell Lawton and Patricia Parmelee, have been conducting since the mid-1980s has examined the legitimacy of this perspective. We studied depression as it occurs among a population of very old individuals who reside in a residential care facility, usually because their needs exceed their abilities

IRA R. KATZ • Department of Psychiatry, University of Pennsylvania, Philadelphia, Pennsylvania 19104.

Handbook of Aging and Mental Health: An Integrative Approach, edited by Jacob Lomranz. Plenum Press, New York, 1998.

and those of their families to keep them in the community. In this context, depression might be an understandable reaction to the indignities, stresses, and losses of institutional life and the diseases that made it necessary; it might be reasonable to view it as an existential response rather than a clinical condition. However, we have argued (Katz & Parmelee, 1994) that depression should be viewed as a clinical syndrome, even in the residential care facility, because it is persistent, associated with increased medical morbidity, and, specifically, responsive to active treatment. Our finding that elderly residential care patients respond to treatment with antidepressant medication but not to placebo (under double-blind conditions) implies that major depression is a (treatable) clinical disorder, and not an existential state, even when it occurs among the frail elderly.

Because the basic assumptions underlying the work outlined here are, in many ways, distinct from those of other manuscripts, it is important to emphasize the similarities. Underlying this work and most of the current research and clinical literature on late-life depression is an optimistic view of the process of aging. We focus on depression as a significant complication of the chronic, disabling medical illnesses that are common in late life, because there is strong evidence that, in its absence, older people have an impressive ability to adapt and compensate for the effects of disease and disability. Moreover, it is important to note that the focus of the research in this chapter is the vulnerable elderly, those with significant, chronic physical illness. In this, we distinguish between the identification of a subgroup of older individuals who are vulnerable to depression and a more general concern for the elderly as a vulnerable group. The weight of the evidence from epidemiological research suggests that, at present, the aged as a group are not more vulnerable to major depression than younger adults; in fact, the cohort that constitutes the current generation of older individuals may be less vulnerable to major depression (though not to less severe but nonetheless clinically significant depressive symptoms) than the generations that follow. Finally, although there is considerable controversy about the extent to which the symptoms of major depression differ across the lifespan, it is interesting to reflect upon the literature suggesting that cognitive and ideational symptoms such as guilt and self-reproach may be less common in late life, while somatic symptoms may be more common. From the perspective of the elderly self that is discussed extensively in this volume, this possible difference in symptoms translates into questions about the extent to which late-life depression is a disease of the self, versus one that, like other illnesses, is experienced by the (more or less intact) self. Further studies of late-life depression from the perspective of the self could lead to advances in both theory and clinical care.

MEDICAL ILLNESS
AND THE CAUSES OF DEPRESSION

Classic studies of depression in older patients, such as those of Stenstedt (1959), Hopkinson (1964), and Mendlewicz (1976), suggest that the pathogenesis of depression differs between those older patients with the initial onset of illness in young adulthood and those for whom it arises *de novo* in late life. Most basically, they suggest that early-onset depressions occur in the context of genetic mechanisms and an excess of mood disorders among first-degree relatives, while those with late onset occur more frequently in the context of chronic medical illness. This generalization has been questioned by research that has not replicated an excess of medical illness in late-onset depressives (Lyness, Conwell, King, et al., 1995), and by the finding that depression in Alzheimer's disease appears to occur primarily among those with positive family histories (Pearlson, Ross, Lohr, et al., 1990). Nevertheless, the weight of the evidence supports the conclusion of the NIH Consensus Statement on the Diagnosis and Treatment of Late-Life Depression (Office of the Medical Applications of Research, 1992) that the hallmark of depression in older people is its comorbidity with medical illness. Therefore, it is reasonable to look at psychiatric medical comorbidity for clues regarding the etiology and pathogenesis of depression in the elderly.

Empirical searches for correlations between depression and specific disorders have identified associations between major depression and frequent/severe headaches, skin infections, respiratory illness, ulcers, hypotension, and diabetes (Moldin, Scheftner, Rice, et al., 1993). However, because multiple paths are involved, understanding of mechanisms is likely to require a more conceptual orientation. General psychosocial factors related to illness that should be considered include self-care disability, impairment of role performance, pain and other distressing symptoms, and reactions to loss, real or symbolic. Biological mechanisms can be divided into those that are specific, occurring in certain diseases or related to certain medications, and those that are more general. Examples of specific mechanisms are those associated with thyroid disease and medications such as reserpine. More recent examples include the relationship between decreased cerebrospinal fluid (CSF) 5-hydroxyindole acetic acid and depression in patients with Parkinson's disease (Mayeux, Stern, & Sano, 1988), presumably as a result of the degeneration of brain-stem serotonergic nuclei, and that between cytopathological lesions of brain-stem aminergic nuclei and major depression occurring in association with Alzheimer's disease (Forstl, Burns, Luthert, et al., 1992; Zubenko & Moossy, 1988; Zweig, Ross, Hedreen, et al., 1988). General mechanisms include those associated with pathology of brain structure and those that follow from disease-related disturbances of the cerebral environment; they may integrate the interacting effects of a number of the common chronic illnesses of late life and could be responsible for significant components of the depressions that occur in association with medical illness in the elderly.

Structural Brain Disease

Current evidence from neuroimaging research suggests that depression may be related to two distinct classes of brain abnormalities: atrophy and clinical–subclinical cerebrovascular disease (Krishnan & Gaddle, 1996).

Atrophy.   As noted earlier, there is evidence suggesting that those depressions occurring in association with both parkinsonism and Alzheimer's disease are associated with pathology of brain-stem aminergic nuclei. At present, it is possible to hypothesize that it arises when disease-related neurodegenerative processes significantly affect monoaminergic systems. It may also be reasonable to ask whether some cases of primary depression arise from isolated neurodegeneration in relevant systems. There are a growing number of computed tomography (CT; e.g., Alexopoulos, Young, & Schindledecker, 1992; Dolan, Calloway, & Mann, 1985; Jacoby, Dolan, Baldy, et al., 1983; Pearlson, Rabins, & Burns, 1991; Pearlson, Rabins, Kim, et al., 1989; Rossi, Stratta, Petruzzi, et al., 1987; Shima, Shikano, Kitamura, et al., 1984) or magnetic resonance imaging (MRI; e.g., Coffey, Wilkinson, Weiner, et al., 1993; Krishnan, McDonald, Escalona, et al., 1992; Rabins, Pearlson, Aylward, et al., 1991; Zubenko, Sullivan, Nelson, et al., 1990) studies demonstrating that atrophy (global or regional) can be observed in patients with major depression (compared to age-matched normals). These findings suggest the importance of a new look at the neuropathology of late-life depression, first to characterize the processes related to the observed atrophy, and then to probe their etiology.

Stroke and Subclinical Cerebrovascular Disease.   Following the pioneering work of Robinson and co-workers, poststroke depression has been intensively investigated. The foundation for subsequent clinical research was a series of studies on experimental cerebral infarction in laboratory animals, which demonstrated that lesions in the distribution of the middle cerebral artery led to profound and widespread depletions of norepinephrine that were associated with behavioral changes (Robinson, 1979; Robinson & Coyle, 1980; Robinson, Schoemaker, & Schlumpf, 1980; Robinson, Schoemaker, Schlumpf, et al., 1975). Together with aminergic theories of the pathogenesis of depression, they suggested a neurochemical model for the pathogenesis of poststroke depression in man. Subsequent clinical studies by Robinson and colleagues demonstrated that poststroke depression was more closely associated with the location of lesions than with the degree of the resulting disability, suggesting that biological mechanisms were operative. More specifically, the finding that depression occurred most often in lesions of the (left) frontal pole was consistent with a model in which affective symptoms arose from disruptions of ascending aminergic fibers on their path to the cortex (Starkstein & Robinson, 1989). Although the extent to which depression is associated with the anatomic localization of cerebral infarctions has been questioned (e.g., Schwartz, Speed, Brunberg, et al., 1993), the key elements of the biological hypotheses may be neurochemical, not anatomic. There are, in fact, data linking poststroke depression with changes in serotonergic systems (Bryer, Starkstein, Votypka, et al., 1992, Mayberg, Robinson, Wong, et al., 1988), but more research in this area, perhaps including the use of pharmacological probes, will be necessary to clarify mechanisms.

Post-stroke depression may serve as a model for a general mechanism that may be more widely operative. Following observations by Krishnan, Goli, Ellinwood, et al. (1988) and Coffey, Figiel, Djang, et al. (1988), a number of investigators (e.g., Coffey, Figiel, & Djang, 1990; Figiel, Krishnan, Doraiswamy, et al., 1991; Fujikawa, Yamawaki, & Touhouda, 1993; Zubenko et al., 1990) have confirmed that patients with late-life depression, especially those with late onset, have greater rates of subcortical and deep white-matter hyperintensities apparent on MRI scans than controls. Studies in elderly medical populations demonstrated that these lesions are associated with risk factors for cerebrovascular disease, including hypertension, diabetes, cardiac disease, and extracerebral carotid artery diseases (Fazekas, Niederkorn, Schmidt, et al., 1988). The histology of the lesions associated with depression is consistent with subclinical cerebrovascular disease or a form of "leukoencephalopathy." Further evidence supporting this hypothesis comes from a study by Miller, Kumar, Yousem, et al. (1994), who found a relative absence of high-intensity signals among those (rather rare) late-life depressives without cerebrovascular risk factors.

These MRI findings may serve as a marker for processes that underlie the increased rates of depression that occur in association with a number of the common medical disorders of the elderly, including hypertension, atherosclerosis, diabetes, and heart diseases of various types. It is important to determine whether depressions with and without high-intensity signals differ in clinical features, natural history, and treatment response, and to investigate the association between white-matter hyperintensities, depression, and subclinical affective symptoms in nonpsychiatric medical populations. Krishnan (1993) has discussed a number of possible neural mechanisms that may underlie the associations of depression with subcortical and deep white-matter hyperintensities and depression. From our perspective, however, the mechanistic questions that are of the greatest interest may be about how these biological lesions (as well as those resulting from neurodegeneration) are transduced or mapped into psychological or behavioral symptoms. One model, related to stress–diathesis theories, could be based upon the hypothesis that cerebral lesions decrease stress tolerance and increase the vulnerability of the individual to experience depression as a consequence of psychosocial or biological stress. Thus, this model predicts that depression should occur as a result of interactions between cerebral lesions and stressful events. Another model, perhaps related to depletion theories, could be based upon the hypothesis that biological lesions cause depression through their effects on the ascending aminergic neural systems that underlie pleasure, motivation, and reinforcement. This model predicts that anhedonia and/or apathy should occur in association with cerebral lesions, either as prodromes for depression or as independent disorders.

Disease-Related Effects on the Cerebral Environment

The hypotheses that depression could result from disturbances of the cerebral environment related to physical illness originated in the 1970s with studies of the regulation of the metabolism of biogenic amine neurotransmitters. Models linking serotonin synthesis to plasma levels of tryptophan and other amino acids suggested that medical illness, subnutrition, tissue injury, muscle wasting, and major changes in physical activity could lead to psychiatric symptoms by affecting plasma levels of amino acids. In addition, studies in our laboratory (Katz, 1982; Katz, Friedman, Parmelee, et al., 1989; Katz, Jain, Muhly, et al., 1985) led to the suggestion that physiological abnormalities associated with secondary aging could lead to mild cerebral hypoxia, and that decreased availability of oxygen and tyrosine or tryptophan (as substrates for the oxygen-requiring enzymes tyrosine and tryptophan hydroxylase in aminergic nerve terminals) could lead to decreased synthesis of monoaminergic neurotransmitters and associated behavioral effects. The behavioral effects of decreased amino acid levels or mild hypoxia (at a level that could affect neurotransmitter synthesis but not energy metabolism) represented a mechanism that could lead to adaptive responses to illness; depression, however, could occur when this homeostatic mechanism went awry. Whether or not these hypotheses were plausible, there was (and remains) little evidence suggesting that they are correct. However, there may be value to the basic idea that systemic illness can lead to the generation of peripheral signals that trigger neural and behavioral responses that can either facilitate adaptation or cause depression. Further research on the central-nervous-system effects of the cytokines that are involved in the regulation of inflammatory processes and immune function is necessary.

Hart (1988), speaking from experience in veterinary practice and research, wrote of the "biological basis of the behavior of sick animals" and stated,

> The most commonly recognized behavioral patterns of animals and people at the onset of febrile infectious diseases are lethargy, depression, anorexia, and reduction in grooming... The behavior of sick animals and people is not a maladaptive response or the effect of debilitation, but rather an organized, evolved behavioral strategy to facilitate the role of fever in combating viral and bacterial infections. The sick individual is viewed as being at a life or death juncture and its behavior is an all-out effort to overcome the disease. (p. 123)

Dantzer and Kelley (1989) noted the similarities between the effects of central or peripheral administration of proinflammatory cytokines and nonspecific symptoms of sickness (sickness behavior) including malaise, decreased social investigation, decreased food and water intake, weight loss, and sleep changes, as well as fever.

There has been considerable interest in the roles of cytokines in the central nervous system (e.g., Plata-Salaman, 1991b); functions being investigated include those related to brain development, neuroregulation, pathological mechanisms in cerebral disease, and the mediation of the central effects of systemic disease that is the focus here. Interleukin-1b, a cytokine secreted primarily by activated macrophages but also by other cells, has central effects when administered intracerebroventricularly in nanogram concentrations and after intravenous or intraperitoneal administration at higher (microgram) levels. Central effects of Il-1b include stimulation of corticotropin-releasing factor (CRF) release (Berkenbosch, van Oers, del Ray, et al., 1987; Sapolsky, Rivier, Yamamoto, et al., 1987); this may be part of a negative feedback system in which leukocyte products such as Il-1b lead to increased cortisol production that can moderate inflammation and immune activity. Other central effects demonstrated in laboratory animals include increases in sleep (Krueger, Walter, Dinarello, et al., 1984), decreased food intake (Plata-Salaman, 1988) and food-motivated behavior (Crestani, Suguy, & Dantzer, 1991), decreased locomotor activity (Dunn, Antoon, & Chapman, 1991), decreased social exploration (Crestani et al., 1991), and, most interesting in this context, effects on behavioral despair, a model for depression (del Cerro & Borrell, 1990). As might be expected from its behavioral effects, II-1b has significant effects on biogenic amines. *In vivo*, there are increases in norepinephrine release or turnover after intracerebroventricular (ICV) (Shintani, Kanba, Nakaki, et al., 1993), intracerebral (IC) (Terao, Oikawa, & Saito, 1993) or intraperitoneal (IP) (Dunn, 1992; Mohankumar & Quadri, 1993) administration, and increases in serotonin release or turnover after ICV (Gemma, Ghezzi, & De Simoni, 1991), IC (Mohankumar, Thyagarajan, & Quadri, 1993; Shintani et al., 1993), and IP (Dunn, 1992) administration. Observed effects on dopaminergic systems have been more variable (Dunn, 1992; Mohankumar, Thyagarajan, & Quadri, 1991, Shintani et al., 1993). II-1b may also play a physiological role in mediating the effects of bacterial endotoxin and lipopolysaccharide (Bluthe, Dantzer, & Kelley, 1992; van Dam, Brouns, Louisse, et al., 1992) as well as those of tumor necrosis factor (Bluthe, Dantzer, & Kelley, 1991).

Although the principle that cytokines can have behavioral effects has been well established, many questions remain about how they are involved in the central effects of systemic illness. While, in general, cytokines cannot cross the blood–brain barrier, they may gain access to the central nervous system though specialized circumventricular organs. Alternatively, they may cause central effects through actions at capillary endothelia that induce a cascade of intracerebral processes leading to behavioral outcomes, or their release in the brain could be induced by actions of substances such as endotoxin or bacterial lipopolysaccharides at the endothelia (van Dam et al., 1992). It is possible that effects result from entry into the brain of activated lymphocytes (Wekerle, Linington, Lassman & Meyerman, 1986) that could then induce subsequent effects. Finally, it is possible that physical illness can lead to central and behavioral effects through mechanisms involving neural signals; evidence for such mechanisms comes from research demonstrating that sickness behavior resulting from peripheral administration of pyrogens or cytokines can be attenuated by vagotomy (Bret-Dibat, Bluthe, Kent, et al., 1995; Fleshner, Goehler, Hermann, et al., 1995).

In summary, this body of literature suggests that symptoms such as easy fatigability, decreased activity, decreased motivation, and anorexia can, at times, be adaptive responses to acute illnesses mediated by activation of cytokine systems. It is reasonable to hypothesize that maladaptive responses such as depression can result when exaggerated responses are triggered by minor infections, injuries, or inflammatory states, or when, once activated, the systems cannot appropriately be turned off; this latter possibility echoes mechanisms that have been proposed for the pathogenesis of chronic fatigue syndrome. A complementary possibility, that some cases of what appear to be primary depression can result from a spontaneous activation of these systems, was suggested by the work of Maes and co-workers. These investigators found that groups of young and middle-aged adults admitted to a psychiatric hospital for depression had decreased levels of visceral plasma proteins, increased levels of acute-phase reactants, increases in mitogen-stimulated production of Il-1b and soluble Il-2 receptors (S-Il2R), and increased plasma levels of S-Il2R (Maes, Bosmans, Suy, et al., 1991a, 1991b; Maes, Scharpé, Bosmans, et al., 1992; Maes, Scharpé, Grootel, et al., 1992; Maes, Scharpé, Meltzer, et al., 1993; Maes, Stevens, Declerk, et al., 1993; Maes, Vandewoude, Scharpé, et al., 1991; Maes, Van der Planken, Stevens, et al., 1992). In depressed patients, they found that increased *ex vivo* rates of mitogen induced Il-1b production in peripheral blood leukocytes was associated with a resistance of plasma cortisol levels to suppression by dexamethasone, suggesting that the hypercortisolemia in depression may, in some cases, be driven by Il-1b (Maes, Bosmans, Meltzer, et al., 1993). A role of cytokines in the pathogenesis of depression was also suggested by Smith (1991), who proposed a "macrophage theory of depression." Based upon these findings, a high priority should be placed upon additional research designed to evaluate the associations between the activation of cytokine systems and both primary depression and mood disorders occurring in association with medical illness.

Considering the phenomenon of sickness behavior suggests the value for re-framing an issue that has long been of concern in both geriatric- and consultation-liaison psychiatry: the overlap in symptoms between major depression and medical illness. This problem has been discussed primarily in terms of the difficulties in diagnosing depression in the presence of significant somatic disease. However, in deciding whether to initiate treatment, it may be important to ask, not whether the symptoms are due to depression or to physical illness, but whether they are adaptive or maladaptive to the patient. Kent, Bluthe, Kelly, et al., (1992) proposed that sickness behavior, defined as including nonspecific symptoms of illness such as anorexia, depressed activity, loss of interest in usual activities, and disappearance of body-care activities, may be appropriate targets for pharmacotherapy, and that an understanding of the mechanisms involved should permit development of new drugs aimed at decreasing sickness or promoting recovery processes. In this, they were referring to research on the behavioral pharmacology of Il-1b receptor antagonists. Based upon findings from laboratory research, other approaches to treatment may involve androgens or either vasopressin or alpha-MSH (melanocyte stimulating hormone) analogues (Dantzer, Bluthe, & Kelley, 1991; Opp, Obal, & Krueger, 1988). It may also be reasonable to propose pharmacotherapy for sickness behavior with more traditional psychopharmacological agents. Given the interactions between Il-1b and the biogenic amines, it would be useful to investigate the effects of antidepressants or stimulants on disease-associated symptoms. Other approaches may also be possible; De Sarro, Masuda, Ascioti, et al. (1990) have reported that sedation resulting from administration of Il-2 can be blocked by naltrexone. Furthermore, sickness behavior models suggest the value of research on novel approaches to the treatment of depression in cases where cytokine systems may be activated. Uehara, Ishikawa, Okumura, et al. (1989), and Crestani et al. (1991) have demonstrated that certain behavioral effects of Il-1b, like its pyrogenic effect, can be antagonized by prostaglandin-synthesis inhibitors, and Plata-Salaman (1991a) has demonstrated that its anorectic effect can be blocked by corticosteroids.

Implications of Multiple Mechanisms

Hypothesized paths to the onset of depression in patients with significant medical illness include specific mechanisms that occur in association with certain disorders or adverse effects to certain medications and two putative general mechanisms, one involving clinical–subclinical cerebrovascular disease and the other, cytokine effects. The possibility that multiple mechanisms may be operative has clear implications for research. Investigators should characterize study populations with respect to risk factors for cerebrovascular disease and the activation of inflammatory processes, as well as the specific drugs and medical illnesses that may directly lead to depression; statistical power for investigating any one mechanism could be improved if experimental approaches are able to control for the other(s). Each of the general mechanisms also suggests research strategies for extending and improving clinical care. Although the associations between subclinical cerebrovascular disease and psychopathology were first suggested in patients with major depression, the specificity of these associations remains to be established. Studies in primary care and medical specialty services may be useful in determining whether subcortical and deep white-matter hyperintensities in MRI scans may also be associated with other forms of mood disorder or disturbances of affective regulation, behavior, and cognition. The activation of cytokine systems, similarly, may induce sickness behavior manifested by vegetative symptoms such as fatigue, decreased motivation, and anorexia, as well as full-blown depressive syndromes. Studies of the phenomenology, natural history, and pathogenesis of these symptoms in relevant patient populations could lead to novel treatments.

CONSEQUENCES OF DEPRESSION

The NIH Consensus Statement on the Diagnosis and Treatment of Depression in Late Life (1992) asked "What are the consequences of failure to recognize and treat depression in elderly people?" and concluded,

> Many of our senior citizens will live their final years in despair and suffering without any appreciation of their affliction or the understanding and comfort of those most dear to them. Professional help is not often sought or offered, and depression is not likely to be brief. The likely consequences are loss of personal happiness and severe strain on living circumstances. Depression may trigger a shift from home to a nursing facility, or may shift the person from a warm and respected friend or loved one to an isolated individual with lost status. Untreated depression costs money because physical illnesses require more medical services, living arrangements become institutional, and employment is lost. These costs should be substantially preventable with presently validated case recognition and treatment techniques. (p. 1023)

Findings presented at the Consensus Conference (Schneider, Reynolds, Lebowitz, et al., 1994), together with more recent data (Katz & Alexopoulos, 1996), indicate that depression in late life is a persistent or recurrent disorder that can result from psychosocial stress or physiological effects of disease, and can lead to excessive disability, cognitive impairment, increased symptoms from

medical illness, physiological deterioration, increased utilization of health
care services, and increased rates of suicide and nonsuicide mortality. Although
the psychiatric morbidity associated with depression includes (preventable)
recurrences, substance abuse, and cognitive impairment, it is suicide that makes
the most compelling case for the importance of recognizing depression in general medical care settings. While suicide in younger populations can be attributed to a number of disorders, including substance abuse, psychoses, and personality disorders, as well as to depression, both psychological autopsy studies
of completed suicides (Conwell, Olsen, Caine, et al., 1991) and psychiatric
evaluations of those surviving attempted suicide (Lyness, Conwell, & Nelson,
1992) demonstrate that suicide in the elderly is more specifically related to
depression. The possibilities for prevention are demonstrated most strongly by
the finding that the majority of patients who commit suicide have seen their
primary care physicians shortly before their deaths. One study investigating a
series of suicides found that half of those over age 65 visited a physician within 1
week of death, and that 90% did so within 3 months (Barraclough, Bunch,
Nelson, et al., 1974); another found that more than one-third visited physicians
within 1 week, and 75% within 1 month (Miller, 1978). Moreover, results from a
study that utilized a somewhat isolated community, the Swedish Island of
Gotland, found that educating primary care regarding the diagnosis and treatment of depression can, in fact, decrease suicide rates (Rutz, von Knorring, &
Walinder, 1989).

Amplifying Medical Morbidity

The general medical consequences of depression in older adults with significant physical disorders can be summarized with the unifying hypothesis that
depression interacts with medical or neurological illness to modify the course of
the disease and to amplify the associated disability, medical symptoms, metabolic effects, health service use, and mortality (Katz, Streim, & Parmelee, 1994).

Disability. The association between depression and disability is a highly
reproducible finding, apparent with summary measures of disability in hetero-
genous samples as well as with disease-specific measures in more homogeneous
populations. Using findings from a community sample, Gurland, Wilder, and
Berkman (1988) demonstrated that the path leading from depression to disability
is comparable in strength to that leading from disability to depression. The
magnitude of the disability attributable to depression in young and middle-aged
adults in medical care settings was evaluated by Wells, Stewart, Hays, et al.,
(1989), who found that patients with depression were associated with poor
physical, social, and role functioning that could not be attributed to psychiatric–
medical comorbidity. The extent of disability related to depression was comparable with or worse than eight major chronic medical conditions. Studies of the
relationships between health status, depression, and functional impairment
demonstrate that depression can lead to increased disability or a negative out-

come from rehabilitation of patients with stroke (Feibel & Springer, 1982; Mayo, Korner-Bitensky, & Becker, 1991; Parikh, Robinson, Lipsey, et al., 1990), myocardial infarction (Schleifer, Macari-Hinson, Coyle, et al., 1989; Stern, Pascale, & McLoone, 1975), chronic obstructive pulmonary disease (Schenkman, 1985; Weaver & Narsavage, 1992), hip fracture (Mossy, Knott, & Craik, 1990; Mossey, Mutran, Knott, et al., 1989), parkinsonism (Starkstein, Mayberg, Leiguarda, et al., 1992), arthritis (Beckham, D'Amico, Rice, et al., 1992), and macular degeneration (Shmuely-Dulitzki, Rovner, Zisselman, et al., 1995). Moreover, there is evidence from randomized clinical trials that depression remains responsive to drug treatment in longer-term-care populations, inpatient rehabilitation facilities, and in patients with parkinsonism, cancer, ischemic heart disease, chronic obstructive pulmonary disease, and rheumatoid arthritis (Katz, 1993). However, the available treatment studies have, in general, focused on the safety and the efficacy of treatment for the alleviation of depressive symptoms. They have been limited, both in design and sample size, in their ability to test for wider benefits of treatment, and the key question, regarding the extent to which treatment of depression reduces disability, has not been answered. A significant exception to this generalization, and a model that should guide future research, is a double-blind, placebo-controlled study of nortriptyline treatment in patients with chronic obstructive pulmonary disease, in which Borson, McDonald, Gayle, et al., (1992) demonstrated that treatment of depression can both reduce depressive symptoms and improve day-to-day functioning.

Pain. Several recent studies have demonstrated associations between pain and depression among elderly patients with chronic medical illness (Cohen-Mansfield & Marx, 1993; Parmelee, Katz, & Lawton, 1991; Williamson & Schulz, 1992). As with disability, the relationships are apparently bidirectional. Williamson and Schulz (1992) have considered pain as a cause of depression; their results indicate that both pain and the severity of medical illness are important contributors to functional disability, which, in turn, contributes to depression. Parmelee et al., (1991), in contrast, have considered the possibility that depression may cause or exacerbate pain. They find that increased pain complaints associated with depression occur primarily in those patients who have medical illnesses that can account for the pain, and propose that depression can amplify the intensity of pain due to diagnosable somatic disease.

Drug Side Effects. Miller, Pollack, Rifai, et al. (1991) evaluated somatic symptoms occurring early in the course of nortriptyline treatment for major depression in a group of elderly patients. They found that the frequency of somatic complaints declined by 50% during the acute phase of treatment, in parallel with the reduction in depression, and suggested that many of the symptoms that are usually attributed to side effects of nortriptyline either result from depression or are amplified by an interaction between depression and drug effects. A dramatic example of this phenomenon is that demonstrated by Costa, Mogos, and Toma (1985), who reported that drug treatment of depression can help cancer patients tolerate side effects of chemotherapy and suggested that it may, in this way, facilitate the administration of adequate courses of treatment and improve survival.

Malnutrition. Morley and Kraenzle (1994) reported that depression was the most common cause of weight loss among the residents of a community nursing home, where it was responsible for 36% of those who lost 5 pounds or more over 6 months. The principle that depression is a common cause of weight loss in nursing home residents was confirmed by Blaum, Fries, & Fiatarone (1995) in analyses that used a (U.S.) multistate database. Associations between depression and biochemical markers of protein-calorie undernutrition (e.g., plasma levels of albumin) in both long-term-care patients and adult psychiatric inpatients suggest that depression may be associated with protein-calorie subnutrition (Katz, Beaston-Wimmer, Parmelee, et al., 1993; Maes, Vandewoude, Scharpé, et al., 1991). However, other findings on acute-phase reactants suggest that these physiological abnormalities may be related to (cytokine-mediated) metabolic effects of disease or inflammation, as well as from decreased food intake (Maes, Scharpé, Bosmons, et al., 1992). Thus, depression may be either a direct cause of subnutrition or an amplifying factor, increasing the extent of catabolism occurring in elderly patients with severe chronic illness. In either case, treatment of depression may be necessary to reverse wasting and deterioration. Neuroendocrine abnormalities associated with depression in late life include hypercortisolemia, decreased feedback regulation of the hypothalamic–pituitary–adrenal axis, and decreased growth-hormone responses to pharmacological stimuli. These findings have usually been discussed as possible diagnostic markers or probes of the neurochemical basis of depression. However, it is possible that these abnormalities may have physiological significance specifically in the frail elderly. Recent research in younger, predominantly premenopausal women, suggests that major depression can be associated with the acceleration of osteoporosis, possibly through the effects of increased cortisol levels (Michelson, Stratoris, Hill, et al., 1996); further study is necessary to confirm these findings in the elderly, and to investigate the extent to which muscle and brain, as well as bone, can be target organs for the effects of hypercortisolemia.

Health Services Use. Increases in the use of general medical health services; both inpatient and outpatient, in patients with depression are readily demonstrated both in adult populations and in the elderly (Barksy, Wyshak, & Klerman, 1986; Conwell, 1996; McFarland, Freeborn, Mullooly, et al., 1985; Waxman, Carner, & Blum, 1983). The major question in this area, however, has been whether this effect remains after controlling for medical comorbidity. One recent investigation suggests that the increased rates of hospitalization associated with nonspecific measures of poor mental health remain significant after controlling for general medical status (Manning & Wells, 1992). Koenig, Shelp, Goli, et al., (1989) find that depressed patients had longer lengths of stay as well as more hospital days subsequent to an index hospitalization (and greater in-hospital mortality) than controls from the same population matched with respect to age, type and severity of illness, and functional status. Finally, Fries, Mehr, Schneider, et al. (1993) report that depression increases the amount of nursing-care time required by nursing home residents, even after controlling for the associations between depression and disability. Together these findings demonstrate that depression can increase general health care costs.

Hinrichsen, Hernandez, and Pollack (1992) have demonstrated that major depression represents a significant source of stress and burden to those who care for older patients. Thus, in evaluating the societal impact of depression, it is important to consider the informal as well as formal components of care, and indirect as well as direct costs.

Gerety, Chiodo, Kanten, et al. (1993) asked older subjects to respond to standardized vignettes describing a series of diseases and treatment, and found that individuals with depression were less likely to opt for treatment, regardless of the probable outcome. This finding confirms concerns that treatment refusal may, at times, be an indirect form of self-destructive behavior related to depression. The report that depressed patients may be reluctant to seek treatment for medical conditions appears, at first, to be at odds with their increased utilization of health care services. Taken together, these findings suggest that general health service use in patients with depression may often be a manifestation of desperation rather than goal-directed behavior; they suggest that treatment of depression could improve the efficiency with which health care is administered. The associations between depression, treatment refusal, and suicidal ideation are also relevant to ongoing debates about treatment refusal and the right to die (Sullivan & Youngener, 1994). Although the issues involved in these debates are complex, it is clear that concerns about treatment refusal, the right to die, assisted suicide, and euthanasia all argue strongly for the importance of facilitating the access of chronically or terminally ill patients to clinical evaluation and treatment for depressive symptoms.

Mortality.   Avery and Winokur (1976) reported a generation ago that elderly depressed patients who received "adequate treatment" survived longer than those who did not, and suggested that treatment of depression in the aged could extend life; however, there must be questions about the extent to which their findings reflected the impact of health status on the delivery of treatment. Recently, Frasure-Smith, Lesperance, and Talajic (1993) reported that depression after a myocardial infarction was associated with increased mortality, even after controlling for the severity of patients' cardiac disease. In long-term care, recent research uniformly demonstrates an association between depression and decreased survival, but there has been controversy about the underlying mechanism. While Rovner, German, Brant, et al. (1991) reported that the increase in mortality related to depression persisted after controlling for the associations between depression and medical illnesses, Parmelee, Katz, and Lawton (1992), who used more comprehensive measures of medical comorbidity, found that it did not. Recently, however, Samuels, Katz, Parmelee, et al. (1997) examined this issue in a sample of depressed older patients from a residential care setting and found that the severity of core depressive symptoms predicted morality even after controlling for measures of comorbid disease and functional disability. Interestingly, while depressive symptoms predicted mortality in this sample, anxiety did not, suggesting that there is specificity to the association between psychiatric symptoms and decreased survival.

Implications.   The research literature reviewed here demonstrates that the diagnosis and treatment of depression occurring in association with significant medical illness can have a major impact on patients' overall health and health care utilization. Our society as a whole, as well as our patients and their families, have a major stake in ensuring that older patients with depression receive appropriate treatment.

CONCLUSIONS

This review has focused primarily on biological causes of depression and on clinical consequences. There are, of course, comparable findings on the social causes of depressions occurring in association with medical illness and on the biological consequences of severe affective disorders. The primary conclusions must be that the interactions between medical illness and psychiatric symptoms are extensive, complex, and bidirectional. Secondary aging is a social and psychiatric as well as physical phenomenon; interventions intended to improve the subjective experience, functional capacity, and physiological status of older patients with chronic illness could target any of these domains. Moreover, what has been learned regarding the interactions between mental and physical health in late life is very likely to be informative about the experience and care of young adult patients who suffer from disease and disability. The findings reviewed here that link depression and related symptoms with the pathophysiology of disease in late life suggest that it is not possible to separate mental and physical health in late life. Geriatric care that fails to recognize the importance of psychiatric–medical comorbidity will not meet patients' needs to minimize distress and optimize function, or society's to provide effective care at reasonable cost.

REFERENCES

Alexopoulos, G. S., Young, R. C., & Schindledecker, R. D. (1992). Brain computed tomography in geriatric depression and primary degenerative dementia. *Biological Psychiatry, 31*, 591–599.
Avery, D., & Winokur, G. (1976). Mortality in depressed patients treated with electroconvulsive therapy and antidepressants. *Archives of General Psychiatry, 33*, 1029–1037.
Barksy, A. J., Wyshak, G., & Klerman, G. L. (1986). Medical and psychiatric determinants of outpatient medical utilization. *Medical Care, 24*, 548–563.
Barraclough, B. M., Bunch, J., Nelson, B., & Sainsburcy, S. (1974). A hundred cases of suicide: Clinical aspects. *British Journal of Psychiatry, 125*, 355–373.
Beckham, J. C., D'Amico, C. J., Rice, R., & Jordan, J. S. (1992). Depression and level of functioning in patients with rheumatoid arthritis. *Canadian Journal of Psychiatry, 37*, 539–543.
Berkenbosch, F., van Oers, J., del Ray, A., Tilders, F., & Besedonsky, H. (1987). Corticotropin-releasing factor-producing neurons in the rat activated by interleukin-1. *Science, 238*, 524–526.

Blaum, C. S., Fries, B. E., & Fiatarone, M. A. (1995). Factors associated with low body mass index and weight loss among nursing home residents. *Journal of Gerontology*, *50*, M162–M168.

Bluthe, R. M., Dantzer, R., & Kelley, K. W. (1991). Interleukin-1 mediates behavioral but not metabolic effects of tumor necrosis factor alpha in mice. *European Journal of Pharmacology*, *209*, 281–283.

Bluthe, R. M., Dantzer, R., & Kelley, K. W. (1992). Effects of interleukin-1 receptor antagonist on the behavioral effects of lipopolysaccharide in rat. *Brain Research*, *573*, 318–320.

Borson, S., McDonald, G. J., Gayle, T., Deffebach, M., Lakeskminarayans, S., Van Tuinen, C. (1992). Improvement in mood, physical symptoms, and function with nortriptyline for depression in patients with chronic obstructive pulmonary disease. *Psychosomatics*, *33*, 190–201.

Bret-Dibat, J. L., Bluthe, R. M., Kent, S., Kelley, K. W., & Dantzer, R. (1995). Lipopolysaccharide and interleukin-1 depress food-motivated behavior in mice by a vagal mediated mechanism. *Brain, Behavior, and Immunity*, *9*, 242–246.

Bryer, J. B., Starkstein, S. E., Votypka, V., Parikh, R. M., Price, T. R., & Robinson, R. G. (1992). Reduction of CSF monoamine metabolites in poststroke depression: A preliminary report. *Journal of Neuropsychiatry and Clinical Neuroscience*, *4*, 440–442.

Coffey, C. E., Figiel, G. S., & Djang, W. T. (1990). Subcortical hyperintensity on magnetic resonance imaging: A comparison of normal and depressed elderly subjects. *American Journal of Psychiatry*, *147*, 187–189.

Coffey, C. E., Figiel, G. S., Djang, W. T., Cress, M., Saunders, W. B., & Weiner, R. D. (1988). Leukoencephalopathy in elderly depressed patients referred for ECT. *Biological Psychiatry*, *24*, 143–161.

Coffey, C. E., Wilkinson, W. E., Weiner, R. D., Parashos, I. A., Djang, W. T., Webb, M. C., Fiegel, G. S. & Spritzer, C. E. (1993). Quantitative cerebral anatomy in depression: A controlled magnetic resonance imaging study. *Archives of General Psychiatry*, *50*, 7–16.

Cohen-Mansfield, J., & Marx, M. S. (1993). Pain and depression in the nursing home: Corroborating results. *Journal of Gerontology*, *48*, P96–P97.

Conwell, T., Olsen, K., Caine, E. D., & Flannery, C. (1991). Suicide in later life: Psychological autopsy findings. *International Psychogeriatrics*, *3*, 59–66.

Conwell, Y. (1996). Outcomes of depression. *American Journal of Geriatric Psychiatry*, *4*, S34–S44.

Costa, D., Mogos, I., & Toma, T. (1985). Efficacy and safety of mianserin in the treatment of depression of women with cancer. *Acta Psychiatrica Scandinavica*, *72*, (Suppl. 320), 85–92.

Crestani, F., Suguy, F., & Dantzer, R. (1991). Behavioral effects of peripherally injected interleukin-1: Role of prostaglandins. *Brain Research*, *542*, 330–335.

Dantzer, R., Bluthe, R. M., & Kelley, K. W. (1991). Androgen-dependent vasopressinergic neurotransmission attenuates interleukin-1-induced sickness behavior. *Brain Research*, *557*, 115–120.

Dantzer, R., & Kelley, K. W. (1989). Stress and immunity: An integrated view of relationships between the brain and the immune system. *Life Sciences*, *44*, 1995–2008.

De Sarro, G. B., Masuda, Y., Ascioti, C., Audino, M. G., & Nistico, G. (1990). Behavioral and ECoG spectrum changes induced by intracerebral infusion of interferons and interleukin 2 in rats are antagonized by naloxone. *Neuropharmacology*, *29*, 167–179.

del Cerro, S., & Borrell, J. (1990). Interleukin-1 affects the behavioral despair responses in rats by an indirect mechanism which requires endogenous CRF. *Brain Research*, *528*, 162–164.

Dolan, R. J., Calloway, S. P., & Mann, A. H. (1985). Cerebral ventricular size: Depressed subjects. *Psychological Medicine*, *15*, 873–878.

Dunn, A. J. (1992). Endotoxin-induces activation of cerebral catecholamine and serotonin metabolism: Comparison with interleukin-1. *Journal of Pharmacology and Experimental Therapeutics*, *261*, 964–969.

Dunn, A. J., Antoon, M., & Chapman, Y. (1991). Reduction of exploratory behavior by intraperitoneal injection of interleukin-1 involves brain corticotropin-releasing factor. *Brain Research Bulletin*, *26*, 539–542.

Fazekas, F., Niederkorn, K., Schmidt, R., Offenbacker, H., Horner, S., Bertha, G., & Lechner, H. (1988). White-matter signal abnormalities in normal individuals: Correlation with carotic ultrasonography, cerebral blood flow measurements, and cerebrovascular risk factors. *Stroke*, *19*, 1285–1288.

Feibel, J. H., & Springer, C. J. (1982). Depression and failure to resume social activities after stroke. *Archives of Physical Medicine and Rehabilitation*, *63*, 276–278.

Figiel, G. S., Krishnan, K. R., Doraiswamy, P. M., Rao, V. P., Nemeroff, C. B., & Boyko, O. B. (1991). Subcortical hyperintensities on brain magnetic resonance imaging: A comparison between late age onset and early onset elderly depressed subjects. *Neurobiology of Aging, 26*, 245–247.

Fleshner, M., Goehler, L. E., Hermann, J., Relton, J. K., Maier, S. F., & Watkins, L. R. (1995). Interleukin-1 beta induced corticosterone elevation and hypothalamic NE depletion are vagally mediated. *Brain Research Bulletin, 37*, 605–610.

Forstl, H., Burns, A., Luthert, P., et al. (1992). Clinical and neuropathological correlates of depression in Alzheimer's disease. *Psychological Medicine, 22*, 877–884.

Frasure-Smith, N., Lesperance, F., & Talajic, M. (1993). Depression following myocardial infarction: Impact on 6-month survival. *Journal of the American Medical Association, 270*, 1819–1825.

Fries, B. E., Mehr, D. R., Schneider, D., Folez, W. J., & Burke, R. (1993). Mental dysfunction and resource use in nursing homes. *Medical Care, 31*, 898–920.

Fujikawa, T., Yamawaki, S., & Touhouda, Y. (1993). Incidence of silent cerebral infarction in patients with major depression. *Stroke, 24*, 1631–1634.

Gemma, C., Ghezzi, P., & De Simoni, M. G., (1991). Activation of the hypothalamic serotonergic system by central interleukin-1. *European Journal of Pharmacology, 209*, 139–140.

Gerety, M. B., Chiodo, L. K., Kanten, D. N., Fuley, M. R., & Cornell, J. E. (1993). Medical treatment preferences of nursing home residents: Relationship to function and concordance with surrogate decision makers. *Journal of the American Geriatric Society, 41*, 953–960.

Gurland, B. J., Wilder, D. E., & Berkman, C. (1988). Depression and disability in the elderly: Reciprocal relations and changes with age. *International Journal of Geriatric Psychiatry, 3*, 163–179.

Hart, B. L. (1988). Biological basis of the behavior of sick animals. *Neuroscience and Biobehavioral Reviews, 12*, 123–137.

Hinrichsen, G. A., Henandez, N. A., & Pollack, S. (1992). Difficulties and rewards in family care of the depressed older adult. *Gerontologist, 32*, 486–492.

Hopkinson, G. (1964). A genetic study of affective illness in patients over 50. *British Journal of Psychiatry, 110*, 244–254.

Jacoby, R. J., Dolan, R. J., Baldy, R., & Levy, R. (1983). Quantitative computed tomography in elderly depressed patients. *British Journal of Psychiatry, 143*, 124–127.

Katz, I. R. (1982). Is there a hypoxic affective syndrome? A contribution from neurochemistry. *Psychosomatics, 23*, 846–853.

Katz, I. R. (1993). Drug treatment of depression in the frail elderly: Discussion of the NIH Consensus Development Conference on the Diagnosis and Treatment of Depression in Late Life. *Psychopharmacology Bulletin, 29*, 101–108.

Katz, I. R., & Alexopoulos, G. (1996). Consensus Update Conference: Diagnosis and treatment of late-life depression. *American Journal of Geriatric Psychiatry, 4* (Suppl. 1), S1–S95.

Katz, I. R., Beaston-Wimmer, P., Parmelee, P. A., Friedman, E., & Lawton, M. P. (1993). Failure to thrive in the elderly: Exploration of the concept and delineation of psychiatric components. *Journal of Geriatric Psychiatry and Neurology, 6*, 161–169.

Katz, I. R., Friedman, E., Parmelee, P., et al. (1989). Amino acid levels in elderly nursing home residents. *Journal of Geriatric Psychiatry and Neurology, 2*(4), 215–222.

Katz, I. R., Jain, A. K., Muhly, C., & Hoeldke, R. (1985). Models for the pathogenesis of psychiatric, affective, and behavioral symptoms in chronic illness: Neurochemistry of secondary aging. In C. Shagass, R. C. Josiassen, E. H. Bridger, et al. (Eds.), New York: Elsevier. *Proceedings of the IVth World Congress of Biological Psychiatry*, pp. 1406–1408.

Katz, I. R. & Parmelee, P. A. (1994). Depression in the residential care elderly. In L. S. Schneider, C. F. Reynolds, B. D. Lebowitz, & A. Friedhoff (Eds.), *Diagnosis and treatment of depression in late life: Results of the NIH Concensus Development Conference*, (pp. 437–461). Washington, DC: American Psychiatric Association Press.

Katz, I. R., Streim, J., & Parmelee, P. (1994). Prevention of depression, recurrences and complications in late life. *Preventive Medicine, 23*, 743–750.

Kent, S., Bluthe, R. M., Kelley, K. W., & Dantzer, R. (1992). Sickness behavior as a new target for drug development. *Trends in the Pharmacological Sciences, 13*, 24–28.

Koenig, H. G., Shelp, F., Goli, V., Cohen, A. J., & Blazer, D. G. (1989). Survival and health care utilization in elderly medical inpatients with major depression. *Journal of the American Geriatric Society*, *37*, 399–606.

Krishnan, K. R. (1993). Neuroanatomic substrates of depression in the elderly. *Journal of Geriatric Psychiatry and Neurology*, *6*, 39–58.

Krishnan, K. R., & Gaddle, K. M. (1996). The pathophysiological basis for late life depression: Imaging studies of the aging brain. *American Journal of Geriatric Psychiatry*, *4*, S22–S33.

Krishnan, K. R., Goli, V., Ellinwood, E. H., France, R. D., Blazer, D. G., & Nemeroff, C. B. (1988). Leukoencephalopathy in patients diagnosed as major depressive. *Biological Psychiatry*, *25*, 519–522.

Krishnan, K. R., McDonald, W. M., Escalona, P. R., Doraiswamy, P. M., & Na, C. (1992). Magnetic resonance imaging of the caudate nuclei in depression: Preliminary observations. *Archives of General Psychiatry*, *49*, 553–557.

Krueger, J. M., Walter, J., Dinarello, C. A., et al. (1984). Sleep promoting effects of endogenous pyrogen (interleukin-1). American Journal of Physiology, *246*, R994–R999.

Lyness, J. M., Conwell, Y., King, C., Cox, C., & Caine, E. D. (1995). Age of onset and medical illness in older depressed inpatients. *International Psychogeriatrics*, *7*, 63–74.

Lyness, J. M., Conwell, Y., & Nelson, J. G. (1992). Suicide attempts in elderly psychiatric inpatients. *Journal of the American Geriatric Society*, *40*, 320–324.

Maes, M., Bosmans, E., Meltzer, H. Y., Scharpe, S., & Suy, E. (1993). Interleukin-1b: A putative mediator of HPA axis hyperactivity in major depression? *American Journal of Psychiatry*, *150*, 1189–1193.

Maes, M., Bosmans, E., Suy, E., Vandervost, C., & DeJonekheere, C. (1991a). Depression-related disturbances in mitogen-induced lymphocyte responses and interleukin-1b and soluble interleukin-2 receptor production. *Acta Psychiatrica Scandinavica*, *84*, 379–386.

Maes, M., Bosmans, E., Suy, E., Vandervost, C., DeJonekheere, C., & Raus, J. (1991b). Immune disturbances during major depression: Upregulated expression of interleukin-2 receptors. *Neuropsychobiology*, *24*, 115–120.

Maes, M., Scharpé, S., Bosmans, E., Vanderwonde, M., & Suy, E. (1992). Disturbances in acute phase plasma proteins during melancholia: Additional evidence for the presence of an inflammatory process during that illness. *Progress in Neuropsychopharmacology and Biological Psychiatry*, *16*, 501–515.

Maes, M., Scharpé, S., Grootel, L. V., Vyttenbroeck, W., Cooreman, W., Vandervorst, C., & Raus, J. (1992). Higher α_1-antitrypsin, haptoglobin, ceruloplasmin, and lower retinol binding protein plasma levels during depression: Further evidence for the existence of an inflammatory response during that illness. *Journal of Affective Disorders*, *24*, 183–192.

Maes, M., Scharpé, S., Meltzer, H. Y., & Cosyns, P. (1993). Relationships between increased haptoglobin plasma levels and activation of cell-mediated immunity in depression. *Biological Psychiatry*, *34*, 690–701.

Maes, M., Stevens, W. J., Declerk, L. S., Bridts, C. H., Peeters, D., Schotte, C., & Cosyns, P. (1993). Significantly increased expression of T-cell activation markers (interleukin-2 and HLA-DR) in depression: Further evidence for an inflammatory process during that illness. *Progress in Neuropsychopharmology and Biological Psychiatry*, *17*, 241–255.

Maes, M., Van der Planken, M., Stevens, W. J., Peeters, D., De Clerq, L. S., Bridts, C. H., Schotte, C., & Cosyns, P. (1992). Leukocytosis, monocytosis, and neutrophilia: Hallmarks of severe depression. *Journal of Psychiatric Research*, *26*, 125–134.

Maes, M., Vandewoude, M., Scharpé, S., De Clercq, L. S., Stephens, W. J., Lepoutre, L., & Schotte, C. (1991). Anthropometric and biochemical assessment of the nutritional state in depression: Evidence for lower visceral protein plasma levels in depression. *Journal of Affective Disorders*, *23*, 25–33.

Manning, W. G., & Wells, K. B. (1992). The effects of psychological distress and psychological well-being on use of medical services. *Medical Care*, *30*, 541–553.

Mayberg, H. S., Robinson, R. G., Wong, D. F., Parikh, R., Bolduc, P., Starkstein, S. E., Price, T., Dannals, R. F., Links, J. M., Wilson, A. A., et al. (1988). PET imaging of cortical S2 serotonin receptors after stroke: Lateralized changes and relationship to depression. *American Journal of Psychiatry*, *4*, 937–943.

Mayeux, R., Stern, Y., & Sano, M. (1988). The relationship of serotonin to depression in Parkinson's disease. *Movement Disorders*, *3*, 237–244.

Mayo, N. E., Korner-Bitensky, N. A., & Becker, R. (1991). Recovery time of independent function post-stroke. *American Journal of Physical Medicine and Rehabilitation*, *70*, 5–12.

McFarland, B. H., Freeborn, D. K., Mullooly, J. P., & Pope, C. R. (1985). Utilization patterns among long-term enrollees in a prepared group practice health maintenance organization. *Medical Care*, *23*, 1221–1233.

Mendlewicz, J. (1976). The age factor of depressive illness: Some genetic considerations. *Journal of Gerontology*, *31*, 300–303.

Michelson, D., Stratoris, C., Hill, L., Reynolds, J., Gallinen, E., Chronsos, G., Gold, P., & Gottlieb, G. L. (1996). Bone mineral density in women with depression. *New England Journal of Medicine*, *336*, 1176–1181.

Miller, D., Kumar, A., Yousem, D., et al. (1994). MRI high intensity signals in late life depression and Alzheimer's disease: A comparison of subjects without cerebrovascular risk factors. *American Journal of Geriatric Psychiatry*, *2*, 332–337.

Miller, M. (1978). Geriatric suicide—the Arizona study. *Gerontologist*, *18*, 488–495.

Miller, M. D., Pollock, B. G., Rifai, A. H., Parades, C. F., Perel, J. M., George, C., Stack, J. A., & Reynolds, C. F. (1991). Longitudinal analysis of nortriptyline side effects in elderly depressed patients. *Journal of Geriatric Psychiatry and Neurology*, *4*, 226–230.

Mohankumar, P. S., & Quadri, S. K. (1993). Systemic administration of interleukin-1 stimulates norepinephrine release in the paraventricular nucleus. *Life Sciences*, *52*, 1961–1967.

Mohankumar, P. S., Thyagarajan, S., & Quadri, S. K. (1991). Interleukin-1 stimulates the release of dopamine and dihydroxyphenylacetic acid from the hypothalamus in vivo. *Life Sciences*, *48*, 925–930.

Mohankumar, P. S., Thyagarajan, S., & Quadri, S. K. (1993). Interleukin-1b increases 5-hydroxy-indoleacetic acid release in the hypothalamus in vivo. *Brain Research Bulletin*, *31*, 745–748.

Moldin, S. O., Scheftner, W. A., Rice, J. P., Nelson, E., Knesevich, M. A., & Skishal, H. (1993). Association between major depressive disorder and physical illness. *Psychological Medicine*, *23*, 755–761.

Morley, J. E., & Kraenzle, D. (1994). Causes of weight loss in a community nursing home. *Journal of the American Geriatric Society*, *42*, 583–585.

Mossey, J. M., Knott, K., & Craik, R. (1990). The effects of persistent depressive symptoms of hip fracture recovery. *Journal of Gerontology*, *45*, M163–M168.

Mossey, J. M., Mutran, E., Knott, K., & Craik, R. (1989). Determinants of recovery 12 months after hip fracture: The importance of psychosocial factors. *American Journal of Public Health*, *79*, 279–286.

Office of the Medical Applications of Research, National Institutes of Health, Bethesda, MD. (1992). Consensus Development Panel on Depression in Late Life: Diagnosis and treatment of depression in late life. *Journal of the American Medical Association*, *268*(8), 1018–1024.

Opp, M. R., Obal, F., & Krueger, F. (1988). Effects of a-MSH on sleep, behavior, and brain temperature: Interactions with Il-1. *American Journal of Physiology*, *255*, R914–R922.

Parikh, R. M., Robinson, R. G., Lipsey, J. R., Starkstein, S. E., Federoff, J. P., & Price, T. R. (1990). The impact of poststroke depression on recovery in activities of daily living over a 2-year follow-up. *Archives of Neurology*, *47*, 786–789.

Parmelee, P. A., Katz, I. R., & Lawton, M. P. (1991). The relation of pain to depression among institutionalized aged. *Journal of Gerontology*, *46*, M15–M21.

Parmelee, P. A., Katz, I. R., & Lawton, M. P. (1992). Depression and mortality among institutionalized aged. *Journal of Gerontology*, *47*, P3–P10.

Pearlson, G. D., Rabins, P. V., & Burns, A. (1991). Centrum semiovale white-matter CT changes associated with normal aging: Alzheimer's disease and late life depression with and without reversible dementia. *Psychological Medicine*, *21*, 321–328.

Pearlson, G. D., Rabins, P. V., Kim, W. S., Speedie, L. J., & Moberg, P. J. (1989). Structural brain changes and cognitive deficits in elderly depressives with and without reversible dementia ("pseudo-dementia"). *Psychological Medicine*, *19*, 573–584.

Pearlson, G. D., Ross, C. A., Lohr, W. D., Rovner, B. W., Chase, G. A., Folstein, M. F. (1990). Association between family history of affective disorder and the depressive syndrome of Alzheimer's disease. *American Journal of Psychiatry, 147*, 452–456.

Plata-Salaman, C. R. (1988). Food intake suppression by immunomodulators. *Neurosciences Research Communications, 3*, 159–165.

Plata-Salaman, C. R. (1991a). Dexamethasone inhibits food intake suppression induced by low doses of interleukin-1 beta administered intracerebroventricularly. *Brain Research Bulletin, 27*, 737–738.

Plata-Salaman, C. R. (1991b). Immunoregulators in the nervous system. *Neuroscience and Biobehavioral Reviews, 15*, 185–215.

Rabins, P. V., Pearlson, G. D., Aylward, E., Kumar, A. J., & Dowell, K. (1991). Cortical magnetic resonance imaging changes in elderly inpatients with major depression. *American Journal of Psychiatry, 148*, 617–620.

Robinson, R. G., & Coyle, J. T. (1980). The differential effect of right versus left hemispheric cerebral infarction on catecholamines and behavior in the rat. *Brain Research, 188*, 63–78.

Robinson, R. G., Schoemaker, W. J., & Schlumpf, M. (1980). Time course of changes in catecholamines following right hemispheric cerebral infarction in the rat. *Brain Research, 181*, 202–208.

Robinson, R. G., Schoemaker, W. J., Schlumpf, M., Volk, D., & Bloom, F. E. (1975). Effect of experimental cerebral infarction in rat brain on catecholamines and behavior. *Nature, 225*, 332–334.

Robinson, R. H. (1979). Differential behavioral and biochemical effects of right and left hemispheric cerebral infarction in the rat. *Science, 205*, 707–710.

Rossi, A., Stratta, P., Petruzzi, C., De Donatis, M., Wistico, R., & Casacchia, M. (1987). A computerized tomographic study in DSM-III affective disorders. *Journal of Affective Disorders, 12*, 259–262.

Rovner, B. W., German, P. S., Brant, L. J., Clark, R., Burton, L., & Foldstein, M. F. (1991). Depression and mortality in nursing homes. *Journal of American Medical Association, 265*, 993–996.

Rutz, W., von Knorring, L., & Walinder, J. (1989). Frequency of suicide on Gotland after systematic post-graduate education of general practitioners. *Acta Psychiatrica Scandinavica, 80*, 151–154.

Samuels, S. C., Katz, I. R., Parmelee, P. A., Boyce, A., & De Filippo, S. (1997). Use of the Hamilton and Montgomery Asberg Depression Scales in the institutional elderly: Relationship to measures of cognitive impairment, disability, physical illness, and mortality. *American Journal of Geriatric Psychiatry, 5*, 172–176.

Sapolsky, R., Rivier, C., Yamamoto, G., Plotsky, P., & Vale, W. (1987). Interleukin-1 stimulates the secretion of hypothalamic corticotropin-releasing factor. *Science, 238*, 522–524.

Schenkman, B. (1985). Factors contributing to attrition rates in a pulmonary rehabilitation program. *Heart and Lung, 14*, 53–58.

Schleifer, S. J., Macari-Hinson, M. M., Coyle, D. A., Slater, W. R., Kahn, M., Gorlin, R., & Zucker, H. D. (1989). The nature and course of depression following myocardial infarction. *Archives of Internal Medicine, 149*, 1785–1789.

Schneider, L. S., Reynolds, C. F., & Lebowitz, B. D. (Eds). (1994). *Diagnosis and treatment of depression in late life: Results of the NIH Consensus Development Conference.* Washington, DC: American Psychiatric Association Press.

Schwartz, J. A., Speed, N. M., Brunberg, J. A., Bremer, T. L., Brown, M., & Greden, J. F. (1993). Depression in stroke rehabilitation. *Biological Psychiatry, 33*, 694–699.

Shima, S., Shikano, T., Kitamura, T., Masuda, Y., Taukumo, T., Kanba, S., & Asai, M. (1984). Depression and ventricular enlargement. *Acta Psychiatrica Scandinavica, 70*, 274–277.

Shintani, F., Kanba, S., Nakaki, T., Nebuza, M., Kinashita, N., Suzuki, E., Yozi, G., Koto, R., & Asai, M. (1993). Interleukin-1b augments release of norepinephrine, dopamine, and serotonin in the rat anterior hypothalamus. *Journal of Neuroscience, 13*, 3574–3581.

Shmuely-Dulitzki, Y., Rovner, B. W., Zisselman, P., et al. (1995). The impact of depression on functioning in elderly patients with low vision. *American Journal of Geriatric Psychiatry, 3*, 325–329.

Smith, R. S. (1991). The macrophage theory of depression. *Medical Hypotheses, 35*, 298–306.

Starkstein, S. E., Mayberg, H. S., Leiguarda, R., Preziosi, T. J., & Robinson, R. G. (1992). A prospective longitudinal study of depression, cognitive decline, and physical impairments in patients with Parkinson's disease. *Journal of Neurology, Neurosurgery, and Psychiatry, 55*, 377–382.

Starkstein, S. E., & Robinson, R. G. (1989). Affective disorders and cerebral vascular disease. *British Journal of Psychiatry, 154*, 170–182.

Stenstedt, A. (1959). Involutional melancholia: An etiologic, clinical and social study of endogenous depression in later life, with special reference to genetic factors. *Acta Psychiatrica et Neurologica Scandinavica, 127* (Suppl.), 5–71.

Stern, M. J., Pascale, L., & McLoone, J. B. (1975). Psychosocial adaptation following myocardial infarction. *Journal of Chronic Disease, 29*, 513–526.

Sullivan, M. D., & Youngner, S. J. (1994). Depression, competence, and the right to refuse lifesaving medical treatment. *American Journal of Psychiatry, 151*, 971–978.

Terao, A., Oikawa, M., & Saito, M. (1993). Cytokine-induced change in hypothalamic norepinephrine turnover: Involvement of corticotrophin-releasing hormone and prostaglandins. *Brain Research, 622*, 257–261.

Uehara, A., Ishikawa, Y., Okumura, T., Okamura, K., Sekiza, C., Takasuzi, Y., & Namiki, M. (1989). Indomethacin blocks the anorexic action of interleukin-1. *European Journal of Pharmacology, 170*, 257–260.

van Dam, A. M., Brouns, M., Louisse, S., & Berkenbosch, F. (1992). Appearance of interleukin-1 in macrophages and in ramified microglia in the brain of endotoxin-treated rats: A pathway for the induction of non-specific symptoms of sickness? *Brain Research, 588*, 291–296.

Waxman, H. M., Carner, E. A., & Blum, A. (1983). Depressive symptoms and health service utilization among the community elderly. *Journal of the American Geriatric Society, 31*, 417–420.

Weaver, T. E., & Narsavage, G. L. (1992). Physiological and psychological variables related to functional status in chronic obstructive pulmonary disease. *Nursing Research, 41*, 286–291.

Wekerle, H., Linington, C., Lassman, H., & Meyerman, R. (1986). Cellular immune reactivity within the CNS. *Trends in Neuroscience, 9*, 271–277.

Wells, K. B., Stewart, A , Hays, R. D., Burnham, M. A., Rogus, W., Daniels, M., Beuy, S., Greenfield, S., & Ware, J. (1989). The functioning and well being of depressed patients. *Journal of the American Medical Association, 262*, 914–919.

Williamson, G. M. & Schultz, R. (1992). Pain, activity, restriction, and symptoms of depression among community-residing elderly adults. *Journal of Gerontology, 47*, P367–P372.

Zubenko, G. S., & Moossy, J. (1988). Major depression in primary dementia. *Archives of Neurology, 45*, 1182–1186.

Zubenko, G. S., Sullivan, P., Nelson, J. P., Belle, S. H., Huff, F. J., & Wolf, G. L. (1990). Brain imaging abnormalities in mental disorders of late life. *Archives of Neurology, 47*, 1107–1111.

Zweig, R. M., Ross, C. A., Hedreen, J. C., Steele, C., Cardillo, J. E., Whitehouse, P. J., Folstein, M. F., & Price, D. L. (1988). The neuropathology of aminergic nuclei in Alzheimer's disease. *Annals of Neurology, 24*, 233–242.

CHAPTER 22

The Variability of Depression in Old Age

Narrative as an Integrative Construct

KEITH G. MEADOR AND DAN G. BLAZER

INTRODUCTION

Although there have been attempts throughout the ages to understand, describe, and treat depression (Jackson, 1986), the word *depression* continues to be used variably according to context and the predisposing biases of the speaker. Our discussion in this chapter embodies a fluid understanding of depression. Inherent to our constructive position is an appreciation for the heterogeneity of depressive disorders in the elderly. While acknowledging the considerable strides made during the last 20 years in delineating major depression using the categorical methods of the third edition of the *Diagnostic and Statistical Manual of Mental Disorders* (DSM-III; American Psychiatric Association, 1980) and subsequent editions of the DSM, we suggest limits to that framework for the optimal understanding of the vicissitudes of depression in old age. We propose that an optimal understanding of depression in general, but particularly in the elderly, requires a biopsychosocial formulation that is derived and interpreted in the context of a particular, contextually and historically contingent, narrative.

DIAGNOSTIC AND DESCRIPTIVE DILEMMAS

In discussing the significance of diversity within theoretical developments regarding aging, Calasanti (1996) provides a useful framework for consideration

KEITH G. MEADOR AND DAN G. BLAZER • School of Medicine and Divinity School, Duke University, Durham, North Carolina 27708.

Handbook of Aging and Mental Health: An Integrative Approach, edited by Jacob Lomranz. Plenum Press, New York, 1998.

of the variability of depression in older persons. While there are a number of significant components within her proposal regarding diversity, central to this discussion are references to the historical context and the fluidity of structures and processes bringing us "face to face with the contextual, dynamic, and social constructed aspects of the social world" (Calasanti, 1996, p. 155). This paradigmatic presentation of diversity by social gerontologists challenges our diagnostic constructions and opens the door for consideration of contextual and historical particularities. Although this is relevant for mental health diagnoses in general, it is particularly significant in the elderly in light of the experiential underpinnings of historical cohorts in conjunction with life-course issues (Pearlin & Skaff, 1996).

Much discussion has occurred in recent years regarding the prevalence of major depression in the elderly when using the criteria stipulated in DSM-III and subsequent editions of the DSM. The Diagnostic Interview Schedule (DIS; Robins, Helzer, Croughan, & Ratcliff, 1981), based on these criteria, was used for determining the most frequently cited 1-year prevalence rate of major depression in those aged 65 and older of .9% compared with a 2.7% rate for adults in general (Robins & Regier, 1990). Follow-up studies using the assumptions and criteria of the original Epidemiologic Catchment Area (ECA) study while adjusting for potential underestimation due to misclassification of somatic symptoms did not significantly alter the original 1-year prevalence rates for major depression in the 65-and-over age group (Heithoff, 1995). While not detracting from the reproducibility and significance of this finding the meaning and implications for policy and intervention in regard to this finding must be carefully considered. Blazer (1993) has pointed out that relatively low rates of major depression do not imply that depression as an entity is a rare phenomenon, but rather that major depression as defined by the specific assumptions of the ECA is only the "tip of the iceberg."

The clinical significance of other variations of depression in old age is a growing concern for mental health professionals and the health care system as a whole. Both Gurland, Curland, and Curiawsky (1983) and Blazer and Williams (1980) recognized the clinically and societally significant distress of depression among older adults using community-based, cross-cultural samples and diagnostic structures not restricted to a DSM-III major depressive disorder diagnosis. Their findings of a prevalence of 10–15% of clinically significant depression is consistent with the findings of more recent studies of the general population (Horwath, Johnson, Klerman & Weissman, 1994; Judd, Rapaport, Paulus, & Brown, 1994). Whether one refers to this depression as minor, subsyndromal, or some other variation, its relevance to the clinical care of patients and challenge to our categorical diagnostic models must be acknowledged (Broadhead, Blazer, George, & Tse, 1990). While allowing for the declining likelihood of qualifying for a diagnosis of major depression among the elderly, Mirowsky and Ross (1992) examined aging as a multidimensional phenomenon, establishing that average levels of depression, as measured with a short form of the Center for Epidemiological Studies Depression Scale (CES-D), are lowest for middle-aged adults and then rise with age after 60. They attribute much of this rise to life-course and social phenomena such as retirement, widowhood, and economic hardship, along with physical deterioration and the loss of personal control. Clearly, there is variability in the construct "depression."

Further complexity is interjected through the particularity and specificity of depression's presentation within core demographic groupings. Gallo, Anthony, and Muthen (1994) reported a decreased endorsement of the dysphoria/anhedonia question within the DIS when elders are compared with younger persons. The presence of this finding, in spite of controlling for multiple other demographic factors, is an example of a variability that must be considered. Others have noted underreporting of depressive symptoms in general by older adults (Lyness et al., 1995), emphasizing the necessity of interpreting negative responses from older adults within a larger clinical context and with corroborating sources. From a cognitive-psychological perspective, older persons have distinguished themselves from younger adults by showing increased differentiation and adaptation, with a decreased propensity toward cognitive distortions, such as excessive personalization, characteristically found with depressed younger persons (Hay-slip, Galt, Lopez, & Nation, 1994).

The varied interracial differences found in the prevalence rates of depressive symptoms using the CES-D across all age groups indicates the importance of sociocultural and economic factors in determining the level of depressive symptoms (Jones-Webb & Snowden, 1993). Callahan and Wolinsky (1994) found differential response tendencies among race–gender groups when using the CES-D, suggesting sociocultural particularity in its applicability. Another study of African American males in an acute care hospital showed that self-rated symptoms are a particularly insensitive measure of depression in elderly African American men (Koenig et al., 1992).

Two potential contributing factors to the variability of depression that are of particular relevance in the elderly are bereavement and the relationship of physical illness and frailty with depression. Although bereavement can occur throughout the life cycle, the likelihood increases in late life. Bereavement does not inevitably lead to depression, but it is frequently related to depressive symptoms and exemplifies the heterogeneity of mood responses in older adults. While Zisook, Schuchter, Sledge, and Mulvihill (1993) found that elderly widows and widowers were less prone to depression than younger persons losing a spouse, De Leon, Kasl, and Jacobs (1994) found that the young-old widows (ages 65–74) retained higher depression scores well after the first year of widowhood compared to their older counterparts. This finding suggests that the context and specific coping capacities (Caserta & Lund, 1993) are central to understanding the bereavement process and the revolution of depressive symptoms within that process. Recent sleep studies challenge an arbitrary delineation between bereavement and depression, finding that the sleep patterns for some persons who would be descriptively designated as experiencing uncomplicated bereavement are more consistent with those of major depression than the sleep patterns of normal controls (Reynolds et al., 1992).

Katz has described the integral relationship of physical illness and frailty with depression in Chapter 21 in this volume, a relationship, however, that is variable and complex. Williamson and Schulz (1992) highlight the intricacy of both objective and subjective physical health in the context of other life circumstances in contributing to the development of depression. Beekman, Criegsman, Deeg, and Van Tilburg (1995) did not find a relationship between physical illness and depression in women and the young-old (ages 55–64), yet a highly significant association was found between them in men and the old-old (75 years and above). Rovner (1993) has reported that 30% of nursing home patients, who are typically among the most physically ill and frail, have major depression or clinically significant depressive symptoms and a substantially increased mortality risk. Although the risk factors for this level of depression in the long-term-care setting are not clear (Parmelee, Katz, and Lawton, 1992), the potential contribution of physical frailty must be considered via direct and indirect effects. While the prevalence rates would indicate a distinctive variant of depression in nursing homes, Zung, Broadhead, and Roth (1993) also found that older persons have increased depressive symptoms in an outpatient primary care clinical context when screened using the Zung Depression Scale (Zung, 1965).

A BIOPSYCHOSOCIAL FRAMEWORK

Having examined the variability of the presentation of depression by context as well as other factors, we propose a biopsychosocial framework within which to further construct a contextually narrative understanding of depression in old age. Light, Grigsby, and Bligh (1996) provide a theoretical construct in which gerontology can engage the biopsychosocial formulation of health care and mental health in particular. Their articulation of heterogeneity within aging as it intersects with a multidimensional understanding of persons challenges reductionistic tendencies and provides a context in which more optimally to incorporate our understanding of depressed older persons for research as well as clinical purposes. Attempts to categorize depression in a less comprehensive fashion limits our understanding of the variability of depression in elders, as well as distorts our interventions, having individual clinical and public health ramifications. An overview of the diversity of possibilities embodied within a biopsychosocial formulation of depression in old age will provide a framework for conceptualizing an integrative understanding and response. As each of these dimensions has been discussed in previous chapters within this volume, we do not to reiterate the breadth of each dimension but rather focus on the variability across dimensions of late-life depression.

Krishnan and McDonald (1993) provide an example of biological variability. They describe structural changes in the brain that are most likely secondary to atherosclerosis as delineating a specific form of late-life depression, distinguishing this from genetically mediated and psychosocially determined depression. Increased apathy may be a unique symptom in persons with this type of depression (Krishnan, Hays, Tupler, George, & Blazer, 1995). Reichman and

Coyne (1995) describe the need for sorting subjective depressive symptoms, anhedonia, and neurovegetative depressive symptoms in the context of Alzheimer's disease and multi-infarct dementia. Genetic significance in influencing depressive symptoms is argued to be primary in a twin study using two samples, with one from the American Association of Retired Persons (AARP) having an average age of 60 years, while the other was much younger (Kendler et al., 1994). The potential biologically mediated contributors to depression are substantive and varied, necessitating careful consideration when evaluating depressive symptoms in the elderly.

The psychological dimension can be conceptualized using a number of different psychological theories. While behavioral, psychodynamic, and cognitive models all contribute to our understanding of depression in older persons, they must concurrently have explanatory power concerning the continuity of personhood while adapting to change and stressors. The heterogeneity of psychological responses and the explanations of those responses challenge categorical attempts to codify those responses independent of the narrative context. While DSM-IV and its predecessors have used Axis II in their diagnostic framework as an attempt to fulfill part of this function, this type of classification of personality fosters reductionistic assumptions regarding the psychological understanding of patients and may give the false security that an adequate psychological assessment has been made.

The value of a historically and contextually sensitive psychological understanding of older patients is reflected in the findings of Andersson and Stevens (1993). Their work is based on attachment theory, as developed by Bowlby (1979). When examining early experiences with parents in relationship to a variety of psychological measures in community residents ages 65–74, poor parental attachments were significantly associated with difficulties with self-esteem, anxiety, and depression in men. The effect was stronger for older persons lacking a current attachment figure in some form of an affectionate partner, and depression was not significantly associated with poor parental attachments for women. While the gender-specific finding may be distorted by the generalized, negative well-being of unattached women irrespective of their parental attachments, the relevance of contextual and historical factors is evident. Hopefulness or the lack thereof, as represented in hopelessness, is frequently considered to be clinically determinative within psychological constructs. The mixed results of a recent study by De Vellis and Blalock (1992) convey the ambiguity and complexity in examining such factors. The self has assumed a position as a primary construct within psychological theorizing and has been defined as "a dynamic system subject to complex psychological and historical processes and as the integrating site of conflictual and multi-valence tendencies" (Labouvie-Vief, Chiodo, Goguen, Diehl, & Orwoll, 1995, p. 412). Although self-representations have been assumed to ascend to higher levels of differentiation and organization during the aging process (Baltes & Staudinger, 1993), Labouvie-Vief et al. (1995) did not find more advanced forms of thinking to be characteristically associated with old age. Rather, they found more advanced self-representations to be most likely to be associated with middle-aged adults. Wisdom and the ability to conceptualize in

terms of complexity and transformation may be more contingent upon particularities of the life course and its narrative than being generalizable expectation
of older adulthood. The capacity for wisdom and accumulated experience to
mitigate against hopelessness is likely to be dependent upon the particular
context in which it is appropriated.

Finally, within the psychological consideration of depression in old age,
one should include existential dynamics or issues of meaning. Frankl (1965),
Yalom (1980), and Erikson, Erikson, and Kivnick (1986), and many others have
contributed to the literature relating depression to existential struggles around
meaning. The clinician should also recognize that meaninglessness not only
manifests itself in depressive symptoms but may also be conveyed in other
symptoms that mask the existential dilemmas of older persons. One example of
this might be compulsive activity. Continual activity with subsequent dissipa-
tion of the older person's energy may serve to alleviate the discomforting experience of reflecting upon one's life. When considering these existential issues,
there is no definition of meaning that will apply to the particular story of each
older adult. The clinician must therefore develop some capacity to elicit the
story and search in a discerning fashion to determine if struggles of meaninglessness are a significant component of the depressive symptoms. Yalom (1980)
states that meaning usually refers to a sense of coherence, with terms such as
purpose, intention, aim, function, and *significance* frequently being used in
relation to these issues. Adequate understanding of these issues requires an
appreciation of the heterogeneity of aging, as well as clinical familiarity and
comfort with the vicissitudes of depression in old age.

The most frequent construct considered within the social dimension of a
biopsychosocial formulation of late-life depression is social support. Oxman,
Berkman, Kasl, Freeman, and Barrett (1992) examined the association between
social support and depressive symptoms in the community elderly and found
that among the social support and network factors, loss of a spouse and adequacy of emotional support and its change during the years of the study were of
the most significant. Other significant characteristics included tangible support
adequacy and its change, loss of confidant, and number of children making
weekly visits, and the change in this number during the course of the study. They
emphasized how their findings indicate the need to consider particular dimensions of social support and networks when looking for mental health outcomes
rather than global measures. As this study's findings convey the need for acknowledging the multiplicity of relevant dimensions of social support and
networks, along with the necessity of considering this multiplicity in order to
gain meaningful interpretation of these factors in relation to depression in late
life, Blazer (1993) provides seven hypotheses for understanding this relationship
as he builds on the tradition of Brown and Harris (1978). His proposed hypotheses are as follows:

1. Demographic factors such as gender, race, and age may be contributing
precipitants to the onset of depression in late life. Prejudices related to age and
loss of social roles would be included in this hypothesis. Differences in depres-

sion by race, not explained by confounding factors such as socioeconomic status, should also be included.

2. Traumatic experiences and/or impoverishment early in the life course may increase the risk for onset of late-life depression. Early developmental deprivations may induce the onset of depression, regardless of age. One should also consider that childhood deprivations will affect adult social relationships, which may in turn indirectly contribute to depression in late life. Demographic factors frequently interact with early developmental experiences.

3. Current social stressors may contribute to the onset of depressive disorders in older adults. Social stressors may in and of themselves complicate the outcome of late-life depression. Many of the studies examining the association between stressful life events and depression are based on this hypothesis.

4. A limited social network, such as few family members, few friends, and/or absence of a spouse, increases the risk for depressive disorders in late life. Most studies associating marital status with depression are based on this hypothesis. This hypothesis relates to the main effects of impaired social support in contrast to Hypothesis 7.

5. Decreased social interaction, perception of social support, and instrumental support lead to late-life depression. Impaired social network and social status, along with poor social integration into the community, may all contribute to decreased social interaction and impairment of one's perceived personal support.

6. Social disintegration is a main effect, with poor social integration leading directly to the onset and perpetuation of late-life depression. A lack of religious affiliation and a generally unstable environment may contribute directly to the induction and outcome of depression in late life.

7. The causal relationship between social stressors and depressive disorders in the elderly may be buffered by both social support and the social network. When both of these are impaired, the impact of social stress is amplified. Buffering hypotheses in regard to late-life depression are based on this hypothesis. While these hypotheses do not specifically address the intersection of social stressors and biological causes of depression, they do provide the conceptual framework for postulating mechanisms of induction, as well as mitigation, of biological factors.

Krause (1995) distinguishes social role (position in a group) from social identity (self-evaluation within a role), pointing out that individuals occupy a number of different roles concurrently within which identities of varying significance develop. The fact that a person values some roles and their respective identities more highly than others plays a significant part in defining the person's self-representation with a hierarchy developing accordingly. The hierarchy that is established with regard to emotional investment in these roles was significant in Krause's findings when he examined stress, alcohol use, and depressive symptoms in late life. His study is relevant to this chapter, as he found that alcohol use reduces the negative impact of events arising in social roles that are not highly valued by the elders, while alcohol use exacerbates the effects of stressors that emerge in relationship to the roles that are most highly valued by the older adults. Krause appropriately argues that these findings encourage continued efforts toward disaggregating stressful life-event checklists in an attempt to develop a theoretically more meaningful way of understanding the particularity to context of life stressors. In yet another study, Finch and Zautra (1992) challenge the view that there is an inverse association between socially supportive relationships and late-life depression. They found that previous methodologies had failed to detect a latent relationship between negative social ties and depression within a longitudinal model. This finding indicates the need for a more careful assessment of the valence of social dynamics within a contextual and historical frame. One final notable variant to be considered within the social dimension of a biopsychosocial model is the finding that providing support to others in the context of informal assistance, but not formal assistance, decreases depressive symptoms and enhances feelings of personal control in later life (Krause, Herzog, & Baker, 1992). The necessity of examining social parameters thoroughly in the clinical setting with an attentiveness to the tremendous potential for variability in significance of impact is evident.

NARRATIVE AS AN INTEGRATIVE
CONSTRUCT

Having discussed the limitations of reductionistically categorical diagnostic models for depression in old age, while presenting the variability within a more comprehensive biopsychosocial framework, one is left with a constructive challenge. We need an operational construct that provides fluid yet substantive structure, along with clinical utility, while retaining a contextual and historical integrity that accommodates the heterogeneity of aging and facilitates formulation of such perturbations within the life course as depression. While allowing that the many disciplines involved in the study and treatment of late-life depression have their inevitable intellectual biases and assumptions, we propose that a narrative approach to assessment and clinical care of older persons can help mitigate the competing forces in order to optimally understand and treat depression. Although narrative has been discussed in previous chapters, we want to build on those discussions in the consideration of depression. Hunter (1991) has challenged the assumption that the practice of medicine is based on scientific, factual knowledge, independent of context and historical narrative. She states that

> medicine is fundamentally narrative and its daily practice is filled with stories.... Patient's stories within medicine are more or less pared-down autobiographical accounts that chronicle the events of illness and sketch out a common sense etiology.... Physicians take such a story, interrogate and expand it, all the while transmuting it into medical information. Sooner or later they will return it to the patient as a diagnosis, an interpretive retelling that points toward the story's ending. In this way, much of the central business of caring for patients is transacted by means of narrative. (p. 5)

While Hunter focuses specifically upon the medical profession in the classical clinical context, the paradigm that she describes can be extrapolated to any interventional setting. The concept of listening to a story and then engaging in an interpretive retelling, looking toward the story's ending or finding a new story, has particular relevance for psychodiagnostic and psychotherapeutic processes. Although perhaps not openly acknowledged, contemporary mental health practitioners working under various constraints, including economic and systemic ones along with unperceived intellectual ones, attempt to avoid this narrative process and extricate the patient's symptomatic presentation out of its historical and contextual contingencies. While this may seem optimal in the immediacy of demands for efficiency, the loss of the intricacies of variability within the biopsychosocial story of the patient will inevitably lead to a more limited understanding of the patient and constrain creativity and specificity in developing interventions. Yet, is a narrative construct functional in practice? Though it may appear time consuming and at times superfluous, to reject a narrative approach, we believe, actually limits the functional viability of comprehensively assessing and caring for the depressed elderly in light of the previously described variability and heterogeneity of presentation.

Alasdair MacIntyre (1981, p. 208) states that "narrative history of a certain kind turns out to be the basic and essential genre for the characterization of human actions." The "characterization of human actions" is an elemental part of knowledge claims and developing interventions for the treatment of clinically significant phenomena. With regard to knowledge claims or epistemological challenges in general, but particularly in the context of human relationships, MacIntyre (1977) states that

> to be unable to render oneself intelligible is to risk to be taken to be mad—is, if carried far enough—to be mad. And madness or death may always be the outcomes which prevent the resolution of an epistemological crisis, for an epistemological crisis is always a crisis in human relationships. When an epistemological crisis is resolved, it is by the construction of a new narrative which enables the agent to understand *both* how he or she could intelligibly have held his or her original beliefs *and* how he or she could have been so drastically misled by them (p. 455; emphasis in original)

The construction of a new narrative is the fundamental goal of the treatment of depression in late life. A narrative construct allows, even demands, examination of the vicissitudes of depression in late life, with all of their contextual and historical contingencies, and allows for creativity and varied alternatives of adaptation in responding to that understanding. Limentani (1995) describes the transforming creative potential within the psychotherapeutic process addressing depression in late life. He states, "My own view is that we should regard old age as the fruit of our own creative actions" (p. 832). George (1996) advocates a similar position from a social–gerontological perspective, challenging social–psychological research to engage individuals as architects of their life-course trajectories. While a hopeful expectancy for a new creative narrative with active participation on the part of elders in designing a new trajectory is legitimate and appropriate, a reminder of the intricacies of the therapeutic process is embodied within the findings of Santor and Zuroff (1994). They found that older persons who describe being unable to accept the past are at an increased risk for depressive symptoms even after accounting for effects due to age, sex, and physical symptoms. A narrative psychotherapeutic model allows for an integration of a constructivist understanding of one's life within a historically, culturally, and developmentally contingent framework.

Depressed older adults may be unable to tell their stories in a way that has coherence and meaning, thereby conveying "acceptability." Acceptability of stories is determined by multiple factors, but the central determinant, both implicitly and explicitly, is the primary community in all of its historicity and cultural contingencies. The practitioner providing care for the depressed older adult should assist the patient in accessing the determinative components of his or her life-course narrative within a biopsychosocial framework with knowledge and appreciation of this community as defined by history and contemporary contextual factors such as social supports and network. It should be emphasized here that the bodily or biologically interpreted determinants of the story are central to an adequate understanding within such a narrative structure (Frank, 1995). There is only one way to gain that knowledge. "Knowledge is stories" (Schank, 1990, p. 1): stories about one's body, one's friends, one's family, and one's life experiences. We must elicit and engage the stories so as to have the particularity of knowledge with which to assist depressed elders in finding a transforming narrative for challenging the depressive symptoms and their frequent embodiment of tragedy and meaninglessness that lure persons toward violence and destructive alternatives. According to Hauerwas and Burrell (1977) a transforming narrative will embody: "(1) power to release us from destructive alternatives; (2) ways of seeing through current distortions; (3) room to keep us from having to resort to violence; and (4) a sense for the tragic: how meaning transcends power" (p. 35). The discernment of transforming narratives is a central skill to be developed by the mental health practitioner caring for the depressed elder.

While a narrative construct can imply an excessive relativity limiting the capacity for discernment to some, this is not a necessary implication. A historically and developmentally construed interpretation of narrative within the context of a particular community can allow one to discern the potential for finding a transforming narrative within the clinical presentation of a life story. It is with the particularity of community that one finds the stories that convey meaning, interpret distortions, and frame the rationalizations for violence and destruction of one's self and others. The intimacy of psychotherapy invites exploration of this particularity. The implementation of such a construct within a biopsychosocial model offers a hope for meeting the needs of older persons with their variable and diverse presentations of depression. The acceptance of one's past and the limitations of the present with affective resolve, while finding hope in working toward a new narrative that embodies a sense of competency and meaningfulness, defies overly reductionistic assumptions and methods in the assessment and treatment of depression in old age.

REFERENCES

American Psychiatric Association. (1980). *Diagnostic and statistical manual of mental disorders* (3rd ed.). Washington DC: Author.

Andersson, L., & Stevens, N. (1993). Associations between early experiences with parents and well-being in old age. *Journal of Gerontology: Psychological Sciences, 48*, P109–P116.

Baltes, P. B., & Staudinger, U. M. (1993). The search for a psychology of wisdom. *Current Directions in Psychological Science, 2*, 75–80.

Beekman, A. T. F., Kriegsman D. M. W., Deeg, D. J. H., & Van Tilburg, W. (1995). The association of physical health and depressive symptoms in the older population: Age and sex differences. *Social Psychiatry Psychiatric Epidemiology, 30*, 32–38.

Blazer, D. G., & Williams, C. D. (1980). Epidemiology of depression and dysphoria in an elderly population. *American Journal of Psychiatry, 137*, 439–443.

Blazer, D. G. (1993). *Depression in late life.* (2nd ed). St. Louis: Mosby.

Bowlby, J. (1979). *The making and breaking of affectional bonds.* London: Tavistock.

Broadhead, W. E., Blazer, D. G., George, L. K., & Tse, C. K. (1990).Depression, disability days and days lost from work in a prospective epidemiologic survey. *Journal of the American Medical Association, 264*, 2524–2528.

Brown, G. W., & Harris, T. O. (1978). *Social origins of depression.* London: Tavistock.

Calasanti, T. M. (1996). Incorporating diversity: Meaning, levels of research, and implications for theory. *Gerontologist, 36*, 147–156.

Callahan C. M., & Wolinsky, F. D. (1994). The effect of gender and race on the measurement properties of the CES-D in older adults. *Medical Care, 32*, 341–356.

Caserta. M. S., & Lund D. A. (1993). Intrapersonal resources and the effectiveness of self-help groups for bereaved older adults. *Gerontologist, 33*, 619–629.

De Leon C. F., Kasl, S. V., & Jacobs, S. (1994). A prospective study of widowhood and changes in symptoms of depression in a community sample of the elderly. *Psychological Medicine, 24*, 613–624.

De Vellis, B. M., & Blalock, S. J. (1992). Illness attributions and hopelessness depression: The role of hopelessness expectancy. *Journal of Abnormal Psychology, 101*, 257–264.

Erikson E. H., Erikson, J. M., & Kivnick H. Q. (1986). *Vital involvement in old age.* New York: Norton.

Finch, J. F., & Zautra A. U. J. (1992). Testing latent longitudinal models of social ties and depression among the elderly: A comparison of distribution-free and maximum likelihood estimates with nonnormal data. *Psychology and Aging, 7*, 107–118.

Frank, A. W. (1995). *The wounded storyteller.* Chicago: University of Chicago Press.

Frankl, V. (1965). *The doctor and the soul.* New York: Knopf.

Gallo, J. J., Anthony, J. C., & Muthen, B. O. (1994). Age differences in the symptoms of depression: A latent trait analysis. *Journal of Gerontology: Psychological Sciences, 49*, P251–P264.

George, L. K. (1996). Missing links: The case for a social psychology of the life course. *Gerontologist, 36*, 248–255.

Gurland, B. J., Copeland, J., & Curiawsky, J. (1983). *The mind and mood of aging.* New York: Haworth Press.

Hauerwas, S., & Burrell, D. (1970). From system to story: An alternative pattern for rationality in ethics. In S. Hauerwas, (Ed.), *Truthfulness and tragedy* (pp. 15–39). Notre Dame, IN: University of Notre Dame Press.

Hayslip G., Galt, C. P., Lopez F. G., Nation P. C. (1994). Irrational beliefs and depressive symptoms among younger and older adults: A cross-sectional comparison. *International Journal of Aging and Human Development, 38*, 307–326.

Heithoff, K. (1995). Does the ECA underestimate the prevalence of late life depression? *Journal of the American Geriatrics Society, 43*, 2–6.

Horwath, E. W., Johnson, J., Klerman, G. L., & Weissman, M. M. (1992). Depressive symptoms as relative and attributable risk factors for first-onset major depression. *Archives of General Psychiatry, 49*, 817–823.

Horwath, E. W., Johnson, J., Klerman, G. L., & Weissman, M. M. (1994). What are the public health implications of subclinical depressive symptoms? *Psychiatric Quarterly, 65,* 323–337.

Hunter, K. M. (1991). *Doctor's stories: The narrative structure of medical knowledge.* Princeton, NJ: Princeton University Press.

Jackson, S. (1986). *Melancholia and depression: From Hippocratic times to modern times.* New Haven, CT: Yale University Press.

Jones-Webb, R. J., & Snowden, L. R. (1993). Symptoms of depression among blacks and whites. *American Journal of Public Health, 83,* 240–244.

Judd L. L., Rapaport, M. D., Paulus, M. P., & Brown, J. L. (1994). Subsyndromal symptomatic depression: A new mood disorder? *Journal of Clinical Psychiatry, 55,* 18–28.

Kendler, K. S., Walters E. E., Truett, K. R., Heath, A. C., Neale, M. C., Martin, N. G., & Eaves, L. J. (1994). Sources of individual differences in depressive symptoms: Analysis of two samples of twins and their families. *American Journal of Psychiatry, 151,* 1605–1614.

Koenig, H. G., Meador, K. G., Goli, V., Shelp, F., Cohen, H. J., & Blazer D. G. (1992). Self-rated depressive symptoms in medical patients: Age and racial differences. *International Journal Psychiatry in Medicine, 22,* 11–31.

Krause, N. (1995). Stress, alcohol use, and depressive symptoms in later life. *Gerontologist, 35,* 296–307.

Krause, N., Herzog, A. R., & Baker, E. (1992). Providing support to others and well-being in later life. *Journal of Gerontology: Psychological Sciences, 47,* 300– 311.

Krishnan, K. R. R., & McDonald, W. M. (1993). Ateriosclerotic depression. *Medical Hypotheses, 44,* 111–115.

Krishnan, K. R. R., Hays, J. C., Tupler, L. A., George, L. K., & Blazer, D. G. (1995). Clinical and phenomenological comparisons of late-onset and early-onset depression. *American Journal of Psychiatry, 152,* 785–789.

Labouvie-Vief, G., Chiodo, L. M., Goguen L. A., Diehl, M., & Orwoll, L. (1995). Representations of Self across the life span. *Psychology and Aging, 10,* 404–415.

Light, J. M., Grigsby, J. S., & Bligh, M. C. (1996). Aging and heterogeniety: Genetics, social structure and personality. *Gerontologist, 36,* 165–173.

Limentani, A. (1995). Creativity and the Third Age. *International Journal of Psycho-Analysis, 76,* 825–833.

Lyness, J. M., Cox, C., Curry, J., Conwell, Y., King, D. A., & Caine, E. D. (1995). Older age and under-reporting of depressive symptoms. *Journal of the American Geriatrics Society, 43,* 216–221.

MacIntyre, A. (1977). Epistemological crisis, dramatic narrative, and the philosophy of science. *Monist, 60,* 453–472.

MacIntyre, A. (1981). *After virtue,* Notre Dame, IN: University of Notre Dame Press.

Mirowsky, J., & Ross, C. E. (1992). Age and depression. *Journal of Health and Social Behavior, 33,* 187–205.

Oxman, T. E., Berkman, L. F., Kasl, S., Freeman, D. H., & Barrett, J. (1992). Social support and depressive symptoms in the elderly. *American Journal of Epidemiology, 135,* 356–368.

Parmelee, P. A., Katz, I. R., & Lawton, M. P. (1992). Incidence of depression in long-term care settings. *Journal of Geriatrics: Medical Sciences, 47,* M189–M196.

Pearlin, L. I., & Skaff, M. M. (1996). Stress and the life course: A paradigmatic alliance. *Gerontologist, 36,* 239–247.

Reichman, W. E., & Coyne A. C. (1994). Depressive symptoms in Alzheimer's disease and multi-infarct dementia. *Journal of Geriatric Psychiatry and Neurology, 8,* 96–99.

Reynolds, C. F., Hoch, C. C., Buysse, D. J., Houck, P. R., Schlernitzauer, M., Frank, E., Mazumdar, S., & Kupfer, D. J. (1992). Electroencephalographic sleep in spousal bereavement and bereavement-related depression of late life. *Biological Psychiatry, 31,* 69–82.

Robins, L. N., Helzer, J. E., Croughan, J., & Ratcliff, K. S. (1981). National Institutes of Mental Health Diagnostic Interview Schedule: History, characteristics, and validity. *Archives of General Psychiatry, 38,* 381–389.

Robins, L. N., & Regier, D. A. (1990). *Psychiatric disorders in America.* New York: Free Press.

Rovner, B. W. (1993). Depression and increased risk of morality in the nursing home patient. *American Journal of Medicine, 94*(5A), 195–225.

Santor, D. A., & Zuroff, D. C. (1994). Depressive symptoms: Effects of negative affectivity and failing to accept the past. *Journal of Personality Assessment, 63*, 294–312.

Schank, R. C. (1990). *Tell me a story: A new look at real and artificial memory.* New York: Scribner's.

Wells, K. B., Stewart A., Hays, R. D., Burnam, M. A., Rogers, W., Daniels, M., Berry, S., Greenfield, S., & Ware, J. (1989). The functioning and well-being of depressed patients. *Journal of the American Medical Association, 262*(7), 914–919.

Williamson, G. W., & Schulz, R. (1992). Physical illness and symptoms of depression among elderly outpatients. *Psychology and Aging, 3*, 343–351.

Yalom, I. (1980). *Existential psychotherapy.* New York: Basic Books.

Zisook S., Shuchter, S. R., Sledge, P., & Mulvihill M. (1993). Aging and bereavement. *Journal of Geriatric Psychiatry and Neurology, 6*, 137–143.

Zung, W. W. K. (1965). A self-rating depression scale. *Archives of General Psychiatry, 12*, 63–70.

Zung, W. W. K., Broadhead, W. E., & Roth M. E. (1993). Prevalence of depressive symptoms in primary care. *Journal of Family Practice, 37*, 337–344.

CHAPTER 23

Aging and Behavioral Medicine

A Triaxial Model

DAVID I. MOSTOFSKY

INTRODUCTION

Research programs in gerontology theory and clinical geriatrics have approached
problems of aging and mental health either as separate areas of inquiry that beg
for integration and conciliation, or as coincident outcomes attributable to both
biological and psychosocial changes. The former approach would have us search
for causes that give rise to the unique physical and psychological characteristics
associated with old age, and would have us focus largely on impairments and
deficits. It would also try to bring to bear the personality and intrapsychic forces
that, together with the social and cultural setting of the specific individual, could
account for the individual differences that are noted in the effectiveness with
which one confronts old age and is often able to exert countercontrolling influence. But the causal links from biology to mental health are less than compelling.
The alterations in perceptions, emotional lability, and reality orientation are not
adequately explained by neurotransmitter chemistry. Mental health concerns
draw attention to conditions of "desertion, disability, dependency, and death"
(Herman, 1988, p. 110) as added negative and unavoidable accompaniments to
the fate of living long. This approach would appear to offer the interested
investigator the choice of investing in either elucidating basic mechanisms of
aging *or* of delineating psychosocial processes that may provide a necessary
condition for the development of mental health pathologies.

The latter approach asserts a concurrent emergence of age-related changes
with mental health problems, an approach that embraces a more promising
holistic and monistic appreciation of both aging and mental health. However, the
hallmark of such an approach is often understood to endow both the expression

DAVID I. MOSTOFSKY • Department of Psychology, Boston University, Boston, Massachusetts 02215.
Handbook of Aging and Mental Health: An Integrative Approach, edited by Jacob Lomranz. Plenum
Press, New York, 1998.

of behavior and physiological homeostasis with common modes of action, if not common or shared mechanisms. Such an assertion is clearly fraught with serious difficulties, not the least of which being that data from our current state of knowledge will not support this view. A major emphasis in this chapter is placed on the need to reconsider our conceptual framework in a way that will be seen as logically convincing and reasonable, and yet not so restrictive as to deny the role of many of the traditional hypothetical constructs and presumed intervening variables that have populated the psychological literature on these topics. In some sense, the issues of aging and mental health bear a strong resemblance to the interdisciplinary activities concerned with chronic illnesses as studied across the developmental spectrum and do not necessarily involve an obvious need for accessing psychological or psychiatric services. There are, however, important differences. Aging is not a disease ("disease: a pathological condition of the body that presents a group of symptoms peculiar to it and which sets the condition apart as an abnormal entity differing from other normal and pathological body states"; *Taber's Cyclopedic Medical Dictionary*, 12th edition). It is not contagious. Its onset is not associated with a bacterial or viral process. While it is recognized to refer to changes in structure and function that are manifest after the passage of many years, it is also acknowledged that, strictly speaking, aging begins at birth. And while structure and function—both physiological and psychological—measured during advanced age is almost always poorer than its optimal level (having occurred years earlier), the elderly are in fact often spared from suffering many of the "diseases of childhood," presumably because their constitution is actually more resistant to such sicknesses. Biological markers for aging have been rather elusive. The condition of progeria, itself a strange pathology whose definition of "precocious aging" does little to explicate matters, shares with its young victims many of the organic characteristics that are visible in geriatric populations along with senility (technically defined as "the stage of being old," but universally accepted to mean dementia associated with old age). Lipofuscin deposits, which have been shown to accompany normal aging in both humans and infrahumans, do not have any notable functional or cognitive attributes (Nandy, 1982). Clearly, aging cannot be reduced to a biological phenomenon alone. And although there may be a risk to "biologize" older people, there is no defense to exclude an examination of biological considerations in aging and gerontology (Kart, Metress, & Metress, 1992).

Mental illness, on the other hand, does in fact represent a pathological condition that presents a group of symptoms peculiar to it, and that sets the condition apart as an abnormal entity differing from other normal and pathological body states, yet the general rule seems to be to refer to many of such conditions as "disorders" rather than diseases. The implication, it appears, is that one is dealing more with some form of dysregulation rather than some truly abnormal intruder in the psychobiological system. If taken seriously, the substitution of a concept of dysregulation in place of the more popular one of deficit might well contribute to a radical shift in the course of geriatric research and in the development of therapeutic strategies appropriate for this population. Advocates of a dysregulation emphasis have noted that pathology associated with dyscontrol is reversible, whereas that associated with deficit is only compensable and not reversible (Freides, 1995). Disorders of mood are seen as disorders because they are either inappropriate, they endanger normal functioning, they aggravate preexisting or concurrent morbidities, they introduce complications in the efficient medical management of the patient's total health objectives, or they are unacceptably painful to the patient or to those who are caregivers and/or to those who comprise the social support machinery for the client/patient. Fantasy in and of itself is not necessarily an "illness." It is only when fantasy interferes with properly executing the affairs of daily living that it calls attention to the need for treatment. Grief, anxiety, thought disorganization, disinterest in vegetative behaviors, and the like are not sufficient indicators by themselves to warrant attention and treatment. When the criteria for the "illness" are met, then and only then does intervention become mandated. But does the "mental health illness" qualify for being a "disease"? The term *major depressive disorder* is largely accepted to describe a constellation of signs and symptoms (i.e., a syndrome rather than a specific pathologic process), even though there are neurobiological substrates that are unique to the condition (Duffy & Coffey, 1997). Is there a process involved? Clearly, there is no contagion. There are no bacterial or viral organisms to be destroyed. The "biological markers," such as they may be found, are not to be confused with the essential nature of the disorder itself, which is after all a disorder of behavior. There is no assurance either logically or empirically that restoring a chemical imbalance will ipso facto repair a behavioral dysfunction. The undeniable fact that certain emotional states will lead to the production or inhibition of selected physiological or neurochemical products in no way establishes that injecting adrenalin will give rise to those same emotional states. Antidepressants alone will mostly fall short of restoring normal functioning to the depressed patient, unless accompanied by a therapy program that does not depend upon drugs or electric shock exclusively.

SCIENTIFIC APPROACHES
TO CLINICAL CONCEPTS

Among the disorders that have been intensively studied and for which an underlying chemistry has been mapped in greatest detail, the problems of depression offer an exemplary model for conceptualizing a mind–body relationship and for understanding the special features of the geriatric patient who suffers from the disorder. Not infrequently, physical complaints (especially of pain) mask conditions of depression, and expressions of depression are often less psychodynamic in origin than they are products of nutritional or pharmacological side effects. More than one author has noted that depression in the elderly has been widely underdiagnosed and undertreated (Capriotti, 1995). Whether disease or not, people suffer from depression, especially older people. Whether disease or not, the disease model emphasizes the Pasteur-motivated search for "cause"—or at least the antecedents—and then proceeds to design a scientific strategy to eliminate the problem or, ideally, to eliminate the antecedent precipitant. To develop an integrated understanding of depression, aging, and treatment requires that we examine in critical yet objective fashion some of the assumptions that we have allowed to serve as the basis of our everyday practice and research. In part, the concern with our current state of prosecuting research and treatment programs for gerontological communities reflects the failure of just such a scientific perspective advocated by Pasteur so many years ago. But in that same distant past, the almost forgotten counterpoint represented by Claude Bernard appears to have resurfaced with a renewed emphasis on both the *milieu internale* and the *milieu externale* as seen in a holistic union. A premise of this chapter is that the impetus that seems to have catapulted the ill-defined area of "behavioral medicine" into much prominence in the recent past will serve well as a model for better integration and understanding within the areas of gerontology and mental health. A derivative of this premise would suggest that we may need to worry less about blazing new creative technological or methodological paths in our research and training activities, and perhaps need to reconsider whether we might have been asking too many incorrect questions. Our search for biopsychosocial "markers," for identifying and correlating "deficits," for plotting developmental trend lines, and for setting social objectives such as independent living, productivity, and the like, may have yielded some insight into narrowly defined parts of the larger system, but for all these heroic efforts, we may have missed an appreciation of the larger model of which aging and mental health comprise but a fraction of the whole.

Perhaps a starting point in our revised thinking would be to affirm a belief that we claim to hold but to which we give little evidence of supporting in our practical activities. While we are aware that our experimental designs represent a compromise between a complex and multifaceted reality that we imagine to exist and analytic technologies that we have available, we continue to pose and to examine isolated, fractionated, and nonoperationally definable questions. In doing so, we neglect opportunities for alternative question–solution protocols that have made their way into the scientific domain. It seems safe to claim that we would find agreement that the world of our existence will not be accurately represented by any linear and univariate model. Yet despite such a consensus, we have yet to attract an interest in colleagues or students to pursue alternative methods of analysis and applications that are already commonplace in the study of many nonlinear dynamic systems. Chaos and catastrophe theories, which are select examples of such nonlinear models, may or may not prove to be appropriate for the problems that we choose for study. Neural network modeling may or may not be effective in our quest to develop improved theoretical formulations of aging and mental health. But we will never know the value of these options unless we attempt to put them to test. While it would be too much to expect that we can begin running from a cold start, a critical reflection on our current conceptualizations of order and disorder may begin to suggest implications that we have not thought of heretofore.

A TRIAXIAL CONTINUUM
IN BEHAVIORAL MEDICINE

Much of the thinking that has evolved in defining the rationale for behavioral medicine—particularly as it relates to the development of rational treatment and intervention strategies—is concerned with a perspective and approach, rather than with any new theoretical or technological innovation. At its best, it is expected to offer scientific rigor to psychosocial and psychobiological interactions by drawing upon findings that are derived from properly executed studies and properly interpreted empirical results. By general agreement, discussions in the area of behavioral medicine are limited to topics and issues in non-mental-health medicine, yet we should anticipate that the methodological shifts introduced in these areas will prove to be valuable when applied to considerations of aging and mental health as well. By adopting a different perspective, we would allow ourselves the luxury to reconsider concepts and relations that we hold dear, and even to be moved to consider posing questions other than the ones we have been accustomed to, or to reevaluate the familiar ones we now favor, but in a different light. At the very least, we would be able to restore and redirect the discussion of both aging and mental health so as to recognize the centrality of *behavior*.

An important document, "Vitality for Life: Psychological Research for Productive Aging" (American Psychological Society, 1993) summarized the consensus of a number of participating organizations and individuals who declared that, first and foremost, aging is a behavioral issue. The report recognized the first among four priorities for funding and research efforts, that of "Health: Understanding and changing health behaviors to promote productive aging," further noting that

> we must develop an understanding of how to change behaviors which damage health
> and how to maintain behaviors which promote health…. Although longevity has in-
> creased in past years, quality of life has not necessarily shown a similar increase. (p. 8)

The business of changing behaviors has preoccupied many scientists and clinicians. Therapists, broadly defined, have opted for a variety of strategies and techniques that have evolved and have been derived from theory, tradition, and temperamental attraction to a particular style. And like the wise but blind men of Hindustan, who disputed the essence of what is an elephant, "each was partly in the right, and all were in the wrong."

In an attempt to provide an alternative I have suggested elsewhere (Mostofsky, 1981, 1997) that any sickness condition can be best evaluated by considering its properties positioned among three different and independently derived factors (although the factors will not necessarily be orthogonal). Although it would probably be more technically accurate to represent such a model in a three-dimensional display, as a practical matter it may be easier to identify the respective characteristics when projected in a continuous and linear fashion, as shown in Figure 23–1.

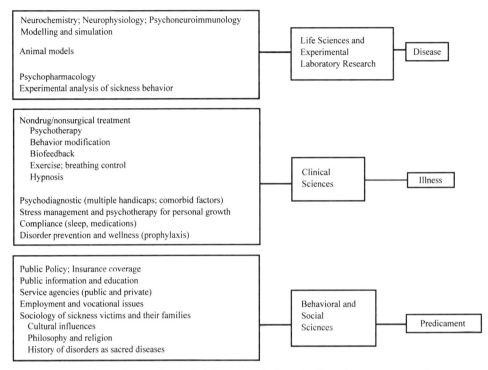

Figure 23–1. Three dimensions of sickness and chronic disorders represented as a continuum of disease, illness, and predicament.

When considering classic health problem, the separate axes refer to "disease," "illness," and "predicament." The progression from top to bottom, corresponding to "hard science" and "soft disciplines," respectively, reflects the correlated stereotyped and parochial strengths offered by the different professions. Each axial may be recognized by its "symptoms" that are common to it alone, and each axis has properties that allow it to undergo change and modification. It is notable that in this conceptual framework, the hunt for "precursors" is not exclusively centered in the brain, any more than it must necessarily be found in the "psyche." As can be seen from Table 23–1, elements of a sickness have different meanings and implications depending on which of the axes are to be considered. Most important is the recognition that the axes do not depend on each other for validation. One can be diagnosed with a disease that does not have any expression of "illness" or restriction of function (e.g., hypertension). Similarly, one may suffer from a "predicament" that may or may not coexist with a disease or illness aspect (e.g., an overbearing personality). The classification scheme leaves open the possibility that any intervention may operate on but a single axis, or that it may interact with one or both of the others. But, above all, the domain of the behavioral medicine activities spans a universe of disciplines and addresses questions that range from micromolecular properties of an or-

Table 23–1. The Dimensions of Sickness

Disease	Illness	Predicament
1. Physical reality not necessarily organ specific.	1. Declaration of disease in symptomatic form; organ specific.	1. Complex of social ramifications with immediate bearing on the individual.
2. Specific change in organ or tissue	2. Social manifestation, usually a limitation	2. Diffuse, multifactorial, personal, but not necessarily unique.
3. May be trivial.	3. May change for better or worse; does not reclassify the "disease."	3. Very unstable structure.
4. Vaild without "illness." Does not depend on implication for its existence.	4. Vaild without discoverable disease.	4. Valid without disease or illness.
5. Amoral.	5. Probably judged "morally." Modified by psychosocial processes.	5. Highly charged with moral implications; dependent on social mores.
6. Diagnosis means discovery: specifies structural functional change.	6. Diagnosis means description and semantic reattribution.	6. Diagnosis means discernment.
7. Spac, place, and time are irrelevant.	7. Space, place, and time are very relevant; modified by developmental processes. Significance expands and contracts.	7. Space, place, and time are paramount.
8. Knowledge grows with investigation.	8. Knowledge grows with classification.	8. Knowledge grows with understanding.
9. Search for specific therapy for reconciliation.	9. Search for palliation and personal change.	9. Search social and political remedies.

Source: Adapted with permission from Mostofsky (1981).

ganic entity, or that concern themselves at various times with psychological and social forces that affect the course and severity of a disorder, and that engage community, social agencies, and governmental policies, all of whom have serious bearing on the status of the individual's health problem. This organizational schema is designed to facilitate a better appreciation of the target complaint and would regard genetic, personality, developmental, and psychosocial processes as modulators of the essential properties that comprise the axis under study. The schema is not designed to provide an explanatory umbrella for all possible variables that may interact with psychological or biological variables. The formulation allows us to better appreciate that mental states may (or may not) aggravate preexisting health and organic states, or that attitudes and reimbursement policies in effect in a given culture and political setting can be major predicament factors in the ability of persons to tolerate or to improve the status of their quality of living.

It should be noted without qualification that conceptualizing the separate dimensions of sickness as different does not preclude the realization that a purely psychological or social (contextual) set of conditions may indeed be the precursor of a structural disease element. We have long appreciated the effect of physiological systems on behavior, but only recently has there been a willingness to consider that behaviors and psychological and/or social states may bring about changes in physiology (Mostofsky, 1976). Of particular importance to clinical management in gerontological settings are findings such as those by Langer (1989), which demonstrate the crucial role played by the perception and activities of exercising control in modulating health, quality of life, and longevity itself. Other reports confirm remarkable neurobiological changes secondary to psychosocial crises (Post, 1992). Given the scientific validity of illness and predicament contributions to disease, it should not be surprising to expect salutary functional and environmental conditions to foster beneficial results at the level of biological organization.

STRUCTURE, FUNCTION, AND CONTEXT

But since aging is hardly a "disorder," the triaxial labels require some translation. Without loss of precision, an equivalent for the coordinate system of disease–illness–predicament can be labeled as a *structure–function* and *contextual* system. And perhaps the much maligned designation of a "biopsychosocial" approach toward a study of aging is comfortably represented by these very same labels of structure–function and context. The behavioral medicine orientation adds a few critical wrinkles, however, including but not limited to the following points:

1. An underlying biological process accompanying advancing years does not by itself serve as a causal factor in any behavioral restriction of function. And while one might speculate that biological changes (e.g., changes in emotional thresholds) may actually serve to *facilitate* or to *improve* personal and interpersonal conduct, one cannot compellingly reach such a correlation on the basis of observed biological change alone. Disease (structure) may exist completely without traces of illness (nontrivial restricted function). And though the elderly may be perceived by themselves and by others as endowed with greater "wisdom," these data, by themselves, cannot compellingly argue for the presence of any concurrent biological changes (Denney, Dew, & Kroupa, 1995; Orwoll & Perlmutter, 1990).

2. A corollary of the independence among the facets of these factors suggests that treatment or intervention at the disease (structure) level does not guarantee changes in behavioral or contextual variables (Birren, Woods, & Williams, 1980; Baddeley, Sunderland, & Harris, 1982). The distinctions, however, do not preclude changes taking place beyond the limited domain for which they are initially targeted.

3. A corresponding corollary would remind us that change in function cannot by itself impute underlying biological alterations in structure. We may briefly examine the classic example of senility as it has been brought to us from much experimentation with infrahumans and to a lesser degree from postmortem sections of human patients. Senility, as it is popularly represented, is not a normal manifestation of the aging process (Besdine et al., 1980). Senility cannot even be accurately called a "disease"; rather, it is a term that is used improperly to describe a wide variety of conditions that arise from an equally wide variety of causes (Larson, Sjögren, & Jacobson, 1963; Perret & Birri, 1982; Siobhan, Semple, Smith, & Swash, 1982). The mere presence of differences in cognitive performance, albeit statistically significant, must be recognized as distinctively different in kind and form from pathological impairments of cognitive systems. The demonstrations, however reliable, that aged animals and/or aged humans have longer response and reaction times or take longer to verbalize their answers to survey questions, respectively, do not by themselves constitute pathology (Birren et al., 1980). The once accepted truism that age-induced memory deficits inevitably result from the aging process, which is typified by hardening of the arteries, was soundly rejected, following numerous studies that indicated that blood flow in healthy elderly subjects was not significantly decreased compared to control subjects, which were as much as 50 years younger. Similar results were found when total brain oxygen consumption was compared between the two groups. Replications of these studies concluded that only 12–17% of age-related cognitive deficits were related to impaired vascular functioning, whereas a full 50% of mentally impaired elderly subjects present with pathological signs in brain autopsies. From the reports appearing in the current literature, one is left with the clear impression that more recent studies that have employed MRI and similar technologies support these findings.

If the progression of aging does not lead to the claimed ravages of cognitive and functional decline, as would be implied by a "disease" process, then we are left with examining the "aging-related" dysfunctions as "illness" conditions. As with physical illnesses, mental health conditions present severe limitations on normal behavior routines and can exist without a predisposing biological substrate. Indeed, as can be seen from Table 23–1, illness does not require a documented disease base for validating its existence. And, as with somatic illness, conditions such as depression force us to search for correlations both intrinsic and extrinsic to the patient. Personality, sex, situational factors, and, above all, age have been justifiably the focus of much research attention over the last few decades. These investigations have enriched our understanding of the nature of illness variations and of the "factor loadings" that might enable us to offer predictions among subgroups of the population at large. Perhaps, therefore, the almost consensual accepted perception that those in later life are particularly vulnerable to depression and suicide (de Leo & Diekstra, 1990) derives from some of this research. Furthermore, there are suggestions that a higher percentage of admissions on the psychiatric units were considered appropriate, and overall psychological assessment was better on the psychiatric unit (Norquist et al.,

1995). Such findings may well bias our expectations to anticipate mental health complications and to regard depression (in particular) as normative among those of advancing age. Without regard to the influence of predicament and culture, we may also perpetuate the bias that it is a natural given for women to be at greater risk for depression than men. While this may be true for those residing in developed countries (where the ratio is about 2:1), the ratio in developing countries varies, with most studies reporting no differences in ratios attributable to gender difference (Culbertson, 1997).

Sadly, it is often the aged themselves that attribute such "normative" states to themselves, and, in doing so, make it difficult for primary care physicians to address somatic complaints, many of which may mask a truly depressive state and/or which, when treated by medication, may adversely affect cognitive behavior and functioning. Common misperceptions of aging and illness that affect the assessment process, and that can be identified as the source of the ways in which many older patients interpret their illnesses and their expectations of treatment including the following:

- Old age is something to be denied or avoided at all costs.
- Age is a legitimate excuse for not being compliant or for poor health practices. After all: "What difference will it make at this point?"
- There should be a remedy for every illness and pain, and it is the physician's responsibility to prescribe one.
- Memory lapses should be concealed, because they might be a sign of senility.
- Chronic illnesses should be approached and dealt with in the same way as any other illness.
- Reducing one's pace or, "taking it easy," is an appropriate response to most complaints of age and illness (Hichey, 1988, p. 63).

ALTERNATIVE HYPOTHESES

There would appear to be an alternative conceptualization to understanding the change in function with the passage of time. One must admit for consideration that the "illness" of depression is in essence a change in function, to be sure, but one that is psychobiologically beneficial. While there can be hardly anything joyful about witnessing one's close friends and family slowly but inexorably disappearing from the ranks of the living, perhaps the response to reflect, to withdraw, and even to grieve may be appreciated as an adaptive and constructive response, strengthened and maintained by positively reinforcing consequences. It was, after all, B. F. Skinner who reminded us that a reinforcer is not to be defined by the physical properties of the item or stimulus event, but rather that the reinforcer represents the relationship enjoyed by the person and his or her history of exposure to the universe of behaviors and consequences that will ultimately define the motivation to pursue or to retract from future exposure with the consequential stimulus.

To turn the question of relating aging to mental health into a search for a conceptual framework that will illuminate our appreciation of a social–biological–psychological entity is no small challenge (Millenson, 1995). It may well come at a cost that will require us to abandon a comfortable set of assumptions that has directed our research and training activities for a long time. And if the price for asking such altered questions brings us into contact with the shady world of "alternative" medicine, with all its herbs, potions, magic elixirs and modern-day versions of exotic techniques and technologies, so be it. If with advancing age comes wisdom—a quality and property of functioning that emerges only at selected segments of the developmental spectrum—might it not require an equally new and different perspective on what is "adaptive" or "age appropriate"? Granting that healthy lifestyles, both physical and emotional, are always to be preferred, might it not be that our definitions and criteria for such targeted objectives will be different, so much so that we may regard some of them as "unhealthy" when they appear at a different stage of development? And even for those healthy objectives, might it not be that conventional psychotherapeutic and behavior modification protocols, which are properly prescribed for similar behavior changes occurring among younger patients/clients presenting with identical symptomatologies, are *inappropriate* with the aging? Not because they will not work, but because they may alter the beneficial contribution of these "illness" conditions that render the survivor *more* resistant to attack. The better question may yet be not *how* to motivate older patients to change, but rather *whether* and *when*, and *why* undertake such a mission (Sennott-Miller & Kligman, 1992). Such a position shares with Ryff (1995) the observation that a conceptual framework built on arbitrary standards of mental health bears little resemblance to extant scientific studies of subjective well-being, in which measures of happiness and life satisfaction are the reigning empirical indicators.

If there is merit to a triaxial conceptualization that embraces structure–function and context, we should be open to consider what we might wish to change at the predicament level *independent* of any illness marker (i.e., even when no apparent limitation on functions seems present). We should also admit to the possibility that while there is no *compelling* reason for the three elements of the continuum to interact with one another, that possibility must be considered as a reasonable outcome. Our efforts at the social management of depression or of the aging populations may yet prove to exert influences at the level of biological substrates, and it goes without saying that we should not be surprised to expect improvements in many areas that constitute "quality of life" and personal functioning. The nature of the behavioral medicine enterprise forces us to consider the inherent interdisciplinarity of approaching disorder problems. Insofar as our professional focus is directed toward social and psychological variables and issues, we are no less free to disregard the world of the immune system (and its responsiveness to behavioral, emotional, and environmental conditions), the central nervous system (and its responsiveness to behavioral, emotional, and environmental conditions) and the associated neurochemistry that is the setting for much of the organic activity that is within us. It may seem odd to involve the social worker and clinical psychologist in topics that heretofore have been considered the exclusive province of the life science specialist, but it is only through such integration of training and cross-disciplinary fertilization of ideas that we can hope to arrive at any innovative theory development for old age and mental health.

EPILOGUE

The chapters of this volume each, in its own way, reflect the considered views of different orientations that are designed to enable us to deliberate and to think out loud about theoretical formulations that concern the various facts, speculations, and predictions with regard to aging and mental health: what they are and how to improve on them for the future. Although theory development in the psychology of aging has not escaped the attention of gerontologists, each of these chapters, by its very inclusion, testifies to the inadequate status by which the social and health sciences have attempted to represent a comprehensive formulation or understanding of aging and mental health (Bengtson, Parrott, & Burgess, 1996; Schroots, 1996). Certainly, we appear to be a far distance from proposing grand theories that can be submitted to experimental verification. The present chapter is no different. It, too, offers its modest message in the hope that current and future scholars and practitioners will direct attention to the need for recognizing more operationalized questions and strategies for effecting change. While such thinking is too often associated with a parochial "behaviorist" orientation, one would hope that it may be seen as a compatible and, indeed, natural ingredient for reliable progress and development when applied to any other theoretical system. A special effort has been made to direct the reader's attention to the need for recognizing a distinction among structure, function, and context. Encouraged by the fact that classical problems of *non*-mental-health disorders and sickness have attracted interest among the social and behavioral sciences as well as the life sciences and medicine, such a distinction should prove to be most valuable for explicating problems in the aging and gerontological areas as well. For example, it liberates one from the constraining demands to demonstrate that psychotherapeutic intervention has any direct effect on a condition for which a presumed (or even established) organic pathophysiology is assumed to predispose the patient/client to suffering. Indeed, the ability to demonstrate such a direct effect is too often seen as a requirement to validate such interventions. The proposed formulation would certainly view such an assertion as erroneous.

The triaxial distinction also allows for the possible interaction of even remote social change to impact disease and illness, and the implications are hardly trivial. Among the obvious implications that derive from a multidimensional nosology in mental health are the need to address more than a single orientation and to design interdisciplinary curricula to attract disciplines that are not yet major players in either the game of aging or of mental health, and to commit ourselves to broaden the base of our thinking and experimentation to include multivariate and nonlinear protocols and analytical models. While we have long toyed with the tongue-twister of "biopsychosocial," we need to move to the next level to create programs—research, training, and clinical—that, when brought to fruition, will be able to offer improved functioning for elderly persons in ways that will be clinically significant.

REFERENCES

Antonovsky, A. (1979). *Health, stress, and coping.* San Francisco: Jossey-Bass.

American Psychological Society. (1993). Vitality for life: Psychological research for productive aging. *APA Observer* [Special Issue], Report No. 2.

Baddeley, A., Sunderland, A., & Harris, J. (1982). How well do laboratory-based psychological tests predict patients' performance outside the laboratory? In S. Corkin, K. L. Davis, J. H. Growdon, E. Usdin, & R. J. Wurtman (Eds.), *Alzheimer's disease: A report of progress in research: Vol. 19: Aging* (pp. 141–148). New York: Raven Press.

Bengtson, V. L., Parrott, T. M., & Burgess, E. O. (1996). Progress and pitfalls in gerontological thinking. *Gerontologist, 36,* 768–772.

Besdine, R. W., Brody, J. A., Butler, R. N., Duncan, L. E., Jarvik, L., & Libow, L. (1980). Senility reconsidered. *Journal of the American Medical Association, 244,* 259–263.

Birren, J. E., Woods, A. M., & Williams, M. V. (1980). Behavioral slowing with age: Causes, organization, and consequences. In L. W. Poon (Ed.), *Aging in the 1980's* (pp. 293–308). Washington, DC: American Psychological Association.

Capriotti, T. (1995). Unrecognized depression in the elderly: A nursing assessment challenge. *Medsurg Nursing, 4*(1), 47–54.

Culbertson, F. M. (1997). Depression and gender. *American Psychologist, 52,* 25–31.

de Leo, D., & Diekstra, R. F. W. (1990). *Depression and suicide in late life.* Toronto: Hogrefe & Huber.

Denney, N. W., Dew, J. R., & Kroupa, S. L. (1995). Perceptions of wisdom: What is it and who has it? *Journal of Adult Development, 2,* 37–47.

Duffy, J. D., & Coffey, C. E. (1997). The neurobiology of depression. In M. R. Trimble & J. L. Cummings (Eds.), *Contemporary behavioral neurology* (pp. 275–288). Boston: Butterworth–Heinemann.

Freides, D. (1995). Autism and other pervasive disorders: Proposal for a paradigmatic shift. Unpublished manuscript.

Hayflick, L. (1988). Why do we live so long? *Geriatrics, 43,* 77–87.

Herman, C. D. (1988). Insights into aging: Desertion, disability, dependency, and death. *Geriatric Medicine Today, 7,* 108–116.

Hickey, T. (1988). Changing health perceptions of older patients and the implications for assessments. *Geriatric Medicine Today, 7,* 59–66.

Hobfoll, S. E. (1989). Conservation of resources. *American Psychologist, 44,* 513–524.

Kart, C. S., Metress, E. K., & Metress, S. P. (1992). *Human aging and chronic disease.* Boston: Jones & Bartlett.

Langer, E. J. (1989). *Mindfulness.* Reading, MA: Addison-Wesley.

Lappe, M. (1994). *Evolutionary medicine: Rethinking the origins of disease.* New York: Sierra Club Books.

Larson, T., Sjögren, T., & Jacobson, G. (1963). Senile dementia: A clinical, socio-medical and genetic study. *Acta Psychiatria Scandinavia, 39*(Suppl. 167), 1–259.

Millenson, J. R. (1995). *Mind matters.* Seattle: Eastland Press.

Mostofsky, D. I. (1976). *Behavioral control and modification of physiological activity.* Englewood Cliffs, NJ: Prentice-Hall.

Mostofsky, D. I. (1981). Recurrent paroxysmal disorders of the central nervous system. In S. M. Turner, K. S. Calhoun, & H. E. Adams (Eds.), *Handbook of clinical behavior therapy* (pp. 447–474). New York: Wiley.

Mostofsky, D. I. (1997). Behavioral treatment. In M. R. Trimble & J. L. Cummings (Eds.), *Behavioral neurology* (pp. 327–336). Oxford, UK: Butterworth Heinemann.

Nandy, K. (1982). Neuronal lipofuscin and its significance. In D. Platt (Ed.), *Geriatrics* (pp. 257–262). Berlin: Springer-Verlag.

Nesse, R. M., & Williams, G. C. (1994). *Why we get sick*. New York: Times Books.

Norquist, G., Wells, K. B., Rogers, W. H., Davis, L. M., Kahn, K., & Brook, R. (1995). Quality of care for depressed elderly patients hospitalized in the specialty psychiatric units or general medical wards. *Archives of General Psychiatry, 52*, 695–XXX.

Orwoll, L., & Perlmutter, M. (1990). The study of wise persons: Integrating a personality perspective. In R. J. Sternberg (Ed.), *Wisdom: Its nature, origins and development* (pp. 160–177). New York: Cambridge University Press.

Perret, E., & Birri, R. (1982). Aging, performance decrements and differential: Cerebral involvement. In S. Corkin, K. L. Davis, J. H. Growdon, E. Usdin, & R. J. Wurtman (Eds.), *Alzheimer's disease: A report of progress in research: Vol. 19, Aging* (pp. 133–140). New York: Raven Press.

Post, R. M. (1992). Transduction of psychosocial stress into the neurobiology of recurrent affective disorder. *American Journal of Psychiatry, 149*, 999–1010.

Ryff, C. D. (1995). Psychological well-being in adult life. *Current Directions in Psychological Science, 4*, 99–104.

Sacher, G. A. (1980). Theory in gerontology: Part 1. In C. Eisdorfer (Ed.), *Annual review of gerontology and geriatrics* (pp. 3–25). New York: Springer.

Schroots, J. J. F. (1996). Theoretical developments in the psychology of aging. *Gerontologist, 36*, 742–748.

Sennott-Miller, L., & Kligman, E. W. (1992). Healthier lifestyles: How to motivate older patients to change. *Geriatrics, 47*, 52–59.

Siobhan, A., Semple, C., Smith, C. M., & Swash, M. (1982). The Alzheimer disease syndrome. In S. Corkin, S. L. Davis, J. H. Growdon, E. Usdin, & R. J. Wurtman (Eds.), *Alzheimer's disease: A report of progress in research, Vol. 19, Aging* (pp. 93–108). New York: Raven Press.

Williams, G. C., & Nesse, R. M. (1991). The dawn of Darwinian medicine. *Quarterly Review of Biology, 66*, 1–22.

Epilogue

Future Perspectives

Jacob Lomranz

The area of mental health is obviously interwoven in, and to a certain extent dependent on, the larger field of gerontology. At the end of the twentieth century, we have to ask: Where is the field of gerontology and the area of mental health in aging at this point, and where are they going? While our achievements have, to a great extent, laid the foundations for future developments in the field in the next century, it may be rather difficult to answer this question, especially in light of theorizing. The implications of the history and multidimensionality of the field precludes us at this time from inferring its exact future course. Achenbaum (1995), asking how far gerontology has become a science, concludes: "Thus by the end of the twentieth century, gerontology has emerged as a field, not a scientific specialty. Indeed, some researchers on aging have begun to subvert the assumption that gerontology should be classified primarily as a 'science'" (p. 253). The field may deepen its specialties and subfields, may become more coherent and integrated, or, to the contrary, it may be come dissolved as the different areas are incorporated in the various specialties and related scientific domains. A prominent founder of gerontology, Neugarten (1994), has predicted "the end of gerontology," since age in itself cannot be maintained as a criterion for theory or research. In fact, a model by which an expert on human cells also functions as a "gerontologist," or a physician or clinical psychologist is able to treat adolescent clients as well as elderly ones, may be rationally defended. Our perhaps hidden assumptions regarding the concept of a "unified science of aging" should be clarified. Being biopsychosocial human beings, we note the inherent multidimensionality of aging, and it has yet to be demonstrated that the quest for gerontology as a unified science can be attained. Psychology, for

JACOB LOMRANZ • Department of Psychology and the Herczeg Institute on Aging, Tel Aviv University, 69978, Tel Aviv, Israel.

Handbook of Aging and Mental Health: An Integrative Approach, edited by Jacob Lomranz. Plenum Press, New York, 1998.

instance, with its different branches, including "hard-core" scientific research applications, seems to be becoming more compartmentalized, and at the same time some of its branches have nearly been incorporated into other disciplines (e.g., the neurosciences). To what extent can we, or do we want to, avoid a similar development in gerontology?

It is my belief, however, that as gerontology and its branch of mental health become truly multidisciplinary in a more meaningful manner than at present, a course that may entail a paradigmatic shift in its research, they will remain unique as a viable major scientific field in the family of science. In order to embark on such a course, a number of future theoretical developments may be required, and certain issues should be highlighted. First and foremost, the various disciplines of the gerontological tree must be deepened and interrelated, and integrative efforts invested in specialized fields without neglecting inter- disciplinary efforts. As Estes, Binney, and Culbertson (1992) note, "We lack an age disciplinary perspective or stronghold, while we also lack the models and support for truly interdisciplinary work" (p. 43). Providing these should lead to novel frameworks that will incorporate existing research, produce new models for future research, and result in more appropriate multidisciplinary construc- tions. Some further projected goals are as follows:

1. *Developmental perspectives in a multidisciplinary framework*: Future multidisciplinary investigations in mental health of the elderly should be increasingly anchored in lifespan models of aging (Baltes, 1987; Schulz & Heckhausen, 1996), and the trap of biological or psychosocial reductionism must be avoided. Biological, psychological, environmen- tal, and behavioral factors should be more successfully integrated into lifespan developmental frameworks and constructed better to fit the multidisciplinary metaphor of mental health. Advances in aging and mental health will require tighter interactions between theory, basic and clinical research, and application (Katz, 1995).

2. *Gerontologists are challenged by questions about the kinds of theories*, in terms of structural organization as well as content and methods of observation that they should adopt, as well as the *kind* of science they strive for. Theorists would have to ask themselves whether they are following "traditional theory" (empirical, predictive, and value free) or "critical theory" (hermeneutic and grounded in values and human interests), and whether theories in clinical gerontology can be con- structed with moral indifference (Moody, 1988). We also have to ask ourselves to what extent the different "theories" in gerontology (e.g., disengagement theory, activity theory, exchange theory) help us to un- derstand mental health and systematically examine the utility of cur- rent conceptualization in explaining various aspects of mental health in the aged.

3. *Theories should be interrelated*: many of the present conceptual frame- works may become integrated in new conceptualizations (e.g., the the- ory of gerotranscendence [Tornstam, 1992] may incorporate disengage-

ment theory as well as Erikson's concept of integrity) and further novel attempts to integrate the bio-psycho-socio-multidimensional components in higher structural theoretical levels should emerge (e.g., gerodynamics/ branching theory—Schroots, 1995; thanatology in a lifespan framework— Kastenbaum, 1985).

4. *Induction and deduction in a dialectic relationship* in gerontological inquiry: Many of the conceptualizations in this volume are based on empirical data, and theory construction in science has often proceeded from induction, observation, and organization of research, enabling the formulation of orderly patterns and sequences to deductive schemata, a conceptual structure with central assumptions and corollaries permit- ting hypothesis testing and prediction. It seems that in the future, research in gerontology will progress in light of a dialectic process be- tween these two models (i.e., the interplay of inductive conceptualiza- tions expanded to deductive formulations continuously being revised as data is further generated in an inductive manner; Riegel, 1976). This trend will gain impetus through the recent innovations in research methodology (Schaie, 1988).

5. *Qualitative* (e.g., Birren, Kenyon, Ruth, Schroots, & Svensson, 1996) *and quantitative research methods need to be unified in the future.* While basically a core methodological endeavor, this will reflect the further, long-awaited theoretical integration between science, the humanities, and the helping professions. Further advancing statistical methods (e.g., structural equation modeling, hierarchical linear modeling, mathemati- cal formulations, event history analysis, etc.) may facilitate conceptual frameworks and raise basic theoretical questions.

The aforementioned issues all have a direct bearing upon the field of mental health and aging, as development strives to "cross frontiers" (Achenbaum, 1995) horizontally (to other related disciplines) as well as vertically (moving a stage up in achieving paradigmatic shifts and progress in science).

Relating specifically to clinical gerontology, we note that the area of mental health for the elderly seems to be heading for a major crisis in the coming years as mental health needs grow but mental health care and Medicare reimburse- ments shrink. It is estimated that the needs of older adults in the year 2020, when 80 million baby-boomers pass the age 65, may triple. Mental health clinicians and researchers will be confronted with members of a cohort who, in addition to the brain diseases, may forcefully retrieve the category of "neuroticism," in the repertoire of geropsychiatry. This is a group with high rates of emotional dis- orders, mainly depression, suicide, anxiety, and drug abuse, despite the fact that these baby-boomers grew up during a time of unprecedented scientific advance, technological growth, and economic prosperity (Koenig, George, & Schneider, 1994). Clinical gerontology does not seem to be ready to meet these challenges. Added to the absence of appropriate policies and organizational settings, the field of *education* is far from equipped to meet scientific and applied needs: One of the most distressing facts is that most students and clinicians do not have much interest in clinical geropsychology or gerontology. While the shortage and growing need for mental health clinicians has continuously been underscored, unfortunately, these remonstrations have not been heeded (Gatz & Finkel, 1995; Santos & VandenBos, 1982). Gutmann (1992) correctly states that "we have to revitalize and redirect teaching, research, and practice.... Paradigm shifts are required to thaw our frozen, biased conceptions of the aging population" (p. 7). Progress in theory construction should attract to the field clinicians who may presently feel that they have no reliable conceptual basis.

To move ahead, the field of gerontological mental health should seek the possible practical applications of theoretical gerontology and consider, among others, the following issues in light of future developments:

Metaphors and models: In an early paradigmatic stage, concepts, ideas, and metaphors may be retained and used, although they may present assumptions and concepts that have been outdated or are irrelevant (Kuhn, 1967). The present metaphors about aging and mental health reinforce continued separation of human entities (e.g., "age," "disability," and "disease") as if they existed in separate realms. At the same time, other basic entities such as ethnicity, gender, and class need to be expanded further and incorporated into clinical gerontology. Mental health metaphors and models may be largely rhetorical and superfluous, many of them initially not created for the aging population (Birren & Lanum, 1991). Various *definitions of abnormality* and clinical diagnostic categories, for instance, may not be relevant to the elderly. Such definitions have always been time-, space- and culture-bound, and have changed accordingly. Various behaviors regarded as psychopathology, such as behaviors grounded in loss, daily stress, or depression, should be reconceptualized in light of the asynchronalized existential predicament of the aged in society. It seems that clinical gerontology should further clarify its relationship to the philosophy of science as well as to its images of human nature and of the elderly. Thus, a future challenge is to reconcile and change our scientific metaphors and images of mental health in the aged in light of present culture and on the basis of clinical observation, conceptualization, and treatment.

SPECIFIC CROSS-FERTILIZATIONS

Bridges between disciplines are weak. The coming years will witness further gains and expansion of the biomedical field. Future gains in basic neurobiology and in human genetics can be expected to afford major opportunities for research advances in geriatric mental health. Gerontologists must take care not to trail behind such developments, but must become part of them in a multidimensional framework. Another such instance regards the cross-fertilization of social psychology and the dynamic life-course perspective, as George (1966) has elaborated in an illuminating exposition. Such a link would enrich the adult developmental mental-health-related areas of personality, identity, self-concept, family relations, cultural meanings, and the notions of well-being, transition, and heterogeneity—all then expanding the conceptual basis of mental health in later life.

Other islands that need to be bridged in relation to clinical gerontology are, to my mind, sociology and psychology. The two disciplines play a prominent role in gerontology. Sociology has supplied a major basis that, in many ways, has made "social gerontology" a viable field and is responsible for our knowledge and awareness of the social, institutional, and cultural aspects of aging. However, while the two disciplines share common research interest (e.g., in concepts such as the self, identity, family, etc.), vast areas of psychology, such as the fields of personality, cognitive psychology, and clinical psychology are underrepresented in sociology and, as a matter of fact, in gerontology in general. While psychology has richly contributed to gerontology and added special areas of investigation, for example, in the domains of research methodology, biological, medical, cognitive, personality, family, social, and environmental influences on behavior, and psychological applications to the individual and to society (see Birren & Schaie, 1977, 1985, 1990, 1996), it is my contention that these do not have a strong enough impact on the basic "psychosocial stream" of gerontology in general and on mental health specifically. Psychology, I believe, has not sufficiently addressed the inner life of the elderly person, and has not succeeded in introducing individuality—intrapsychically as well as interpersonally—into gerontology. Elderly individuals need more to be viewed as active, meaning searching, creative, self-structuring, energetic organisms, as dynamic travelers on the life course. Such an impact would also substantially enhance our knowledge in the more sociological-emphasized research areas such as heterogeneity, role of gender, transitions, and life-course trajectories, which would all benefit from the supplementation of individual differences and the comprehension of the processes of individuation and personal dynamics. Such cross-fertilization would certainly enrich the behavioral basis of the field of mental health in the aged.

Theories of human nature, change processes, and personality should be the sources of clinical methodology. We should further seek to bridge biology, medical approaches, sociology, and social theory with the psychology of mental health and aging in order to provide a firmer basis for clinical gerontology.

CLINICAL PSYCHOLOGY AND AGING

Clinical psychology in itself will have to expand and increase its impact when it comes to the aged. Elderly people should benefit from all the existing helping modalities available to other age groups, including the modality of psychotherapy (Zarit & Knight, 1996), the need for which is expected to increase for future elderly cohorts. Psychodynamic theory is rather circumscribed when it comes to aging. For its impact to be materialized, an appropriate conceptual basis is crucial. There is a wealth of diverse theoretical sources to be modified and incorporated in clinical geropsychology, and the initial blending of conceptualizations is underway (e.g., Lomranz, 1986; Nemiroff & Colarusso, 1990; Woods, 1996); however, further impetus is required. Theoretical formulations of psychic organization, ego processes, age-related psychodynamic conflicts and adjustment, self-identity and coping mechanisms, reformulating the impact of loss, family and gender, as well as the basic concepts of integration and adaptation, establishing unique diagnostic categories, elaborated personality dimensions, and further cognitive and neurological testing are only some of the challenges for clinical geropsychologists. A concentrated effort should be made to bring to the fore those elaborations of object-relation theorists who have theoretically and clinically modified infant and child-centered concepts. For instance, the Kleinian "positions" (e.g., paranoid–schizoid, or depressive), analyzed in light of different notions of time, space, dialectics, and intersubjectivity, can be understood as appropriate lifespan concepts (Ogden, 1994). Additional concepts elaborating differentiated processes revealing the personal, interpersonal, and psychosociological levels of adjustment and creativity (Rosow, 1994), as well as unique descriptive categories, are needed to explain the novel abilities, resilience, and mental capacities required in light of the challenges to adults in modern society (Kegan, 1994).

CLINICAL GERONTOLOGY
IN A COMMUNITY–CULTURAL PERSPECTIVE

Sciences may be defined as a subsystem of culture and is always embedded in a changing, dynamic cultural context. Scientific activity as a form of human activity is regulated by the rules that govern groups and communities at large. A science–culture interplay is continuously operating. The construction of theories, formulations of clinical treatment approaches and techniques, and investments or prevention of specific research efforts are all inherently related to cultural dimensions as portrayed by the Zeitgeist. Gerontology and its branch of mental health, just like any other discipline, falls under the thumb of the Zeitgeist; moreover, just as the Zeitgeist may influence trends of activity in mental health, these trends may also in turn bring about change in the Zeitgeist. The question to be dealt with is what impact does modern society and its Zeitgeist have on the study and treatment of the elderly person? Scientific and clinical language, paradigms, norms, and ideologies, as well as the personalities and unchecked tendencies and fears of researchers, may all lead to "knowledge traps" (Hazan, 1980) blocking the advancement of clinical gerontology.

In the science–culture interplay, interactive community–individual aspects may be noted. Merton (1973) and Polanyi (1958) expand on the concept of the "scientific community" as a collective that evolves its own norms, pressures, and policies, the major pursuits of the community being determined, to a large extent, by communally shared images of knowledge and beliefs. The history of science reveals that theories that were initially rejected eventually gained acceptance with time as they squared with cultural values (Conant, 1952), and that theoretical positions and beliefs often exert a negative influence by standing in the way of progress and dominating a discipline, so that investigation is preempted (Schultz, 1981). Are the modes and morals of clinical gerontology perhaps directed or circumscribed by such predicaments? Mental health approaches can be understood not only in relation to the significance of research results or even treatment gains, but also in a sociopsychocultural perspective, revealing the impact of the clinical approach and research on the culture, and demonstrating how the quest for mental health in the elderly portrays the image of aging, which in turn influences the general cultural ethos.

As to the individual aspects, the creation of a body of knowledge is often a melting pot for different personal, autobiographical, scientific, ethical, and cultural needs (Lubow, 1977). "Science as scientist" (Robinson, 1976) presents a perspective from which we can understand how scientists use tacit knowledge (Polanyi, 1958) to form their inquiries. Merton (1973) explores the ways in which knowledge is shaped by scientists' existential conditions, their personal interests and values. The scientific and professional presentations of mental health in aging cannot be understood without considering these processes. Such individual–scientific dynamics deserve even more attention due to the fact that the scientific community of clinical gerontologists, being multidisciplinary in its core, presents a greater variability of mental health professionals and scientists than is found in any other specific discipline (e.g., psychiatry). In addition, dealing with a population and culture so immersed in stigmatization and false beliefs, gerontologists should be highly sensitive as scientists in checking their covert assumptions in theory building, research, and treatment.

The cultural–individual interplay and its impact on theory building is not easy to capture. People and social structures may change in different ways, and keeping the two synchronized may be an unending task (Riley, Kahn, & Foner, 1994). Therefore, scientific activity itself, as it operates within the community of clinical gerontologists, needs to be an object of investigation: What are our ways of "searching for the truth," what are our hidden assumptions, our images of aging, our relation to time and death (Kastenbaum, 1985)? What criteria do we apply to what is "knowledge" (Knorr-Centina & Mulkay, 1983)? What are our professional and intellectual alliances? Why do the areas of mental health and aging not receive a more prominent place in the structural and political frameworks of gerontological societies (at present, e.g., clinical geropsychology or the area of mental health as a whole is minimally represented in the Gerontological Society of America meetings)? How is the mental health of the aged, theoretically and politically, embedded in the power structure of science and society?

As clinicians and scientists, we have to foster openness and be more attentive to the separate and social voices of elderly persons. It seems that despite the growing proportion of older people, they have yet to contribute to defining the discourse of aging, adaptation, and well-being through their own vision and language.

We approach a fascinating era that provides challenges, presents opportunities, and invites creative gerontologists to the area of mental health. The future course of clinical gerontology will largely determine the quality of life of the aged and the nature of our society. Many theoretical and practical questions await answers to which the developmental and multidisciplinary domains offer a rich repertoire that holds the potential for imaginative theory building, opens new frontiers of knowledge, treatment, and education, and sustains the gerontologist's excitement. If this volume, with its seven parts spanning a wide range of cogent issues in the field of mental health and aging, will be thought provoking, increase elaborated thinking, encourage more self-critical tendencies, indicate further research directions, and, especially, lead to conceptualizations, it will have served a useful purpose.

REFERENCES

Achenbaum, W. (1995). *Crossing frontiers: Gerontology emerges as a science.* New York: Cambridge University Press.

Baltes, P. (1987). Theoretical propositions of life-span developmental psychology. *Developmental Psychology, 23,* 610–617.

Birren, J., & Lanum, J. (1991). Metaphors of psychology and aging. In G. Kenyon, J. Birren, & J. Schroots (Eds.), *Metaphors of aging in science and the humanities* (pp. 115–126). New York: Springer.

Birren, J., & Schaie, W. (Eds.). (1977, 1985, 1990, 1996). *Handbook of the psychology of aging.* New York: Van Nostrand.

Birren, L., Kenyon, G., Ruth, J.-E., Schroots, J., & Svensson, T. (Eds.). (1996). *Aging and biography: Explorations in adult development.* New York: Springer.

Conant, J. (1952). *Modern science and modern man.* New York: Columbia University Press.

Estes, C., Binney, E., & Culbertson, R. (1992). The gerontological imagination. *International Journal of Aging and Human Development, 50,* 40–53.

Frank, L. K. (1956). Analysis of various types of boundaries. In R. Grinker (Ed.), *Towards a unified theory of human behavior* (pp. 354–357). New York: Basic Books.

Gatz, M., & Finkel, S. (1995). Education and training of mental health service providers. In M. Gatz (Ed.), *Emerging issues in mental health and aging* (pp. 282–302). Washington, DC: American Psychological Association.

George, L. (1966). Missing links: The case for a social psychology of the life course. *Gerontologist, 36*(2), 248–255.

Gutmann, D. (1992). The disappearing geropsychologist. *Northwestern Center on Aging, 8,* 7.

Hazan, H. (1980). *The limbo people: A study of the constitution of the time universe among the aged.* London: Routledge & Kegan Paul.

Kastenbaum, R. (1985). Dying and death. In J. Birren & W. Schaie (Eds.), *Handbook of the psychology of aging* (pp. 619–643). New York: Van Nostrand.

Katz, I. (1995). Infrastructure requirements for research in late-life mental disorders. In M. Gatz (Ed.), *Emerging issues in mental health and aging* (pp. 256–281). Washington, DC: American Psychological Association.

Kegan, R. (1994). *In over our heads: The mental demands of modern life.* Cambridge, MA: Harvard University Press.

Knorr-Centina, K., & Mulkay, M. (1983). *Science observed: Perspectives on the social study of science.* Beverly Hills, CA: Sage.

Koenig, H., George, L., & Schneider, R. (1994). Mental health care for older adults in the year 2020: A dangerous and avoided topic. *Gerontologist, 34*(5), 674–679.

Kuhn, T. (1967). *The structure of scientific revolutions.* Chicago: University of Chicago Press.

Lomranz, J. (1986). Personality theory: A position and derived teaching implications in clinical psychology. *Professional Psychology: Research and Practice, 14,* 215–218.

Lubow, R. (1977). *The war animals.* New York: Doubleday.

Merton, K. (1973). *The sociology of science.* Chicago: University of Chicago Press.

Moody, R. (1988). Towards a critical gerontology: The contribution of the humanities to theories of aging. In J. Birren & V. Bengtson (Eds.), *Emergent theories of aging* (pp. 19–40). New York: Springer.

Nemiroff, R., & Colarusso, C. (1990). *New dimensions in adult development.* New York: Basic Books.

Neugarten, B. (1994). The end of gerontology. Chicago: Northwestern University, Center on Aging, *10* (Spring), 1.

Ogden, T. (1994). *Subjects of analysis*. London: Karnac Books.

Polanyi, M. (1958). *Personal knowledge*. Chicago: University of Chicago Press.

Riegel, K. (1976). *Psychology of development and history*. New York: Plenum.

Riley, M., Kahn, R., & Foner, A. (1994). *Age and structural lag*. New York: Wiley.

Robinson, D. (1976). *An intellectual history of psychology*. New York: Macmillan.

Santos, J., & VandenBos, G. (1982). *Psychology and the older adult*. Washington, DC: American Psychological Association.

Schaie, W. (1988). The impact of research methodology on theory building in the developmental sciences. In J. Birren & V. Bengtson (Eds.), *Emergent theories of aging* (pp. 41–57). New York: Springer.

Schroots, J. (1995). Gerodynamics: Towards a branching theory of aging. *Canadian Journal of Aging, 14*, 74–81.

Schultz, D. (1981). *A history of modern psychology*. New York: Academic Press.

Schulz, R., & Heckhausen, J. (1996). A life span model of successful aging. *American Psychologist, 51*(7), 702–714.

Tornstam, L. (1992). The *quo vadis* of gerontology: On the scientific paradigm of gerontology. *Gerontologist, 32*, 318–326.

Woods, R. (1996). *Handbook of the clinical psychology of aging*. New York: Wiley.

Zarit, S., & Knight, B. (Eds.). (1996). *A guide to psychotherapy and aging*. Washington, DC: American Psychological Association.

Index

ISBN 0-306-45750-4

90000